Cardiac Surgery of the Neonate and Infant

ALDO R. CASTAÑEDA, M.D., Ph.D.

Surgeon-in-Chief
Department of Cardiac Surgery
The Children's Hospital Boston
William E. Ladd Professor of Surgery
Harvard Medical School
Boston, Massachusetts

RICHARD A. JONAS, M.D.

Department of Cardiac Surgery
The Children's Hospital Boston
Associate Professor of Surgery
Harvard Medical School
Boston, Massachusetts

JOHN E. MAYER, Jr., M.D.

Department of Cardiac Surgery
The Children's Hospital Boston
Associate Professor of Surgery
Harvard Medical School
Boston, Massachusetts

FRANK L. HANLEY, M.D.

Department of Cardiac Surgery
The Children's Hospital Boston
Assistant Professor of Surgery
Harvard Medical School
Boston, Massachusetts
Chief, Cardiothoracic Surgery
University of California, San Francisco
San Francisco, California

With illustrations by Rebekah Dodson

W.B. SAUNDERS COMPANY

A Division of Harcourt Brace & Company

Philadelphia
London   Toronto   Montreal   Sydney   Tokyo

Cardiac Surgery of the Neonate and Infant

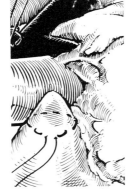

W.B. SAUNDERS COMPANY
A Division of
Harcourt Brace & Company

The Curtis Center
Independence Square West
Philadelphia, Pennsylvania 19106

Library of Congress Cataloging-in-Publication Data

Cardiac surgery of the neonate and infant /
Aldo R. Castañeda . . . [et al.].

p.   cm.

Includes bibliographical references and index.

ISBN 0–7216–4301–9

1. Heart—Surgery.   2. Infants—Surgery.   3. Infants
(Newborn)—Surgery.   I. Castañeda, Aldo R.
[DNLM: 1. Heart Surgery—in infancy & childhood.
2. Infant, Newborn, Diseases—surgery.   WS 290 C26658
1994]

RD598.C3527 1994   617.4′12′00832—dc20

DNLM/DLC   93–22880

Cardiac Surgery of the Neonate and Infant   ISBN 0–7216–4301–9

Printed in the United States of America.

Last digit is the print number: 9   8   7   6   5   4   3   2

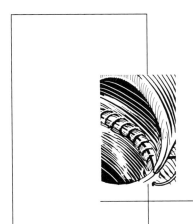

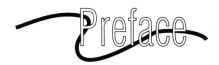

A number of books and monographs on cardiac surgery have appeared in recent years, but most reflect the views of a number of different authors representing diverse institutional philosophies. Our aspirations in writing this book were to assemble the experience gained by four surgeons working in a single institution guided by a cohesive philosophy and to focus the text on cardiac surgery in the neonate and infant, since the treatment philosophy that has been pursued at the Children's Hospital in Boston for the last two decades has centered on definitive neonatal and infant repair.

An additional intent was to expand the text beyond the conventional subjects of pathology and pathophysiology of congenital heart disease, indications for surgery, and descriptions of surgical techniques and to include chapters on developmental biology of the heart, the lungs, and the cental nervous system, information on cardiopulmonary bypass, hypothermia and circulatory arrest, and protection of the neonatal myocardium. Most of the discussions on these subjects are supported by information obtained during recent experimental laboratory studies. We trust that these chapters will prove interesting and will kindle the curiosity and the desire for investigative work, particularly in upcoming generations of pediatric cardiac surgeons.

The chapters dealing with important future developments (at least as we see them) in myocardial and cerebral protection during open heart surgery in neonates and infants and future use of clinical fetal cardiac surgery are intended not only to inform but also to stimulate others to contribute new ideas to the development of these rapidly expanding fields.

Optimal treatment of congenital heart disease,

perhaps more than any other disease entity, requires the harmonious interaction of a number of different medical specialists, nurses, and paramedical personnel. To attain excellence in this field, an intimate, mutually respectful, intellectually focused, and committed interaction of all members of this multidisciplinary team is essential. Surgical results reflect not only the competence of the surgical team but also the quality of pediatric cardiologists, anesthesiologists, radiologists, and pathologists, of specialized nurses in the operating room, intensive care unit, and on the floor, and of a team of experienced and highly specialized cardiopulmonary perfusionists. The stimulating intellectual environment provided by the Children's Hospital of Boston and Harvard Medical School has greatly enhanced these efforts.

This is an appropriate opportunity to thank all of our colleagues and collaborators at Children's Hospital for their professionalism and dedication to excellence and friendship. Without every component of this large team, this work could not have been accomplished.

Special thanks are due to our colleagues who graciously contributed the following chapters to this book: Dr. James Lock on Interventional Cardiology, Dr. Paul Hickey and Dr. Dolly Hansen on Anesthesia for Cardiovascular Surgery in the neonate and infant, Dr. David Wessel for perioperative management of the neonate and young infant in the cardiac intensive care unit, and Dr. Edward Walsh for management of postoperative cardiac arrhythmias.

Over the last two decades, our Department of Cardiac Surgery has had the good fortune to attract a large number of superb trainees both to our clinical service and to our research laboratory. Many of them have continued working in pediatric cardiac surgery, and many now lead their own divisions or departments of pediatric cardiac surgery in this country and abroad. To all of our trainees, we express our sincere thanks for their dedication and hard work and also for the important intellectual input they provided during their stay in our department. Through their probing questions, they helped us to challenge dogmas and either directly or indirectly they stimulated us to pursue new ideas.

Thanks are also due to Mr. Edward Wickland, our initial contact with the W.B. Saunders Company, and to Ms. Avé McCracken, Acquisitions Editor; Ellen B. Zanolle, Designer; and Paula Shargel-Green, Production Manager, for seeing the project through to its completion. We are especially grateful to Ms. Becky Dodson, who with her artistry and her patience in dealing with the ever-changing demands of the four authors produced outstanding illustrations that help clarify the intricate technical details of the many operations discussed in this book better than words. We also gratefully acknowledge the editorial assistance of Mrs. Marcia Lawson and a special appreciation to Ms. Laura Young, who so expertly assisted in preparing the manuscripts for this book.

ALDO R. CASTAÑEDA, M.D.
RICHARD A. JONAS, M.D.
JOHN E. MAYER, JR., M.D.
FRANK L. HANLEY, M.D.

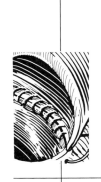

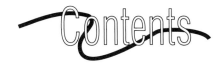

Contents

☐

3

Part

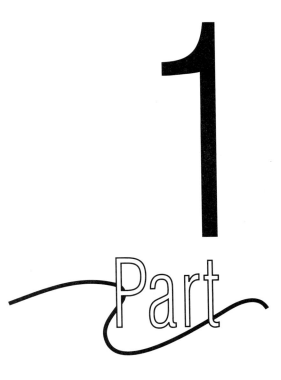

Part

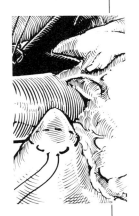

General Considerations

Chapter

Developmental Biology

HEART

Immediately after the umbilical cord is tied, the fetus ceases its dependent existence and the neonate becomes independent, at least from a cardiorespiratory standpoint. An understanding of the transition from the fetal to the postnatal and, eventually, the adult type of circulation offers an insight into the reason most congenital heart defects, including very complex malformations, are well tolerated in utero, while postnatally these same conditions become life threatening. An appreciation of the unique growth potential of the fetal and neonatal myocardium and coronary bed offers further insight into the benefits of correcting congenital heart defects early in life.

FETAL CIRCULATION

It must be understood that almost all current knowledge about fetal circulation has been acquired from studies in sheep. Despite the obvious species differences, including the length of gestation, there seem to be sufficient similarities to warrant extrapolation of lamb data to humans. It is beyond the scope of this chapter to exhaustively review past and present contributions in this field, but much is owed to Sir Geoffrey Dawes[7] and Dr. Abraham Ru-

dolph[25] for their pioneering and scholarly work in this area.

After oxygenation in the placenta (facilitated by the increased affinity of fetal hemoglobin for oxygen), umbilical venous blood (Po_2, 35 mm Hg; O_2 saturation, 80%) proceeds either to bypass the liver through the ductus venosus, entering the right atrium directly, or to traverse the liver before entering the inferior vena cava (Fig. 1–1). Little is known about what regulates the amount of blood shortcircuited through the ductus venosus. Inferior vena cava (IVC) blood, which contains umbilical, lower body, and portal venous blood, represents approximately 70% of the total systemic venous return to the heart. Within the right atrium, approximately 25% of the IVC blood (mostly O_2-rich blood that has traversed the ductus venosus) passes directly into the left atrium through the foramen ovale, where it mixes with pulmonary venous blood. Left atrial blood (Po_2, 27 mm Hg; O_2 saturation, 65%) passes into the left ventricle and supplies the coronary arteries, the head (including the brain), and the upper extremities. Only 10% of this blood ejected from the left ventricle crosses the aortic isthmus to contribute to flow in the descending thoracic aorta. Superior vena cava (SVC) blood contributes only about

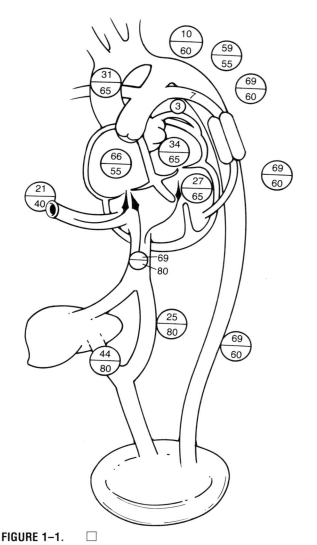

FIGURE 1–1. ☐

Diagram of the fetal circulation of the late gestational lamb (modified from Rudolph). Upper figures within the circles represent percentages of blood flow through the various components of the fetal circulation; lower figures represent oxygen saturation values (%). (Modified from Rudolph AM. Changes in the circulation after birth. In Rudolph AM (ed). Congenital Disease of the Heart. Chicago, Year Book Medical, 1974, p 3).

Late in gestation, pressures in the fetal left and right ventricles are the same (approximately 70 mm Hg systolic). This pressure is transmitted into the pulmonary arteries and ascending and descending thoracic aorta. The left and right sides of the fetal circulation function more or less "in parallel," a major distinction from the postnatal "in series" circulation. Combined ventricular output (CVO), a term coined by Rudolph[26] to describe the total volume of blood ejected by both left and right ventricles in the fetus, also includes pulmonary and coronary flow. The amount of CVO passing through the placenta is approximately equal to the volume of right ventricular blood that passes through the lungs after birth. The myocardium receives a large proportion of the CVO, commensurate with the metabolic rate of this organ. In the fetus the right ventricle ejects approximately 65% and the left ventricle only about 35% of the CVO. Because 8% flows through the lungs, about 60% of the total CVO crosses the ductus arteriosus into the descending thoracic aorta.

CHANGES IN THE CARDIOPULMONARY CIRCUIT IMMEDIATELY AFTER BIRTH

Interruption of the umbilical cord causes an immediate increase in systemic vascular resistance and also a reduction in the return of IVC blood to the heart. Concurrent with these changes is a rapid decrease in pulmonary vascular resistance, accompanied by an increase in pulmonary blood flow. The ductus arteriosus constricts primarily in response to the increased arterial Po_2, but removal of circulating placental prostaglandin E_2 (PGE_2) may also influence this process. In the mature infant, the ductus usually becomes functionally closed within the first 12 to 24 hours after birth. This process depends primarily on systemic arterial Po_2 levels and is reversible with PGE_1. Usually, within approximately 2 weeks, a fibrosing process in the ductus results in anatomic closure. In addition to Po_2 levels, the ductus is also responsive to prostaglandins, bradykinin, and other vasoactive substances. As pointed out by Rudolph, the primary change in the circulation after birth is "a shift of the blood flow for gas exchange from the placenta to the lungs."[25] After birth, with the elimination of the placental circulation, closure of the ductus, and a decrease in pulmonary vascular resistance, the right ventricle ejects all of its blood into the pulmonary circulation. The ductus venosus also closes soon after birth; this structure does not appear to be sensitive to varying levels of Po_2, Pco_2, or pH, and its regulation in utero and postnatally continues to be poorly understood.

The parallel configuration of the fetal circulation

25% of total venous return to the heart and has a significantly lower Po_2 and oxygen saturation (14 mm Hg and 40%, respectively). Practically all SVC blood flows into the right ventricle and the pulmonary trunk. Only about 8% is diverted into the high-resistance pulmonary vascular circuit; the rest is ejected through the ductus arteriosus into the descending thoracic aorta, with a Po_2 of 21 mm Hg and an O_2 saturation of 60%. Because of the crossing streams of IVC and SVC blood in the right atrium, organs distal to the ductus arteriosus are supplied with blood that has a lower Po_2 and O_2 saturation than that in the brain and upper extremities. Thus the placenta receives blood with low O_2 saturation, maximizing the efficiency of placental gas exchange.

explains why most complex congenital cardiac lesions are well tolerated in utero. Transposition of the great arteries is an example. In the normal fetus, ascending aortic blood is slightly better oxygenated (approximately 10%) than the blood entering the descending thoracic aorta. In transposition this difference is reversed; otherwise, the effect of transposition of the great arteries on the fetal circulation is of little consequence. The abnormal blood flow to and from the lungs in this condition, and in other complex malformations that may be fatal soon after birth, is unimportant in the fetus as long as the placenta provides gaseous exchange. Also, because right and left ventricular pressures are essentially identical in the fetus, the presence of an interventricular communication is functionally unimportant. However, there are congenital cardiac defects in the fetus that lead to important secondary anatomic and physiologic abnormalities. An extreme example is premature closure of the foramen ovale, which most likely causes left ventricular hypoplasia; it is reasonable to assume that the normal size of the left ventricle is very much dependent on the volume of blood that enters and leaves its cavity during fetal development. Nevertheless, even this lesion is well tolerated in utero. Lesions that are poorly tolerated in utero (albeit not well understood) include those in which there is regurgitation of the atrioventricular or semilunar valves and also congenital heart block, all lesions that compromise combined ventricular output.

In addition to these physiologic and anatomic differences and changes in the fetal, neonatal, and adult circulation, there are important developmental considerations concerning normal and pathologic cardiac growth. Significant progress has been made in identifying developmental changes of the heart at a cellular and subcellular level.

DEVELOPMENTAL CONSIDERATIONS

Normal Cardiac Growth

In the embryo and early fetus, the heart grows by increasing the number of myocytes (hyperplasia). Near term, mitotic activity declines, and cardiac growth occurs mostly by enlargement of pre-existing myocytes (hypertrophy)[31] (Fig. 1–2). Hemodynamic factors seem to provide the principal stimulus for both hypertrophy and hyperplasia of myocytes, while early stages of cytodifferentiation and looping are probably intrinsic myocyte properties. Some degree of mitotic activity in cardiac myocytes (hyperplastic phase of myocardial growth) persists during early neonatal life. For example, in rats the mitotic

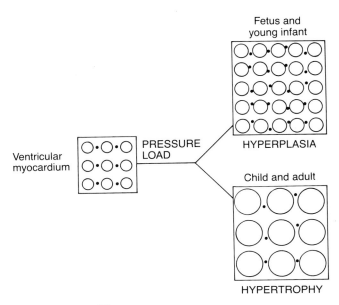

FIGURE 1–2. □

Schema of cross section of a segment of ventricular myocardium before and after exposure to pressure overload. In the fetus, neonate, and young infant, the increase in myocardial mass is due to myocyte hyperplasia and moderate hypertrophy and is accompanied by increased coronary angiogenesis. In the older infant, child, and adult, myocardial hypertrophy is due only to massive myocyte hypertrophy without accompanying coronary angiogenesis. Large circles represent myocytes. Small dots represent coronary arteries.

phase is responsible for a twofold increase in the number of myocytes during the first 3 weeks of life.[2] Although not definitely proved in the human, myocyte mitotic activity and the potential for hyperplasia allegedly persist for 3 to 6 months after birth, after which all myocytes become terminally differentiated cells.[3] Curiously, although the capacity for hyperplasia is lost, mature myocytes may nevertheless retain some capacity for DNA replication. For example, at birth, virtually all myocardial cells are mononucleated, whereas close to 25% of adult human cardiac myocytes are binucleated.[23] Polyploidy increases with advancing age and particularly with pathologic hypertrophy.[27] Myocyte binucleation may be caused by fusion of mononucleated cells, amitotic nuclear division, or mitotic division of nuclei without cytoplasmic separation (i.e., karyokinesis without cytokinesis).[5] After mitotic activity of myocytes ceases, hyperplasia of the nonmuscular components of the heart nevertheless continues. Hypertrophy is characterized by lengthening as well as thickening of the myocyte, whose volume can increase 30- to 40-fold during normal postnatal growth and maturation.[23]

Coronary angiogenesis in the neonate occurs even more rapidly than myocyte hyperplasia.[22] During physiologic hypertrophy, capillary units continue to proliferate in proportion to myocardial mass, maintaining a constant intercapillary distance.[1]

Regulation of Postnatal Cardiac Growth

Regulation of postnatal cardiac growth is not completely understood. Most likely, hemodynamic factors play the most important role in the regulation of physiologic growth of the heart after birth. Other factors may include increasing demands of the rapidly growing animal, including hypoxia, the stage of myocardial maturity, and stimulation of alpha$_1$-adrenergic receptors.

As previously mentioned, the acute transition from intrauterine to extrauterine circulation results in important changes. Interruption of the placental circulation increases peripheral resistance and the left ventricular afterload, while expansion of the lungs and the increase in pulmonary arteriolar Po$_2$ decrease the pulmonary vascular resistance, thereby reducing the right ventricular afterload.[26] Hence, postnatal right ventricular growth is mostly determined by volume load, whereas left ventricular growth becomes more dependent on both volume and pressure overload. These hemodynamic changes lead to a rapid increase in left ventricular mass and a much slower increase in right ventricular mass.[2] Subcellular and microvascular changes also occur more rapidly in the left ventricle than in the right. By 1 month of age, the left ventricle significantly outweighs the right in human infants.[10]

Myocardial Response to Chronic Stress

Myocytes

In the neonate and young infant, the heart responds to stress by a combination of hyperplasia and hypertrophy, analogous to normal postnatal growth.[4] Intensification of myocardial hyperplasia in immature hearts exposed to chronic stress was identified as early as 1966, and subsequent studies have demonstrated increased DNA synthesis and mitosis in immature hearts subjected to chronic stress.[6, 9] In contrast, chronic stress in adult hearts induces hypertrophy of pre-existing myocytes rather than hyperplasia.[31] Although mitosis of adult cardiac myocytes has not been reported, nevertheless it has been suggested that adult myocytes may divide by amitotic division of multinucleated myocytes when a certain "critical" size is attained.[19] Also, with advancing age or senescence, the capacity to develop myocardial hypertrophy decreases, probably because of a reduced capacity to synthesize proteins.[15]

Coronary Circulation

In adult hearts, hypertrophy caused by pressure overload is commonly associated with a decrease in myocardial perfusion reserve, which may result in myocardial ischemia during periods of acute stress. The difference between the resting and the maximally vasodilated coronary blood flow represents the coronary flow reserve.[14] The coronary flow may be increased by recruitment of "reserve" coronary vascular beds or by a decrease in coronary vascular resistance.[20] However, in immature animals with pressure overload hypertrophy, coronary vascular reserve may be normal. Flanagan and associates[11] found that the coronary flow reserve in lambs with left ventricular hypertrophy caused by pressure overload was normal, while a similar pressure overload induced in adult sheep resulted in an impaired coronary perfusion reserve. This suggests that a pressure overload in immature hearts induces enhanced microvascular growth, or angiogenesis, in addition to myocyte hyperplasia. When pressure overload hypertrophy is not accompanied by coronary angiogenesis, intercapillary distance increases, and capillary density decreases.

Reduced coronary flow reserve in the hypertrophied ventricle has been attributed to a decrease in capillary density,[21] inadequate caliber of the large coronary arteries,[18] coronary ostial obstruction,[30] or increased extravascular forces impeding blood flow within the intramural coronary vessels.[13] In experimental pressure overload hypertrophy, coronary vascular resistance correlates with capillary density. During acute stress, however, other factors come into play. The importance of a reduced coronary perfusion reserve has yet to be clearly established. Furthermore, other factors, in addition to age, that may influence the coronary response to hypertrophy include (1) the nature of the ventricle, with the right ventricle capable of augmenting resting myocardial blood flow more consistently than the left (77% to 137% versus 30%, respectively); (2) the duration of the mechanical overload; (3) the abruptness of onset of the hypertrophy-inducing stimulus; and (4) the presence of ventricular failure.

Functional Consequences of Myocardial Hypertrophy

The functional consequences of myocardial hypertrophy are the result of adaptive and nonadaptive changes induced by the overloading stimulus. Thus, the distinction between normal cardiac growth and function and abnormal ventricular hypertrophy and dysfunction is not clear-cut. For example, in adult hearts, overload hypertrophy of the left ventricle induced by systemic hypertension causes significant functional consequences,[17] whereas most studies in larger animals and humans with stable left ventricular hypertrophy have demonstrated essentially normal afterload and global left ventricular function.[12, 28] However, over time, left ventricular myocardial failure and damage develop if the pressure overload is not relieved. Pressure overload hypertrophy induced in adult animals is associated with a depressed ventricular myocardial contractile state,[8] whereas hypertrophy induced in immature animals is associated with a normal contractile state when comparisons are made with age-matched controls. In light of present knowledge, interpretation of these data is difficult. It is possible that these changes in ventricular contractility may be due either to shifts in myosin isoenzymes or to a decreased responsiveness to beta-adrenergic receptor agonists.

Perhaps the most striking feature of the cardiac hyperplastic and hypertrophic response of immature hearts to pressure overload is the rapidity with which these changes develop. Although few data exist regarding the effect of age on the capacity of the left ventricle to hypertrophy in response to an increase in afterload, senescent rats have been found to have a diminished capacity to develop hypertrophy and to synthesize DNA in response to pressure overload.[15] Thus, available data suggest that the capacity for hypertrophy decreases with increasing age. Molecular studies have demonstrated the rapidity with which the rat myocyte responds quickly to pressure overload. Gene expression of c-*myc* and c-*fos* proto-oncogenes occurs in rat cardiac cells within 1 hour after imposing an acute pressure load.[16] Similarly, HSP70, the gene of a major heat shock protein that protects the cell under various conditions, is also induced within an hour. Transcription of c-*myc*, c-*fos*, and HSP70 messenger RNAs (mRNAs) ceases within 24 to 48 hours, but the presence of the related proteins in the nucleus may play a permissive role in facilitating the continuous hypertrophic response. Thus, an acute left ventricular pressure overload elicits a rapid change in the gene expression, including reinduction of protein synthesis and activation of the proto-oncogenes responsible for both cell hyperplasia and hypertrophy. These alterations in gene expression and the capacity of the cell machinery to respond to these signals ultimately seem to determine the functional capacity of the hypertrophied myocardium.[24, 29]

CONCLUSION

The effect of age on the development of myocardial hypertrophy and the functional difference between normal growth (physiologic hyperplasia and hypertrophy) and pathologic hypertrophy have yet to be fully determined. Clearly, there is an important interaction among the effects of gene switches,

structural alterations induced by hemodynamic and autonomic factors, and nutrient availability on ventricular function, both at rest and during additional stress. Experimental data suggest that age is indeed a very important factor in determining type, rapidity, and functional features of myocardial response to pressure overload. In neonatal hearts, pressure overload induces mostly hyperplasia of myocytes and coronary angiogenesis. In adult hearts, pressure overload induces only hypertrophy of myocytes without coronary angiogenesis. In light of this, repair during the early hyperplastic phase of cardiac growth is expected to yield normal or near-normal left and right ventricular function and also to decrease the potential for electrical instability of the myocardium. Thus, early repair (during the hyperplastic phase) should not only eliminate the many adverse effects of the unrepaired congenital cardiac defect on important organs (such as the heart itself, lungs, and brain), but also eliminate the reduced capacity of the myocardium to respond to chronic stress.

REFERENCES

1. Anversa P, Loud AV, Giacomelli F, et al. Absolute morphometric study of myocardial hypertrophy in experimental hypertension. II. Ultrastructure of myocytes and insterstitum. Lab Invest 38:597, 1978.
2. Anversa P, Olivetti G, Loud AV. Morphometric study of early postnatal development in the left and right ventricular myocardium of the rat. I. Hypertrophy, hyperplasia, and binucleation of myocytes. Circ Res 46:495, 1980.
3. Brown AL. Morphologic factors in cardiac hypertrophy. In Alpert NR (ed). Cardiac Hypertrophy. New York, Academic Press, 1971, p 11.
4. Bujaisky L, Zak R. Biological mechanisms of hypertrophy. In Fozzard HA, Haber E, Jennings RB, et al (eds). The Heart and Cardiovascular System. New York, Raven Press, 1986, p 1491.
5. Clubb FJ Jr, Bishop SP. Formation of binucleated myocardial cells in the neonatal rat: An index for growth hypertrophy. Lab Invest 50:571, 1984.
6. Crane WAJ, Dutta LP. Utilization of tritiated thymidine for desoxyribonucleic acid synthesis by the lesions of experimental hypertension in the rat. J Pathol Bacteriol 86:83, 1963.
7. Dawes GS. Fetal and Neonatal Physiology. Chicago, Year Book Medical, 1968.
8. Dowell RT, Haithcoat JL, Hasser EM. Pressure-induced cardiac enlargement in neonatal and adult rats. Left ventricular weight and hemodynamic responses during the early adaptive period. Tex Rep Biol Med 39:139, 1979.
9. Dowell RT, McManus RE. Pressure-induced cardiac enlargement in neonatal and adult rats. Left ventricular functional characteristics and evidence of cardiac muscle cell proliferation in the neonate. Circ Res 42:303, 1978.
10. Emery JL, Mithal A. Weights of cardiac ventricles at and after birth. Br Heart J 23:313, 1961.
11. Flanagan MF, Fujii AM, Colan SD, et al. Myocardial angiogenesis and coronary perfusion in left ventricular pressure overload hypertrophy in the young lamb: Evidence for inhibition with chronic protamine administration. Circ Res 68:1458, 1991.
12. Fujii AM, Gelpi RJ, Mirsky I, et al. Systolic and diastolic

dysfunction during atrial pacing in conscious dogs with left ventricular hypertrophy. Circ Res 62:462, 1988.

13. Harrison DG, Barnes DH, Hiratzka LF, et al. The effect of cardiac hypertrophy on the coronary collateral circulation. Circulation 71:1135, 1985.

14. Hoffman JIE. Maximal coronary flow and the concept of coronary vascular reserve. Circulation 70:153, 1984.

15. Isoyama S, Wei JY, Izumo S, et al. Effect of age on the development of cardiac hypertrophy produced by aortic constriction in the rat. Circ Res 61:337, 1987.

16. Izumo S, Nadal-Ginard B, Mahdavi V. Protooncogene induction and reprogramming of cardiac gene expression produced by pressure overload. Proc Natl Acad Sci USA 85:339, 1988.

17. Kannel WB. Implications of Framingham study data for treatment of hypertension: Impact of other risk factors. In Laragh JH, Buhler FR, Seldin SW (eds). Frontiers in Hypertension Research. New York, Springer-Verlag, 1981, p 17.

18. Linzbach AJ. Heart failure from the point of view of quantitative anatomy. Am J Cardiol 5:370, 1960.

19. Linzbach AJ. Hypertrophy, structural dilatation and chronic failure of the human heart. Folia Fac Med Univ Comenianae Bratisl 10:75, 1973.

20. Lombardo TA, Rose L, Taeschler M, et al. The effect of exercise on coronary blood flow, myocardial oxygen consumption, and cardiac efficiency in man. Circulation 7:71, 1953.

21. Mueller TM, Marcus ML, Kerber RE, et al. Effect of renal hypertension and left ventricular hypertrophy on the coronary circulation in dogs. Circ Res 42:543, 1978.

22. Olivetti G, Anversa P, Loud AV. Morphometric study of early postnatal development in the left and right ventricular myocardium of the rat. II. Tissue composition, capillary growth, and sarcoplasmic alterations. Circ Res 46:503, 1980.

23. Oparil S. Pathogenesis of ventricular hypertrophy. J Am Coll Cardiol 5:57B, 1985.

24. Re RN. Cellular mechanisms of growth in cardiovascular tissue. Am J Cardiol 60:104, 1987.

25. Rudolph AM. Changes in the circulation after birth. In Rudolph AM (ed). Congenital Disease of the Heart. Chicago, Year Book Medical, 1974, p 17.

26. Rudolph AM. The changes in the circulation after birth. Their importance in congenital heart disease. Circulation 41:343, 1970.

27. Sandritter W, Scomazzoni G. Desoxyribonucleic acid content (Feulgen photometry) and dry weight (interference microscopy) of normal and hypertrophic heart muscle fibers. Nature 202:100, 1964.

28. Sasayama S, Franklin D, Ross J Jr. Hyperfunction with normal inotropic state of the hypertrophied left ventricle. Am J Physiol 232:H418, 1977.

29. Simpson PC. Role of proto-oncogenes in myocardial hypertrophy. Am J Cardiol 62:13G, 1988.

30. Vogelberg K. Die lichtungsweite der coronarostein an normalen und hypertrophen herzen. Ztschr Kreislafforsch 46:101, 1957.

31. Zak R. Development and proliferative capacity of cardiac muscle cells. Circ Res 35(suppl II):17, 1974.

CENTRAL NERVOUS SYSTEM

RELATIONSHIP BETWEEN DEVELOPMENT OF THE CENTRAL NERVOUS SYSTEM AND REPAIR OF CONGENITAL HEART DISEASE

Undoubtedly the most complex and least well understood system in the body is the central nervous system. One fact that does appear to be clear is that after birth the body does not have the ability to replace neurons. Therefore, loss of neurons related to congenital heart disease—whether from cyanosis, inadequate substrate supply as a result of congestive heart failure, or injury during repair secondary to the deleterious effects of cardiopulmonary bypass or circulatory arrest—is likely to compromise the ultimate potential of the individual. Study of injury to the central nervous system in the adult with heart disease has been hampered by the generalized nature of arteriosclerotic disease, which affects the majority of adults undergoing cardiac surgery. Atheromatous disease of the extracranial carotid arterial system or intracranial arterial tree may have resulted in pre-existing cerebral injury before cardiac surgery or can contribute to localized areas of inadequate perfusion during cardiopulmonary bypass. The risk of particulate embolism is increased during maneuvers such as aortic cannu-

lation. In contrast, the child with heart disease who is essentially free of arterial disease presents a unique opportunity to study perioperative factors that might compromise the central nervous system. However, before generalizations can be made, careful consideration must be given to the developmental changes that occur in the central nervous system during the first years of life. It seems more than likely that these changes may work to the advantage of the cardiac surgeon by offering windows of opportunity when the individual will be maximally resistant to the stresses of cardiac repair. It is also likely that this understanding will provide a rational basis for improved methods of protecting the central nervous system during cardiac repair.

BASIC STRUCTURAL EMBRYOLOGY OF THE CENTRAL NERVOUS SYSTEM

The first divisions of the fertilized egg result in a hollow sphere termed the *blastula*. Subsequently, an invagination of cells begins at a specific point on the surface of the blastula, the blastopore. This invagination, termed *gastrulation*, results in an internal layer of cells, the *endoderm*, and an external layer, the *ectoderm*. Next an intermediate layer of cells, the *mesoderm,* forms from migration of cells from the ectoderm and endoderm. Development of the central nervous system begins on the seventeenth day of intrauterine life with the formation of a longitudinal groove in the ectoderm that eventually invaginates itself to form a complete tube, the *neural tube.*[21] Adjacent mesodermal tissue becomes segmented into *somites,* which contribute to the vertebrae as well as to the ribs, skeletal muscle, and dermis. Ectodermal tissue adjacent to the neural tube forms the *neural crest.* Neural crest cells give rise to the spinal and autonomic ganglia, the glial cells of the peripheral nervous system, and a variety of non-neural tissues, including melanocytes and chromaffin cells of the adrenal medulla.

At about the 25th day of intrauterine life, three dilatations appear at the rostral (cephalic) end of the neural tube. These vesicles give rise to the forebrain, including the cerebral hemispheres, optic nerves, and retinae; the midbrain; and the hindbrain, including the pons, cerebellum, and medulla oblongata. The caudal portion of the neural tube gives rise to the spinal cord. As a result of unequal growth of these different components, three flexures appear. Cavities form within the vesicles; these will eventually form the ventricular system of the brain.

CENTRAL NERVOUS SYSTEM DEVELOPMENT AT THE CELLULAR LEVEL

Cellular Proliferation

Initially, the ectodermal cells lining the neural tube are arranged as simple columnar epithelium. As cellular proliferation proceeds, the columnar epithelium is converted to pseudostratified epithelium in which mitotic figures are found exclusively at the luminal (ventricular) surface.[2] There are multiple synonyms for this epithelium, including the germinal epithelium, neuroepithelium, germinal matrix, ventricular layer, and ependymal layer.

Assuming that the fully developed human brain contains approximately 100 billion neurons and that these do not divide after birth, the developing brain must add an average of 250,000 neurons per minute of early development[6] (Fig. 1–3). However, the brain is not composed solely of neurons. Virchow coined the term *neuroglia* (nerve glue) for the numerous cells other than neurons that make up the central nervous system. Glia outnumber neurons by about 10 to 1 and make up about half the bulk of the nervous system. Although they were previously thought to have a simple supportive role, they are now known to interact with neurons in a highly interdependent fashion, influencing development, differentiation, and physiologic function. One specialized function previously attributed to glia is no longer attributed to them: namely, the function of the blood-brain barrier. This is now believed to be the role of endothelial cells alone.[27]

Although the full-term fetus is born with a full complement of neurons, there is a rapid proliferation of glial cells after birth. The human neonatal brain weighs 350 gm, while the adult brain weighs 1400 gm. Much of this growth occurs during the first year of life, with brain weight increasing to 500 gm by 3 months of age, 660 gm by 6 months of age, and 925 gm by 1 year of age.[1] Not all of this increase in weight is related to proliferation of glial cells. There are also the laying down of myelin, an increase in the size of neurons, and the development of complex neuronal processes (axons and dendrites), including the formation of synapses.

Cellular Differentiation

Development of an organism with any degree of complexity requires generations of specialized cells from less specialized ancestors. A superficial analysis would suggest that all that is required for this process is the genetic code with the requisite switching genes to control the timing of various steps of differentiation. However, the cytoplasm clearly contains factors that regulate development.[26] For example, somatic cells synthesize mainly RNA. When the nucleus of a somatic cell is transplanted to an enucleated but fertilized egg, the hybrid cell synthesizes primarily DNA; only at later stages of development does it resume RNA synthesis. Another example of an epigenetic influence is the phenomenon of *induction.* For example, the formation of the neural tube is induced by tissue in the dorsal lip of the blastopore. Spemann[24] demonstrated in 1938 that portions of the dorsal lip could induce the formation of the neural tube in unusual locations when transplanted from one gastrula to another. This observation and others suggested that certain cells in such a transplant serve as an organizer for future differentiation of the tissue around them. Thus the progressive specialization of cell types arises from complex interactions between genetic instructions, influences arising from the cell cytoplasm, and influences from the extracellular environment.

Influence of Neurotransmitters on the Differentiation of Neurons. Another example of the role of extrinsic factors, rather than direct genetic programming of a cell's fate, can be observed in the acquisition of transmitter properties by the neuron.

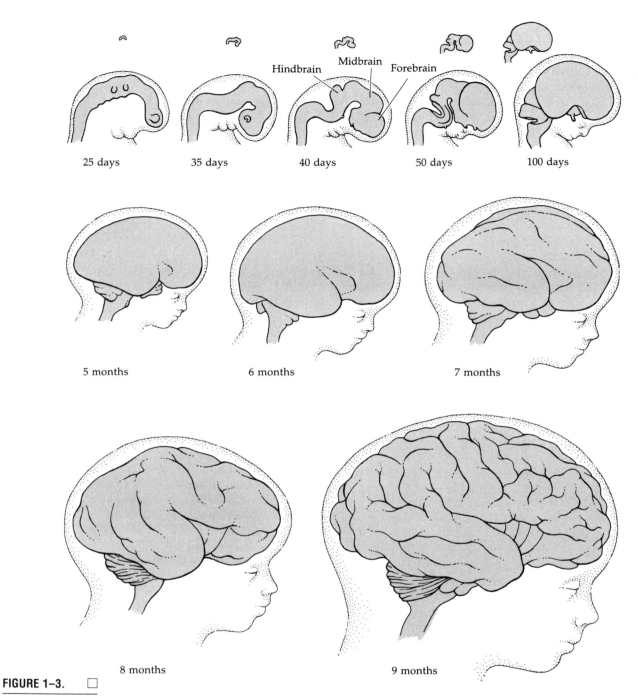

Hindbrain Midbrain Forebrain

25 days   35 days   40 days   50 days   100 days

5 months   6 months   7 months

8 months   9 months

FIGURE 1–3. ☐

Development of the human brain. Assuming that the fully developed human brain contains approximately 100 billion neurons and that these do not divide after birth, the fetal brain must add an average of 250,000 neurons per minute of early development. (From Purves D, Lichtman JW. Principles of Neural Development. Sunderland, MA, Sinauer Associates, 1985, p 18.)

A number of studies using cultured neurons have demonstrated that neurons can switch from adrenergic to cholinergic transmission under the influence of different culture media.[20] A similar result has been found in transplant experiments using sympathetic and parasympathetic ganglion cells transplanted to the vagal region of the chick embryo.[16]

Differentiation of Neuronal Ion Channels. Study of the amphibian *Xenopus* has demonstrated that in the early neural tube phase of development, the depolarization current is primarily a result of calcium influx.[25] Later in development there is a brief spike of depolarization as a result of rapid sodium influx, followed by a slower influx of calcium. In the mature *Xenopus* larva the depolarization spike is wholly related to sodium influx. Similar studies of developing skeletal and cardiac muscle suggest that a gradual transition from calcium-dependent to sodium-dependent action potentials may be a rather general feature of excitable cells during development.

Cellular Migration

As described in the section "Cellular Proliferation," neuronal mitoses occur predominantly in the germinal matrix adjacent to the lumen of the neural tube. For these cells to be precisely located for their ultimate function, neuronal migration is required. An important feature of this migratory process is that cells undergoing their final mitosis early in development are found in deep cortical layers, whereas later-forming cells are found in progressively more superficial layers. This "inside-out" gradient means that later-forming cells migrate past neurons that are already in place.[2] This may have important implications for the subsequent development of intracortical connections. Intracortical circuitry is characterized by a columnar organization.

There are probably several mechanisms that help to direct cells to their ultimate location. Some cells clearly have an inherent directional predilection, as has been demonstrated for neuroblastoma cells. Cells tend to cling to solid surfaces and move along them. For example, embryonic epithelial cells, when cultured on a glass plate scored with fine grooves, tend to move along the grooves.[22] Cell adhesion molecules (CAMs) play a major role in assisting the aggregation of like cell types and the establishment of patterns of cellular positioning.[27] Antibodies to neural CAMs have been found to disrupt morphogenesis in a manner consistent with the hypothesis that CAMs play a role in pattern formation.

Programmed Cell Death

The total number of neurons in any given brain region is remarkably constant from individual to individual. While some of the regulation of neuronal number is accomplished during the phases of cellular proliferation and migration, another mechanism also plays an important role in this process of regulation. The process of programmed cell death has been studied most closely in the simple soil-dwelling nematode, *Caenorhabditis elegans*. This simple organism consists of 959 cells, 302 of which are neurons. During development, 118 neurons die in a highly specific, preprogrammed fashion.[14] Specific genes have been isolated that have been described

as "suicide" genes, because activation of these genes results in inexorable cell death. The CED3 gene causes massive calcium influx into the cell, while the CED4 gene causes cell death by protein phosphorylation.[29] The CED9 gene appears to be in control of the activation of these two suicide genes. While it is activated, the suicide genes remain inactive. If the CED9 gene becomes inactive, the two suicide genes are activated, and the cell dies.[11]

It is important not to extrapolate too freely from simple invertebrate organisms to the embryology of complex vertebrates. Invertebrate cells must differentiate after very few cell divisions, because the total number of cell divisions before development is completed is small. In contrast, cells at early stages in the development of vertebrates have a much broader range of potential fates. Nevertheless the existence of cell death as part of vertebrate development has been clearly demonstrated. For example, in the lateral motor columns of the spinal cord, there are initially more cells than will be found at maturity. During a defined temporal window, the total number of neurons in the lateral motor column decreases by about 40%.[10] The same is true of the cells in the sensory ganglia. Cell death, in part, involves competition for available targets. Cells that are unsuccessful in the competition for target tissue are eliminated. One of the mechanisms that accomplishes this elimination is the complex protein, nerve growth factor (NGF). An understanding of the significance of NGF as well as its purification led to a Nobel Prize for Levi-Montalcini in 1986.[17] NGF is produced by the targets of NGF-sensitive neurons (sympathetic and sensory neurons in the periphery and some populations of central nervous system neurons, including the cholinergic cells of the basal forebrain). The NGF-sensitive cells have specific NGF receptors on their axon terminals that take up NGF from the target cell. The NGF is then transported back to the neuronal cell bodies, where it promotes cell survival and differentiation. In the absence of NGF, the neurons die. Currently it is not known whether there are other trophic substances that operate on other cell types in a manner similar to that of NGF. It is assumed that such molecules exist, and much current research is seeking such substances.

Cellular Maturation: Axons, Dendrites, Synapses, and Energy Metabolism

Directional Growth of Axons

The growth of an axon to a specific target cell to which the neuron can then rapidly communicate is a uniquely neuronal property. The means by which axons are able to traverse long distances and accurately locate target cells are as yet poorly understood. Most likely a number of influences act together to ensure accurate navigation. The mechanisms that lead axons to their targets may be quite different from those that signal arrival at an appropriate target.[21]

Although, in general, axonal growth is specific, in some areas there is a refinement of axonal projections as the organism matures. Initially there may be a considerable overproliferation of axons projecting to areas where they do not project in the mature animal. These ectopic projections are then withdrawn during the course of development.

The revision of axonal connections during development could involve either the death of cells that project inappropriately or the withdrawal of axonal branches. In fact, both cell death and axon withdrawal seem to occur outside of the cerebral cortex, although within the cerebral cortex, the mechanism seems to be primarily axon withdrawal.

Before an axon is able to establish synaptic connection with the target cell, it is necessary for that target to have established an appropriate receptive surface—that is, to have elaborated its dendritic tree.[27]

Dendritic Development

One of the most striking characteristics of differentiated neurons is the immense diversity of the dendritic branching patterns. A useful generalization is that dendrites are less sensitive to the environment than axons and that many aspects of dendritic form are determined by factors that are intrinsic to the neurons themselves. Nevertheless, although neurons from the same class show broad similarities of shape when grown in tissue culture, there are also multiple individual differences.

Dendrites often develop at the same time that incoming axons targeting that cell are arriving and establishing synaptic connections. This is particularly true in cortical areas. For example, in the dentate gyrus of the rat adjacent to the hippocampus, growth of dendrites begins around birth and is essentially complete by about 30 days of age[7] (Fig. 1–4). Axonal ingrowth and synaptogenesis occur over this same period. A similar pattern of dendritic differentiation occurs in the case of Purkinje cells of the cerebellar cortex. In other regions of the brain, parallel development of dendrites and axons is not invariably seen. Studies of the auditory system of the chicken reveal that some cells develop a system of dendrites that is considerably more extensive than that that is maintained in the adult.

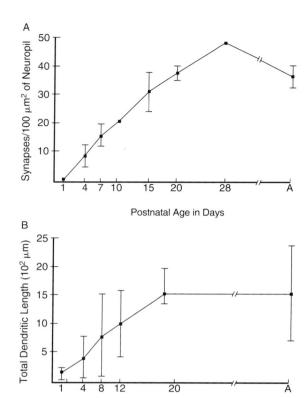

FIGURE 1–4. ☐

The mean total dendritic length of individual neurons according to age in the rat. (From Steward O. Principles of Cellular, Molecular, and Developmental Neuroscience. New York, Springer-Verlag, 1989, p 182.)

Although some cells appear to be capable of developing dendrites in the absence of axonal innervation, for many neurons the final form of the dendrite seems to depend not only on the presence, but also on the functional activity of the synapses that innervate them. For example, sensory deprivation can lead to dramatic alterations in the size and orientation of dendrites in sensory structures (e.g., visual deprivation leads to a redistribution of dendrites of stellate cells in the visual cortex). Normally the dendrites of stellate cells arborize extensively within the fourth layer of the cortex, where thalamic axons terminate; if animals are raised in the dark, the dendrites arborize predominantly in other layers and appear to avoid the fourth layer. Nevertheless, the dendrites are still easily recognizable as typical of stellate cells. It may be that intrinsic factors determine the initial form of the dendrite, while extrinsic factors maintain dendrites, preventing their deterioration.[27]

Synapses

Synapse Formation. An understanding of synapses is fundamental to an understanding of the computational powers of the central nervous system, as well as to an understanding of information storage and behavior modification. Much of the information that is known about synapse formation has been gained from a study of neuromuscular junctions. Only relatively recently has more direct study of central synapses begun.

It appears that synaptogenesis begins very early in development and continues for a long time. Synapse formation usually starts as soon as axons reach the vicinity of postsynaptic cells. Spontaneous miniature end plate potentials can be recorded from individual *Xenopus* muscle fibers within a day of fertilization and within only a few hours of neural tube closure. Postsynaptic potentials can be evoked in muscles by nerve stimulation just a few hours later.[3] Similarly, synapses between neurons in the mammalian autonomic nervous system begin to form within hours of axon arrival in the neighborhood of the target cells.

Although synaptogenesis begins very early in intrauterine life, the process continues for a considerable period of time. The number of synapses that can be counted in electron microscopic sections in many areas of the mammalian brain continues to increase for weeks to months after birth (Fig. 1–5). Furthermore, a plateau does not necessarily indicate that synapse formation has stopped; synapses might still be turning over at a steady rate.

Once a synapse has formed, the attainment of fully mature characteristics still takes many days or even several weeks. For example, the metabolism and function of acetylcholine (ACh) receptors change with time. The half-life of both junctional and extrajunctional receptors in the chick 1 week after hatching is about 30 hours; by several weeks later, the half-life of receptors has increased to 5 days.[4] A similar stabilization occurs at newly formed synapses in mammalian muscle.

Neurotransmitter Receptors and Synaptogenesis. Neurotransmitters are not inherently excitatory or inhibitory. The action of a neurotransmitter depends on its postsynaptic receptor and the intracellular processes that are influenced by the receptor. There are two general classes of receptors: those that function through their actions on ion channels and those that induce the activation of a separate system of activators within the cell, the so-

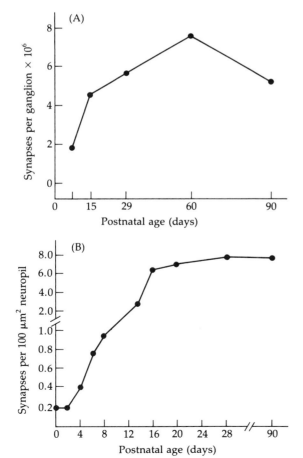

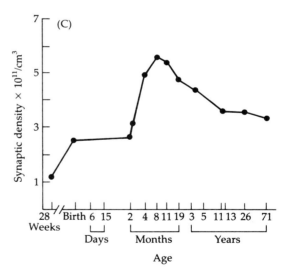

FIGURE 1–5. □

Synaptogenesis measured by synapse counts in electron microscopic sections in the rat superior cervical ganglion *(A)*, the rat visual cortex *(B)*, and the human visual cortex *(C)*. (From Purves D, Lichtman JW. Principles of Neural Development. Sunderland, MA, Sinauer Associates, 1985, p 209.)

called *second messenger system.* A second messenger system may involve the induction of genes or the transcription of RNA.[18]

The best understood receptor is the nicotinic receptor for ACh. In response to the binding of ACh, a cation-specific ion channel is rapidly opened, leading to an increase in sodium and potassium conductance and then to rapid depolarization of the membrane. The structure of the receptor protein has been defined. It is a protein consisting of five subunits. The ion channel is essentially a pore, the sides of which are formed by portions of the membrane-spanning domains of each of the subunits. The binding of ACh to the receptor is thought to cause a change in the conformation of the receptor. Other properties of receptors are also likely to be the result of conformational changes. For example, the phenomenon of desensitization is probably caused by a change of the receptor between a resting activatable conformation and an inactive conformation in response to prolonged exposure to ACh.

Gamma-aminobutyric acid (GABA) and glycine receptors are ionophore-linked receptors like ACh. They differ from ACh in that they open anion-specific membrane channels, leading to an increase in chloride conductance. There are a number of similarities in structure between the subunits of the GABA and ACh receptors.

The amino acid neurotransmitters (e.g., glutamate, aspartate) also use ionophore-linked receptors. There are three major types of excitatory amino acid receptors. The quisqualate and kainate receptors open both cation and anion channels. The *N*-methyl-D-aspartate (NMDA) receptor opens a calcium channel. It is thought that the calcium that enters the neuron in response to the opening of the NMDA channel may serve as an intracellular second messenger. In this way the NMDA receptor is thought to function as both an ionophore-linked receptor and a second messenger–linked receptor.

A number of other neurotransmitters, including dopamine, serotonin, norepinephrine and histamine, function as second messenger–linked receptors, generally through activation of the enzyme adenylate cyclase. Resultant increases in intracellular cyclic adenosine monophosphate (cAMP) activate cAMP-dependent protein kinase, which in turn phosphorylates a particular set of enzyme substrates within the cell. Another important second messenger system, as described in relation to the NMDA receptor, is the calcium-dependent system. Calcium stimulates calmodulin-dependent protein kinase, resulting in phosphorylation of the proteins that are normally the substrates of this kinase. Recent work has suggested that the calcium/calmodulin second messenger system plays an important

role in the phenomenon of "long-term potentiation" of synaptic transmission. This phenomenon was initially discovered in the hippocampus, which has a high concentration of NMDA receptors and is thought to play a role in memory formation. Short periods of high-frequency stimulation of afferent pathways induce increases in synaptic potency that persist for days and sometimes weeks.

For almost 100 years neuroembryologists have believed that one of the mechanisms by which neurons establish contact and form a synapse with an appropriate target cell is through the recognition of specific molecular surface markers on the target cell. In 1895 Langley suggested that axons grew more or less randomly throughout targets, exploring the suitability of cells that they happened to contact. Currently it is thought that membrane receptor sites may function at least in part in this role.[8] For example, glutamate recognition sites are widely distributed in human fetal brain in a pattern that is distinct from that observed in the adult brain. In adult humans and rats, there are few glutamate binding sites in the globus pallidus region of the basal ganglia. However, in the first week of life there is a very rapid increase in the number of glutamate binding sites in the rat (Fig. 1–6); this increase occurs parallel to the known establishment of synapses in this area over the same time frame.[9] A similar result has been suggested by the study of two human brains, 2 and 6 weeks old. This high concentration of glutamate receptors in the globus pallidus during the perinatal period raises the possibility that glutamate excitotoxicity[23] may be involved in the pathogenesis of cerebral palsy, a com-

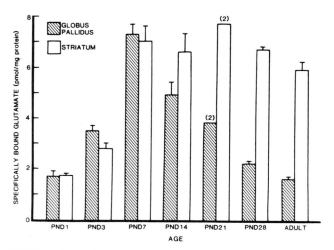

FIGURE 1–6. ☐

Glutamate binding in globus pallidus and striatum in the developing rat brain. This figure illustrates the rapid increase in glutamate binding receptor sites in the first weeks of life. (From Greenamyre T, Penney JB, Young AB, et al. Evidence for transient perinatal glutamatergic innervation of globus pallidus. J Neurosci 7:1022, 1987.)

mon outcome of perinatal hypoxia and ischemia, although rare at older ages.

Maturation of Cellular Energy Metabolism

There is currently much interest in the rapid changes that occur in high-energy phosphate metabolism in the first weeks of life. Increasing sophistication in both in vitro and in vivo methods of nuclear magnetic resonance (NMR) spectroscopy allows for noninvasive measurement of phosphocreatine and adenosine triphosphate as well as the flux between these two compounds.[5] The concentration of phosphocreatine relative to total nucleoside triphosphate concentration, as measured by NMR spectroscopy, doubles in the first 40 days of life in the mouse brain (Fig. 1–7).[12] This ratio also doubles in the human brain over a period beginning at 30 weeks of gestation and continuing after birth. In contrast to the gradual increase in phosphocreatine concentration over 40 days, there is a sudden increase in the rates of aerobic and anaerobic metabolism during a narrow time window lasting 3 to 5 days in the middle of the first month of life of the rat. Holtzman and associates[13] studied potassium-stimulated respiration in cerebral cortical slices taken from rats 2 to 60 days old. They found a 300% to 500% increase in tissue respiration with exposure to potassium in animals 15 days and older but not in animals 10 days old and younger. This is consistent with the relatively abrupt increase in the maximal respiratory capacity of the cerebral cortical tissue of the immature rat as measured by stimulation with the uncoupling agent 2,4-dinitrophenol (DNP). There is a similar change in the ability to produce lactate. More recent work by the same group at Children's Hospital in Boston has demonstrated that there is a rapid increase in phosphorous fluxes catalysed by creatine-kinase over the same narrow time frame which can facilitate rapid conversion of phosphocreatine to adenosine triphosphate. Adenosine triphosphate synthesis catalyzed by creatine kinase increases about four times in the rat brain in the narrow time frame between 10 and 15 days of age.[12] This allows the maturing animal to respond more rapidly to increasing energy demands. Whether this is advantageous in protecting the animal from a hypoxic ischemic insult remains unclear. Although it may be useful to be able to instantly couple energy production to demand in the more mature animal, it is also possible that in the fetus facing the stress of the birth process, a lack of energy coupling to demand is protective against excitotoxic neuronal injury. The same argument can be applied to the low density of neurotransmitter receptors in the neonate; thus, this may be a useful protective mechanism.

Early studies by Norwood and coworkers[19] at Children's Hospital in Boston, using NMR spectroscopy and perfused neonatal rat brain, examined the rate of disappearance of phosphocreatine and adenosine triphosphate during total ischemia at two different temperatures. The half-life of phosphocreatine in the isolated neonatal rat brain was 7.5 and 9.5 minutes, whereas that of adenosine triphosphate was 9.0 and 70 minutes at 37°C and 20°C, respectively. While the pH dropped 0.5 units at 37°C, it was unchanged during ischemia at 20°C. After ischemia at 20°C, adenosine triphosphate and phosphocreatine returned to preinsult levels within 20 minutes, while at 37°C, the recovery of adenosine triphosphate and phosphocreatine was incomplete. Norwood and colleagues also demonstrated that total ischemia resulted in a slower depletion of phosphocreatine in the neonatal rat as compared with adult rats, while the half-life for adenosine triphosphate depletion in adult and neonatal rats was the same. This may well be related to the change in creatine kinase activity with age, as demonstrated by Holtzman and associates.[12]

Apart from assessment of phosphocreatine and adenosine triphosphate, there are several other metabolites and lipids that are detectable by ^{31}P or ^{1}H magnetic resonance spectroscopy and that show substantial changes during early development, al-

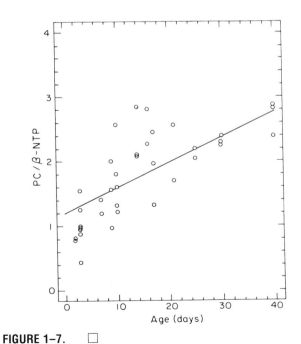

FIGURE 1–7. □

The concentration of phosphocreatine relative to total nucleoside triphosphate concentration as measured by NMR spectroscopy doubles in the first 40 days of life in the mouse brain. (From Holtzman D, McFarland EW, Jacobs D, et al. Maturational increase in mouse brain creatine kinase reaction rates shown by phosphorous magnetic resonance. Brain Res Dev Brain Res 58:181–188, 1991.)

though the exact significance of these changes as yet remains unclear.[5] Phosphoethanolamine (PEth) comprises the bulk of the phosphomonoester (pme) peak in neonatal pigs and rats, but only 40% to 50% of the pme peak in adult rats and humans. PEth may be related in some way to myelin production. N-Acetylaspartic acid (NAA), which may serve as a precursor to NAA glutamate (a neuroexcitatory compound), shows a fivefold increase in rat brain between birth and 20 days.[15] NAA produces an extremely powerful ^{1}H NMR signal and may prove to be a useful marker of neuronal viability. It is currently being used to follow the progress of neurodegenerative conditions such as Alzheimer's disease. It is possible that it will be a useful marker of developmental progress. In contrast to the fivefold increase observed with NAA, taurine, which facilitates synaptic connections in developing neuronal tissue, undergoes a fourfold decrease from birth to adulthood. Glutamate, the excitatory amino acid neurotransmitter, is the most abundant amino acid in adult brain. It has been shown to double in concentration between birth and 21 days in rats.

NMR spectroscopy has also demonstrated probable differences in the buffering capacities of adult and neonatal brain. This buffering difference may help to account for the ability of the neonatal brain to survive longer periods of hypoxia or anoxia when compared with adults of the same species.[5, 28]

PRENATAL BRAIN PERFORMANCE

The earliest detectable reflex in the nervous system appears at about the eighth week of intrauterine life.[1] If a stimulus is applied to the lip region at this time, the hand region exhibits a withdrawal reflex. Touching the lips at 11 weeks of gestation elicits swallowing movements. At 14 weeks of gestation, the reflexogenic zones spread so that touching the face of the embryo results in a complex sequence of movements consisting of head rotation, grimacing, stretching of the body, and extension of the extremities. At 22 weeks, the embryo exhibits stretching movements and pursing of the lips; at 29 weeks, sucking movements become apparent. At birth almost all reflexes are of brain stem origin; cortical control of such reflexes is minimal.

POSTNATAL GROSS STRUCTURAL DEVELOPMENT

As described previously, there is an enormous increase in the size of the human brain during the first year of life. Virtually no neurons are added after birth, but there is a large increase in the number of glial cells, the size and complexity of the neurons, the amount of myelin, and the number and complexity of neuronal connections. The color of the cortex at birth is uniformly pale, similar to the color of white matter. Although the newborn brain shows the same six-layered cellular lamination of the adult cerebral cortex, the cells of the neonatal cortex are tightly packed together, with few, if any, processes to separate them. Nissl bodies (RNA ribosomes attached to flattened vesicles) are sparse in cortical neurons, although they are abundant in brain stem and spinal cord neurons.[1]

At 3 months of age there is still poor differentiation between gray and white matter, and cortical Nissl substance remains scanty, but neurons are not as closely packed as in the newborn brain. By 6 months, Nissl material is more prominent, and the distinction between gray and white matter can be easily made. By 1 year of age, the density of cortical neurons has been further reduced as a result of an increase in neuronal and glial processes separating neuronal cell bodies. The Nissl substance within the cell bodies is well developed.

CHANGES IN CEREBRAL BLOOD FLOW AND OXYGEN CONSUMPTION

Cerebral blood flow in the human newborn is low. It increases to reach a maximum of 105 ml/100 gm/min between the ages of 3 and 5 years and then decreases to reach the adult rate of 54 ml/100 gm/min. Oxygen consumption in the newborn brain is also low and increases with maturation, reflecting the changes in energy metabolism at a cellular level as described earlier. Oxygen consumption peaks at 5 ml/100 gm/min, which is equivalent to 50% of the child's total oxygen consumption. With further development it reaches the adult level of 3.5 ml/100 gm/min. The low cerebral oxygen consumption in the brain at birth mirrors the low levels of creatine kinase activity at that time.[1]

DEVELOPMENT OF BEHAVIOR

In the past, the study of behavior and its development by psychologists and ethologists has been quite a separate discipline from neurobiology. However, more recently the gap between these fields has narrowed. Ethologists have shown that much animal activity is innate and not subject to modification by environmental influences. This is also true for humans, in whom much inherent behavior results from neural connections that ensure survival and reproduction and that remain quite outside the sphere of consciousness. Indeed, consciousness is just a small corner of the human "neural universe."[21] Nevertheless, there are behaviors that can be modified by the environment. The most graphic examples are the imprinting in some newly hatched birds. Newly hatched ducklings will crouch and run away when a human attempts to pick them up, but goslings will follow the first moving object they see after birth and will persist indefinitely in this maladaptive behavior. However, this permanent imprinting effect occurs most powerfully soon after hatching and is lost completely within 1 to 2 days. Another example of behavioral modification by environmental influences can be found in the development of bird song. Young finches raised in isolation develop a song that, although quite poor in quality, is recognizable as the song of that species. However, the fully formed song must be learned from mature finches during a critical period early in life. Sparrows' preconception of what constitutes a proper song is so acute that they will not learn the songs of other sparrow species when exposed to them in the laboratory. However, they are able to learn their own song even when it is spliced together with songs of other species in what would seem to be a confusing sequence. Indeed, many observations confirm that the neonatal nervous system contains detailed information about what behaviors to learn and when to learn them.

COMPLETION OF NEURAL DEVELOPMENT

It is difficult to define the point at which neural development ends, if indeed it ever does. The ability of higher animals to modify their behavior as a result of experience implies that the nervous system changes continually throughout life. It seems most likely that synapses represent the sites of continuing neural evolution. The study of "synaptic plasticity" is currently an area of intense interest. Whether synaptic plasticity is based primarily on continuous turnover of synapses—with new synapses being continuously formed while older synapses are broken—or on modification of the efficacy of established, permanent synapses remains unclear.

CONCLUSION

Clearly there are many unanswered questions regarding neural development at all levels: molecular, cellular, anatomic and physiologic. In some ways, the neural development of complex animals resem-

bles the development of a closed ecosystem in which individual neurons behave like separate organisms. What happens to an individual nerve cell cannot be foretold with any exactness, because its role in life depends on competitive interactions with similar cells. Exploring this field of "neuroecology," as Purves and Lichtman[21] have termed it, may provide the best hope of understanding the remarkable properties of the human nervous system.

REFERENCES

1. Afifi AK, Bergman RA. Basic Neuroscience. Baltimore, Urban & Schwartzberg, 1986.
2. Bayer SA, Altman J. Neocortical Development. New York, Raven Press, 1991.
3. Blackshaw SE, Warner AE. Low resistance junctions between mesoderm cells during development of trunk muscles. J Physiol (Lond) 255:209, 1976.
4. Burden S. Development of the neuromuscular junction in the chick embryo: The number, distribution, and stability of acetylcholine receptors. Dev Biol 57:317, 1977.
5. Corbett RJT. In vivo multicenter magnetic resonance spectroscopy investigation of cerebral development. Sem Perinatol 14:258, 1990.
6. Cowan WM. Aspects of neural development. In Porter R (ed). Neurophysiology III. International Review of Physiology. Vol 17. Baltimore, University Park Press, pp 149–191.
7. Cowan WM, Stanfield BB, Kishi K. The development of the dentate gyrus. Curr Top Dev Biol 15:103, 1980.
8. Edelman GM. Cell adhesion molecules. Science 219:450, 1983.
9. Greenamyre T, Penney JB, Young AB, et al. Evidence for transient perinatal glutamergic innervation of globus pallidus. J Neurosci 7:1022, 1987.
10. Hamburger V. Cell death in the development of the lateral motor column of the chick embryo. J Comp Neurol 160:535, 1975.
11. Hengartner MO, Ellis RE, Horvitz HR. C. elegans gene CED-9 protects cells from programmed cell death. Nature 356:494, 1992.
12. Holtzman D, McFarland EW, Jacobs D, et al. Maturational increase in mouse brain creatine kinase reaction rates shown by phosphorus magnetic resonance. Dev Brain Res 22:58, 1991.
13. Holtzman D, Olson J, Zamvil S, et al. Maturation of potassium stimulated respiration in rat cerebral cortex slices. J Neurochem 39:274, 1982.
14. Horvitz HR, Ellis HM, Sternberg PW. Programmed cell death in nematode development. Neurosci Comment 1:56, 1982.
15. Koller KJ, Coyle JT. Ontogenesis of N-acetyl-aspartate and N-acetyl-glutamate in rat brain. Dev Brain Res 15:137, 1984.
16. LeDouarin NM. Migration and differentiation of neural crest cells. Curr Top Dev Biol 16:31, 1980.
17. Levi-Montalcini R, Levi G. Selective growth-stimulating effects of mouse sarcoma, producing hyperplasia of sympathetic ganglia and hyperneurotization of viscera in the chick embryo. J Exp Zool 123:223, 1953.
18. McGeer PL, Eccles JC, McGeer EG. Molecular Neurobiology of the Mammalian Brain. New York, Plenum Press, 1987.
19. Norwood WI, Norwood CR, Ingwall JS, et al. Hypothermic circulatory arrest: 31-phosphorous nuclear magnetic resonance of isolated perinatal neonatal rat brain. J Thorac Cardiovasc Surg 78:823, 1979.
20. Patterson PH, Chun LL. The induction of acetylcholine synthesis in primary cultures of dissociated rat sympathetic neurons. I. Effects of conditioned medium. Dev Biol 56:263, 1977.

21. Purves D, Lichtman JW. Principles of Neural Development. Sunderland, MA, Sinauer Associates, 1985.
22. Rovensky YA, Slavnaja IL, Vasiliev JM. Behaviour of fibroblast-like cells on grooved surfaces. Exp Cell Res 65:193, 1971.
23. Simon RP, Swan JH, Griffith T, et al. Blockade of N-methyl-D-aspartate receptors may protect against ischemic damage in the brain. Science 226:850, 1984.
24. Spemann H. Embryonic Development and Induction. New York, Yale University Press, 1938.
25. Spitzer NC. Development of membrane properties in vertebrates. Trends Neurosci 4:169, 1981.
26. Stent GS. Explicity and implicit semantic content of the genetic information. In Butts RE, Hintikka J (eds). Foundational Problems in the Special Sciences. Dordrecht, Holland, D. Reidel, 1977, pp 131–149.
27. Steward O. Principles of Cellular, Molecular, and Developmental Neuroscience. New York, Springer-Verlag, 1989.
28. Volpe JJ. Hypoxic-ischemic encephalopathy: Basic aspects and fetal assessment. In Volpe JJ (ed). Neurology of the Newborn. Philadelphia, WB Saunders, 1987, pp 160–195.
29. Yuan JY, Horvitz HR. The Caenorhabditis elegans genes CED-3 and CED-4 act cell autonomously to cause programmed cell death. Dev Biol 138:33, 1990.

RESPIRATORY SYSTEM

An understanding of the developmental features of the respiratory system is relevant to surgical repair of congenital heart disease for a number of reasons. First, many cardiac defects (e.g., tetralogy of Fallot with pulmonary atresia and truncus arteriosus) involve not only the heart, but also the lungs and the pulmonary circulation. Second, the success of reparative or palliative cardiac operations is often highly dependent on the status of the lungs and pulmonary circulation, and in the extreme case, pulmonary vascular obstructive disease (PVOD) precludes intracardiac repair. Third, the development of the gas-exchanging apparatus in the lung and the pulmonary circulation are interrelated, and therefore, it is important that conditions in the pulmonary circulation be optimized to optimize the development of the gas-exchanging units. Finally, and perhaps most importantly, a significant fraction of the final development of both the gas-exchanging apparatus and the pulmonary circulation occurs postnatally, and therefore, interventions that alter the hemodynamics of the pulmonary circulation can have a significant effect on the overall development of the entire cardiorespiratory system.

DEVELOPMENT OF THE GAS-EXCHANGING APPARATUS

The tracheobronchial tree begins as a ventral outpouching from the primitive foregut at approximately 4 weeks of gestation, with endodermal ingrowth into the surrounding mesenchymal tissue. This ingrowth initiates the pseudoglandular phase of lung development, which continues up to 16 to 17 weeks of gestation. During this time the tubules branch out to give rise to successive generations of the tracheobronchial tree, and during these first 16 to 17 weeks, the architecture of the entire tracheobronchial tree is determined.[1] The majority (65% to 75%) of the bronchi are formed between the tenth and fourteenth week of gestation.[3] This development is believed to depend on interactions between the epithelium and the mesenchymal tissue that involve the release of soluble factors, as well as on direct contact between the epithelium and the mesenchyme.[7] During this stage, the mesenchymal tissue is also differentiating to initiate the formation of cartilage, connective tissue, muscle, blood vessels, and lymphatics.[6] After birth, the conducting airways increase in both length and diameter, but the number of conducting airways does not change. The early gestational age at which airway development occurs explains the finding of reduced numbers of airway generations in those with congenital diaphragmatic hernia, as the intestines migrate back into the abdomen at approximately 10 weeks of gestation.[12]

Beginning at 17 weeks of gestation, the lung enters the canalicular stage, during which the initial formation of respiratory bronchioles and acinar units begins and the lumens of the airways begin to widen, with thinning of the epithelium. The epithelium of the distal airways begins to differentiate into cells that are recognizable as type I (flat pneumocytes) and type II (cuboidal) cells. There is evidence that the type I cells arise by differentiation from type II cells[1] and that this differentiation is modulated by direct cellular contacts between the epithelium and mesenchymal fibroblasts. Rearrangement of the interstitium and a relative slowdown in mesenchymal growth occur, resulting in a reduction of the distance between the lumen of the distal airways and the lumen of the adjacent blood vessels.[2]

The saccular (or terminal sac) stage begins at 26 weeks of gestation and is characterized by an enormous enlargement of the peripheral air spaces.[3]

Some terminal bronchioles are transformed into respiratory bronchioles, and clusters of airways called *saccules* appear. The saccules are not true alveoli, because they are larger and do not have the smooth outline of true alveoli.[6] It has been thought that in humans this developmental stage lasts until full-term birth, and the formation of true alveoli is generally believed to be a postnatal event.[3, 12] Others have suggested that true alveoli may be found at as early as 32 to 34 weeks of gestation.[2] However, surfactant production by the type II pneumocytes occurs late in gestation (generally around 32 to 34 weeks) and appears to be at least partially governed by the level of corticosteroids in the fetal circulation.[1] Interestingly, differentiation of the respiratory epithelial cells in the acinus appears to depend on the extent of contact between interstitial fibroblasts and respiratory epithelial cells and the type of collagen in proximity to the epithelial cells.[1]

The alveolar phase of development involves the formation of secondary septa within the terminal saccules along with the deposition of elastin.[2] The saccules are partitioned into alveolar ducts and sacs, and each terminal saccule develops into an alveolar duct proximally and an atrium distally. One to four alveolar sacs form distal to the atrium of each terminal saccule, and each sac consists of many alveoli.[6] There is some dispute about the duration of this phase, with some authors concluding that alveolarization is complete by 24 months,[2] while others contend that adult numbers of alveoli are not reached until 8 years of age.[6, 12] Studies in rats show that, in conjunction with alveolarization, the volume of the air space increases by a factor of 6.2 and capillary volume increases by a factor of 7.6, while the total volume of lung tissue increases by a factor of only 2.6.[2] Similar changes seem to occur in humans during the first 18 months of life. Thereafter, these various compartments appear to grow more proportionately.[2]

From a clinical perspective, a few experimental observations on the development of the gas-exchanging apparatus seem worthy of emphasis. The first is that elevated concentrations of inspired oxygen result in reduced postnatal septation of alveoli and a decrease in the normal increase in alveolar surface area.[7] The second is that although corticosteroids cause an increase in surfactant production by type II pneumocytes, they also cause a generalized enhancement of lung maturation by reducing cell division and increasing differentiation. As a result, the lungs of neonatal animals from mothers treated with steroids late in pregnancy are somewhat smaller than normal at birth.[1] Postnatal administration of corticosteroids to rats during the period of alveolar septation results in markedly impaired septation.[7]

DEVELOPMENT OF THE PULMONARY VASCULATURE

The development of the preacinar pulmonary arterial system is closely related to the development of the air-conducting system. The primitive heart anlage with systemic arterial and venous connections is present by the third week of gestation, and the sixth branchial arches, which will ultimately form the central pulmonary arteries, appear at 32 days.[3] Within the lung parenchyma, the intrapulmonary blood vessels develop from the mesenchymal tissue during the pseudoglandular phase of airway development. Before the connection of the sixth branchial arch to the intrapulmonary vasculature, the developing lung buds receive their arterial supply from paired segmental arteries that arise from the dorsal aorta. Normally, by 50 days, these segmental arteries have regressed and no longer supply the lung.[3] However, these vessels do persist in certain circumstances, such as lobar sequestration and some cases of tetralogy of Fallot with pulmonary atresia, and in these situations they become the large systemic arteries that supply the lung parenchyma. The normal pulmonary arteries continue to develop and branch alongside the emerging tracheobronchial tree, and additional preacinar arteries (including the "supernumerary" arteries that do not follow the tracheobronchial tree but supply the acinus directly) continue to appear up to the time that terminal bronchioles are forming (16 weeks).[6, 15] Thereafter, these arteries increase in length and diameter, but new preacinar arteries do not appear. All subsequent arterial branches that form in the lung are within the acinus. There is a marked increase in the number of these intra-acinar arteries in the first 2 months after birth, and the majority of the new arterial branches that appear postnatally are formed within the first year of life as new alveoli are forming.[3] The walls of the preacinar pulmonary arteries normally change from elastic to muscular in nature as the vessel progresses from a proximal to a distal location. Normally this transition occurs at the level of the bronchiolus (seventh generation of branching of the tracheobronchial tree). This "adult" pattern of elastic arteries to the seventh generation and muscular arteries in successive generations of the pulmonary arterial tree is achieved by the nineteenth week of gestation.[3] Just before birth, the wall thickness of the preacinar arteries is significantly greater than it is shortly after birth;

this prenatal morphology appears to be due to thickened and overlapping endothelial and smooth muscle cells in the vessel wall.[15] In utero the wall thickness of these vessels is 14% to 20% of the external arterial diameter.[6] These thick-walled arteries are thought to be responsible for the high pulmonary vascular resistance in utero. Within minutes after birth, the endothelial cells lining the nonmuscular arteries of the alveolar walls become remarkably thinner, apparently in association with inflation of the lung and the consequent "stretching" of the vascular tree.[15] Similar thinning of the smooth muscle cells in the media also occurs, along with reduced overlapping between adjacent cells.[3, 15] Within the first month, the ratio of wall thickness to external diameter reaches the "adult" level of 6%.

Development of the intra-acinar vessels begins later in gestation, and a significant proportion of this development continues after birth. This postnatal development is heavily influenced by hemodynamic conditions in the pulmonary vascular bed, including both pulmonary blood flow and pulmonary artery pressure. In the normal pulmonary artery tree, there is a progressive decrease in the muscularization of the muscular pulmonary arteries as the more distal generations of the pulmonary artery tree are encountered. In the normal newborn, the intra-acinar arterial branches are mostly nonmuscular, but after birth there is a gradual muscularization of the intra-acinar vessels until the adult pattern is reached. In some conditions in which there is markedly elevated pulmonary vascular resistance in the neonate, such as persistent fetal circulation and (interestingly) the meconium aspiration syndrome, the normal neonatal pattern of nonmuscularized intra-acinar arteries is not present,[12] and there is an abnormal distal extension of arterial musculature into the acinar vessels. Similar excessive muscularization of the peripheral arterial branches is also found in patients with the hypoplastic left heart syndrome.[3] In the postnatal period, the extension of muscle into the acinar vessels occurs at an accelerated pace in patients with lesions that result in increased pulmonary blood flow, such as ventricular septal defect or patent ductus arteriosus.[3, 9, 11, 12] In addition, the amount of muscle in the normally muscularized preacinar arteries is increased in conditions in which there is increased pulmonary artery pressure[9, 11, 12] and the numbers of intra-acinar vessels are reduced, implying that the normal postnatal proliferation of intra-acinar vessels is impaired.[3, 9, 11, 12] Similar findings have been noted after experimentally created systemic-to-pulmonary artery shunts in growing pigs, and the severity of the changes increased with longer periods of increased pulmonary blood flow and pressure.[13]

The most important issue in situations of increased pulmonary blood flow and pulmonary artery pressure is the development of PVOD. This disorder clearly represents a postnatal developmental problem in the pulmonary vasculature, and it is essentially always fatal once it progresses beyond a certain stage.[8, 11] Because PVOD is not present at birth and early correction (at <9 months of age) of the underlying cardiac or great vessel lesion that causes the increased pulmonary blood flow and pressure prevents the occurrence of PVOD,[11] there continues to be a strong motivation to repair these cardiovascular defects before PVOD develops. The pathologic features of PVOD were described by Heath and Edwards,[5] who first proposed a scheme for classification of the stages of this disorder. The six stages of this classification are based primarily on changes in the media and intima of the pulmonary arteries in the "earlier" stages and are shown in Table 1–1. Patients with lesions beyond grade II have a high likelihood of persistent pulmonary hypertension if the repair is carried out after 2 years of age.[11] An additional morphologic/morphometric classification, subsequently described by Rabinovitch and associates,[9] focused on the extent of muscularization of the pulmonary arterial tree, the degrees of extension of muscularization into the peripheral arterioles, and the number of peripheral arterial branches at the acinar level (see Table 1–1). Unfortunately, the exact links between increased pulmonary blood flow and pressure and the development of PVOD remain incompletely understood, but some initial efforts to understand this process have been made by Rabinovitch and coworkers.[8] In one study, abnormalities were found in the luminal surfaces of pulmonary artery endothelial cells of patients with pulmonary hypertension. There was also increased density of microfilament bundles and rough endoplasmic reticulum in these same endothelial cells from these patients. In the subendothelium, degradation and neosynthesis of the internal elastic lamina were identified.[8] In an experimental model of pulmonary hypertension in the rat, an increased

TABLE 1–1. □ CLASSIFICATION OF PVOD

AUTHOR	STAGE	DESCRIPTION
Heath and Edwards[5]	I	Medial hypertrophy
	II	Intimal proliferation
	III	Intimal fibrosis
	IV	Medial atrophy with dilatation
	V	Angiomatoid malformation
	VI	Fibrinoid necrosis
Reid and Rabinovitch[9]	A	Abnormal distal extension of smooth muscle into normally nonmuscularized arteries
	B	Medial hypertrophy of muscular arteries
	C	Reduced number of arterioles

number of breaks in the internal elastic lamina of large muscular arteries were identified.[8] The synthesis of elastin was increased, but the elastin was abnormally distributed as fragments, which was suggestive of lysis of the elastin, presumably caused by production of an elastase.[8] These abnormalities were associated with "migration" of smooth muscle cells from the media to the subendothelial layers.[8] In light of recent advances in the understanding of interactions between the endothelium and the smooth muscle of blood vessel walls, it is also interesting to note that in the intra-acinar pulmonary arteries, the internal elastic lamina (which separates the endothelium from the media) is patchy and thin. It is in these same arteries that intimal proliferation occurs in response to the pulmonary hypertension associated with congenital heart defects.[3]

There are also changes in the smooth muscles themselves in the early weeks after birth. The smooth muscle cells initially assume the morphologic characteristics of a secretory cell, and, associated with this, there is an increase in the numbers and thickness of the elastic laminae in the vessel wall. This deposition of connective tissue in the wall of the vessel is thought to stabilize the structure of the wall.[3] Relatively soon thereafter (within weeks in the rat), the morphology of the smooth muscle cells changes to that of mature contractile cells.

At the microvascular level, additional changes occur in the first 1.5 years after birth; these have been termed *microvascular maturation* by Burri.[2] In this phase there is a change from a double to a single capillary network in the secondary septa of the alveolar wall, and this change appears to result from a fusion of the two capillary networks.[2] The result of this alteration of the microvascular bed is to reduce the amount of interstitial tissue in the alveolar wall and to reduce the thickness of the interalveolar septa. As a consequence of these changes in the interalveolar septa, there is a marked increase in the alveolar surface area.[2]

The bronchial arterial circulation, which supplies systemic arterial blood to the walls of the major airways of the tracheobronchial tree, develops quite separately from the pulmonary arteries. Bronchial arteries arise from the descending aorta and do not appear until the ninth to twelfth week of gestation. They appear to be embryologically quite distinct from the primitive systemic arteries that supply the lung parenchyma during the first 6 weeks of gestation. The true bronchial arterial circulation does interconnect with the pulmonary artery circulation by capillary anastomoses proximal to the level of the terminal bronchiole,[6] but the frequency and size of these connections normally decreases during the first years of life.[3]

The development of the pulmonary veins seems to occur more or less parallel with the development of the pulmonary arterial system chronologically. The intrapulmonary veins develop from the mesenchymal tissue in the developing lung, and they initially connect to the systemic venous system until 28 to 30 days of gestation. At this time the more proximal (cardiac end) pulmonary vein develops as an outpouching from the left atrium and connects with the previously developed intrapulmonary veins. Some connections between the pulmonary and systemic venous systems do persist in humans, and in cases in which there is a failure of the development of the normal connections between the heart and the intrapulmonary veins, these connections become the only pathway for the pulmonary venous blood.[3] Normally the pulmonary veins have relatively thin musculature in their walls, but in certain conditions, such as the hypoplastic left heart syndrome and obstructed anomalous pulmonary venous return, there is a marked increase in muscularization of the pulmonary veins. It seems likely that these excessively muscularized veins may contribute to pulmonary vascular resistance in these conditions.[3]

DEVELOPMENTAL INTERACTIONS BETWEEN THE AIRWAYS AND THE VASCULATURE

Both experimental and clinical observations support the concept that development in the vasculature influences development in the gas-exchanging apparatus. As noted earlier, congenital heart defects that result in excessive pulmonary blood flow and pulmonary artery pressure are associated with reduced numbers of intra-acinar vessels and abnormal distal extension of muscle into the intra-acinar vessels.[3, 8] Experimentally, the construction of a systemic-to-pulmonary artery shunt results in similar changes in the arterial musculature, but also in decreased lung compliance.[13] Even more interestingly, after removal of these shunts, there was multiplication of both arteries and alveoli at a faster than normal rate.[14] In contrast, ligation of the left pulmonary artery in neonatal pigs resulted in alveoli that were normal in number but smaller than normal in size, while the hyperperfused right lung had reduced numbers of alveoli that were of normal size.[4] In patients with tetralogy of Fallot with or without pulmonary atresia, however, decreased numbers of alveoli that were normal in size have been found.[10] Although the experimental and clinical observations of the effects of either increased or decreased pulmonary blood flow on alveolar development have not been entirely consistent, it is clear that development of the airways and development of the vasculature are linked.

CONCLUSIONS

This review of the development of the lung has emphasized that an important fraction of the development of the lung occurs after birth, particularly within the first 1 to 2 years, and that the presence of congenital cardiac defects has an important impact on this postnatal phase of lung development. The obvious inference from these two points is that early interventions to address congenital heart defects are likely to result in the optimal opportunity for normal development in the lung vasculature and in the gas-exchanging apparatus.

REFERENCES

1. Adamson IYR. Development of lung structure. In Crystal RG, West JB, Barnes PJ, et al (eds). The Lung. New York, Raven Press, 1991, pp 663–670.
2. Burri PH. Postnatal development and growth. In Crystal RG, West JB, Barnes PJ, et al (eds). The Lung. New York, Raven Press, 1991, pp 677–687.
3. Haworth SG. Pulmonary vascular development. In Long WA (ed). Fetal and Neonatal Cardiology. Philadelphia, WB Saunders, 1990, pp 51–63.
4. Haworth SG, McKenzie SA, Fitzpatrick M. Alveolar development after ligation of left pulmonary artery in newborn pig: Clinical relevance to unilateral pulmonary artery. Thorax 36:938–943, 1981.
5. Heath D, Edwards JE. The pathology of hypertensive pulmonary vascular changes in the pulmonary artery with special reference to congenital cardiac septal defect. Circulation 18:533–547, 1958.
6. Inselman LS, Mellins RB. Growth and development of the lung. J Pediatr 98:1–15, 1981.
7. Massaro D, Massaro GD. Regulation of the architectural development. In Crystal RG, West JB, Barnes PJ, et al (eds). The Lung. New York, Raven Press, 1991, pp 689–698.
8. Rabinovitch M. Developmental biology of the pulmonary vascular bed. In Freedom RF, Benson LN, Smallhorn JF (eds). Neonatal Heart Disease. Springer Verlag, London, 1992, pp 45–64.
9. Rabinovitch M, Haworth SG, Castaneda AR, et al. Lung biopsy in congenital heart disease: A morphometric approach to pulmonary vascular disease. Circulation 58:1107–1122, 1978.
10. Rabinovitch M, Herrera-deLeon V, Castaneda AR, Reid LM. Growth and development of the pulmonary vascular bed in patients with tetralogy of Fallot with or without pulmonary atresia. Circulation 64:1234–1249, 1981.
11. Rabinovitch M, Keane JF, Norwood WI, et al. Vascular structure in lung tissue obtained at biopsy correlated with pulmonary hemodynamic findings after repair of congenital heart defects. Circulation 69:655–667, 1984.
12. Reid LM. Lung growth in health and disease. Br J Dis Chest 78:113–134, 1984.
13. Rendas A, Lennox S, Reid L. Aorta-pulmonary shunts in growing pigs. J Thorac Cardiovasc Surg 77:109–118, 1979.
14. Rendas A, Reid L. Pulmonary vasculature of piglets after correction of aorta-pulmonary shunts. J Thorac Cardiovasc Surg 85:911–916, 1983.
15. Riley DJ. Vascular remodeling. In Crystal RG, West JB, Barnes PJ, et al (eds). The Lung. New York, Raven Press, 1991, pp 1189–1198.

2

Chapter

Cardiopulmonary Bypass, Hypothermia, and Circulatory Arrest

It is difficult to argue with the basic premise that complete repair in the first days of life will result in the best long-term outlook for the neonate with a congenital heart anomaly. Why, then, is it only now, nearly 40 years since the introduction of the heart-lung machine, that this goal is beginning to be realized? In 1953, Lillehei and coworkers[48] undertook corrective cardiac procedures in infants with remarkably low morbidity and mortality. However, their method of support for the patient was cross circulation, with the parent functioning as a human oxygenator. When others attempted to duplicate these results using the cumbersome heart-lung machines of the early 1950s, extremely high morbidity and mortality resulted. Despite some refinements of the cardiopulmonary circuit in the 1960s, it was not until 1972, with the refinement of hypothermic circulatory arrest for repair of complex anomalies in infancy by Barratt-Boyes et al.,[6] and subsequently by Castaneda et al.,[18] that improved results were achieved. Hypothermic circulatory arrest, particularly as described by Barratt-Boyes and coworkers, with predominantly surface cooling, limited core cooling, and rewarming using cardiopulmonary bypass (CPB), limited exposure of the infant to CPB to less than 20 minutes. However, by this time the concept of two-stage repair, with an initial palliative procedure (which avoided CPB early in infancy) followed later by a corrective procedure, had become entrenched. Continuing technologic refinements in CPB during the 1980s further reduced the morbidity associated with bypass in neonates and young infants. Although a corrective operation such as an arterial switch currently can be undertaken with a mortality risk of less than 2% in the first month of life, morbidity continues to be significant. This chapter will examine the sources of that morbidity.

MORBIDITY OF CARDIOPULMONARY BYPASS

There are multiple potential sources of organ injury associated with the use of CPB. Large numbers of microemboli, both particulate and gaseous, have been documented by techniques such as retinal fluorescein angiography[13] and specific histochemical methods.[55] These studies have demonstrated the important role of arterial filters and oxygenator design in minimizing the incidence of microemboli.[14] Activation of various humoral cascades by blood contact with synthetic surfaces has been cited as the cause of the whole-body inflammatory response to CPB.[83] In 1983, Kirklin and colleagues[46] described activation of the complement system as a consequence of CPB. The concentration of the complement degradation product C3a was related to the duration of CPB. In a separate study, this group demonstrated

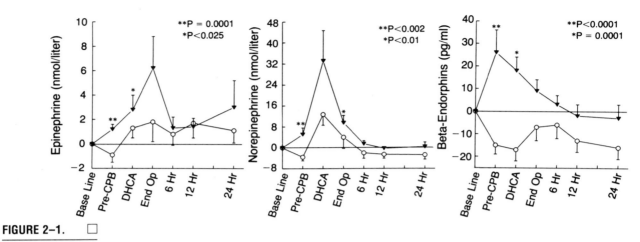

FIGURE 2–1. □

Perioperative changes in plasma epinephrine, norepinephrine, and beta-endorphin in neonates undergoing deep hypothermic circulatory arrest. The solid triangles indicate patients under halothane anesthesia, while the open circles indicate patients under sufentanil anesthesia. The response to the stress of cardiopulmonary bypass, hypothermia, and circulatory arrest can be markedly attenuated by the anesthesia technique. (From Anand KJS, Hickey PR. Halothane-morphine compared with high-dose sufentanil for anesthesia and postoperative analgesia in neonatal cardiac surgery. N Engl J Med 326:1–9, 1992.)

that microvascular permeability is increased by 120 minutes of CPB.[70] C3a has been shown to increase microvascular permeability in the cheek pouch of hamsters.[10]

Both coagulation and fibrinolytic cascades are strongly activated during CPB, resulting in a risk of coagulation factor consumption during CPB and postoperative bleeding. Activation of kallikrein cascades results in elevated levels of bradykinin during and soon after CPB. Other mediators of the whole-body inflammatory response that currently are subjects of investigation include the arachidonic acid cascade (which can result in the release of platelet-activating factor), thromboxane A_2, and interleukin-1.[26] Interleukin-1, which is produced by activated white cells, mediates fever, changes in endothelial cell function and permeability, and a decrease in vascular resistance.

Activation of the cellular components of blood as well as endothelial cells throughout the body further contributes to the whole-body response to CPB. Expression of binding sites or ligands (intercellular adhesion molecule [ICAM] 1–3) on endothelial cells is associated with the extravascular migration of activated neutrophils.[74] These cells are a potent source of oxygen free radicals, which can cause tissue injury.[49] Neutrophil elastase, a connective tissue proteinase and a product of neutrophil activation that appears in plasma, is increased by CPB[84]; peak concentration correlates with the duration of bypass. Platelets activated during CPB both aggregate and adhere to synthetic surfaces, contributing to thrombus formation.

CPB results in a profound metabolic and endocrinologic response.[40] This is an exaggeration of the usual response of the body to the stress of surgery or injury and is importantly influenced by the method of anesthesia[3] (Fig. 2–1), as well as by CPB variables such as the constituents of the prime fluid.[61] Even with a glucose-free prime, blood glucose levels rise secondary to increased glycolysis and gluconeogenesis. There is catabolism of proteins, which contributes amino acids for gluconeogenesis as well as mobilization of fat stores, resulting in increased levels of free fatty acids and ketone bodies. Growth hormone (GH), cortisol, and epinephrine levels increase, contributing particularly to the increased rate of carbohydrate metabolism. In spite of the increase in blood glucose levels, insulin may be decreased initially, but subsequently there is a gradual rise in insulin level. However, insulin is less effective than usual in promoting glucose utilization, indicating some degree of insulin resistance. Vasopressin secretion by the posterior pituitary increases in addition to increased secretion of virtually all the hormones secreted by the anterior pituitary, including adrenocorticotropic hormone (ACTH), thyroid-stimulating hormone (TSH), GH, and prolactin. Most studies have revealed a massive increase in catecholamines, particularly epinephrine. Reves and associates[63] found a ninefold increase in epinephrine and a doubling of norepinephrine during moderately hypothermic bypass in adults (Fig. 2–2). This is almost certainly related to decreased breakdown of catecholamines by the lungs,[34] as well as to increased secretion by the adrenal medulla and the sympathetic nervous system.

The particular significance of these pathologic sequelae of CPB for the infant and child relates to the small blood volume of the pediatric patient relative to the priming volume and synthetic surface area of

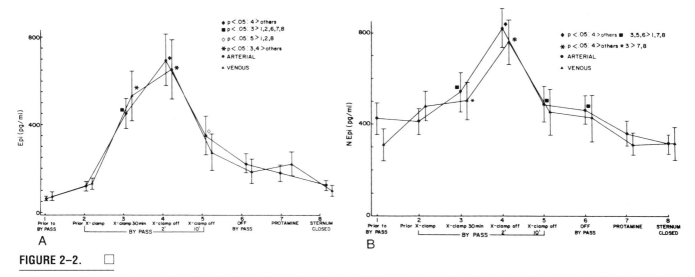

FIGURE 2–2. ☐

Continuous cardiopulmonary bypass with moderate hypothermia is associated with a ninefold increase in epinephrine *(A)* and a doubling of norepinephrine *(B)*. (From Reves JG, Karp RB, Buttner EE, et al. Neuronal and adrenomedullary catecholamine release in response to cardiopulmonary bypass in man. Circulation 66:49–55, 1982.)

the CPB circuit. The average neonate weighing 3.5 kg has a blood volume of 280 ml, while the total priming volume for a standard pediatric oxygenator including filters and tubing is more than 700 ml. Within the oxygenator, the blood is exposed to the huge surface area of a membrane (in membrane oxygenators) or to bubbles (in bubble oxygenators), where gas transfer occurs.

The most visibly obvious morbidity of CPB in the neonate and infant after cardiac surgery is the development of whole-body edema, which is sometimes massive. In a prospective study of 100 neonates with a mean weight of 3.4 kg undergoing corrective cardiac surgery employing approximately 2 hours of CPB, the average fluid accumulation was greater than 600 ml.[87] In their study of complement activation, Kirklin and colleagues[46] demonstrated that young age was an important predictor of pulmonary and hemorrhagic dysfunction as well as overall postoperative morbidity. Young age, per se, is associated with increased capillary permeability and lymph flow.[37, 66]

Decreased Tissue Perfusion During Pediatric Cardiac Surgery

In adults, most cardiac surgical procedures can be performed with the CPB pump perfusing the body at close to a low-normal flow index (2.4 L/min/m²). Often this is not possible in children with congenital heart disease. Most corrective procedures are intracardiac, and the presence of systemic-to-pulmonary collateral blood vessels can result in a high volume of blood returning to the left side of the heart, ob-

scuring surgical exposure. This "left heart return" can be reduced by decreasing the whole-body perfusion rate. Complex anomalies of the aorta or of systemic venous return often mandate complete cessation of bypass during certain phases of the procedure (for example, neonatal surgery for the hypoplastic left heart syndrome). As previously described, deep hypothermic circulatory arrest also serves to decrease the total duration of bypass, thereby decreasing the deleterious effects of long CPB times although adding the effects of hypothermic whole-body ischemia.

In addition to deliberate reduction of flow rate (and, therefore, systemic perfusion) to improve intracardiac exposure, there is an ever-present risk, when dealing with many congenital heart anomalies, that there will be an unrecognized "steal" away from the systemic circulation, resulting in inadequate systemic organ perfusion. The most common cause of this problem is diffuse systemic-to-pulmonary collateral formation in the lungs. These multiple small collaterals have the same effect as discrete, large, aortopulmonary collaterals; an unrecognized patent ductus arteriosus; or a patent systemic-to-pulmonary arterial shunt such as a Blalock shunt. Blood that is pumped into the aorta never reaches the systemic capillary bed but simply passes from the aorta to the pulmonary artery. It then passes into the pulmonary veins, to the left atrium and, if an atrial septal defect (ASD) is present, it returns to the oxygenator through the venous cannula. If an ASD is not present, the blood passes into the left ventricle, through the ventricular septal defect (VSD), and—depending on the degree of tricuspid regurgitation—back into the right atrium, and from there to the oxygenator. If there is neither an ASD nor a VSD, and if cardiac action has been reduced by hypothermia so that the blood returning to the left heart cannot be ejected, there is a high risk of distention of the pulmonary capillaries, resulting in injury to the lungs and distention of the left ventricle, which causes significant myocardial injury. While placement of a vent into the left atrium will decompress the left heart and avoid the damage caused by distention, it will also provide direct return to the oxygenator, which may result in inadequate systemic perfusion. Some other specific clinical situations are described later. In summary, it is essential that the surgeon give careful consideration to the specific perfusion risks secondary to the particular anatomy of a given patient. Many cases of postoperative lung dysfunction that have been attributed to "pump lung," as well as many cases of low cardiac output attributed to postischemic myocardial dysfunction, may actually be the result of failure to avoid left heart distention. Likewise, postoperative dysfunction of other organs may well be a result of inadequate systemic perfusion, despite the fact that the recorded pump flows, and perhaps even the recorded blood pressure, during perfusion appear satisfactory.

In conclusion, as a result of either deliberate reductions in flow rate or unrecognized inadequate systemic perfusion owing to "runoff," there are periods of decreased tissue perfusion that place organs at risk of ischemic injury. The organ most sensitive to ischemic injury is the brain. In Chapter 32, mechanisms of neurologic morbidity associated with pediatric cardiac surgery are discussed in greater detail.

RATIONALE FOR THE USE OF HYPOTHERMIA DURING CARDIOPULMONARY BYPASS

Full-flow CPB at 2 to 2.4 L/min/m^2 provides just enough flow to maintain a low-normal cardiac index. Any further reduction in flow, either as a result of the mechanisms previously described or secondary to temporary technical malfunction of the heart-lung machine, may compromise substrate supply to tissues, resulting in irreversible cellular injury. The best protection against such injury is achieved with hypothermia. While there is some evidence that severe degrees of hypothermia (<10°C) can result in tissue injury,[11] there is little evidence that milder degrees of hypothermia are injurious, despite anecdotal reports.[24]

Protective Mechanisms of Hypothermia

Hypothermia is the key strategy employed to reduce ischemic injury. This section will focus on mechanisms of cerebral protection afforded by hypothermia; myocardial protection afforded by hypothermia is described in Chapter 3. The protective effect of hypothermia is derived in part from a reduction in metabolic rate reflected in decreased oxygen consumption, as was emphasized in early studies undertaken by Bigelow et al.[9] Metabolic rate is determined by the activity of many enzyme systems. The relationship between the activity of an enzyme at temperature t_1 and its activity at temperature t_2 was described by van't Hoff as

$$Q10 = (k_2/k_1)10/t_2\text{-}t_1$$

where Q10 is the van't Hoff coefficient for a 10° change in temperature, and k_1 and k_2 are the reaction velocities at absolute temperatures t_1 and t_2.[73] Thus, if an enzyme has a Q10 of 2, its reaction velocity will be halved after a 10°C decrease in temperature. The whole-body Q10 for humans has been estimated at 2.2.[58] There may be a difference between the Q10 for adults and the Q10 for children, which has recently been estimated at 3.7.[35]

If a reduction in metabolic rate were the sole protective effect of hypothermia and if Q10 is approximately 2.5, then the 20°C reduction in temperature employed during clinical deep hypothermic circulatory arrest (DHCA) should extend the safe period for the brain from 3 to 5 minutes at 37°C to 15 to 25 minutes at 17°C.[58] Survival studies in animals and the clinical application of DHCA have both suggested that the safe duration of DHCA is, in fact, extended to more than 25 minutes (although probably less than 60 minutes with current techniques)[42] at a tympanic membrane temperature of 17°C.

Hypothermia and pH

Intracellular pH plays a critical role in facilitating continuing intracellular metabolic activity. Many metabolic intermediate substrates are weak acids with low molecular weight either innately or at the expense of intracellular phosphorylation. At physiologic intracellular pH, these metabolic intermediates exist principally in the ionized state and, as such, are highly hydrophilic. While hydrophilic, they are restricted to exiting the cell at specific channels. As intracellular pH becomes progressively more acidotic, less of the metabolic intermediate is dissociated. In the nonionized lipophilic state, they are free to passively diffuse across cellular membranes, resulting in loss of metabolic substrates.[57]

The dissociation constant of water (pK) is highly temperature dependent such that the pH of water at 37°C is 6.8, while at 20°C it is 7.40 (Fig. 2–3).

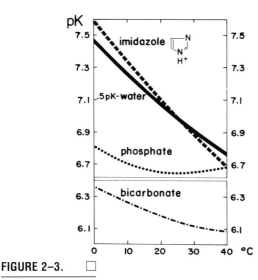

FIGURE 2–3. ☐

Cooling of either water or blood in a closed system is associated with an alkaline shift in pH. (From Rahn H, Reeves RB, Howell BJ. Hydrogen ion regulation, temperature, and evolution. Am Rev Resp Dis 112:165–172, 1975.)

Thus, hypothermia will decrease the ratio of nonionized to ionized metabolic intermediates, reducing their loss by passive diffusion through the lipid (hydrophobic) cell membrane. Furthermore, reducing the rate of anaerobic glycolysis occurring under conditions of ischemia results in a decrease in the production of hydrogen ions. In addition, intracellular enzyme systems function most efficiently at a higher pH during hypothermia.[62]

Hypothermia and the No-Reflow Phenomenon

In 1968, Ames and associates[2] described the phenomenon of the no-reflow lesion. If a biologic suspension of colloidal carbon is infused into the cerebral circulation after a 15-minute period of normothermic arrest, white areas of variable size, representing regions with no microcirculatory perfusion, are visible. In 1979, Norwood and coworkers[57] studied the no-reflow lesion as a function of the duration of ischemia or anoxia, the pH of the perfusate, and the cerebral temperature. This study confirmed that the no-reflow lesion was abated by hypothermia (90 minutes at 20°C) and a more alkaline extracellular pH. The no-reflow lesion was demonstrated to be a function of anoxia rather than arrested circulation, because it could be reproduced by perfusion with blood exposed to pure nitrogen.

More recent work has demonstrated the diverse role of endothelial cells in regulating vascular tone through vasoconstricting substances such as endothelin and vasodilating substances such as the endothelium-derived relaxing factor or nitric ox-

ide.[50] In part, the no-reflow lesion may represent hypoxic injury upsetting the normal balance of these competing dilating and constricting influences.

Hypothermia, Cerebral Blood Flow, and Cerebral Metabolic Rate

Under normothermic conditions, cerebral blood flow (CBF) is maintained over a wide range of perfusion pressure, so-called *pressure flow autoregulation*. This is achieved by a combination of cerebral vasodilatation and peripheral vasoconstriction. In studies by Greeley and colleagues,[36] CBF, as estimated by the xenon clearance method, in children undergoing CPB was found to be linearly associated with temperature. It was theorized that during and after moderately hypothermic CPB (25°C to 32°C), autoregulation was preserved, but after deep hypothermia (18°C to 22°C), autoregulation was lost. More recently, these authors calculated the cerebral metabolic rate from oxygen extraction using jugular venous oxygen content and arterial oxygen content in a similar group of patients with concomitant measurements of CBF.[35] This study revealed that at a pump flow rate of 100 ml/kg/min, CBF was in excess of that needed for metabolic requirements at all temperatures, in spite of loss of autoregulation.

Studies at Children's Hospital in Boston[43] using a miniature piglet model of hypothermic circulatory arrest also showed that both CBF and cerebral metabolic rate as determined by oxygen and glucose consumption were depressed at 45 minutes of reperfusion, by which time normothermia had been achieved. However, after 3 more hours of reperfusion, both blood flow and metabolic rate returned to normal (Fig. 2–4). A similar result was found in animals undergoing continuous low-flow (50 ml/kg/min) hypothermic bypass. It is possible that temporary depression of blood flow and metabolic rate reflects incomplete, nonhomogeneous rewarming of the brain.

Hypothermia and High-Energy Phosphate Stores

The development of nuclear magnetic resonance spectroscopy has enabled in vivo assessment of high-energy phosphate stores within the brain. Early magnets had a narrow bore, and studies were restricted to perfused rodent brains; however, current high-intensity (e.g., 4.7 T), wide-bore horizontal magnets allow assessment of the brain of intact anesthetized animals. Norwood and coworkers[58] reported the results of studies using crystalloid-perfused neonatal rat brain. They found that levels of phosphocreatine and adenosine triphosphate (ATP) decreased coordinately during normothermic ischemia and increased coordinately on resumption of perfusion. This is in contrast to adult *myocardium,* in which the decrease in phosphocreatine significantly precedes that of ATP, and the recovery of phosphocreatine precedes recovery of ATP. Hypothermia to 20°C resulted in complete preservation of ATP stores for 20 minutes of ischemia, while phosphocreatine fell rapidly. Phosphocreatine returned to control levels within 20 minutes of reperfusion.

At Children's Hospital in Boston, studies of miniature piglets undergoing hypothermic circulatory arrest have included assessment of cerebral high-energy phosphates and intracellular pH using magnetic resonance spectroscopy. In contrast to Norwood's finding in the isolated neonatal rat brain, it was found that in the 1-month-old intact piglet cooled to 15°C (nasopharyngeal temperature), both phosphocreatine and ATP deteriorated and became undetectable within 32 minutes of the onset of circulatory arrest. After 45 minutes of reperfusion rewarming, phosphocreatine had returned to 92% of baseline and ATP to 61% of baseline. After 3 more hours of reperfusion, phosphocreatine was 99% of baseline and ATP was 90% of baseline (Fig. 2–5).

DEEP HYPOTHERMIC CIRCULATORY ARREST

The technique of DHCA has been widely employed since the 1970s for repair of both simple and complex congenital heart anomalies in neonates, small infants, and, occasionally, older children. In the early 1970s, when CPB hardware and techniques were still particularly injurious to small infants, DHCA held the important advantage of decreasing total CPB time. With refinement in CPB for infants, reduction in CPB time has become a less important rationale for continued application of DHCA. Nevertheless, DHCA provides unparalleled surgical exposure in the small heart by eliminating the need for multiple cannulae within the field. In some anomalies of arterial and venous anatomy, its use is unavoidable.

Technique

The current technique of DHCA employed at Children's Hospital in Boston has been refined over the 20 years it has been in use. During that time the number of surgical procedures performed each year

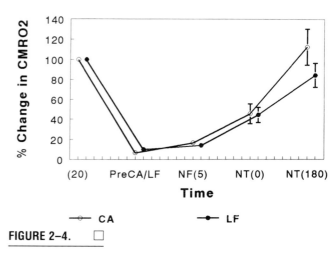

FIGURE 2–4. □

Cerebral metabolism as determined from oxygen consumption (CMRO2) remains depressed after both deep hypothermic circulatory arrest (CA) and low-flow bypass (LF) after 45 minutes of rewarming to normothermia. After 3 more hours of normothermic perfusion, cerebral metabolism has returned to baseline. NF(5), 5 minutes after beginning; NT(0), 45 minutes after reperfusion; NT(180), 3 hours after normothermic reperfusion; (20), baseline after 20 minutes normothermic bypass for stabilization. (From Kawata H, Fackler JC, Aoki M, et al. Hypothermic circulatory arrest versus low flow bypass in piglets: Acute recovery of cerebral blood flow and metabolism. J Thorac Cardiovasc Surg. In press.)

using circulatory arrest has increased because of the trend toward earlier repair of many lesions, including neonatal repair of both transposition of the great arteries and tetralogy of Fallot. Other centers have refined methods of continuous perfusion for small infants and neonates and prefer this approach.

Cooling Phase

Although the technique is predominantly one of core cooling using CPB, some spontaneous surface cooling is allowed during the induction of anesthesia and during the introduction of an arterial line (usually percutaneously in the radial artery) and at least one secure intravenous line. Generally, a central venous line is not placed. It is important that room temperature be maintained at less than 20°C (68°F) throughout the procedure and that overhead lighting be reduced to a minimum to avoid radiant heating of the myocardium. Illumination should be predominantly by the surgeon's headlight using a xenon (low levels of infrared and red) light source. Surface cooling is aided by the placement of ice bags on and around the head as the skin is being prepared, and the cooling/warming blanket on which the child lies is recirculated at 3°C to 4°C.

The perfusate consists of a pH-balanced crystalloid solution (Normosol-R pH 7.4) with the addition of citrated blood to achieve a hematocrit level of 20% on bypass. The ionized calcium level is not corrected, so it is usually very low (<0.4 mmol/L; nor-

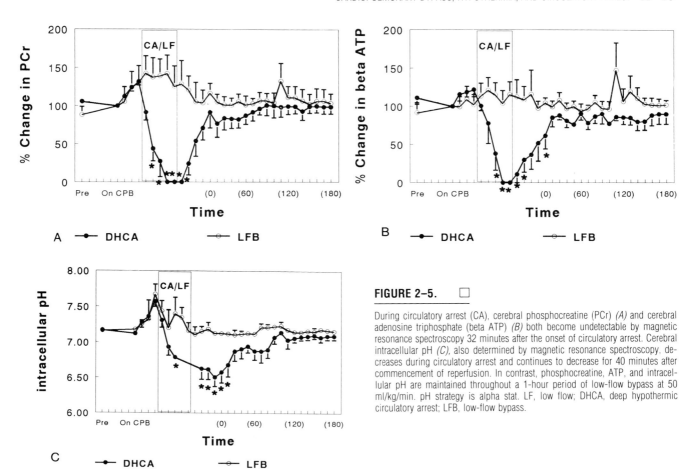

FIGURE 2–5. ☐

During circulatory arrest (CA), cerebral phosphocreatine (PCr) *(A)* and cerebral adenosine triphosphate (beta ATP) *(B)* both become undetectable by magnetic resonance spectroscopy 32 minutes after the onset of circulatory arrest. Cerebral intracellular pH *(C)*, also determined by magnetic resonance spectroscopy, decreases during circulatory arrest and continues to decrease for 40 minutes after commencement of reperfusion. In contrast, phosphocreatine, ATP, and intracellular pH are maintained throughout a 1-hour period of low-flow bypass at 50 ml/kg/min. pH strategy is alpha stat. LF, low flow; DHCA, deep hypothermic circulatory arrest; LFB, low-flow bypass.

mal, 1.0 mmol/L). Heparin is added to the prime to achieve 2.5 U/ml. (The patient is also heparinized directly with 2 mg/kg.) The activated clotting time is maintained at greater than 400 seconds. The perfusate is recirculated at room temperature through the circuit, which includes a variable prime membrane oxygenator (Cobe; Lakewood, CO) and a 40-μm arterial filter (Pall Ultipor No. LPE-1440 [Pall Biomedical Products Corporation; Glen Cove, NY]). An ascending aortic arterial cannula and a single right atrial venous cannula (C.R. Bard; Billerica, MA) are placed. CPB and core cooling are begun as soon as the cannulae are in place. Typically, by this time spontaneous surface cooling secondary to room temperature cooling and the cooling blanket has decreased the rectal temperature to 33°C. As soon as bypass is initiated, cooling of the water passing through the heat exchanger is begun, reducing the temperature by 5°C over 5 minutes. There are important differences in the efficiency of heat exchangers. At Children's Hospital in Boston, chilled wall water is available, which allows for relatively rapid cooling. Extremely rapid cooling (e.g., rectal temperature less than 18°C in less than 10 to 12 minutes) is best avoided, although maximal cooling with the

heat-exchanging system in use at Children's Hospital can achieve this degree of hypothermia in the average neonate within 7 to 8 minutes. Esophageal, tympanic, and rectal temperatures are monitored in all patients. The machine flow rate during cooling for patients weighing between 2.5 and 10 kg is 150 ml/kg. (The same flow rate is also used for rewarming.) The alpha stat method of acid-base management is used at present; i.e., the pH is maintained at 7.40 as measured at 37°C and is not corrected for patient temperature (see later discussion). It is important to avoid prebypass alkalosis induced by hyperventilation, as well as exceeding alpha stat in an alkaline direction. Within the first minute of bypass, phentolamine (Regitine), 0.2 mg/kg; furosemide, 0.25 mg/kg; and methylprednisolone (Solu-Medrol), 30 mg/kg, are administered. Cooling is continued until both rectal and tympanic membrane temperatures are less than 18°C. Pentothal, 10 mg/kg, is given approximately 10 minutes after initiation of bypass. The ascending aorta is crossclamped inferior to the arterial cannula, and a cardioplegic solution (oxygenated Plegisol [Abbott Laboratories, North Chicago, IL]) 20 ml/kg, is administered into the aortic root. Bypass is discontinued. Blood is drained from the patient through the venous cannula, aided by gentle rhythmic compression of the abdomen combined with sustained gentle inflation of the lungs. For most procedures the venous line is then clamped and removed.

During the circulatory arrest period, the perfusate is recirculated at 18°C.

Rewarming Phase

The heart is filled with saline to exclude air, with particular attention paid to displacing air from the left ventricle, left atrium, and pulmonary veins. The venous cannula is reinserted, and bypass is recommenced with the perfusate at 18°C. Water temperature is maintained at no more than 10°C higher than the temperature of the venous blood return, with a maximum water temperature of 42°C. Generally, the crossclamp is removed shortly after recommencing bypass. Mannitol, 0.5 gm/kg, is given at the time the aortic crossclamp is removed. At a rectal temperature of 30°C, calcium gluconate is given in a dose of 1.0 gm for the first unit of whole blood used in the prime and 0.5 gm for each additional unit. Thereafter, calcium gluconate is given as needed to maintain normal ionized calcium levels. Mean perfusion pressure is maintained between 30 and 70 mm Hg during rewarming using phentolamine, 0.1 mg/kg, or phenylephrine (Neosynephrine), 5 μg/kg, as needed. At a rectal temperature of 32°C, arterial blood gases, electrolytes, calcium, glucose, and osmolarity are measured and adjusted to normal. When effective cardiac action is regained, usually close to the time that calcium is administered, the perfusionist slightly retards venous return, which shifts perfusate from the reservoir into the patient (raising central venous pressure a few millimeters) and results in pulsatile ejection by the heart. Ventilation should be begun at this time. This will aid in the elimination of any residual intracardiac air before the discontinuation of bypass and also allow a decision to be made regarding the level of inotropic support to be used when weaning from bypass. There may be additional advantages (e.g., catabolism of norepinephrine). When first weaning from bypass, a low-dose dopamine infusion at 5 μg/kg/min is routinely used in all small neonates and infants undergoing circulatory arrest, although it is often possible to reduce or discontinue this before they leave the operating room.

Despite two decades of use, at least three important controversies regarding the technique of DHCA remain to be resolved: pH and Pco_2 management, surface cooling versus core cooling, and duration of circulatory arrest.

pH and Pco_2 Management. Management of ar-
terial pH and Pco_2 during CPB remains controversial even in the adult undergoing moderately hypothermic (25°C) CPB. When adding the variables of young age, profound levels of hypothermia, and low-flow states or DHCA, there are few experimental or clinical data on which to base a rational decision for optimal neurologic protection by appropriate acid-base management. As already described, intracellular and membrane-based enzyme systems function most efficiently at a pH of 7.4 at 37°C.[72] Under normal circumstances, both metabolic and respiratory compensatory mechanisms function to maintain this pH. Cooling results in a shift of the dissociation constant of water such that neutral pH at a body temperature of 20°C is approximately 7.7.[60] Several cellular enzyme systems have been demonstrated to function more efficiently at this pH.[92] Certainly, the "alpha," or the ratio of dissociated to nondissociated imidazole groups of histidine, an essential component of the protein buffer system, remains constant by allowing an increase in pH parallel to the natural increase in pH of water with a decrease in temperature. This is the "alpha stat" strategy of acid-base management. Because no compensation has been made, blood from an individual undergoing alpha stat management, when warmed by a blood gas analyzer to 37°C (as is usually done), will register an arterial pH of 7.40 and a Pco_2 of 40. It is important at all times to specify whether the stated pH and Pco_2 values are "corrected to 37°C" or "corrected to patient temperature." The concept of alpha stat regulation was popularized only relatively recently and has come into widespread clinical practice since the 1980s. Clinical and laboratory evidence support its continued use; for example, whole-body oxygen consumption is greater with alpha stat than with pH stat.[82] More importantly, alpha stat is associated with more appropriate CBF than is a more acidotic strategy.[39, 56]

CBF flow in excess of the metabolic requirement, so-called "luxuriant" CBF, exposes the patient on continuous CPB to an increased risk of microemboli. In contrast to the child, whose greatest risk of cerebral injury is probably a hypoxic or ischemic injury related to low-flow or no-flow states, microembolic injury is probably the greatest risk for the adult patient on continuous CPB with mild or moderate hypothermia.[54] However, there are several arguments in favor of the alternative philosophy of "pH stat" management for the young patient exposed to deep hypothermia and low-flow bypass or circulatory arrest. The addition of carbon dioxide to the gas mixture in the oxygenator during cooling results in a "patient temperature–corrected" pH and Pco_2 profile unchanged from that seen at 37°C. This relative acidosis serves as a stimulus for cerebral vasodilation, resulting in increased CBF under conditions of very low cerebral perfusion pressure.[39] Furthermore, hypothermia causes a leftward shift of the oxygen-hemoglobin dissociation curve. Relative alkalosis induces a further shift to the left, thereby possibly decreasing oxygen availability at the tissue level,[30] while relative acidosis shifts the curve to the right, resulting in greater availability of oxygen at the tissue level. Interestingly, work with magnetic resonance spectroscopy by Swain and coworkers,[78] as well as in the laboratory at Children's Hospital in Boston,[4] suggests that cerebral intracellular pH shifts in an alkaline direction during hypothermia, even when blood pH is managed by the pH stat strategy. Thus, it is possible that the advantages of the alpha stat system for intracellular enzyme systems may hold with the pH stat system, along with the advantage of better preservation of CBF during periods of borderline perfusion.

In a small retrospective study of 16 neonates and young infants who underwent Senning procedures for transposition of the great arteries under DHCA at Children's Hospital in Boston (mean duration, 43 minutes; range, 35 to 60 minutes),[41] 10 underwent pH stat management and six underwent alpha stat management. The pH ($P = .05$) and Pco_2 ($P = .002$) measured immediately before circulatory arrest were important predictors of developmental outcome, with a worse outcome at the alpha stat end of the pH/Pco_2 spectrum (i.e., more alkaline pH was associated with a worse outcome) (Fig. 2–6). The mean duration of core cooling on CPB for these patients was 14.5 ± 6.2 minutes ($P = .1$). Duration of circulatory arrest was not associated with develop-

mental outcome ($P = .49$). These data can be interpreted to suggest that with a relatively short cooling time, use of a more alkaline strategy may result in less effective brain cooling owing to cerebral vasoconstriction or less adequate delivery of oxygen because of the leftward shift of the oxygen-hemoglobin dissociation curve.

Much of the discussion as to which pH strategy should be applied to humans during hypothermic bypass has been derived by extrapolation from comparative physiologic studies of various animals that become hypothermic during their normal existence. Generally, cold-blooded animals (ectotherms, poikilotherms), whose body temperature follows ambient temperature, apply the alpha stat strategy. However, hibernating animals, which are warm-blooded endotherms at times other than when they are hibernating, apply the pH stat strategy by hypoventilating and allowing a respiratory acidosis to develop. Rahn and associates,[60] Reeves,[62] Swan,[80] and White[88] have argued persuasively that optimizing enzyme function at low temperatures, as is done by ectotherms, is the more appropriate strategy for humans on CPB. This argument, more than any other, has been the deciding factor in convincing many centers to adopt the alpha stat approach, but a good argument can be made that the hibernating animal is much more closely analogous to the infant undergoing circulatory arrest or low-flow perfusion than is the cold-blooded vertebrate that must remain active at low temperatures. The goal of the hibernating animal is to *minimize* whole-body oxygen consumption and energy expenditure and to preserve flow to essential organs such as the brain while minimizing flow to nonworking areas such as skeletal muscle. It is clear that a prospective randomized study of pH strategy in infants undergoing deep hypothermic bypass, with or without circulatory arrest, is warranted. Such a study is currently under way at Children's Hospital in Boston. Prospective studies of pH strategy have already been reported in adults undergoing moderately hypothermic continuous perfusion (25°C to 28°C) and have shown no important differences in neuropsychometric outcome.[65] The pH strategy is much less critical when moderate, rather than deep, hypothermia is used, as the difference between the two strategies is much less at higher temperatures. In addition, when there is no need to reduce perfusion throughout the procedure, as is usually the case for adults undergoing surgery for acquired heart disease, it is less likely that blood flow to the brain will be compromised.

Surface Cooling Versus Core Cooling. Early in DHCA development, cooling was accomplished primarily by surface cooling using ice bags and a

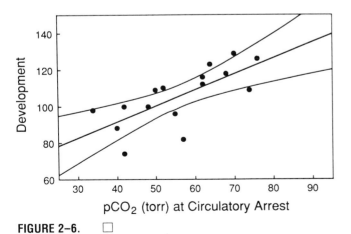

FIGURE 2–6. ☐

In a retrospective study of cognitive development after a mean circulatory arrest duration of 43 minutes, a more alkaline pH during cooling before circulatory arrest (alpha stat) was associated with worse cognitive outcome ($r = 0.071$, $P = .002$). (From Jonas RA, Bellinger DC, Rappaport LA, et al. pH strategy and developmental outcome after hypothermic circulatory arrest. J Thorac Cardiovasc Surg 106:362–368, 1993.)

cooling blanket with a short period (less than 5 minutes) of core cooling on CPB. Proponents of surface cooling argue that not only does it shorten the total duration of CPB, but it also results in more uniform total-body cooling with elimination of temperature gradients.[89] Exclusive use of CPB for cooling has been shown to result in skeletal muscle remaining at a relatively high temperature.[1] Disadvantages of surface cooling are its duration (often requiring as long as 90 minutes to achieve a rectal temperature of less than 25°C in a child weighing 6 to 8 kg), the difficulty of maintaining adequate tissue perfusion as cardiac output decreases (resulting in lactic acidosis),[38] and the risk of ventricular fibrillation at temperatures below 30°C. During surface cooling in piglets with a left-to-right shunt, an increased shunt and diminished systemic perfusion with altered cellular metabolism has been noted.[51] The differences between the two modes of cooling are blurred by the common practice of starting informal surface cooling in infants by using a cooling blanket as soon as anesthesia is established, by the cool ambient temperature of the operating room, and by unheated breathing circuits and intravenous fluids. Although the operation is not delayed to allow cooling, most infants have cooled to a rectal temperature of approximately 32°C by the time core cooling with CPB is instituted.

The duration of core cooling is also controversial. Early descriptions of the technique of DHCA suggested cooling to a rectal temperature of 22°C.[5] In general, both rectal and tympanic membrane temperatures currently are lowered to less than 18°C before instituting DHCA.[45] However, because the efficiency of heat-exchanging systems used as part of the CPB circuit varies widely, these temperatures can be achieved with less than 10 minutes of cooling with some systems or may require as long as 30 minutes with others. In a small retrospective study of 28 children who underwent the arterial switch procedure for correction of transposition of the great arteries with a mean circulatory arrest period of 64 minutes (range, 49 to 109 minutes), the intraoperative variable most strongly associated with intellectual development was the duration of cooling on CPB before DHCA.[7] In children subjected to a cooling duration of less than 20 minutes, the relationship between intellectual development and duration of cooling was positive and highly significant ($r = 0.85; P < .001$). Within this range of cooling duration, an increase of 5 minutes of core cooling was associated with a 26-point increase in the developmental score. Most of these patients underwent alpha stat management of pH and Pco_2, unlike the Senning patients previously described who mainly underwent pH stat management. It could be in-

ferred that the arterial switch patients required longer periods of cooling to achieve homogeneous brain hypothermia (and, thereby, protection) because of the cerebral vasoconstriction induced by their more alkaline pH management. The critical importance of very small temperature gradients (2°C) within the brain in ameliorating or exacerbating cerebral ischemic injury has been demonstrated in a rodent model.[17]

Duration of Circulatory Arrest. There is unlikely to be a single specific duration of DHCA that is appropriate for all individuals. This is partly because of individual biologic variability but is also a reflection of the diverse techniques that go together to make up DHCA as it is employed at various centers. For example, the studies by Rossi and Ekroth and their coworkers[29, 67] (in which serum creatine kinase-BB was measured after DHCA) employed the pH stat method of acid-base control. Control groups were patients who did not undergo CPB. They concluded that the serum level of creatine kinase-BB corresponded to the duration of DHCA. However, in a subsequent study by the same authors[68] in which alpha stat management was employed and the control group of patients underwent low-flow cardiopulmonary bypass, identical elevations in creatine kinase-BB were seen in patients who had not undergone DHCA.

Even this last study, however, suffers from the disadvantage of heterogeneity of the study and control groups. Since the late 1980s, Children's Hospital in Boston has been undertaking (ongoing for life of patients) a prospective study of circulatory arrest using a homogeneous patient population (i.e., patients undergoing the arterial switch operation for transposition in the first 3 months of life) (The Boston Circulatory Arrest Study).[42] During the enrollment phase of the study, patients randomly underwent either circulatory arrest or continuous low-flow bypass. A total of 171 patients were enrolled, and the mean duration of circulatory arrest was 55 minutes. Analysis of the perioperative results demonstrated that assignment to circulatory arrest was associated with a significantly greater release of creatine kinase-BB and that the release increased with an increasing duration of circulatory arrest (Fig. 2–7).

Experimental studies of brain structure and function after DHCA have suggested that at a rectal temperature of 15°C to 20°C, a 30-minute total arrest time is "safe" with respect to central nervous system damage.[31, 32, 47] Conflicting results have been reported with circulatory arrest times between 45 and 60 minutes.[53, 81] The reappearance latency and latency to continuous electroencephalogram (EEG) activity have been related to duration of circulatory

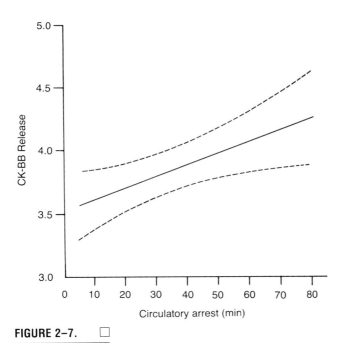

FIGURE 2–7. □

In a prospective study of circulatory arrest versus continuous low-flow bypass conducted at Children's Hospital, Boston, there was a linear association between duration of circulatory arrest and total creatine kinase-BB (CK-BB) release during the first 6 hours postoperatively.

arrest[20]; this has been confirmed by the Boston Circulatory Arrest Study. Functional disturbances after circulatory arrest include transient choreoathetosis, which has been reported to occur in between 1% and 19% of patients on the second to sixth postoperative day. One patient in the Boston Circulatory Arrest Study had transient choreoathetosis. Although usually transient, severe choreoathetosis may result in permanent abnormalities of movement.[15, 16, 77, 90] Transient seizures have been reported to occur in 4% to 10% of infants in the immediate postoperative period,[16, 19, 28] although these are rarely seen in adults.[22] Definite clinical seizures were seen in 12% of the patients undergoing circulatory arrest but in only 1% of patients undergoing continuous hypothermic bypass in the Boston Circulatory Arrest Study. Seizures, as determined from EEG activity in the first 48 hours after surgery, were seen in 26% of patients undergoing circulatory arrest and in 13% of patients undergoing continuous hypothermic bypass. There was a strong association ($P = .004$) between the duration of circulatory arrest and the occurrence of seizures (Fig. 2–8).

There are a large number of studies of cognitive development after DHCA, but in general they are marred by methodologic limitations, including lack of an appropriate control group, small sample size, limited power, diverse cardiac defects, age at repair, retrospective study design, and comparison of techniques used during different time frames.[12, 19, 25, 86, 91] Preliminary analysis of the developmental outcome at 1 year of age, which is being undertaken as part of the Boston Circulatory Arrest Study, suggests an important association between the occurrence of postoperative seizures and a worse-than-normal outcome for the Psychomotor Development Index, primarily a measure of motor skills (Newburger JW, Jones R-A, unpublished data). To date, the Mental Development Index, which is primarily an assessment of cognitive abilities, does not appear to be affected by the occurrence of perioperative seizures or assignment to circulatory arrest or continuous bypass.

Examining differences between patients and their siblings, Wells and associates[86] found that patients who had undergone DHCA in infancy had scores on the McCarthy Developmental Scale that were significantly worse than those of their siblings. These differences were positively associated with the duration of circulatory arrest. Children who had undergone similar cardiac procedures and were operated on under moderate hypothermia and continuous CPB had scores comparable to those of their siblings. Other studies of cognitive, behavioral, and linguistic development have also shown deficits in these areas, sometimes related to the duration of DHCA.[12, 19, 25] Other reports have shown no significant differences in children after DHCA when com-

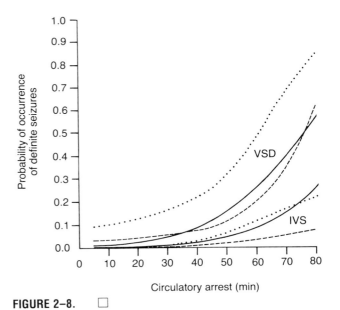

FIGURE 2–8. □

In a prospective study of circulatory arrest versus low-flow bypass conducted at Children's Hospital, Boston, longer duration of circulatory arrest was associated with a greater probability of occurrence of definite clinical seizures ($P = .004$). The association was stronger with patients who had an associated ventricular septal defect (VSD), who were also older, than with patients who had an intact ventricular septum (IVS).

pared with controls, including one study in which patients were tested preoperatively and used as their own controls.[64, 75]

HYPOTHERMIC LOW-FLOW BYPASS

Although it might seem intuitively obvious that some CBF, no matter how little, is better than no blood flow at all, there is considerable evidence that this is not necessarily the case. An analogy can be drawn with myocardial protection, in which a single dose of cardioplegic solution and a single period of myocardial ischemia appear to give better protection, particularly in the neonate, than continuing myocardial perfusion. A number of rodent models of cerebral ischemia have been used to examine the differences between partial and complete ischemia. Several studies have suggested that because of continuing substrate supply during a period of partial ischemia, a greater level of acidosis develops, with a resultant greater potential for cellular injury.[8] This may be particularly relevant in the brain because of the difficulty with which lactate crosses the blood-brain barrier and because of the dependence of neurons on glucose for metabolism. Cerebral injury from partial ischemia has been shown to be exacerbated by hyperglycemia when this is present before the insult.[59, 69] This has also been suggested clinically when DHCA is employed.[29] Steward and colleagues[76] found that only one of six patients with a glucose level less than 216 mg/dl developed neurologic impairment after DHCA, while six of 25 with levels of 216 to 432 mg/dl and two of three with levels higher than 432 mg/dl showed impairment. Ratcliffe and coworkers[61] also cautioned against the use of glucose in the prime fluid for children weighing less than 15 kg, noting hyperlactemia in children when glucose solutions were employed. The high glucose content of citrate/phosphate/dextrose (CPD) bank blood used to maintain hematocrit when employing the large prime volume required in conventional circuits for small children is emphasized by this study. However, there is some evidence that preischemic and postischemic hyperglycemia may be less of a problem in the neonate than in more mature animals.[21] This may be related to differences in energy metabolism in the very immature animal.

Technique

The technique of hypothermic low-flow bypass employed at Children's Hospital in Boston has evolved since the late 1980s. The technique was de-

veloped in response to the problems of children with complex forms of transposition who were undergoing repair during the neonatal period. For example, children with severe hypoplasia or interruption of the aortic arch associated with transposition of the great arteries and a VSD require excessive periods of DHCA (at least 80 to 90 minutes) if the entire procedure of arch reconstruction, arterial switch, and VSD closure is performed under circulatory arrest. It was found that with appropriate placement of a single venous cannula in the right atrium, bypass could be continued while the arterial switch component of the procedure was undertaken. Often, if the VSD is a high subarterial defect, it can also be closed by working through the anterior semilunar valve or, if the right ventricle requires enlargement, by working through an infundibular incision in the right ventricle. Familiarity with this technique has enabled its extension to other anomalies such as truncus arteriosus and tetralogy of Fallot. The use of a single atrial venous cannula rather than two caval cannulae carries certain advantages in the neonate. There is the obvious advantage of less cluttering of the surgical field with two cannulae and associated tourniquets. Because the right atrium is in full view of the surgeon, it is obvious at all times whether adequate drainage is being achieved. This is particularly useful information, because the neonate will often require a large (sometimes massive) amount of fluid in response to the capillary leak induced by CPB.[85] If individual caval cannulae have been placed, a high fluid requirement may be falsely attributed to poor cannula placement. Often, bicaval cannulation does not allow adequate right atrial decompression, particularly when the aorta is not clamped and there is coronary sinus return to the right atrium. Furthermore, in the neonate with transposition of the great arteries, a balloon atrial septostomy will usually have been performed. The resulting ASD will allow venting of the left heart return directly to the venous cannula, without the need for a left atrial vent. For this reason it is important that intracardiac defects should not be closed until the final stages of the procedure.

Apart from the continuation of bypass at a reduced flow rate, all other aspects of perfusion using hypothermic low-flow bypass in the neonate are identical to the protocol described for circulatory arrest. The primary rationale for hypothermic low-flow bypass is that many such procedures will also entail a period of circulatory arrest for the performance of deep intracardiac procedures or aortic arch reconstruction. One of the most important decisions that must be made when employing continuous hypothermic bypass is the selection of a flow rate during the period of "low flow." The flow rate currently employed at Children's Hospital in Boston is 50 ml/kg/min, which is a flow index of approximately 0.71 $L/min/m^2$ in the average neonate.

Hypothermic Low-Flow Perfusion Rate

A number of studies have examined the lower limit of blood flow that is tolerated at hypothermic temperatures. In 1984, Fox and colleagues[33] examined regional and total cerebral flow using microspheres in monkeys. Arteriovenous oxygen extraction was also measured to assess adequacy of cerebral flow. The authors found that oxygen consumption by the brain remained the same at all flow rates down to 0.5 $L/min/m^2$, despite a decrease in total brain blood flow. The oxygen consumption was maintained in part by increased oxygen extraction and in part by redistribution of perfusate from the rest of the systemic circulation to the brain. Using an argon saturation and desaturation method in adult patients undergoing CPB at 27°C, Soma and colleagues[71] found that cerebral blood flow was maintained despite hypotension (mean arterial pressure, 34 to 50 mm Hg) as long as the perfusion flow rate was maintained at more than 40 ml/kg/min. Miyamoto and coworkers[52] examined cerebral blood flow by direct measurement of superior sagittal flow in dogs on bypass at 20°C. They concluded that the optimal perfusion flow rate for the brain during deep hypothermic CPB at 20°C was 30 ml/kg/min, with a possible oxygen debt in the brain resulting in anaerobic metabolism if the perfusion flow rate was kept at 15 ml/kg/min or less. In a clinical study by Kern and associates,[44] it was suggested that a cellular oxygen debt occurs between 5 and 30 ml/kg/min at 18°C and between 30 and 35 ml/kg/min at 27°C to 28°C. A study by Swain and colleagues[78] employing phosphorous nuclear magnetic resonance spectroscopy in adult sheep suggested that high-energy phosphate stores were maintained by flow rates as low as 10 ml/kg/min. A flow rate of 5 ml/kg/min resulted in progressive deterioration of both creatine phosphate and ATP, as well as development of intracellular acidosis.

COMPARISON OF DEEP HYPOTHERMIC CIRCULATORY ARREST AND LOW-FLOW BYPASS

As previously described, at Children's Hospital in Boston there has been a transition from the exclusive use of DHCA to frequent application of low-flow hypothermic bypass. Within a short time of this transition, it became clear that neonates subjected to the extra duration of bypass were likely to be more edematous at the conclusion of the procedure. This suggested the desirability of a prospective randomized study (i.e., the Boston Circulatory Arrest Study). The study has confirmed that a 25% to 50% greater volume of fluid must be added to the bypass circuit for patients undergoing low-flow bypass when compared with that required for DHCA, and there is a correspondingly greater weight gain in the operating room in these patients when compared with patients undergoing DHCA. However, this additional weight gain and fluid accumulation have not been associated with extra time in the intensive care unit or total duration of hospitalization. Analysis of the perioperative results to date has found an important increased risk of seizures with circulatory arrest, increased release of creatine kinase-BB, and greater latency before return of EEG activity. The long-term significance of these findings remains to be determined, although preliminary analysis suggests an association between seizures and a worse-than-normal outcome on the Psychomotor Development Index.

SPECIAL SITUATIONS

Pulmonary Atresia

When pulmonary blood flow is not derived directly from a ventricle (and assuming that a cavopulmonary shunt has not been performed), pulmonary blood flow must be derived from a connection between the systemic arterial system and the pulmonary arteries. This may take the form of a systemic-to-pulmonary arterial shunt, a patent ductus arteriosus, or natural aortopulmonary collateral vessels. In these circumstances there is an important risk of runoff from the systemic arterial tree into the pulmonary arteries and, from there, back to the oxygenator, without oxygen and substrates being supplied to systemic tissues.

With the introduction of interventional catheterization methods at Children's Hospital in Boston in 1984 came an increasing interest in the management of complex forms of tetralogy of Fallot accompanied by pulmonary atresia, often with severe hypoplasia of the true pulmonary arteries and correspondingly large collateral vessels. In addition, patients with complex forms of single ventricle with pulmonary atresia have increasingly undergone Fontan operations. For many years, no cases of choreoathetosis had been seen at Children's Hospital, but between 1986 and 1990, 19 new cases of choreoathetosis were noted.[90] In all but one of these cases, the underlying anomaly included pulmonary atresia. It was also noted on review of the preoperative angiograms that in five of 11 cases, large collateral vessels were fed by head vessels such as the vertebral arteries. Since recognition of this problem, care has been taken to coil embolize such vessels preoperatively whenever possible. In addition, changes have been made to the perfusion methods. Attention is given to avoiding alkalosis before bypass as well as during perfusion, because a lower P_{CO_2} causes a decrease in CBF and an increased flow to the lungs. If possible, continuous perfusion is used rather than DHCA.

An operation that is frequently performed in this setting is placement of an allograft conduit from the right ventricle to the severely hypoplastic central pulmonary arteries. Currently we prefer to perform the distal anastomosis with the tiny pulmonary arteries controlled with a C clamp. Most of the proximal anastomosis also can be performed before bypass, including placement of much of the pericardial hood used to supplement the anastomosis. A very short period of bypass is all that is required to perform the right ventriculotomy and to complete the proximal anastomosis. Under these circumstances, when it is important that the heart keep beating, the prime should be maintained at 37°C, and the ionized calcium level in the perfusate should be normalized. Once again it should be emphasized that under usual circumstances, when cooling is to be undertaken to deep hypothermic temperatures, it may be advantageous for myocardial protection to maintain the ionized calcium level at very low levels (secondary to the citrated blood added to the prime). Since adopting these various modifications, the incidence of choreoathetosis in complex forms of pulmonary atresia has been markedly diminished.

Bidirectional Cavopulmonary Shunt, Senning Procedure, and Venous Anomalies

Although much attention has been focused on providing adequate arterial perfusion of the brain and other organs, little attention has been given to ensuring that venous drainage is always totally unobstructed. While total venous return to the pump is clearly apparent to the perfusionist, the distribution of that flow is unknown. For example, consider the situation in which a single venous cannula is inserted in the common atrium of a child with single-ventricle physiology after a previous bidirectional cavopulmonary shunt. When bypass is begun and the venous clamps are fully open, the pressure in the common atrium will fall to 0 mm Hg or less. However, blood returning from the upper body, including the brain, must pass through the entire pulmonary circulation before it reaches the common atrium and returns to the oxygenator. If there is increased resistance in the lungs—which is likely if the lungs are completely collapsed—the distribution of arterial blood flow is likely to be preferentially directed to the lower body, where venous pressure is very low, and away from the upper body and brain, where the venous pressure is higher, perhaps much higher. Therefore, we are always very careful to place a cannula, usually a right-angled, steel-tipped cannula (DLP, Inc.; Grand Rapids, MI), either in the innominate vein or high in the superior vena cava to be sure that there is low cerebral venous pressure.

A common technique of venous cannulation after a Senning operation is placement of a single venous cannula in the anatomic right atrial appendage (i.e., the functional pulmonary venous atrium). As with the bidirectional cavopulmonary shunt, systemic venous return must pass through the lungs before reaching the venous cannula. However, unlike the bidirectional cavopulmonary shunt, distribution of flow should be uniform, because both the superior and inferior vena caval blood must take the same pathway. If, however, there is some obstruction of superior vena cava return, then maldistribution of flow may occur. Thus, in the past when the Senning operation was commonly performed, a need to revise the baffle because of superior vena cava obstruction resulted in a high risk of brain injury.

There are many venous anomalies, particularly in children with heterotaxia, that increase the risk of inadequate venous drainage. In such children, careful consideration must be given to complete venous drainage of all organs, particularly the brain. It may be that ancillary monitoring methods, such as on-line monitoring of jugular venous bulb saturation by a fiberoptic catheter[23] or near-infrared spectroscopy of the brain,[27] will prove useful means of confirming the adequacy of cerebral venous flow in the presence of the venous and arterial anomalies described.

SUMMARY

There can be little doubt that future generations of cardiac surgeons will look back with amazement at current techniques of CPB and circulatory arrest. They will probably marvel that patients could even survive the methods employed, let alone do apparently well clinically in the overwhelming majority of cases, given the remarkably inadequate knowledge about the deleterious effects of CPB, hypothermia, and circulatory arrest. Perhaps we will be viewed in the same light as the barber-surgeons of the eighteenth century who boasted of their ability to amputate a leg in 30 seconds. However, until there is considerable improvement in the fundamental understanding of the pathology of CPB, it will continue to be necessary to undertake open cardiac operations both expeditiously as well as accurately.

REFERENCES

1. Almond CH, Jones JC, Snyder HM, et al. Cooling gradients and brain damage with deep hypothermia. J Thorac Cardiovasc Surg 48:890, 1964.
2. Ames A, Wright RL, Koward M, et al. Cerebral ischemia. II. The no-reflow phenomenon. Am J Pathol 52:437, 1968.
3. Anand, KJS, Hickey PR. Halothane-morphine compared with high-dose sufentanil for anesthesia and postoperative analgesia in neonatal cardiac surgery. N Engl J Med 326:1, 1992.
4. Aoki M, Nomura F, Stromski ME, et al. Effects of pH on brain energetics after hypothermic circulatory arrest. Ann Thorac Surg 55:1093–1103, 1993.
5. Barratt-Boyes BG. Complete correction of cardiovascular malformations in the first two years of life using profound hypothermia. In Barratt-Boyes BG, Neutze JM, Harris EA (eds). Heart Disease in Infancy. Edinburgh, Churchill Livingston, 1973, p 35.
6. Barratt-Boyes BG, Neutze JM, Harris EA (eds). Heart Disease in Infancy. Edinburgh, Churchill Livingstone, 1973.
7. Bellinger DC, Wernovsky G, Rappaport LA, et al. Cognitive development following repair as neonates of transposition of the great arteries using deep hypothermic circulatory arrest. Pediatrics 87:701, 1991.
8. Bengtsson F, Siesjo BK. Cell damage in cerebral ischemia: Physiological, biochemical and structural aspects. In Schurr A, Rigor BM (eds). Cerebral Ischemia and Resuscitation. Boca Raton, FL, CRC Press, 1990, pp 215–223.
9. Bigelow WG, Lindsay WK, Harrison RC, et al. Oxygen transport and utilization in dogs at low body temperatures. Am J Physiol 160:125, 1950.
10. Bjork J, Hugli TE, Smedegard G. Microvascular effects of anaphylatoxins C3a and C5a. J Immunol 134:1115, 1985.
11. Bjork VO, Hultquist G. Brain damage in children after deep hypothermia. Thorax 15:284, 1960.
12. Blackwood M, Haka-Ikse K, Steward D. Developmental outcome in children undergoing surgery with profound hypothermia. Anesthesiology 65:437, 1986.
13. Blauth CI, Arnold JV, Schulenberg WE, et al. Cerebral microembolism during cardiopulmonary bypass. J Thorac Cardiovasc Surg 95:668, 1988.
14. Blauth CI, Smith PL, Arnold JV, et al. Influence of oxygenator type on the prevalence and extent of microembolic retinal ischemia during cardiopulmonary bypass. J Thorac Cardiovasc Surg 99:61, 1990.
15. Brunberg JA, Doty DB, Reilley EL. Choreoathetosis in infants following cardiac surgery with deep hypothermia and circulatory arrest. J Pediatr 84:232, 1974.
16. Brunberg JA, Reilly EL, Doty DB. Central nervous system consequences in infants of cardiac surgery using deep hypothermia and circulatory arrest. Circulation 49:62, 1974.
17. Busto R, Dietrich WD, Globus MYT, et al. Small differences in intraischemic brain temperature critically determine the extent of ischemic neuronal injury. J Cereb Blood Flow Metab 7:729, 1987.
18. Castaneda AR, Lamberti J, Sade RM, et al. Open heart surgery during the first three months of life. J Thorac Cardiovasc Surg 68:719, 1974.
19. Clarkson PM, MacArthur BA, Barratt-Boyes BG, et al. Developmental progress following cardiac surgery in infancy using profound hypothermia and circulatory arrest. Circulation 62:855, 1980.
20. Coles JG, Taylor MJ, Pearce JM, et al. Cerebral monitoring of somatosensory evoked potentials during profoundly hypothermic circulatory arrest. Circulation 70(suppl I):I-96, 1984.

21. Corbett RJT. In vivo multinuclear magnetic resonance spectroscopy. Sem Perinatol 14:258–271, 1990.
22. Coselli JS, Crawford ES, Beall AC, et al. Determination of brain temperature for safe circulatory arrest during cardiovascular operations. Ann Thorac Surg 45:638, 1988.
23. Croughwell N, Frasco P, Blumenthal JA, et al. The effect of temperature on cerebral metabolism and blood flow in adults during cardiopulmonary bypass. J Thorac Cardiovasc Surg 103:549–554, 1992.
24. DeLeon S, Ilbawi M, Arcilla R, et al. Choreoathetosis after deep hypothermia without circulatory arrest. Ann Thorac Surg 50:714, 1990.
25. Dickinson D, Sambrooks J. Intellectual performance in children after circulatory arrest with profound hypothermia in infancy. Arch Dis Child 54:1, 1979.
26. Edmunds H. Inflammatory/immune response. In Jonas RA, Elliott ME (eds). Cardiopulmonary Bypass in the Neonate, Infant and Child. London, Butterworth-Heinemann, 1993.
27. Edwards AD, Wyatt JS, Richardson C, et al. Cotside measurement of cerebral blood flow in ill newborns with near infrared spectroscopy. Lancet 2:770, 1988.
28. Ehyai A, Fenichel GM, Bender HW. Incidence and prognosis of seizures in infants after cardiac surgery with profound hypothermia and circulatory arrest. JAMA 252:3165, 1984.
29. Ekroth R, Thompson RJ, Lincoln C, et al. Elective deep hypothermia with total circulatory arrest: Changes in plasma creatine kinase BB, blood glucose, and clinical variables. J Thorac Cardiovasc Surg 97:30, 1989.
30. Finlayson DC, Kaplan JA. Cardiopulmonary bypass. In Kaplan JA (ed). Cardiac Anesthesia. New York, Grune & Stratton, 1979, pp 393–340.
31. Fisk GC, Wright JS, Turner BB, et al. Cerebral effects of circulatory arrest at 20°C in the infant pig. Anesth Intensive Care 2:33, 1974.
32. Folkerth TL, Angell WW, Fosburg RH, et al. Effect of deep hypothermia, limited cardiopulmonary bypass and total arrest on growing puppies. In Roy PE, Rorek G (eds). Recent Advances in Studies on Cardiac Structure. Vol 10. Baltimore, University Park Press, 1975, pp 411–421.
33. Fox LS, Blackstone EH, Kirklin JW, et al. Relationship of whole body oxygen consumption to perfusion flow rate during hypothermic cardiopulmonary bypass. J Thorac Cardiovasc Surg 83:239, 1982.
34. Gillis CN, Greene NM, Cronau LH, et al. Pulmonary extraction of 5-hydroxytryptamine and norepinephrine before and after cardiopulmonary bypass in man. Circ Res 30:666, 1972.
35. Greeley WJ, Kern FH, Ungerleider RM, et al. The effect of hypothermic cardiopulmonary bypass and total circulatory arrest on cerebral metabolism in neonates, infants, and children. J Thorac Cardiovasc Surg 101:783–794, 1991.
36. Greeley WJ, Ungerleider RN, Kern FH, et al. Effects of cardiopulmonary bypass on cerebral blood flow in neonates, infants, and children. Circulation 80(suppl I):I-209, 1989.
37. Harake B, Power GG. Thoracic duct lymph flow: A comparative study in newborn and adult sheep. J Dev Physiol 8:87, 1986.
38. Harris EA. Metabolic aspects of profound hypothermia. In Barratt-Boyes BG, Neutze JM, Harris EA (eds). Heart Disease in Infancy. Edinburgh, Churchill Livingstone, 1973, pp 65–74.
39. Henriksen L. Brain luxury perfusion during cardiopulmonary bypass in humans. J Cereb Blood Flow Metab 6:366, 1986.
40. Jonas RA. Flow reduction and cessation. In Jonas RA, Elliott ME (eds). Cardiopulmonary Bypass in the Neonate, Infant and Child. London, Butterworth-Heinemann, 1993.
41. Jonas RA, Bellinger DC, Rappaport LA, et al. pH strategy and developmental outcome after hypothermic circulatory arrest. J Thorac Cardiovasc Surg 106:362–368, 1993.
42. Jonas RA, Wernovsky G, Ware J, et al. The Boston Circulatory Arrest Study: Perioperative neurologic outcome after the arterial switch operation. Circulation 86(suppl I):I-360, 1992.
43. Kawata H, Fackler JC, Aoki M, et al. Recovery of cerebral blood flow and energy state after hypothermic circulatory arrest versus low flow bypass in piglets. J Thorac Cardiovasc Surg. In press.

44. Kern FH, Ungerleider RM, Reves JG, et al. The effect of altering pump flow rate on cerebral blood flow and cerebral metabolism in neonates, infants, and children. J Thorac Cardiovasc Surg. In press.

45. Kirklin JW, Barratt-Boyes BG. Cardiac Surgery. 2nd ed. New York, Churchill Livingstone, 1993, pp 61–128.

46. Kirklin JK, Westaby S, Blackstone EH, et al. Complement and the damaging effects of cardiopulmonary bypass. J Thorac Cardiovasc Surg 86:845, 1983.

47. Kramer RS, Sanders AP, Lesage AM, et al. The effect of profound hypothermia on preservation of cerebral ATP content during circulatory arrest. J Thorac Cardiovasc Surg 56:699, 1968.

48. Lillehei CW, Varco RL, Cohen M, et al. The first open-heart corrections of ventricular septal defect, atrioventricular communis, and tetralogy of Fallot utilizing extracorporeal circulation by cross-circulation. A thirty year follow-up. Ann Thorac Surg 41:4, 1986.

49. Lucchesi BR. Neutrophil-derived oxygen radicals in myocardial reperfusion injury. In Zelenock GB, D'Alecy LG, Fantone JC, et al (eds). Clinical Ischemic Syndromes. St Louis, CV Mosby, 1990, pp 257–275.

50. Luscher TF, Vanhoute FM. The Endothelium: Modulator of Cardiovascular Function. Boca Raton, FL, CRC Press, 1990.

51. Mavroudis C, Brown GL, Katzmark SL, et al. Blood flow distribution in infant pigs subjected to surface cooling, deep hypothermia, and circulatory arrest. Deleterious effects in pigs with left to right shunts. J Thorac Cardiovasc Surg 87:665, 1984.

52. Miyamoto K, Kawashima Y, Matsuda H, et al. Optimal perfusion flow rate for the brain during deep hypothermic cardiopulmonary bypass at 20°C. J Thorac Cardiovasc Surg 92:1065, 1986.

53. Molina JE, Einzig S, Mastri AR, et al. Brain damage in profound hypothermia. Perfusion versus circulatory arrest. J Thorac Cardiovasc Surg 87:596, 1984.

54. Moody DM. A new role for radiologists in the development of cardiac surgery. Am J Neuroradiol 12:815, 1991.

55. Moody DM, Bell MA, Challa VR, et al. Brain microemboli during cardiac surgery or aortography. Ann Neurol 28:477, 1990.

56. Murkin JM, Farrar JK, Tweed WA, et al. Cerebral autoregulation and flow/metabolism coupling during cardiopulmonary bypass. The influence of $PaCO_2$. Anesth Analg 66:825, 1987.

57. Norwood WI, Norwood CR, Castaneda AR. Cerebral anoxia: Effect of deep hypothermia and pH. Surgery 86:203, 1979.

58. Norwood WI, Norwood CR, Ingwall JS, et al. Hypothermic circulatory arrest: 31-Phosphorous nuclear magnetic resonance of isolated perfused neonatal rat brain. J Thorac Cardiovasc Surg 78:823, 1979.

59. Pulsinelli WA, Waldman S, Rawlinson D, et al. Moderate hyperglycemia augments ischemic brain damage: A neuropathologic study in the rat. Neurology 32:1239, 1982.

60. Rahn H, Reeves RB, Howell BJ. Hydrogen ion regulation temperature and evolution. Am Rev Resp Dis 112:165, 1975.

61. Ratcliffe JM, Wyse RKH, Hunter S, et al. The role of the priming fluid in the metabolic response to cardiopulmonary bypass in children of less than 16 kg body weight undergoing open-heart surgery. Thorac Cardiovasc Surg 36:65, 1988.

62. Reeves RB. An imidazole alphastat hypothesis for vertebrate acid-base regulation: Tissue carbon dioxide content and body temperature in bullfrogs. Resp Physiol 14:219, 1972.

63. Reves JG, Karp RB, Buttner EE, et al. Neuronal and adrenomedullary catecholamine release in response to cardiopulmonary bypass in man. Circulation 66:49, 1982.

64. Richter JA. Profound hypothermia and circulatory arrest: Studies on intraoperative metabolic changes and late postoperative development after correction of congenital heart disease. In Delange S, Hennis PJ, Kettler D, et al (eds). Cardiac Anesthesia: Problems, Innovations. Boston, Martinus Nijhoff, 1986, pp 121–142.

65. Rogers AT, Prough DS, Roy RC. Cerebrovascular and cerebral metabolic effects of alterations in perfusion flow rate during hypothermic cardiopulmonary bypass in man. J Thorac Cardiovasc Surg 103:363, 1992.

66. Rosenthal SM, LaJohn LA. Effect of age on transvascular fluid movement. Am J Physiol 228:134, 1975.

67. Rossi R, Ekroth R, Lincoln C, et al. Detection of cerebral injury after total circulatory arrest and profound hypothermia by estimation of specific creatine kinase isoenzyme levels using monoclonal antibody techniques. Am J Cardiol 58:1236, 1986.

68. Rossi R, van der Linden J, Ekroth R, et al. No flow or low flow? A study of the ischemic marker creatine kinase BB after deep hypothermic procedures. J Thorac Cardiovasc Surg 98:193, 1989.

69. Siemkowez E, Gjedde A. Postischemic coma in the rat: Effect of different preischemic blood glucose levels on cerebral metabolic recovery after ischemia. Acta Physiol Scand 110:225, 1980.

70. Smith EEG, Naftel DC, Blackstone EH, et al. Microvascular permeability after cardiopulmonary bypass. J Thorac Cardiovasc Surg 94:225, 1987.

71. Soma Y, Hirotani T, Yozu R, et al. A clinical study of cerebral circulation during extracorporeal circulation. J Thorac Cardiovasc Surg 97:187, 1989.

72. Somero GN, White FN. Enzymatic consequences under alphastat regulation. In Rahn H, Prakash O (eds). Acid-Base Regulation and Body Temperature. Boston, Martinus Nijhoff, 1985, pp 55–80.

73. Southard JH. Temperature effects and cooling. In Zelenock GB, D'Alecy LG, Fantone JC, et al. Clinical Ischemic Syndromes. St Louis, CV Mosby, 1990, pp 303–325.

74. Staunton DE, Marlin SD, Stratowa C, et al. Primary structure of ICAM-1 demonstrates interaction between members of the immunoglobulin and integrin supergene families. Cell 52:925, 1988.

75. Stevenson J, Stone E, Dillard D, et al. Intellectual development of children subjected to prolonged circulatory arrest during hypothermic open heart surgery in infancy. Circulation 49(suppl II):54, 1974.

76. Steward DJ, Da Silva CA, Flegel T. Elevated blood glucose levels may increase the danger of neurological deficit following profoundly hypothermic cardiac arrest. Anesthesiology 68:653, 1988.

77. Stewart RW, Blackstone EH, Kirklin JW. Neurological dysfunction after cardiac surgery. In Parenzan L, Crupi G, Graham G (eds). Congenital Heart Disease in the First Three Months of Life: Medical and Surgical Aspects. Bologna, Italy, Patron Editore, 1981, p 431.

78. Swain JA, McDonald TJ, Griffith PK, et al. Low flow hypothermic cardiopulmonary bypass protects the brain. J Thorac Cardiovasc Surg 102:76, 1991.

79. Swain JA, McDonald TJ, Robbins RC, et al. Relationship of cerebral and myocardial intracellular pH to blood pH during hypothermia. Am J Physiol 260:H1640, 1991.

80. Swan H. The importance of acid-base management for cardiac and cerebral preservation during open heart operations. Surg Gynecol Obstet 158:391, 1984.

81. Treasure T, Naftel DC, Conger KA, et al. The effect of hypothermic circulatory arrest time on cerebral function, morphology, and biochemistry. J Thorac Cardiovasc Surg 86:761, 1983.

82. Tuppurainen T, Settergren G, Stensved P. The effect of arterial pH on whole body oxygen uptake during hypothermic cardiopulmonary bypass in man. J Thorac Cardiovasc Surg 98:769, 1989.

83. Utley JR. Pathophysiology of cardiopulmonary bypass: Current issues. J Cardiac Surg 5:177, 1990.

84. Wachtfogel YT, Kulich J, Greenplate J, et al. Human neutrophil degranulation during extracorporeal circulation. Blood 69:324, 1981.

85. Walsh AZ, Wernovsky G, Wypij D, et al. Postoperative course following the arterial switch operation. Circulation 86(suppl I):I-501, 1992.

86. Wells F, Coghill S, Caplan H, et al. Duration of circulatory arrest does influence the psychological development of children after cardiac operation in early life. J Thorac Cardiovasc Surg 86:823, 1983.

87. Wernovsky G, Jonas RA, Newburger JW, et al. The Boston

Circulatory Arrest Study: Hemodynamics and hospital course after the arterial switch operation. Circulation 86(suppl I):I–237, 1992.

88. White FN. A comparative physiological approach to hypothermia. J Thorac Cardiovasc Surg 82:821, 1981.

89. Wolfson SK, Yalav EH, Eisenstat S. An isothermic technique for profound hypothermia and its effect on metabolic acidosis. J Thorac Cardiovasc Surg 45:466, 1963.

90. Wong PC, Barlow CF, Hickey PR, et al. Factors associated with choreoathetosis after cardiopulmonary bypass in children with congenital heart disease. Circulation 86(suppl II):II-118, 1992.

91. Wright J, Hicks R, Newman D. Deep hypothermic arrest: Observations on later development in children. J Thorac Cardiovasc Surg 77:466, 1979.

92. Yancey PH, Somero GN. Temperature dependence of intracellular pH: Its role in the conservation of pyruvate apparent Km values of vertebrae lactate dehydrogenase. J Comp Physiol 125:129, 1978.

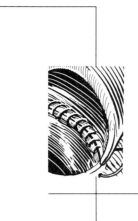

3

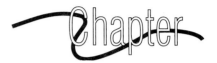

Myocardial Preservation in the Immature Heart

Essentially all repairs of intracardiac malformations in the neonate and infant require a period of myocardial ischemia to provide satisfactory operating conditions for conduction of the repair. There have been extensive efforts to improve the preservation of the heart during these periods of surgically induced ischemia, and although great strides have been made, the need for further improvement in the entire area of myocardial preservation remains. The vast majority of the experimental efforts have involved mature heart models, but, as outlined later, there are reasons to believe that myocardial ischemia in the immature heart may differ in some ways from that in the mature heart, and therefore, different strategies for myocardial preservation during ischemia might be desirable. This discussion will focus primarily on preservation of the immature heart, although it must be understood that the precise definition of the term *immature* remains unclear. Furthermore, the crossover point from immature to mature for the human species is also unknown.

ANATOMIC AND FUNCTIONAL CHARACTERISTICS OF THE IMMATURE HEART

A variety of data suggest that the immature myocardium differs in important ways from the mature myocardium, and some of these differences have potential implications for the preservation of the immature heart during ischemia. The anatomic and functional characteristics of the immature myocardium have been extensively reviewed by Anderson.[1] From a structural standpoint, the heart does change during development, although the rate and timing of these developmental changes vary among different species. Remarkably, relatively little human data are available; in animal data, the level of development seems to be related to the level of maturation and function at birth.[1] The myocytes become larger and more oblong and develop a more complex external shape during development,[63] and the myofibrils become larger and are reoriented along the longitudinal direction of the cell.[75] The number of mitochondria, their orientation to the myofibrils, and the complexity of the cristal structure also evolve during development.[52, 75] These changes in the numbers of myofibrils and mitochondria imply that the demand for oxygen increases with development. The structure and relative amounts of sarcoplasmic reticulum (SR) also change, and the transverse tubular system,[65] which functionally connects the sarcolemma to the SR, develops at varying rates in different species.[1] Because the SR and the transverse tubular system are intimately involved in calcium control during normal contraction and during ischemia, the immature myocardium may be expected to differ in its sensitivity to extracellular calcium concentration associated with these anatomic changes in the organelles known to be involved in calcium homeostasis.

Biochemical changes also occur during myocardial maturation, and the understanding of these changes may have significant importance in the area of myocardial preservation. In general, the fetal mammalian myocardium has the ability to use various substrates, including carbohydrates, medium- and short-chain fatty acids, ketones, and amino acids,[1] but the oxygen consumption of the left ventricle of the fetal lamb is entirely the result of oxidation of glucose, lactate, and pyruvate.[29] In general, there appears to be a greater glycolytic capacity in the fetal heart than in the adult.[39] In the mature heart, long-chain fatty acids are the principal substrate,[39] and oxidation of fatty acids by the myocyte is associated with development of a more complex mitochondrial cristal pattern and the maturation of several enzymes involved in fatty acid metabolism.[1] In most mammals, the enzymatic machinery that allows long-chain free fatty acids to become the primary energy substrate of the heart is in place within a few days or weeks after birth.[1] However, this shift from glucose to fatty acids as the major substrate source occurs at different times in different species, making extrapolation to the developing human heart difficult.[39] The relatively increased ability of the immature heart to utilize anaerobic glycolysis to generate energy has been related to the "resistance" of the immature myocardium to anoxic ischemia.[1]

An important additional area of biochemical and functional differences between immature and mature myocardium involves the control of intracellular calcium concentration. As noted previously, the SR, which is the major source of "activator" calcium for myocardial contraction and the primary site of calcium sequestration during relaxation in the mature heart, is found in increasing amounts as development proceeds.[1, 56] In addition, the calcium-sequestering capacity of the SR and the activity of calcium-dependent adenosine triphosphatase (ATPase) both increase during development.[56, 58] Fabiato found that during the development of the ventricular cell of the rat, there is also a progressive maturation of calcium-induced release of calcium from the SR.[27] Jarmakani and coworkers found that the newborn rabbit heart requires a higher external concentration of calcium than does the adult rabbit heart to achieve a maximal contractile response to calcium,[43, 56, 60] and there has been general agreement (including in experiments with human myocardium) that immature hearts have a greater dependence on the trans-sarcolemmal movement of calcium (i.e., the movement of calcium from the ex-

tracellular to intracellular space) as a source of "activator" calcium for contraction.[1] Finally, there are maturational increases in Na^+/K^+ ATPase activity with development that affect intracellular calcium concentrations through the Na^+-Ca^{++} exchange mechanism.[1] All of these changes in the control of intracellular calcium are consistent with the observations that the immature myocardium has a lower intracellular Ca^{++} concentration,[60] develops less force, and has a lower velocity of shortening and re-extension than the mature myocardial cell.[1, 56] These developmental differences in the ways in which calcium is handled by the immature myocyte are quite likely to have important implications in the response to ischemia because of the role of calcium in irreversible cardiac injury after ischemia and reperfusion.[47]

TOLERANCE OF THE IMMATURE HEART TO HYPOXIA OR ISCHEMIA

The question of whether the immature heart is less sensitive or more sensitive to the effects of hypoxia or ischemia and reperfusion remains unsettled despite numerous investigations. On the theoretical grounds of greater glycolytic capacity as discussed earlier, it has been thought that the immature heart would be better able to tolerate hypoxia or ischemia than the mature heart. Numerous studies in rabbits,[5, 12, 13, 35, 44] rats,[4, 85] and puppies[55] have shown an increased tolerance to normothermic hypoxia or ischemia in the immature animal when compared with the mature animal. In addition to increased glycolytic capacity, a second potential mechanism involved in this improved ischemic tolerance may be better preservation of intracellular, high-energy phosphates.[44, 55, 59, 86] The increase in high-energy phosphates may be related to lower levels of 5-nucleotidase,[55] an enzyme that catalyzes the breakdown of adenosine monophosphate (AMP) to adenosine. It has been hypothesized that lower levels of this enzyme would be associated with higher end-ischemic levels of AMP, which would then be available for rephosphorylation to adenosine triphosphate (ATP) when blood flow was restored.[55] Other investigators have noted that the neonatal rabbit heart has less calcium uptake during ischemia[61] and greater lactate production during anoxic perfusion[44] than the adult heart. Nakanishi and coworkers[57] showed that neonatal rabbits had less accumulation of H^+ intracellularly in response to extracellular acidosis, but had an equivalent accumulation of Ca^{++}. Julia and colleagues[45] also demonstrated an increased ability of the puppy heart to utilize amino acids as substrate during normothermic ischemia when compared with the adult dog heart. These studies demonstrate that a variety of mechanisms may be involved in the tolerance of the neonatal heart to ischemia.

In contrast, experiments in rats[19, 83] and pigs[64] have shown a lower tolerance to ischemia in the neonatal heart than in the mature heart, particularly when assessed by the time to ischemic contracture under normothermic conditions. The greater intracellular accumulation of lactic acid as a result of anaerobic (i.e., glycolytic) metabolism has been hypothesized as the injurious mechanism.[19] Clinically, the most widely quoted study regarding the susceptibility of immature myocardium to ischemia is that by Bull and associates,[16] who found that myocardial ischemic times (>85 minutes) that seem to be well tolerated in adults with adjunctive hypothermic cardioplegia were associated with a significant mortality risk in infants, despite the use of cardioplegia. A subsequent ultrastructural study by Sawa and associates[71] found more mitochondrial injury in human neonates undergoing cardiac repairs than in older children. Thus, the basic issue of the relative susceptibilities of immature versus mature myocardium to ischemia and reperfusion remains unsettled, but there are sufficient data to suggest that the immature myocardium has certain characteristics that distinguish it from mature myocardium and that may have an important effect on its response to ischemia.

EXPERIMENTAL DATA ON PRESERVATION OF THE IMMATURE HEART

Preischemic Interventions

Relatively little information is available on the effects of preischemic interventions on the outcome of a subsequent period of ischemia. Experimental results in lambs and rabbits have suggested that augmentation of myocardial glycogen improved the tolerance of the neonatal heart to anoxia, and results of other experiments in mature dogs and rats have suggested that myocardial function is better preserved during normothermic anoxia when myocardial glycogen stores had been augmented before the insult.[41] More recent experiments in puppies have suggested that the provision of aspartate and glutamate just before ischemia, as part of a warm "induction" cardioplegic solution, results in better tolerance to a subsequent ischemic insult.[48]

The use of corticosteroids as a pretreatment just before the onset of ischemia has been shown to enhance the myocardial tolerance to normothermic ischemia in both pigs[26] and dogs.[42] The mechanism

has been thought to involve "membrane stabilization"[42] or the prevention of phospholipase activation to prevent sarcolemmal injury during reperfusion.[26] No studies appear to have been carried out regarding the value of the use of steroids specifically for the immature myocardium.

Interventions During Ischemia

Hypothermia

Since the time of Bigelow's experiments in the 1950s demonstrating that hypothermia improved the tolerance of the entire organism to ischemia,[7] this physical intervention of reducing the temperature of the tissue during ischemia has remained the mainstay of almost all strategies of myocardial protection. A number of studies have shown that ischemic periods of 1 to 2 hours can be followed by nearly complete recovery of function in immature hearts protected by hypothermia alone.[5, 13, 31] Although it has generally been assumed that this protection results from the reduced metabolic demand of the tissues produced by hypothermia, it is not completely clear that this metabolic effect is the only mechanism of action of hypothermia. There is a large body of evidence that suggests that ischemia causes alterations in sarcolemmal permeability to ions such as sodium, potassium, and calcium.[15] Ferrari and coworkers showed that a major effect of hypothermia is to reduce the accumulation of calcium in the mitochondria during ischemia, presumably through effects on the mitochondrial membrane.[28] It has been hypothesized that hypothermia induces physical changes in the sarcolemma that alter the effects of ischemia on membrane permeability to ions such as sodium and calcium and thereby reduce the likelihood of cell death after a period of ischemia.[69] Nishioka and associates[61] found that newborn rabbit hearts exposed to hypothermic global ischemia had less accumulation of calcium during ischemia and reperfusion than adult rabbit hearts and the postischemic ATP levels were inversely related to intracellular calcium accumulation. This same group demonstrated improved recovery of mechanical function with hypothermic protection in young rabbits when compared with an adult rabbit heart population.[59]

The potential for a deleterious effect of hypothermia induced before the onset of ischemia has been suggested by the report of Reybeka and coworkers.[68] In this experiment in adult rabbit hearts, hypothermia before the onset of cardioplegia-protected ischemia resulted in worse recovery of function than if the heart was kept warm up to the time of onset of

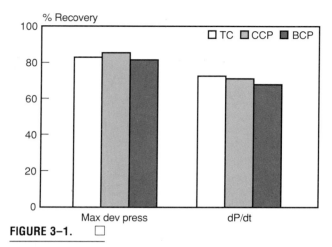

FIGURE 3–1. ☐

Effect of myocardial preservation technique on recovery of systolic function after 2 hours of 15°C ischemia in isolated, blood-perfused, neonatal lamb hearts. BCP, blood cardioplegia; CCP, crystalloid cardioplegia (glucose-K+); Max Dev Press, maximum developed pressure; TC, topical cooling.

ischemia and the cardioplegia itself was used to both cool and arrest the heart. The proposed mechanism of this cold-induced exacerbation of an ischemic injury is hypothermia-induced calcium accumulation in the myocardial cells before the onset of ischemia;[68] data from isolated papillary muscle experiments suggest that hypothermia has a positive inotropic effect through an increase in intracellular calcium. Williams and coworkers[82] reported clinical data supporting this hypothesis by comparing a group of patients in whom hypothermia preceded ischemia with a group in whom normothermic conditions were maintained before the infusion of cold cardioplegic solution. Improved patient survival and better myocardial function were reported in the patients in whom preischemic hypothermia was avoided. These findings were in marked contrast to the usual practice of perfusion cooling on bypass before the application of the aortic crossclamp and without recognizing the cold contracture phenomenon. Stimulated by this discrepancy, experiments have been completed that suggest that, in the isolated neonatal lamb heart, reduced ionized calcium levels during preischemic cooling (accomplished by adding citrate to the perfusion circuit) result in improved recovery of mechanical function after protected ischemia when St. Thomas cardioplegic solution is utilized.[3] Interestingly, the use of an acalcemic glucose-potassium carioplegic solution also prevented the deleterious effects of preischemic hypothermia, despite normal calcium levels during cooling (Mayer JE, unpublished data). The precise explanation for these differences remains unclear, but it is likely that calcium accumulation during ischemia is involved.

Cardioplegia

Debate continues regarding the efficacy of cardioplegia added to hypothermia in enhancing protection of the immature myocardium. The studies of Fujiwara[31] (Fig. 3–1), of Laks and associates[51] in neonatal lambs, and of Baker and colleagues[5, 6] in neonatal rabbits all suggest that in the normal heart there may be no additional benefit of adding cardioplegia to hypothermia. Clark and coworkers[20] reported similar results in the neonatal piglet. However, other studies have shown that the addition of cardioplegia to hypothermia is beneficial. Diaco and coworkers[23] and Konishi and Apstein[49] showed that cardioplegia and hypothermia provided added protection over hypothermia alone (20°C) in neonatal rabbits. Two other experiments have suggested that in a "stressed" neonatal heart subjected to an ischemic insult, a beneficial effect of cardioplegia can be demonstrated that may not be apparent in an otherwise normal neonatal heart. Bove and coworkers[14] demonstrated an additive effect of cardioplegia and hypothermia over hypothermia alone in rabbit hearts undergoing ischemia at moderate levels of hypothermia (28°C). At Children's Hospital in Boston,[32] in the hearts of neonatal lambs with pre-existing cyanosis, cardioplegia and hypothermia did provide additional protection when compared with hypothermia (15°C) alone (Fig. 3–2). The importance of species variation when interpreting these types of experiments is demonstrated by the findings of Baker and associates,[6] who found worse recovery when cardioplegia (using St. Thomas cardioplegic solution) was added to hypothermia in neonatal rabbits; however, a significant benefit was

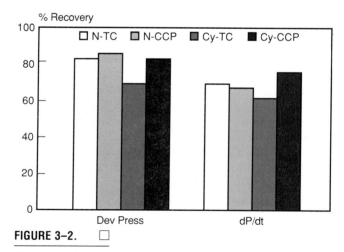

FIGURE 3–2. ☐

Effect of cardioplegia on recovery of systolic function after 2 hours of 15°C ischemia in isolated, blood-perfused, neonatal lamb hearts from normoxemic and cyanotic animals. CCP, crystalloid cardioplegia; Cy, cyanotic; N, normoxemic; TC, topical cooling.

demonstrated in the neonatal piglet. Unfortunately, no clinical studies comparing hypothermia with hypothermic cardioplegia have been reported other than that of Bull and coworkers,[16] nor is it clear whether the immature human heart more closely resembles the rabbit, the lamb, or the piglet in its response to ischemia and reperfusion. We have found in our laboratory that excessively cold cardioplegia (<2°C) results in depressed recovery of mechanical and endothelial function in the neonatal lamb heart.[2]

Cardioplegic Additives

Blood. Although there are multiple studies regarding the use of blood versus crystalloid solutions in the mature heart, few studies have been done in the immature heart. Fujiwara et al.[31] found no benefit of blood cardioplegia over crystalloid cardioplegia or hypothermia in the normal neonatal lamb (Fig. 3–1), but Corno and coworkers found that in the neonatal piglet model, cardioplegic solutions containing blood were associated with improved recovery of function when compared with crystalloid cardioplegic solutions or hypothermia alone.[21] Kofsky and coworkers reported complete recovery of mechanical function and high-energy phosphate levels after 2 hours of hypothermic ischemia with blood cardioplegic solution enriched with aspartate and glutamate.[48] In vitro studies have shown that the amount of oxygen delivered by deeply hypothermic, oxygenated, crystalloid solutions and by hypothermic oxygenated blood do not differ significantly.[25] Other evidence suggests that the presence of red blood cells in these solutions may provide better perfusion at the microcirculatory level during hypothermic perfusion,[78] but this issue has not been addressed in the immature heart. There are other mechanisms by which the addition of blood to cardioplegic solutions may be beneficial, including provision of free-radical scavenging capacity through the catalase in red blood cells and provision of buffering capacity of blood proteins.

Oxygen. There are convincing data that in mature heart systems, the oxygenation of crystalloid cardioplegic solutions is associated with significant improvements in the recovery of postischemic function.[9, 67] No studies on the effects of oxygenation of cardioplegic solutions in the immature heart have been carried out, although Baker et al. reported experimental data that suggest that the level of preischemic oxygenation can influence the outcome of a period of hypothermic ischemia in Krebs-Henseleit–perfused rabbit hearts.[5]

Calcium Content. The optimal concentration of calcium in various cardioplegic solutions remains unknown. Because the intracellular accumulation of calcium during ischemia and reperfusion has been associated with cellular injury, an argument can be made for minimizing the calcium in the extracellular environment during ischemia to prevent intracellular calcium accumulation. However, the "calcium paradox" phenomenon of massive calcium accumulation and rapid cell death occurring after perfusion with acalcemic solutions in normothermic rat hearts has been described,[69] and thus there is a theoretical potential for this phenomenon to occur with acalcemic cardioplegic solutions. Subsequently, it has been shown that hypothermia prevents this phenomenon from occurring in some models,[69] but Hendren and coworkers showed that highly alkaline acalcemic cardioplegic solutions can cause ischemic contracture whereas solutions with lower pH do not in the adult rat heart.[40] A rigorous study of the question of optimal calcium concentration was carried out using St. Thomas solution; a nearly normal calcium concentration was determined to be "optimal" when ischemia was induced at normothermic levels in the adult rat heart.[84] Robinson and Harwood[70] determined that a reduced calcium concentration (0.6 mmol/L) provided optimal recovery when the ischemia was induced at 20°C in the adult rat heart. An important point to consider, however, is that there are high magnesium concentrations in St. Thomas cardioplegic solution that likely compete with calcium at entry points through the cell membrane. Therefore, an optimal calcium concentration determined for a solution containing magnesium may not be applicable if the magnesium is not present. In the adult dog heart, normal levels of calcium in cardioplegic solutions that do not contain magnesium have been found to adversely affect high-energy phosphates and to induce ventricular contraction during ischemia.[79] The recovery of function after ischemia with cardioplegic solutions having a "normal" calcium content (1.2 mmol/L) has been markedly worse in some experiments[10, 34] but not in others.[8] Other studies have shown that the presence of minimal amounts of calcium is associated with excellent recovery of function after prolonged ischemic intervals.[67] Two studies of calcium concentrations in blood cardioplegia in neonatal piglets have reached opposite conclusions. Caspi and coworkers[17] found better recovery of postischemic function when a hypocalcemic blood cardioplegic solution was used, while Corno and associates[21] found that normal calcium levels were associated with better recovery. The report of Kofsky and colleagues[48] supported the use of hypocalcemic blood cardioplegia in the puppy. In a study providing correlative evidence for a deleterious effect of calcium during ischemia, Konishi and Apstein showed that exposure of the neonatal heart to ouabain before hypothermic ischemia was associated with significantly worse recovery of function, presumably because ouabain increases the intracellular calcium concentration through inhibition of Na+/K+ ATPase.[50] As noted earlier, we have found that there are significant interactions between preischemic hypothermia and the calcium content of cardioplegic solutions (Aoki M, unpublished data).

Magnesium. There are no direct data concerning variations in magnesium concentration in cardioplegic solutions for the immature myocardium. The only direct comparison between magnesium-free and magnesium-containing solutions in the immature heart was carried out by Konishi and Apstein[49] in an isolated, blood-perfused rabbit heart system. In this study two magnesium-containing crystalloid cardioplegic solutions (St. Thomas solution and a magnesium-potassium-glutamate solution used at Hôpital Lariboisiere) were found to provide better recovery of function than an acalcemic glucose-potassium solution.[49] Similar results showing greater benefit when magnesium is added to cardioplegic solutions have been reported for the adult rat heart.[34, 79] Yano and coworkers provided data suggesting that the magnesium-containing St. Thomas solution provided good protection of the neonatal and immature heart[85] in a normothermic neonatal rat model.

Calcium channel blockade. In view of the generally deleterious effects of calcium during ischemia and the greater influence of the extracellular concentration of calcium on the function of the immature myocardium, pharmacologic blockade of calcium channels provides a theoretically attractive means of improving myocardial protection during ischemia. Starnes and coworkers found that verapamil improved the recovery of systolic and diastolic function and ATP levels in puppies subjected to normothermic ischemia;[76] a subsequent study from the same laboratory suggested that verapamil added to a potassium cardioplegic solution enhanced the recovery of function after normothermic ischemia.[53] In our studies in isolated neonatal lamb hearts subjected to 2 hours of hypothermic ischemia, nifedipine led to improved recovery of function, but verapamil did not (Fujiwara T, unpublished data). This effect appeared to be due to the more negative inotropic effects of verapamil, despite the equipotent doses used. A clinical trial of a newer calcium channel blocker (nicardipine) by Mori and coworkers noted that postischemic performance was improved with nicardipine when compared with a standard potassium cardioplegic solution.[54] The negative inotropic effects of most other calcium channel blocking agents have limited their application in the clinical setting.

Dosing Regimens for Cardioplegia. In hypothermic models of ischemia in immature hearts, four separate studies all suggest that a single dose, rather than multiple doses, of cardioplegic solution results in improved recovery of function after ischemia. Bove and associates found no additional protection when multiple doses of St. Thomas cardioplegia solution were compared with a single dose in the neonatal rabbit,[14] while Baker and colleagues, working with a similar neonatal rabbit heart model, found worse recovery of function with multiple, rather than single, doses of St. Thomas cardioplegic solution.[5] Sawa and coworkers also found worse outcomes after multiple doses of potassium cardioplegia solution,[72] and Clark and coworkers found that the best recovery of function occurred after a single dose of potassium cardioplegic solution at 4°C in the newborn piglet heart.[20] DeLeon and coworkers reported no advantage to multiple doses of blood cardioplegia in children undergoing arterial switch operations.[22] These studies seem to indicate that as long as the heart remains arrested and hypothermic, additional doses of cardioplegic solution seem to be unnecessary and may even be detrimental.

Reperfusion

There is increasing evidence that events occurring during reperfusion may be equally as important as those occurring during ischemia in determining the ultimate outcome of an episode of ischemia and reperfusion. Interventions in the areas of substrate enhancement, free-radical scavenging, control of the introduction of oxygen, and control of perfusion pressure have all been reported to enhance the recovery of function during reperfusion after ischemia.

Substrate Enhancement

Ischemia clearly reduces the level of high-energy phosphates in the myocardial cell, and there is some correlation between the levels of ATP and subsequent recovery during the reperfusion period, both experimentally[20, 44, 55, 76] and clinically.[16, 38] Therefore, it has seemed logical to attempt to enhance the levels of high-energy phosphate precursors so that ATP levels can be readily restored or to provide metabolic substrates from which the high-energy phosphates can be generated. The approach of preserving high-energy phosphate precursors, such as AMP or adenosine, has not been evaluated in the immature heart, although there is evidence that AMP levels are better preserved during ischemia in the immature heart than in the adult heart.[55] This better preservation of AMP during ischemia has been associated with the finding of a lower level of 5'-nucleotidase, the enzyme that catalyzes the conversion of AMP to the much more diffusible metabolite adenosine, which can then be lost from the cell into the interstitial space. In mature hearts, there is some evidence that the addition of adenosine to cardioplegic solutions[11, 81] or its administration during reperfusion[66] may result in better recovery of ATP levels and function during postischemic recovery. In our laboratory at Children's Hospital in Boston, Nomura et al. found that an infusion of adenosine during the first 20 minutes of reperfusion in isolated neonatal lamb hearts subjected to 2 hours of hypothermic ischemia resulted in marked improvement in both coronary blood flow and recovery of mechanical function.[62] In an alternative approach reported in a mature heart model, ribose and adenine were provided during the postischemic period to serve as the substrate from which adenine nucleotides could be resynthesized through the de novo pathway.[30, 77, 80] The rationale for the use of glucose in many cardioplegic solutions was to provde substrate that could be utilized by the ischemic cell, but, as pointed out previously, multiple doses of cardioplegia solution have been associated with either no improvement or a worse outcome in the immature heart, despite the fact that they provide more substrate for metabolism during ischemia. The approach of providing metabolic substrates that can then be metabolized to generate ATP has not been well studied in the immature heart until relatively recently. Experiments in which the amino acids glutamate and aspartate were added to the initial reperfusate after normothermic hypoxia in puppies demonstrated improvement in high-energy phosphate levels and mechanical function,[46] and the addition of glutamate and aspartate to hypothermic blood cardioplegia solutions during 2 hours of ischemia has also been found to improve postischemic recovery.[48] These amino acids enter into the tricarboxylic acid (Krebs) cycle, and ATP is then generated through oxidative phosphorylation.

Free-Radical Scavengers

The observation that highly reactive oxygen species (free radicals), which have destructive effects on the cellular membrane, are generated during reperfusion after ischemia has led to experiments in which free-radical formation is prevented or free-radical "scavenger" interventions are used. No experiments have been reported in which these types of interventions have been employed in the neonatal heart subjected to hypothermic ischemia. In the laboratory at Children's Hospital in Boston, the recov-ery of isolated neonatal lamb hearts after hypothermic ischemia was not improved by the free-radical scavenging enzymes superoxide dismutase and catalase (Sawatari K, unpublished data). However, Otani and associates[64] reported data from neonatal piglet hearts subjected to 60 minutes of normothermic ischemia that suggested that free-radical formation was an important factor in the injury occurring after this type of ischemia/reperfusion insult. The source of the free radicals in ischemia/reperfusion injury is also not completely resolved; there has been recent interest in this regard in both white blood cells and the endothelium (see Chapter 31). The role of any or all of these free-radical reducing strategies on the outcome of ischemia and reperfusion in the immature heart remains uncertain.

Control of the Introduction of Oxygen

It is clear that oxygen must be reintroduced after ischemia to make the transition back into an oxidative metabolic state. In most cases of surgically induced myocardial ischemia in which cardiopulmonary bypass is used, restoration of blood flow to the heart after ischemia is accompanied by hyperoxia, because the gas provided to the oxygenator of the cardiopulmonary bypass circuit is generally 95% to 100% oxygen. Experiments in our laboratory have raised concerns about reperfusion under conditions of hyperoxia.[74] Isolated, blood-perfused, neonatal lamb hearts underwent 2 hours of deeply hypothermic ischemia with cardioplegia and were then reperfused with either normoxic ($Po_2 = 200$ mm Hg) or hyperoxic ($Po_2 = 540$ mm Hg) blood for the first 10 minutes after ischemia. The hearts reperfused with normoxic blood achieved remarkably better recovery of mechanical function and, interestingly, also showed much better recovery of endothelial function as assessed by vasodilator response to acetylcholine (Fig. 3–3). The mechanisms underlying these effects of varying oxygen tension during reperfusion are not clear, but potential mechanisms may involve free-radical formation by myocytes or leukocytes or a direct vascular effect of hyperoxia, a known vasoconstrictor. The potential clinical significance of this finding remains to be investigated.

Control of Perfusion Pressure

Stimulated by anecdotal clinical observations that high initial reperfusion pressures may be deleterious to the recovery of function after ischemia, a series of experiments in our laboratory have shown that in the isolated, blood-perfused, neonatal lamb heart model, a protocol of low initial reperfusion pressure (20 mm Hg for the first 10 minutes) fol-

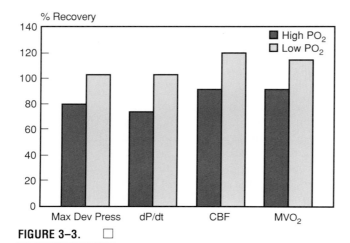

FIGURE 3–3. ☐

Effect of Po2 during initial reperfusion after 2 hours of 15°C ischemia in isolated, blood-perfused, neonatal lamb hearts. CBF, coronary blood flow; Max Dev Press, maximum developed pressure; MVO2, oxygen consumption.

lowed by a gradual increase of pressure up to 60 mm Hg during the remainder of reperfusion was associated with significant improvement in the recovery of mechanical function[33] and coronary endothelial function[73] (Figs. 3–4 and 3–5). Interestingly, this phenomenon of "high-pressure" reperfusion and mechanical dysfunction could be blocked by the administration of either nitroglycerine or nifedipine during the early reperfusion period.[33] This observation, along with the finding that coronary blood flow was extremely high in the first few minutes of high-pressure reperfusion,[73] raises the possibility that the deleterious effect of high reperfusion pressure was related to excessive shear forces on endothelium made vulnerable by the period of ischemia. Possibly, the use of vasodilator agents could offset this effect by inducing maximal vasodilation and thereby reducing shear stress at the arteriolar and microcirculatory levels. Interestingly, a number of pharmacologic agents that have been reported to improve the recovery of mechanical function after ischemia also have vasodilator activity. The mechanisms involved in high-pressure reperfusion injury remain under investigation, but it seems likely that preservation of the vascular bed in general and of the endothelium in particular will be important issues in the future (see Chapter 31).

Calcium

Although no studies have been carried out in the immature heart, an interesting study on calcium-induced reperfusion injury was reported by Hamasaki and coworkers.[36] After 90 minutes of hypothermic arrest in isolated adult rat hearts, reperfusion at 37°C with normal calcium levels resulted in de-

pressed functional recovery and significant creatine kinase losses. These effects were offset by initial reperfusion with hypocalcemic perfusate or by lowering the temperature of the reperfusate.

CURRENT CLINICAL APPLICATIONS OF MYOCARDIAL PRESERVATION TECHNIQUES

The methods employed clinically to protect the immature myocardium during periods of surgically induced ischemia have been borrowed from advances made in the protection of the adult heart and have consisted primarily of hypothermia combined with either potassium-based or potassium- and magnesium-based cardioplegic solutions. In the most widely quoted clinical study, Bull and coworkers found that the addition of St. Thomas cardioplegic solution did not change the overall mortality rate in a series of 200 consecutive patients when compared with the previous 200 patients in whom intermittent hypothermic ischemia was used.[16] However, it was also clear that the patients undergoing cardioplegia had longer ischemic times than those receiving intermittent hypothermia, and the mortality risk did not appear to increase until the clamp times were greater than 85 minutes.[16] The myocardial preservation techniques currently in use at Children's Hospital in Boston are outlined in the following sections.

Preischemic Management

Interventions Before Operation. Several aspects of management of the patient before ischemia

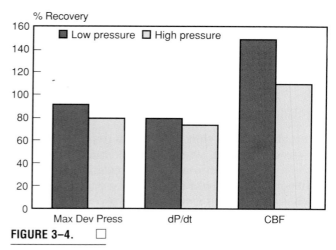

FIGURE 3–4. ☐

Effect of initial reperfusion pressure on recovery after 2 hours of 15°C ischemia in isolated, blood perfused, neonatal lamb hearts. CBF, coronary blood flow; Max Dev Press, maximum developed pressure.

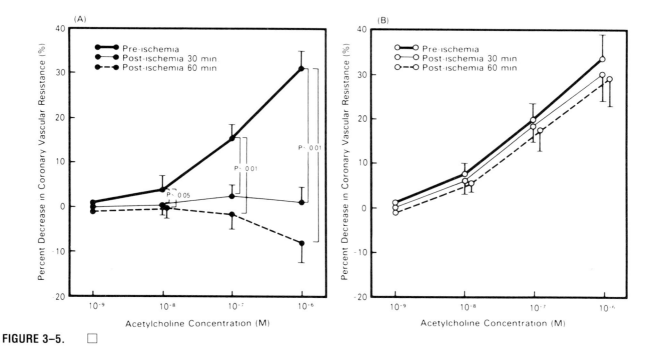

FIGURE 3–5. ☐

Effect of initial reperfusion pressure on endothelial function measured by response to acetylcholine after 2 hours of 15°C ischemia in isolated, blood-perfused, neonatal lamb hearts. *A*, High reperfusion pressure (60 mm Hg). *B*, Low initial reperfusion pressure (20 mm Hg for 10 minutes, 40 mm Hg for the next 10 minutes, and then 60 mm Hg). (From Sawatari K, Kadoba K, Bergner KA, Mayer JE. Influence of initial reperfusion after hypothermic cardioplegic ischemia on endothelial modulation of coronary tone in neonatal lambs. Impaired coronary vasodilator response to acetylcholine. J Thorac Cardiovasc Surg 101:777–782, 1991.)

may have an impact on the outcome after ischemia. Every attempt is made to "resuscitate" the patient before operation and establish a metabolic state as close to normal as possible. Most neonates with critical defects (except for those with obstructed total anomalous pulmonary venous connection) can be restored to a normal metabolic state with the use of prostaglandin E_1 to re-establish ductal patency. The re-establishment of ductal patency allows for adequate pulmonary blood flow in patients with atresia or stenosis of the source of pulmonary blood flow or for perfusion of the descending aorta in patients with various forms of obstruction of the left ventricular outflow tract or the aortic arch. A normal pH level, normal renal and hepatic function, and reversal of other manifestations of tissue hypoxia and ischemia are generally readily achieved and maintained through the use of prostaglandin E_1. The myocardial dysfunction that frequently accompanies the "shock-like" state before resuscitation is generally reversible with temporary inotropic support as well. During this resuscitative phase, the heart (as well as the remainder of the body) should also be nutritionally supported. Generally, in the neonate this support is provided with parenteral nutrition high in glucose and amino acids, although the enteral route can also be used if the mesenteric blood supply is not threatened by runoff from the systemic arterial circulation into the pulmonary

bed. As mentioned previously, experimental reports suggest that augmentation of myocardial glycogen stores before the onset of anoxia is associated with an improved outcome,[41] and our clinical impression that patients who are well resuscitated before operation generally have a better outcome may be partially explained by these experimental observations.

Intraoperative Interventions Before Ischemia. One obvious and important consideration in management of the patient in the operating room before surgically induced ischemia is avoidance of a reduction in myocardial blood flow. Therefore, it is important to prevent runoff from the systemic circulation into the pulmonary circulation when connections between the two circulations exist (e.g., in the child with truncus arteriosus). With induction of anesthesia and mechanical ventilation, there is generally a decrease in pulmonary vascular resistance, and systemic hypotension and hypoperfusion can result. The simple maneuver of temporarily occluding the right pulmonary artery will increase the resistance to pulmonary blood flow and generally restore systemic perfusion pressure, thereby avoiding a myocardial insult. Similar considerations apply to neonatal patients with the hypoplastic left heart syndrome, an aortopulmonary window, or a large ductus arteriosus and also to patients with tetralogy of Fallot with pulmonary atresia and multiple aortopulmonary collaterals. It is also important to note that the possibility of a systemic-to-pulmonary "run-off" as a source of myocardial ischemia (or ischemia of other systemic organs) is not eliminated simply by instituting bypass.

A second important preischemic consideration is the avoidance of ventricular distention. It is clear that myocardial distention increases the myocardial demands for oxygen, and thus it should be avoided by minimizing the amount of blood reaching the left ventricle by controlling the sources of pulmonary blood flow and venting the left ventricle. Distention may also have a particularly disruptive effect on the immature myocardium, perhaps because of developmental changes in the interstitial connective tissues. The reduced ability of the immature left ventricle to respond to afterload stress[1] may also be a function of these differences in the interstitial connective tissues.

A third preischemic consideration that is currently the source of some controversy is the effect of preischemic hypothermia on the outcome of a subsequent period of ischemia. As mentioned previously, based on experimental work by Rebeyka, Williams and coworkers currently advocate the avoidance of hypothermia before ischemia and utilize their cardioplegic solution as both an arresting and hypothermia-inducing vehicle.[82] In contrast, at Children's Hospital in Boston, we have routinely induced hypothermia with core cooling on bypass for periods of 10 to 30 minutes before the application of the aortic crossclamp and have not recognized the "cold contracture" that Williams et al. described. The reasons for this remain speculative, but we have recently measured the ionized calcium concentrations during the preischemic cooling phase of bypass in some of our patients. Because an acalcemic crystalloid priming solution is used and the calcium concentration of the citrated blood added to the bypass prime is not "corrected," calcium concentrations before ischemia are low (0.2 mmol/L). The effect of calcium concentrations during preischemic cooling on the outcome of a subsequent period of ischemia in the neonatal lamb has been investigated in our laboratory, as described previously, and it seems that hypocalcemia during preischemic hypothermia may be protective against the phenomenon of "cold contracture."[3]

A final preischemic intervention is the administration of corticosteroids (methylprednisolone, 30 mg/kg) at the initiation of bypass. The original rationale for the use of methylprednisolone was to prevent the deleterious effects of the "shock-like" state of cardiopulmonary bypass by its vasodilating action.[24] More recent experiments have shown that corticosteroids prevent or reduce membrane injury[26] and may also help to reduce complement and neutrophil activation.[18, 37]

Management During Ischemia

Cardioplegia. Some form of hypothermic cardioplegia is utilized in almost all cases in which the intended repair requires a period of myocardial ischemia. Two different solutions are currently employed, depending on the surgeon's preference and on the bypass technique to be employed. Because of the experimental work showing a benefit with oxygenation of crystalloid cardioplegic solutions,[9] all cardioplegic solutions are currently oxygenated.

Circulatory Arrest. Currently, a single dose of oxygenated St. Thomas cardioplegic solution (Plegisol) at a dose of 20 ml/per kilogram of body weight is utilized. Oxygenation is carried out by instilling filtered 100% oxygen into the plastic bag containing cold (4°C) cardioplegic solution and thoroughly mixing the gas and the solution for several minutes. Then the excess gas is aspirated. The use of a single dose rather than multiple doses is based on the experimental data outlined previously. Because circulatory arrest is utilized, washout of the cardioplegia solution will not occur, and deep hypothermic temperatures (15°C) are used so that significant myocardial rewarming is not likely to occur from surrounding mediastinal tissues. The ambient temperature in the operating room is also reduced to 15°C to 18°C to prevent warming of the heart from the external environment.

Continuous Bypass. Multiple doses of cardioplegia solution are utilized for all cases in which aortic crossclamping is required. Two different cardioplegic solutions are used, depending on the preference of the surgeon. The first is oxygenated St. Thomas solution as previously described. This solution is infused into the aortic root using an infusion system that continuously recirculates the solution through a heat-exchanging reservoir and then into the surgical field to prevent warming of the solution in the infusion line from the ambient temperature. The second solution is an acalcemic, oxygenated, glucose-potassium-bicarbonate solution to which blood from the oxygenator is added. The constituents of this solution are given in Table 3–1. The rationale for the addition of the dilute blood to the solution is based on the observations of Suaudeau and coworkers[78] that the addition of blood may improve the delivery of the solution to the microcirculation. An additional theoretical benefit from the addition of blood is that the blood provides small amounts of calcium to reduce the possibility of "cal-

TABLE 3–1. ☐ GLUCOSE-POTASSIUM-BICARBONATE BASE SOLUTION

Dextrose, 2.5%
Sodium chloride, 0.45%
Potassium chloride, 20 mEq/L
Sodium bicarbonate, 5 mEq/L

cium paradox." It seems unlikely that the addition of these small amounts of blood (hematocrit <5%) significantly increases the oxygen delivery to the myocardium.

Management After Ischemia

Reperfusion Pressure. Based on the experimental work from our laboratory discussed previously,[33, 73] reperfusion pressures are kept low during the initial 5 to 10 minutes after blood flow to the myocardium is restored. With the currently used techniques of cardiopulmonary bypass, which include the use of the alpha-adrenergic antagonist phentolamine (Regitine), there is generally little need to manipulate bypass flows to maintain these low initial reperfusion pressures. No other specific postischemic interventions have been employed thus far, although the concepts of substrate enhancement as reported by investigators at University of California, Los Angeles,[46] and the question of optimal levels of oxygen from our own studies[74] seem to be fruitful areas for investigation.

Calcium. As noted previously, levels of ionized calcium before ischemia are markedly subnormal, and these levels are not normalized until esophageal temperatures reach 28°C to 30°C during reperfusion. This delay in restoration of normal calcium levels during reperfusion may be important in preventing calcium accumulation during the early reperfusion period.[36]

RESULTS

There have been relatively few studies of the impact of various protective measures on the outcome of cardiac operations in neonates and infants. In one retrospective review of 200 consecutive patients at Children's Hospital in Boston, primary myocardial failure in the absence of a residual anatomic problem was not found to be the cause of any deaths. However, the need for inotropic support in the postoperative period has not been eliminated. As part of a study of neurologic outcome of the arterial switch operation in our institution, data on cardiac output have been obtained at 6-hour intervals after sur-

gery. Interestingly, almost all patients have shown a decrease in cardiac output at about 6 hours after operation when compared with the values obtained either immediately after arrival in the intensive care unit or 24 hours after surgery (Newburger J, unpublished data). Although multiple factors may be involved, it is not unrealistic to conclude that this reduced cardiac output is related to imperfect myocardial preservation.

SUMMARY

Although primary surgical repair of a variety of defects is routinely carried out in neonates and infants, our understanding of the mechanisms of ischemic injury and its prevention in the immature heart remains incomplete. Advances in preservation of the adult heart, especially hypothermic cardioplegic arrest, have provided remarkable improvement in the results of adult cardiac surgery, and all of these advances have been adopted, in one form or another, for use in the immature heart. However, as pediatricians are fond of saying, "The child is not a small adult." Efforts must continue toward understanding the effects of ischemia on the immature heart and the effects of the interventions used in attempting to protect it.

REFERENCES

1. Anderson PAW. Immature myocardium. In Moller JH, Neal WA (eds). Fetal Neonatal and Infant Cardiac Disease. Norwalk, CT, Appleton & Lange, 1990, pp 35–71.
2. Aoki M, Kawata H, Mayer JE Jr. Coronary endothelial injury by cold crystalloid cardioplegic solution in neonatal lambs. Circulation 84(suppl II):II-716, 1991.
3. Aoki M, Nomura F, Kawata H, et al. Effect of calcium and preischemic hypothermia on recovery of myocardial function after cardioplegic ischemia in neonatal lambs. J Thorac Cardiovasc Surg 1993; 105:207–213.
4. Avkiran M, Hearse DJ. Protection of the myocardium during global ischemia: Is crystalloid cardioplegia effective in the immature myocardium? J Thorac Cardiovasc Surg 97:220, 1989.
5. Baker JE, Boerboom LE, Olinger GN. Age-related changes in the ability of hypothermia and cardioplegia to protect ischemic rabbit myocardium. J Thorac Cardiovasc Surg 96:717, 1988.
6. Baker JE, Boerboom LE, Olinger GN. Is protection of ischemic neonatal myocardium by cardioplegia species dependent? J Thorac Cardiovasc Surg 99:280, 1990.
7. Bigelow WG, Callaghan JC, Hopps JA. General hypothermia for experimental intracardiac surgery. Ann Surg 132:531, 1950.
8. Bing OHL, LaRaia PJ, Franklin A, et al. Myocardial protection utilizing calcium containing and calcium free perfusates. Basic Res Cardiol 80:399, 1985.
9. Bodenhamer RM, DeBoer WV, Geffin GA, et al. Enhanced myocardial protection during ischemic arrest. J Thorac Cardiovasc Surg 85:769, 1983.
10. Boggs BR, Torchiana DF, Geffin GA, et al. Optimal myocar-

dial preservation with an acalcemic crystalloid cardioplegic solution. J Thorac Cardiovasc Surg 93:838, 1987.

11. Bolling SF, Bies LE, Gallagher KP, et al. Enhanced myocardial protection with adenosine. Ann Surg 47:809, 1989.

12. Bove EL, Gallahger KP, Drake DH, et al. The effect of hypothermic ischemia on recovery of left ventricular function and preload reserve in the neonatal heart. J Thorac Cardiovasc Surg 95:814, 1988.

13. Bove EL, Stammers AH. Recovery of left ventricular function after hypothermic global ischemia: Age-related differences in the isolated working rabbit heart. J Thorac Cardiovasc Surg 91:115, 1986.

14. Bove EL, Stammers AH, Gallagher KP. Protection of the neonatal myocardium during hypothermic ischemia: Effect of cardioplegia on left ventricular function in the rabbit. J Thorac Cardiovasc Surg 94:115, 1987.

15. Buja LM, Chien KR, Burton KP, et al. Membrane damage in ischemia. Adv Exp Med Biol 161:421, 1982.

16. Bull CM, Cooper J, Stark J. Cardioplegic protection of the child's heart. J Thorac Cardiovasc Surg 88:287, 1984.

17. Caspi J, Herman SL, Coles JG, et al. Effects of low perfusate Ca2+ concentration on newborn myocardial function after ischemia. Circulation 82 (suppl V):IV-371, 1990.

18. Cavarocchi NC, Pluth JR, Schaff HV, et al. Complement activation during cardiopulmonary bypass. J Thorac Cardiovasc Surg 91:252, 1986.

19. Chiu CJ, Bindon W. Why are newborn hearts vulnerable to global ischemia? Circulation 76(suppl V):V-146, 1987.

20. Clark BJ III, Woodford EJ, Malec EJ, et al. Effects of potassium cardioplegia on high-energy phosphate kinetics during circulatory arrest with deep hypothermia in the newborn piglet heart. J Thorac Cardiovasc Surg 101:342, 1991.

21. Corno AF, Bathencourt DM, Laks H, et al. Myocardial protection in the neonatal heart. J Thorac Cardiovasc Surg 93:163, 1987.

22. DeLeon SY, Idriss FS, Ilbawi MN, et al. Comparison of single versus multidose blood cardioplegia in arterial switch procedures. Ann Thorac Surg 45:548, 1988.

23. Diaco M, DiSesa VJ, Sun SC, et al. Cardioplegia for the immature myocardium. J Thorac Cardiovasc Surg 100:910, 1990.

24. Dietzman RH, Castaneda AR, Lillehei CW, et al. Corticosteroids as effective vasodilators in the treatment of low output syndrome. Chest 57:440, 1970.

25. Digerness SB, Vanini V, Wideman FE. In vitro comparison of oxygen availability from asanguinous and sanguinous cardioplegic media. Circulation 64(suppl II):II-80, 1981.

26. Engelman RM, Prasad MR, Rousou JA, et al. Steroid-induced myocardial preservation is associated with decreased cell membrane microviscosity. Circulation 80(suppl III):III-36, 1989.

27. Fabiato A. Calcium release in skinned cardiac cells: Variations with species, tissues, and development. Fed Proc 41:2238, 1982.

28. Ferrari R, Raddino R, DiLisa F, et al. Effects of temperature on myocardial calcium homeostasis and mitochondrial function during ischemia and reperfusion. J Thorac Cardiovasc Surg 99:919, 1990.

29. Fisher DJ, Heymann MA, Rudolph AM. Myocardial oxygen and carbohydrate consumption in fetal lambs in utero and in adult sheep. Am J Physiol 238:H399, 1980.

30. Foker JE, Einzig S, Wang T, et al. Adenosine metabolism and myocardial preservation. J Thorac Cardiovasc Surg 80:506, 1980.

31. Fujiwara T, Heinle J, Britton L, et al. Myocardial preservation in neonatal lambs: Comparison of hypothermia with crystalloid and blood cardioplegia. J Thorac Cardiovasc Surg 101:703, 1991.

32. Fujiwara T, Kurtts T, Anderson W, et al. Myocardial protection in cyanotic neonatal lambs. J Thorac Cardiovasc Surg 96:700, 1988.

33. Fujiwara T, Kurtts T, Silvera M, et al. Physical and pharmacological manipulation of reperfusion conditions in neonatal myocardial preservation. Circulation 78(suppl II):II-444, 1988.

34. Geffin GA, Love TR, Hendren WG, et al. The effects of calcium and magnesium in hyperkalemic cardioplegic solutions on myocardial preservation. J Thorac Cardiovasc Surg 98:239, 1989.

35. Grice WN, Konishi T, Apstein CS. Resistance of neonatal myocardium to injury during normothermic and hypothermic ischemic arrest and reperfusion. Circulation 76(suppl V):V-150, 1987.

36. Hamasaki T, Duroda H, Mori T. Temperature dependency of calcium-induced reperfusion injury in the isolated rat heart. Ann Thorac Surg 45:306, 1988.

37. Hammerschmidt DE, White JG, Craddock PR, et al. Corticosteroids inhibit complement-mediated granulocyte aggregation: A possible mechanism for their efficacy in shock states. J Clin Invest 63:798, 1979.

38. Hammon JW Jr, Graham TP Jr, Boucek RJ Jr, et al.: Myocardial adenosine triphosphate content as a measure of metabolic and functional myocardial protection in children undergoing cardiac operation. Ann Thorac Surg 44:467, 1987.

39. Haray I. Biochemistry of cardiac development. In Berne RM (ed). Handbook of Physiology. Vol 1. The Heart. 2nd ed. Baltimore, Williams & Wilkins, 1979, pp 43–60.

40. Hendren WG, Geffin GA, Love TR, et al. Oxygenation of cardioplegic solutions. J Thorac Cardiovasc Surg 94:614, 1987.

41. Hewitt RL, Lolley DM, Adrouny GA, et al. Protective effect of myocardial glycogen on cardiac function during anoxia. Surgery 73:444, 1973.

42. Hicks GL, Hill AA, DeWeese JA. Subendocardial protection during cardiopulmonary bypass: Its use with methylprednisolone and glucose-insulin-potassium. Arch Surg 114:302, 1979.

43. Jarmakani JM, Nakanishi T, George BL, et al. Effect of extracellular calcium on myocardial mechanical function in the neonatal rabbit. Dev Pharmacol Ther 5:1, 1982.

44. Jarmakani JM, Nakazawa M, Nagatomo T, et al. Effect of hypoxia on mechanical function in the neonatal mammalian heart. Am J Physiol 235(5):H469, 1978.

45. Julia PL, Kofsky ER, Buckberg GD, et al. Studies of myocardial protection in the immature heart. J Thorac Cardiovasc Surg 100:879, 1990.

46. Julia P, Young HH, Buckberg GD, et al. Studies of myocardial protection in the immature heart. IV. Improved tolerance of immature myocardium to hypoxia and ischemia by intravenous metabolic support. J Thorac Cardiovasc Surg 101:23, 1991.

47. Katz AM, Reuter H. Cellular calcium and cardiac cell death. Am J Cardiol 44:188, 1979.

48. Kofsky ER, Julia P, Buckberg GD, et al. Studies of myocardial protection in the immature heart. V. Safety of prolonged aortic clamping with hypocalcemic glutamate/aspartate blood cardioplegia. J Thorac Cardiovasc Surg 101:33, 1991.

49. Konishi T, Apstein CS. Comparison of three cardioplegic solutions during hypothermic ischemic arrest in neonatal blood-perfused rabbit hearts. J Thorac Cardiovasc Surg 98:1132, 1989.

50. Konishi T, Apstein CS. Deleterious effects of digitalis on newborn rabbit myocardium after simulated cardiac surgery. J Thorac Cardiovasc Surg 101:337, 1991.

51. Laks H, Milliken J, Haas G. Myocardial protection in the neonatal heart. In Mancelletti C (ed). Pediatric Cardiology. 6th ed. Edinburgh, Churchill Livingstone, 1986, pp 13–26.

52. Legato MJ. Cellular mechanisms of normal growth in the mammalian heart. II. A quantitative and qualitative comparison between the right and left ventricular myocytes in the dog from birth to five months of age. Circ Res 44:263, 1979.

53. Lupinetti FM, Hammon JW, Huddleston CB, et al. Global ischemia in the immature canine ventricle: Enhanced protective effect of verapamil and potassium. J Thorac Cardiovasc Surg 87:213, 1984.

54. Mori F, Miyamoto M, Tsuboi H, et al. Clinical trial of nicardipine cardioplegia in pediatric cardiac surgery. Ann Thorac Surg 49:413, 1990.

55. Murphy CE, Salter DR, Morris JJ, et al. Age-related differences in adenine nucleotide metabolism during in vivo global ischemia. Surg Forum 37:288, 1986.

56. Nakanishi T, Jarmakani JM. Developmental changes in myocardial mechanical function and subcellular organelles. Am J Physiol 246:H615, 1984.
57. Nakanishi T, Seguchi M, Tsuchiya T, et al. Effect of acidosis on intracellular pH and calcium concentration in the newborn and adult rabbit myocardium. Circ Res 67:111, 1990.
58. Nayler WG, Fassold E. Calcium accumulating and ATPase activity of cardiac sarcoplasmic reticulum before and after birth. Cardiovasc Res 11:231, 1977.
59. Nishioka K, Jarmakani JM. Effect of ischemia on mechanical function and high-energy phosphates in rabbit myocardium. Am J Physiol 242:H1077, 1982.
60. Nishioka K, Nakanishi T, George BL, et al. The effect of calcium on the inotropy of catecholamine and paired electrical stimulation in the newborn and adult myocardium. J Mol Cell Cardiol 13:511, 1981.
61. Nishioka K, Nakanishi T, Jarmakani JM. Effect of ischemia on calcium exchange in the rabbit myocardium. Am J Physiol 247:H177, 1984.
62. Nomura F, Aoki M, Mayer JE. Effect of adenosine infusion during reperfusion after cold cardioplegic ischemia in neonatal lambs. Circulation 1993; Suppl. II:II380–II386.
63. Olivetti G, Anversa P, Loud AV. Morphometric study of early postnatal development in the left and right ventricular myocardium of the rat. Circ Res 46:503, 1980.
64. Otani H, Engelman RM, Rousou JA, et al. The mechanism of myocardial reperfusion injury in neonates. Circulation 76(suppl V):V 161, 1987.
65. Page E, Earley J, Power B. Normal growth of ultrastructures in rat left ventricular myocardial cells. Circ Res 34 & 35(suppl II):II-12, 1974.
66. Pitarys CJ, Virmani R, Vildibill HD, et al. Reduction of myocardial reperfusion injury by intravenous adenosine administered during the early reperfusion period. Circulation 83:237, 1991.
67. Randolph JD, Toal KW, Geffin GA, et al. Improved myocardial preservation with oxygenated cardioplegic solutions as reflected by on-line monitoring of intramyocardial pH during arrest. J Vasc Surg 3:216, 1986.
68. Rebeyka IM, Hanan SA, Borges MR, et al. Rapid cooling contracture of the myocardium. J Thorac Cardiovasc Surg 100:240, 1990.
69. Rich TL, Langer GA. Calcium depletion in rabbit myocardium: Calcium paradox protection by hypothermia and cation substitution. Circ Res 51:131, 1982.
70. Robinson LA, Harwood DL. Lowering the calcium concentration in St. Thomas' Hospital cardioplegic solution improves protection during hypothermic ischemia. J Thorac Cardiovasc Surg 101:314, 1991.
71. Sawa Y, Matsuda H, Shimazaki Y, et al. Ultrastructural assessment of the infant myocardium receiving crystalloid cardioplegia. Circulation 76(suppl V):V 141, 1987.
72. Sawa Y, Matsuda H, Shimazaki Y, et al. Comparison of single dose versus multiple dose crystalloid cardioplegia in neonate: Experimental study with neonatal rabbits from birth to 2 days of age. J Thorac Cardiovasc Surg 97:229, 1989.
73. Sawatari K, Kadoba K, Bergner KA, Mayer JE Jr. Influence of initial reperfusion pressure after hypothermic cardioplegic ischemia on endothelial modulation of coronary tone in neonatal lambs. Impaired coronary vasodilator response to acetylcholine. J Thorac Cardiovasc Surg. 101:777, 1991.
74. Sawatari K, Kawata H, Assad RS, et al. Effects of Po_2 level during initial reperfusion after hypothermic cardioplegia in neonatal lambs. Circulation 82(suppl III):III-146, 1990.
75. Sheldon CA, Friedman WF, Sybers HD. Scanning electron microscopy of fetal and neonatal lamb cardiac cells. J Mol Cell Cardiol 8:853, 1976.
76. Starnes VA, Hammon JW Jr, Lupinetti FM, et al. Functional and metabolic preservation of immature myocardium with verapamil following global ischemia. Ann Thorac Surg 34:58, 1982.
77. St Cyr JA, Bianco RW, Schneider JR, et al. Enhanced high energy phosphate recovery with ribose infusion after global myocardial ischemia in a canine model. J Surg Res 46:157, 1989.
78. Suaudeau J, Shaffer B, Daggett WM, et al. Role of procaine and washed red cells in the isolated dog heart perfused at 5 degrees C. J Thorac Cardiovasc Surg 84:886, 1982.
79. Torchiana DF, Love TR, Hendren WG, et al. Calcium-induced ventricular contraction during cardioplegic arrest. J Thorac Cardiovasc Surg 94:606, 1987.
80. Ward HB, St Cyr JA, Cogorgan JA, et al. Recovery of adenine nucleotide levels after global myocardial ischemia in dogs. Surgery 96:284, 1984.
81. Willem de Jong J, Vandermeer P, vanLoon H, et al. Adenosine as adjunct to potassium cardioplegia: Effect on function, energy metabolism, and electrophysiology. J Thorac Cardiovasc Surg 100:445, 1990.
82. Williams WG, Rebeyka IM, Tibshirani RJ, et al. Warm induction blood cardioplegia in the infant. J Thorac Cardiovasc Surg 100:896, 1990.
83. Wittnich C, Peniston C, Ianuzzo D, et al. Relative vulnerability of neonatal and adult hearts to ischemic injury. Circulation 76(suppl V):V-156, 1987.
84. Yamamoto F, Braimbridge MV, Hearse DJ. Calcium and cardioplegia: The optimal calcium content for the St. Thomas' Hospital cardioplegic solution. J Thorac Cardiovasc Surg 87:908, 1984.
85. Yano Y, Braimbridge MV, Hearse DJ. Protection of the pediatric myocardium. J Thorac Cardiovasc Surg 94:887, 1987.
86. Young HH, Shimizu T, Nishioka K, et al. Effect of hypoxia and reoxygenation on mitochondrial function in neonatal myocardium. Am J Physiol 245:H998, 1983.

Anesthesia for Cardiovascular Surgery

In the past, the conventional approach to the infant and neonate with complex congenital heart disease (CHD) was palliative treatment in infancy followed later by repair in childhood. The current philosophy of repairing CHD as early as possible, preferably in the neonatal period, has had significant implications for the anesthetic care of these critically ill infants during cardiac surgery. To meet this challenge, a clear understanding of neonatal respiratory and cardiac physiology, neonatal responses to anesthesia and surgery, and the pathophysiology of complex congenital heart defects is necessary. This understanding must be applied to the important interactions occurring among the infant's ventilatory management, pulmonary blood flow, and cardiac function before, during, and after cardiac surgical procedures.

Neonates and infants have different functions and restricted reserves in almost all organ systems, resulting in a more labile homeostasis. From an anesthesiologist's point of view, the neonate's heart is of particular concern, as many anesthetic agents can adversely affect an already compromised myocardial function.

The small size of these patients also makes maintenance of intraoperative metabolic and thermal homeostasis more difficult, because the large surface area/body mass ratio of the infant favors heat transfer to the environment. Also, the large ratio of blood surface area to blood volume in infants amplifies surface-induced damage to blood components, magnifying the deleterious effects of cardiopulmonary bypass (CPB). Furthermore, because small airways also have a large surface area-to-volume ratio, a small amount of airway edema has a significant effect on airway patency, and hence on lung compliance, after cardiac operations. Whenever water content of the lungs and edema of the airway mucosa increase as a result of surgical CPB and airway trauma, gas exchange, lung compliance, and mediastinal volume are all unfavorably affected.

In general, the challenge is to administer sufficient amounts of anesthetic drug to minimize oxygen consumption, attenuate stress responses, reduce myocardial work and pulmonary vascular reactivity, and control arterial blood pressure. At the same time anesthetic-related hemodynamic depression must be avoided. These goals can be accomplished best when close communication and cooperation exist between the anesthetic and surgical teams.

The differences between neonates or infants and older children in their responses to anesthetic agents, metabolic homeostasis, and the stress of cardiac surgery and cardiopulmonary bypass, and the close interactions between the developing heart and lungs, will each be considered separately in this chapter.

ANESTHETIC TECHNIQUES AND THEIR HEMODYNAMIC EFFECT ON INFANTS WITH CONGENITAL HEART DISEASE

The specific cardiac lesion and the type of operative procedure largely dictate the anesthetic management for any particular patient. A variety of different anesthetic techniques provide good cardiovascular stability in children with CHD.[29] However, cardiovascular stability is not the only criterion for a successful anesthetic. Stress responses to pain and other noxious stimulation are profound in the neonate, regardless of conceptual age.[1, 2, 6] Extreme responses to hormonal and metabolic stress during cardiac surgery and CPB can indeed be very significant and have been correlated with poorer outcome, despite hemodynamic stability, in neonates undergoing cardiac surgery.[3, 5] Lactic acidemia, hyperglycemia, high levels of catabolic hormones, a negative nitrogen balance during the postoperative period, and also a greater incidence of sepsis, disseminated intravascular coagulation, metabolic acidosis, and even death have been demonstrated in premature and term neonates who have undergone cardiac surgical procedures with anesthetic techniques that fail to suppress stress responses.

Anesthetic Plans and Goals

Virtually all infants with CHD can tolerate a well-managed anesthetic without cardiovascular collapse. However, the infant with complex disease is very intolerant of loss of airway patency and resultant hypoventilation, inappropriate amounts and choices of anesthetics, and major intraoperative surgical trauma. Induction of anesthesia is a particularly vulnerable period. Because resuscitation may prove very difficult in infants with complex CHD, the chief emphasis in these patients is on the prevention of circulatory collapse. Therefore, anesthetic techniques must be selected that provide a broad margin of safety based on the pathophysiology anticipated for each specific diagnostic category.

Anesthetic Techniques and Agents

Although inhalational anesthesia is still the most commonly used technique in general pediatric anesthesia, because of the significant myocardial depressant effect of most inhalational agents on the infant and neonatal myocardium, pure inhalational anesthetic techniques are rarely used in infants with complex CHD.

The postnatal myocyte has relatively less contractile mass and poorly organized myofibrils and is less compliant than the myocyte in older children. The incompletely developed sarcoplasmic reticulum and transverse tubulular systems[7] decrease the capacity to store and release calcium. As a group, potent inhalational agents tend to inhibit the normal functioning of calcium pumps in membranes. These differences, taken together, may partially explain the specially potent depressant effects of inhalation anesthetic agents seen in the developing heart.[25]

Inhalation Anesthetics

Because of the previously discussed limitations, inhalation anesthetic agents must be used cautiously, if at all, in infants with CHD. However, occasionally these agents are useful in small, titrated concentrations to control hypertensive responses after induction, when the airway is secure and monitoring and hemodynamic stability are established. In cyanotic infants with good functional cardiac reserve, anesthesia can be cautiously induced with halothane and oxygen, and even with 50% nitrous oxide, without clinically significant decreases in arterial oxygen saturation.[33] However, a decrease in arterial blood pressure frequently occurs with these techniques, and significant systemic hypotension can develop. Importantly, at least in the case of halothane, the levels of inhalation agent tolerated by the sick infant provide inadequate suppression of the stress responses to cardiac surgery and CPB.[3]

Numerous studies have shown that even infants who do not have CHD do not tolerate halothane or isoflurane well; approximately 50% of infants without CHD develop substantial hypotension and bradycardia during induction with these agents unless cardiovascular function is supported.[19, 26, 27] Ventricular function declines during both halothane and isoflurane induction, and stroke volume and ejection fraction decrease by as much as 38%, although such depression may be somewhat less with isoflurane than with halothane.[47] These clinical observations are supported by experimental findings in immature animals, both in vitro, with isolated atrial and ventricular muscle, and in vivo, with some species of young animals.[10, 15] Furthermore, isoflurane is contraindicated in cyanotic infants because it can cause laryngospasm, breath holding, and coughing, resulting in hypoventilation and an increase in pulmonary vascular resistance. Halothane may also cause loss of normal sinus rhythm; this is particularly critical in infants with CHD.

The use of nitrous oxide in patients with intracardiac shunts is controversial, primarily because of its potential for enlarging air emboli, which can interfere with blood flow even without systemic embolization.[51] In infants with intracardiac shunts there exists (theoretically) a potential for systemic shunting of micro- and macrobubbles of air introduced either through central venous lines or after opening the left side of the heart while on CPB. Nitrous oxide, if used at all in the presence of intracardiac shunts, requires meticulous attention to its potential for expanding air emboli.

The use of inhalational agents in children with intracardiac shunting is further complicated by potential differences in uptake and distribution. In a computer model, inhalation induction was slowed in the presence of a central right-to-left shunt, less so with mixed shunts, and showed almost no change in exclusively left-to-right shunts.[62] The model assumed a constant cardiac output; the findings were more significant when insoluble gases such as nitrous oxide were used, but were less significant with more soluble gases such as halothane. Also, clinically, the speed of inhalation induction seems to be affected very little in the presence of a left-to-right shunt.[61] In summary, inhalational anesthetics must be used cautiously in infants with CHD and individually are rarely suitable as the sole anesthetic agent for cardiac surgical procedures in infants who are critically ill.

Intravenous and Intramuscular Anesthetics

Some intravenous anesthetics, such as ketamine and high-dose opiates, can provide improved safety margins for induction of anesthesia in the compromised cardiovascular system of neonates and infants with complex CHD. However, very high transient concentrations of intravenous agents in the arteries, heart, and central nervous system can result from conventional intravenous doses given as a bolus in the presence of a right-to-left shunt, because during the first passage, pulmonary mixing, uptake, and metabolism are bypassed. For example, 1 mg/kg of lidocaine given intravenously as an antiarrhythmic bolus to dogs with surgically created right-to-left shunts resulted in arterial concentrations higher than those reported to cause irreversible myocardial toxicity.[9] In planning intravenous anesthesia, the potential for transiently high arterial levels of intravenously injected anesthetic agents in patients with intracardiac mixing and right-to-left shunts must be considered.

Ketamine. When intravenous access is a problem, intramuscular ketamine (3 to 5 mg/kg) is well tolerated in critically ill infants with cyanosis or congestive heart failure.[46] In fact, ketamine has been shown to have a positive inotropic effect in some experimental studies.[14] Concomitant intramuscular succinylcholine is used to facilitate control of the airway. Atropine or glycopyrrolate helps to decrease the excessive airway secretions often produced by ketamine, and midazolam (0.1 mg/kg) attenuates ketamine's dysphoric effects. Although increases in pulmonary vascular resistance have been reported in adults after administration of ketamine,[28] in sufficiently premedicated children, ketamine causes no change in pulmonary vascular resistance when the airway is maintained and ventilation is supported.[37] The ejection fraction has also been shown to be preserved during ketamine anesthesia.[8] When intravenous access is available in patients with marginal cardiac reserve, intravenous ketamine (1 to 2 mg/kg) is an excellent induction agent for most forms of CHD. Relative contraindications to the use of ketamine are an anomalous coronary artery, critical aortic stenosis, or the hypoplastic left heart syndrome with aortic atresia and hypoplasia of the ascending aorta. Patients with these conditions are prone to the development of ventricular fibrillation because of suboptimal coronary perfusion; also, tachycardia and catecholamine release after ketamine administration may theoretically predispose these patients to ventricular fibrillation, although we have not observed this as a clinical problem.

Opiates. High-dose intravenous opiates, given together with pancuronium and 100% oxygen or air and oxygen, are excellent induction agents in critically ill infants with all forms of CHD; currently this technique is widely used. High-dose opiates in neonates and infants provide reliable hemodynamic stability and suppression of hormonal and metabolic stress responses,[3, 5, 6] including hyperglycemic responses to cardiac surgery.[21] Doses of fentanyl as low as 10 μg per kilogram of body weight may be sufficient for effective baseline anesthesia in neonates, but larger doses are necessary for prolonged anesthesia. In high-risk, full-term neonates and older infants with complex CHD, fentanyl doses as high as 75 μg/kg, given with pancuronium, result in minimal hemodynamic changes on induction and intubation, although mild hemodynamic responses to surgical incision generally occur.[35] Additional doses or infusions of potent opiates may be necessary, as narcotic levels decrease significantly in children during CPB. In addition, there is increasing evidence that suppression of stress responses and more profound amnesia is better accomplished if another anesthetic agent, such as a benzodiazepine, is added to fentanyl.

When high-dose opiate anesthetic techniques are used, oxygen saturation levels are maintained and often improve during induction, intubation, and surgical manipulation, even in cyanotic children. Changes in cardiac output and in systemic and pulmonary vascular resistance in infants given 25 μg/kg of fentanyl have been insignificant.[38] The addition of pancuronium to high-dose fentanyl is recommended, as the vagolytic effects of pancuronium offset the vagotonic effects of fentanyl. Sufentanil (5 to 20 μg/kg) is an alternative to fentanyl and provides roughly equivalent hemodynamic stability, suppression of stress responses, and postoperative analgesia.[16, 42] The use of high-dose fentanyl or sufentanil usually requires continuous overnight postoperative ventilatory support after the operation. Alfentanil, a shorter acting potent opiate used as a continuous infusion (20 μg/kg bolus followed by an infusion rate of 1 μg/kg/min) provides adequate hemodynamic stability and stress suppression intraoperatively in infants for whom postoperative ventilatory support is not needed[18] and in whom early postoperative extubation is desired.

High-dose opiate anesthesia, particularly with fentanyl, increases the ventricular fibrillation threshold; in patients with hypoplastic left heart syndrome, fentanyl significantly decreases the incidence of ventricular fibrillation during operations.[36]

Thiopental. Intravenous induction with thiopental is not used in infants with complex CHD, but a 1 to 2 mg/kg dose used in conjunction with other anesthetic agents is safe for induction in patients with uncomplicated CHD. This technique also results in improved arterial oxygen saturation in cyanotic patients.[43] Propofol, aside from its short duration of action, does not seem to have properties suitable for pediatric cardiac operations in infants because of its known myocardial depressant properties.

Muscle Relaxants. When administered to infants with complex CHD, conventional doses of pancuronium produce no changes in heart rate or blood pressure. A bolus dose of pancuronium, through its vagolytic effects, can produce tachycardia and hypertension, which may, in fact, be desirable to support cardiac output in infants with relatively fixed stroke volumes.[13] If tachycardia is undesirable, Metocurine iodide (Metubine iodide) does not cause tachycardia, hypertension, or dysrhythmias in infants, even at doses of 0.5 mg/kg.[31] In those patients for whom a short-acting, nondepolarizing muscle relaxant is desirable, atracurium besylate or vecuronium bromide, when used at the lower end of their dose ranges, also have few cardiovascular side effects in children.[30, 32] However, use of these two muscle relaxants may cause significant bradycardia in infants when used in conjunction with high-dose opiates such as fentanyl. Bradycardia, or even sinus arrest, can also occur with succinylcholine in infants with CHD. Therefore, atropine should be used in conjunction with intravenous succinylcholine. How-

ever, if potent opiates are used with succinylcholine, severe bradycardia may nevertheless occur, despite the use of atropine.

METABOLIC HOMEOSTASIS AND STRESS RESPONSES: ANESTHETIC EFFECTS

Contrary to previous beliefs, the neonate has a major metabolic and humoral response to stress, particularly the stress of cardiac surgery and CPB.[3–6] Extremely high levels of serum catecholamines, beta-endorphins, cortisol, glucagon, and growth hormone, as well as low levels of insulin, result from such stress. Such extreme catecholamine responses to CPB have also been documented in older infants.[23] The metabolic responses to this neurohumoral stress and the associated hormonal imbalances are characterized by hyperglycemia, high blood lactate levels, protein breakdown, and a negative nitrogen balance. These catabolic changes tend to be severe in the metabolically fragile neonate and often extend for days into the postoperative period.[5, 6, 23] It is precisely at this time that metabolic resources are most needed for wound healing and function of the immune system. Fortunately, these hormonal and metabolic stress responses to CPB can be attenuated by anesthetic management without adversely affecting cardiovascular stability.[4, 6] As mentioned previously, potent inhalational anesthetic agents such as halothane do not effectively attenuate these neurohumoral stress responses.[5, 6] In older infants, high-dose opiate techniques have been shown to reduce catecholamine-induced stress responses to CPB more effectively than inhalational anesthesia alone.[53] Substantial evidence is accumulating that anesthetic management aimed at minimizing these stress responses helps decrease morbidity in neonates undergoing cardiac surgery.[5, 6]

In the premature neonate, extreme stress responses can occur even during a simple procedure such as surgical closure of a patent ductus arteriosus. Experimentally, in the fetal animal undergoing cardiac surgery in the third trimester of gestation, stress responses to CPB are so extreme that placental flow is substantially compromised, leading to fetal death and spontaneous abortion. Use of an anesthetic technique directed at ablation of stress responses—namely, total spinal anesthesia—has significantly contributed to survival after experimental fetal cardiac surgery in animals on CPB by preventing decreases in placental blood flow and gas exchange after bypass.[22]

In the postoperative period, stress responses tend to continue in infants; therefore, anesthetic and analgesic techniques designed to minimize postoperative stress responses can be important in preventing complications. After major cardiac surgery in infants, critical hemodynamic crises may be triggered by inadequate pain control. Also, high-risk infants who have had complex intracardiac repairs and high pulmonary vascular resistance frequently have pulmonary hypertensive crises in the early postoperative period; these result in severe systemic hypotension and sometimes death. These crises most often respond to sedative and analgesic agents that block the stress of tracheal suctioning.[17, 34] Thus, control of pain and stress in the postoperative period can prevent or significantly minimize deleterious hemodynamic crises in addition to attenuating metabolic and hormonal stress responses.

Glucose and Calcium Homeostasis

In the infant, metabolic homeostasis of glucose and calcium is particularly critical during cardiac surgery. Before major surgical manipulation, hypoglycemia may occur during placement of arterial and venous lines, preparation for surgery, and induction, mostly because of limited metabolic reserves, immaturity of the liver, and inadequate oral intake. In contrast, the stress of surgical manipulation, CPB, and profound hypothermia often result in severe hyperglycemia caused by the release of catabolic hormones such as catecholamines and glucagon and decreased levels of insulin. Therefore, glucose levels must be carefully monitored to avoid both hypoglycemia and hyperglycemia. The neurologic sequelae associated with prolonged and severe hypoglycemia are well known, whereas only recently has neurologic damage associated with severe hyperglycemia before episodes of central nervous system ischemia (e.g., hypothermic circulatory arrest) been suggested experimentally.[44, 45] In a preliminary study hyperglycemia was observed to increase the risk of neurologic deficits in small children after deep hypothermic circulatory arrest.[59] Use of high-dose opiate anesthesia markedly reduces the hyperglycemic stress response to CPB in neonates by increasing the insulin-glucagon molar ratio, thus potentially decreasing the risk of injury to the central nervous system.[3, 5]

Because of their minimally calcified skeleton and immature organ function, neonates and infants have difficulty buffering changes in ionized serum calcium when given citrated blood products. Therefore, during transfusion of citrated blood or blood products after CPB, ionized calcium levels must be monitored, and incremental doses of calcium must be given to maintain normal ionized calcium levels. Despite some previous concerns that calcium ad-

ministration may increase pulmonary vascular resistance and cause right ventricular dysfunction, more recent studies fail to show any effect of calcium on either pulmonary vascular resistance or right ventricular function.

The citrated blood used to prime the CPB circuit usually results in circulating ionized calcium levels of less than 0.3 mmol/L during bypass. Consequently, calcium must be added to the pump circuit at some point to restore normal ionized calcium levels before weaning from CPB. However, normal to high circulating calcium levels during reperfusion after myocardial ischemia have been associated with reperfusion injury, myocardial stunning, and even "stone heart" in neonates. Therefore, at Children's Hospital in Boston, we wait until the patient's temperature reaches 32°C before restoring normal ionized calcium levels on CPB.

Because of parathyroid insufficiency, athymic patients such as those with DiGeorge's syndrome may require higher calcium doses during and after cardiac operations.

Coagulation Problems With Cardiac Operations in Infants

Coagulation is abnormal in the young infant, particularly in neonates, and coagulopathies associated with CPB are a particular problem. This is due in part to dilution of coagulation factors and platelets by the large pump-priming volume relative to the infant's circulating blood volume and to more extensive CPB-related damage to all formed elements of blood in these small patients.[40] This, together with extensive surgical suture lines and porous prosthetic materials used for intra- and extracardiac repairs, frequently requires transfusion of relatively large amounts of citrated blood or blood products after CPB operations. Fresh whole blood (less than 48 hours old) has been shown to be preferable to individual blood components for minimizing bleeding problems after cardiac operations in infants.[49] If fresh whole blood is unavailable, platelet concentrates and cyroprecipitates (rather than fresh frozen plasma, to avoid excessive hemodilution) are preferred when coagulopathies are present in infants.[40]

Although desmopressin acetate and aprotinin have been recommended to minimize coagulation problems related to CPB and hypothermia, desmopressin acetate (1-deamino-(8-D-arginine)-vasopressin, or DDAVP) has been shown not to reduce blood loss after cardiac operations in infants with normal coagulation systems.[57] However, DDAVP is effective in children with hemophilia A and von Willebrand's disease. Aprotinin's effectiveness in adults has been demonstrated, but preliminary results from an ongoing study of aprotinin use for children undergoing cardiac surgery are less encouraging.[11]

PULMONARY VASCULAR RESISTANCE AND BALANCE OF SYSTEMIC AND PULMONARY BLOOD FLOW

The higher basal pulmonary vascular resistance and more labile pulmonary circulation, the greater interdependence of left and right ventricles, and the presence of intracardiac shunts all combine to make the pulmonary circulation critical in neonates with complex congenital heart disease. Because pulmonary vascular resistance is also very much dependent on the amount and pattern of ventilation, the inspired oxygen concentration, the pH, and the P_{CO_2}, the anesthetic management of ventilation strongly influences cardiopulmonary function. Right ventricular afterload and systemic arterial oxygen saturation can be manipulated by adjusting ventilation; this will directly affect cardiac performance. In a parallel circulation with a single source of systemic and pulmonary flow, as in truncus arteriosus or aortic atresia, ventilation is very important in influencing pulmonary vascular resistance and, hence, in determining the Qp/Qs ratio and the net systemic blood flow.[34] Although the exact mechanisms underlying the interdependent function of the heart and lungs are poorly understood, the impact of intraoperative ventilation on cardiac function cannot be overemphasized, particularly in the neonate undergoing cardiac surgery. These considerations make close cooperation between the anesthesiologist and cardiac surgeon essential.

In lesions such as the hypoplastic left heart syndrome, pulmonary atresia, and truncus arteriosus[53, 56] and their variants, the widely patent ductus arteriosus (or its equivalent, the common arterial trunk) makes it necessary to carefully balance pulmonary and systemic vascular resistances so that both hypoxemia (from insufficient pulmonary blood flow) and decreased systemic cardiac output (from excessive pulmonary blood flow) are avoided. In truncus arteriosus, for example, torrential pulmonary blood flow can divert or "steal" enough systemic flow to cause ischemia of the myocardium and other organs, which can be reversed by increasing pulmonary vascular resistance.

Pulmonary vascular resistance can best be manipulated by altering ventilation and blood pH. Specifically, changing the pulmonary vascular resistance in the young infant is mostly a matter of regulating Pa_{CO_2}, pH, pulmonary alveolar oxygen

(Pa_{O_2}), and ventilatory mechanics. Arterial carbon dioxide tension is a potent mediator of pulmonary vascular resistance in the newborn. Drummond and coworkers[20] demonstrated that reducing Pa_{CO_2} to 20 mm Hg and increasing the pH to 7.60 produces a consistent and reproducible reduction in pulmonary vascular resistance in infants with pulmonary hypertension. Increasing serum bicarbonate to achieve a pH of 7.5 to 7.6 while maintaining a Pa_{CO_2} of 40 mm Hg has a similar effect on pulmonary vascular resistance.[48, 54] Both Pa_{O_2} and Pa_{O_2} decrease pulmonary vascular resistance. However, in the presence of an intracardiac shunt, changes in Fi_{O_2} have little effect on the Pa_{O_2}. Thus, by inference, a reduction of pulmonary vascular resistance induced by increasing the inspired oxygen concentration probably represents a direct pulmonary vasodilatory effect of Pa_{O_2} rather than Pa_{O_2}.

Ventilatory mechanics also play a major role in controlling shunt flow. Newborns have a closing capacity above functional residual capacity (FRC): therefore, at the end of a normal breath, some airway closure occurs.[50] This results in areas of lung that are perfused yet underventilated. These segments of lung become increasingly hypoxemic, and secondary vasoconstriction occurs. The result is an elevated pulmonary vascular resistance and reduced pulmonary blood flow. Therefore, maintaining lung volumes with large tidal volume ventilation and the addition of positive end-expiratory pressure (PEEP) may restore FRC and decrease pulmonary vascular resistance.[33] However, when excessive PEEP is added or mean airway pressure is high, alveolar overdistention may occur, compressing capillaries in the alveolar wall and interstitium, resulting in elevated pulmonary vascular resistance and reduced pulmonary blood flow. This may be advantageous when pulmonary blood flow is excessive or detrimental when pulmonary blood flow is marginal. These ventilatory management principles are extended into the operative and postoperative periods. Typically, the prebypass management of patients with excessive pulmonary blood flow is aimed at reducing pulmonary blood flow. After induction of anesthesia, oxygen saturation increases. Although this may be caused by reduced oxygen consumption related to anesthesia, excessively high levels of arterial saturation (>90%) usually reflect a decrease in pulmonary vascular resistance, resulting in increased pulmonary blood flow.[35, 37] High oxygen saturations (>90%) caused by high pulmonary flows are managed by maintaining the Fi_{O_2} at 21% and reducing the ventilatory rate to allow the Pa_{CO_2} to rise to 40 to 45 mm Hg. With surface cooling, oxygen consumption and carbon dioxide production decrease, and systemic vascular resistance increases, resulting in further shunting of blood to the pulmonary circulation. Management is directed at increasing pulmonary vascular resistance by reducing ventilatory rates, using smaller tidal volumes to allow lung volumes to fall, and increasing pulmonary vasoconstriction with lower FiO_2. The addition of carbon dioxide to ventilating gas in the postoperative period also has been used to prevent excessive decreases in pulmonary vascular resistance in patients with the hypoplastic left heart syndrome.[39] Careful attention is paid to pulse oximetry to balance systemic and pulmonary blood flow by maintaining oxygen saturations in the 80% to 85% range. Sudden decreases in oxygen saturations are initially treated by increasing tidal volume, ventilatory frequency, and FiO_2. Balancing of the shunt flow is most often required in neonates with a single source of pulmonary and systemic flow; this includes all patients with single ventricle physiology or truncus arteriosus. Neonates who may require increases in pulmonary blood flow include those with tetralogy of Fallot physiology or those needing improved mixing of systemic and pulmonary blood, such as in transposition of the great arteries.

MANAGEMENT OF THE LUNGS DURING CARDIOPULMONARY BYPASS

Management of the lungs during CPB is controversial, primarily because it has not been sufficiently studied. In fact, management of the lungs during CPB in children has not been studied at all. Clearly, management of the lungs during repair of congenital heart defects, particularly in patients with aortopulmonary shunts, must be important. Large aortopulmonary collaterals increase pulmonary venous return to the left heart, effectively decreasing systemic flow. Pulmonary collaterals, particularly those arising from the head vessels and the vertebral arteries, may effectively "steal" flow from the cerebral circulation, contributing to neurologic injury. In one study of adults without CHD, systemic-to-pulmonary bronchial blood flow measured during total CPB was decreased by 40% when 14 cm H_2O of continuous positive airway pressure was used.[63] However, bronchial flow was only 2% to 3% of total pump output. Whether this technique would be useful in decreasing flow through the large aortopulmonary collaterals seen, for example, in patients with tetralogy of Fallot and pulmonary atresia is unknown.

The traditional approach to lung management during total bypass has been to allow the lungs to collapse. Alternative approaches are to maintain continued oxygen flow through the lungs or even to inflate the lungs with a modest amount of continuous positive airway pressure (CPAP) of 5 to 10 cm H_2O). The weight of human and animal evidence available does not support any particular advantage for keeping the lungs inflated; one study showed that CPAP during bypass actually decreased subsequent to arterial oxygenation.[12]

There is also controversy about the management of ventilation during periods of left ventricular ejection on CPB. The concern is that desaturated left ventricular blood will reperfuse a postischemic heart that is being warmed. Depending on whether high oxygen tensions are deleterious to the myocardium during reperfusion, this could be damaging or beneficial. In adult patients undergoing bypass and maintained at zero end-expiratory pressure and no ventilation but connected to a source of 100% oxygen during left ventricular ejection, arterial pH and oxygen tensions are lower and carbon dioxide tensions are higher than when ventilation at 10 breaths per minute is used. However, values in the nonventilated state are well within normal limits on bypass with 100% saturation of arterial blood.[52]

Ventilation of nonperfused lungs during total CPB with no evidence of left ventricular ejection is an altogether different issue and may be quite deleterious. In a study of adult patients, such ventilation of nonperfused lungs in one group resulted in increased intrapulmonary shunting compared with that seen in nonventilated lungs of another group.[60] Experimental studies in calves also showed decreased pulmonary compliance after bypass and increased intrapulmonary shunting when animals were ventilated during total bypass. In an experimental study, spontaneous ventilation associated with total CPB led to massive pulmonary infarctions, probably because of extremely high pH and very low PCO_2 values induced in alveolar and capillary endothelial cells by ventilation in the absence of pulmonary blood flow.[41] From these data, the practice of ventilating nonperfused lungs during total bypass appears to confer no benefits and is potentially harmful.[58]

WEANING FROM BYPASS AND VENTILATION

Management of lung ventilation during weaning from CPB is critical to a successful outcome. To determine whether changes in the pulmonary circulation are contributing to difficulties with weaning from CPB, left and right ventricular function must be assessed by direct visualization or by two complementary approaches. An intraoperative cardiac catheterization allows measurement of pressures within all cardiac chambers and great vessels, together with catheter pullback measurements to uncover any residual pressure gradients across valves or repaired sites of stenosis and conduits. To exclude residual shunts, blood samples from the right and left chambers are also analyzed to detect any increase or decrease in oxygen saturation. More recently, epicardial or transesophageal Doppler echo studies are being used to uncover any residual structural or functional abnormalities and assist in the evaluation of the postoperative cardiac repair.[55] If structural abnormalities are identified, the patient is placed back on CPB and residual defects are repaired. If functional sequelae of the primary lesion or CPB (i.e., pulmonary hypertension and an increase in pulmonary vascular resistance) are identified, the preceding ventilatory maneuvers are employed.

A new, and largely untried, technique that is potentially useful when high pulmonary vascular resistance owing to pulmonary vasoconstriction is a problem during weaning from bypass consists of administration of the specific pulmonary vasodilator nitric oxide via the lungs (see Chapter 5A). Although intraoperative use of nitric oxide has been very limited, it offers promise in situations in which pulmonary vascular resistance is very high but reversible. Nitric oxide has also been shown experimentally in sheep to reverse or prevent the pulmonary vasoconstriction produced by heparin-protamine interactions, making it potentially useful if severe, idiosyncratic pulmonary vasoconstrictive reactions owing to protamine are identified in patients.[24]

MAINTENANCE OF ANESTHESIA AFTER WEANING FROM BYPASS AND DURING TRANSPORT

When the infant has been successfully weaned from bypass, anesthetic management is aimed at maintaining the hemodynamic state that has resulted from the operative repair. Support for the "stunned" myocardium recovering from intraoperative ischemia must be continued. Appropriate ventricular filling pressures must be maintained during the period of labile hemostasis early after bypass when transfusion requirements may be high. It is during this period also that calcium levels must be replenished and anesthesia levels kept sufficiently deep to continue suppression of deleterious hormonal and metabolic stress responses.

During sternal closure, edema of the heart, lungs, and mediastinum after CPB may cause either abrupt or subtle decrements in cardiac and pulmonary functions. Therefore, during and after closure

of the sternum, attention should be paid to detecting subtle evidence of such problems. Because of the infant's ability to maintain an adequate systemic blood pressure in the presence of a declining cardiac output until cardiovascular collapse ensues rather suddenly, a high index of suspicion is in order. Any evidence of decreasing cardiac output or increasing ventricular filling pressures must be analyzed. Inotropic and pressor support during this period should be withdrawn only when all evidence indicates an appropriate cardiac output and ventricular function.

Finally, transport of infants to the intensive care unit after extensive cardiac surgery is hazardous. There are many opportunities for mishap in infants who are intubated and who commonly receive inotropic or pressor support through various central lines. A heightened alertness on the part of all staff is critical to successful transport. Ideally, any suggestion of hemodynamic instability must be resolved in the operating room before transport. Communication with the staff of the intensive care unit before transport concerning details of the infant's cardiopulmonary status and the anticipated time of arrival is important.

It is the anesthesiology staff's responsibility to participate in transfer of the infant onto the intensive care unit bed and to once more review in detail with the intensive care unit staff the pertinent and early postoperative events, the hemodynamic and pulmonary condition of the infant, and the intravenous fluid and drug requirements. The anesthetic management of neonates and infants with complex CHD is as intellectually and technically demanding as that for any patient faced by the anesthesiologist. However, when these cases are managed in a collegial environment, together with surgical colleagues in a cooperative team approach, the results are both professionally and personally rewarding.

REFERENCES

1. Anand KJS, Aynsley-Green A. Metabolic and endocrine effects of surgical ligation of patent ductus arteriosus in the human preterm neonate: Are there implications for further improvement of postoperative outcome? Mod Probl Paediatr 23:143, 1985.
2. Anand KJS, Brown MJ, Bloom SR, et al. Studies on the hormonal regulation of fuel metabolism in the human newborn infant undergoing anaesthesia and surgery. Hormone Res 22:115, 1985.
3. Anand KJ, Hansen DD, Hickey PR. Hormonal-metabolic stress responses in neonates undergoing cardiac surgery. Anesthesiology 73:661, 1990.
4. Anand KJS, Hickey PR. Pain and its effects in the human fetus and neonate. N Engl J Med 317:1321, 1987.
5. Anand KJS, Hickey PR. Halothane-morphine compared with high dose sufentanil for anesthesia and postoperative analgesia in neonatal cardiac surgery. N Engl J Med 326:1, 1992.
6. Anand KJS, Sippell WG, Aynsley-Green A. Randomized trial

of fentanyl anaesthesia in preterm babies undergoing surgery: Effects on the stress response. Lancet I:243, 1987.

7. Anversa P, Olivetti G, Loud AV. Morphometric study of early postnatal development in the left and right ventricular myocardium of the rat. I. Hypertrophy, hyperplasia, and nucleation of myocytes. Circ Res 46:495, 1980.

8. Bini M, Reves JG, Berry D, et al. Ejection fraction during ketamine anesthesia in congenital heart disease patients. Abstract. Anesth Analg 63:186, 1984.

9. Bokesch PM, Castaneda AR, Ziemer G, et al. The influence of a right-to-left cardiac shunt on lidocaine pharmokinetics. Concentrations in intracardiac right-to-left shunts. Anesthesiology 67:739, 1987.

10. Boudreaux JP, Schieber RA, Cook DR. Hemodynamic effects of halothane in the newborn piglet. Anesth Analg 63:731, 1984.

11. Burrows FW. Personal communication, Sept, 1992.

12. Byrick RJ, Kolton M, Hart JT, et al. Hypoxemia following cardiopulmonary bypass. Anesthesiology 53:172, 1980.

13. Cabal LA, Siassi B, Artal R, et al. Cardiovascular and catecholamine changes after administration of pancuronium in distressed neonates. Pediatrics 75:284, 1985.

14. Cook DJ, Carton EG, Housmans PR. Mechanism of the positive inotropic effect of ketamine in isolated ferret ventricular papillary muscle. Anesthesiology 74:880, 1991.

15. Cook DR, Brandom BW, Shiu G, et al. The inspired median effective dose, brain concentration at anesthesia, and cardiovascular index for halothane in young rats. Anesth Analg 60:182, 1981.

16. Davis PJ, Cook DR, Siffler RL, et al. Pharmacodynamics and pharmokinetics of high-dose sufentanil in infants and children undergoing cardiac surgery. Anesth Analg 66:203, 1987.

17. Del Nido PJ, Williams WG, Villamater J, et al. Changes in pericardial surface pressure during pulmonary hypertensive crises after cardiac surgery. Circulation 76(suppl III):93, 1987.

18. den Hollander JM, Hennis PJ, Burm AGL, et al. Alfentanil in infants and children with congenital heart defects. J Cardiothorac Anesth 2:12, 1988.

19. Diaz JH, Lockhart CH. Is halothane really safe in infancy? Anesthesiology 51:S3–S13, 1979.

20. Drummond WH, Gregory GA, Heyman MA, et al. The independent effects of hyperventilation, tolazoline, and dopamine in infants with persistent pulmonary hypertension. J Pediatr 98:603, 1981.

21. Ellis DJ, Steward DJ. Fentanyl dosage is associated with reduced blood glucose in pediatric patients after hypothermic cardiopulmonary bypass. Anesthesiology 72:812, 1990.

22. Fenton KN, Heinemann MK, Hickey PR, et al. The stress response during fetal surgery is blocked by total spinal anesthesia. Surg Forum 43:631–634, 1992.

23. Firmin RK, Bouloux P, Allen P, et al. Sympathoadrenal function during cardiac operation in infants with the technique of surface cooling, limited cardiopulmonary bypass, and circulatory arrest. J Thorac Cardiovasc Surg 90:729, 1985.

24. Fratacci MD, Frostell CG, Chen TY, et al. Inhaled nitric oxide: A selective pulmonary vasodilatory of heparin-protamine vasoconstriction in sheep. Anesthesiology 75:990, 1991.

25. Friesen RH, Henry DB. Cardiovascular changes in preterm neonates receiving isoflurane, halothane, fentanyl and ketamine. Anesthesiology 64:238, 1986.

26. Friesen RH, Lichtor JL. Cardiovascular depression during halothane induction in infants: A study of three induction techniques. Anesth Analg 61:42, 1982.

27. Friesen RH, Lichtor JL. Cardiovascular effects of inhalation induction with isoflurane in infants. Anesth Analg 62:411, 1983.

28. Gassner S, Cohen M, Aygen M, et al. The effect of ketamine on pulmonary artery pressure: An experimental and clinical study. Anaesthesia 29:141, 1974.

29. Glenski JA, Friesen RH, Berglund NL, et al. Comparison of the hemodynamic and echocardiographic effects of sufentanil, fentanyl, isoflurane, and halothane for pediatric cardiac surgery. J Cardiovasc Anesth 2:147, 1988.

30. Goudsouzian NG, Liu LMP, Cote CJ, et al. Safety and effi-

31. Goudsouzian NG, Liu LMP, Savarese JJ. Metocurine in infants and children. Anesthesiology 49:266–269, 1978.

32. Goudsouzian NG, Martyn JJA, Liu LMP, et al. Safety and efficacy of vecuronium in adolescents and children. Anesth Analg 62:1083, 1983.

33. Hammon JW, Wolfe WG, Moran JF, et al. The effect of positive end expiratory pressure on regional ventilation and perfusion in the normal and injured primate lung. J Thorac Cardiovasc Surg 72:680, 1976.

34. Hansen DD, Hickey PR. Anesthesia for hypoplastic left heart syndrome: Use of high dose fentanyl in 30 neonates. Anesth Analg 65:127, 1986.

35. Hickey PR, Hansen DD: Fentanyl and sufentanyl-oxygen-pancuronium anesthesia for cardiac surgery in infants. Anesth Analg 63:117, 1984.

36. Hickey PR, Hansen DD. High dose fentanyl reduces intraoperative ventricular fibrillation in neonates with hypoplastic left heart syndrome. J Clin Anesth 3:295, 1991.

37. Hickey PR, Hansen DD, Cramolini MD, et al. Pulmonary and systemic responses to ketamine in infants with normal and elevated pulmonary vascular resistance. Anesthesiology 62:287, 1985.

38. Hickey PR, Hansen DD, Wessel D, et al. Pulmonary and systemic hemodynamic responses to fentanyl in infants. Anesth Analg 64:483, 1985.

39. Jobes DJ, Nicolson SC, Steven JM, et al. Carbon dioxide prevents pulmonary overcirculation in hypoplastic left heart syndrome. Ann Thorac Surg 54:150, 1992.

40. Kern FH, Morana NJ, Sears J, et al. Coagulation defects in neonates during cardiopulmonary bypass. Ann Thorac Surg 54:541, 1992.

41. Kolobow T, Spragg RG, Pierce JE. Massive pulmonary infarction during total cardiopulmonary bypass in unanesthetized spontaneously breathing lambs. Int J Artif Organs 4:76, 1981.

42. Koren G, Goresky G, Crean P, et al. Pediatric fentanyl dosing based on pharmokinetics during cardiac surgery. Anesth Analg 63:577, 1984.

43. Laishley RS, Burrows FA, Lerman J, et al. Effect of anesthetic induction regimens on oxygen saturation in cyanotic congenital heart disease. Anesthesiology 65:673, 1986.

44. Lanier WL. Glucose management during cardiopulmonary bypass: Cardiovascular and neurologic implications. Anesth Analg 72:423, 1991.

45. Lanier WL, Stangland KJ, Scheithauer BW, et al. The effects of dextrose infusion and head position on neurologic outcome after complete cerebral ischaemia in primates: Examination of a model. Anesthesiology 66:39, 1987.

46. Levin RM, Seleny FL, Streczyn MV. Ketamine-pancuronium-narcotic technique for cardiovascular surgery in infants—a comparative study. Anesth Analg 54:800, 1975.

47. Lichtor JL, Beker BE, Ruschhaupt DG. Myocardial depression during induction in infants. Abstract. Anesthesiology 59:A452, 1983.

48. Lyrene RK, Welch KA, Godoy G, et al. Alkalosis attenuates hypoxic pulmonary vasoconstriction in neonatal lambs. Pediatr Res 19:1268, 1985.

49. Manno CS, Hedberg KW, Kim HC, et al. Comparison of the hemostatic effects of fresh whole blood, stored whole blood and components after open heart surgery in children. Blood 77:930, 1991.

50. Mansell A, Bryan C, Levinson H. Airway closure in children. J Appl Physiol 33:711, 1972.

51. Mehta M, Sokoll MD, Gergis SD. Effects of venous air embolism on the cardiovascular system and acid base balance in the presence and absence of nitrous oxide. Acta Anaesthesiol Scand 28:266, 1984.

52. Moore RA, Gallagher JD, Kingsley BP, et al. The effect of ventilation on systemic blood gases in the presence of left ventricular ejection during cardiopulmonary bypass. J Thorac Cardiovasc Surg 90:287, 1985.

53. Morgan P, Lynn AM, Parrot C, et al. Hemodynamic and

metabolic effects of two anesthetic techniques in children undergoing surgical repair of acyanotic congenital heart disease. Anesth Analg 66:1028, 1987.

54. Morray JP, Lynn AM, Mansfield PB. Effects of pH and P_{CO_2} on pulmonary and systemic hemodynamics after surgery in children with congenital heart disease and pulmonary hypertension. J Pediatr 113:474, 1988.

55. Muhiudeen IA, Roberson DA, Silverman NH, et al. Intraoperative echocardiography for evaluation of congenital heart defects in infants and children. Anesthesiology 76:165, 1992.

56. Nicolson SC and Jobes DR. Hypoplastic left heart syndrome. In Lake CL (ed). Pediatric Cardiac Anesthesia. Norwalk, CT, Appleton & Lange, 1988.

57. Reynolds LM, Nicolson SC, Jobes DR, et al. DDAVP does not decrease bleeding after bypass in young children undergoing extensive reparative procedure. Anesthesiology 77:A1139, 1992.

58. Stanley TH, Liu WS, Gentry S. Effects of ventilatory techniques during cardiopulmonary bypass on post-bypass and postoperative pulmonary compliance and shunts. Anesthesiology 46:391, 1977.

59. Steward DJ, DaSilva CA, Flegel T. Elevated blood glucose levels may increase the danger of neurological deficit following profoundly hypothermic cardiac arrest. Letter. Anesthesiology 68:653, 1988.

60. Svennevig JL, Lindberg H, Gelran O, et al. Should the lungs be ventilated during cardiopulmonary bypass? Clinical, hemodynamic and metabolic changes in patients undergoing elective coronary artery surgery. Ann Thorac Surg 37:295, 1984.

61. Tanner G, Angers D, Barash PG, et al. Does a left to right shunt speed the induction of inhalational anesthesia in congenital heart disease? Abstract. Anesthesiology 57:A427, 1982.

62. Tanner GE, Angers DG, Barash PG, et al. Effect of left-to-right, mixed left-to-right, and right-to-left shunts on inhalational anesthetic induction in children. Anesth Analg 64:101, 1985.

63. Ungerleider RM, Greeley WJ, Sheikh KH, et al. Routine use of intraoperative epicardial echo and Doppler color flow imaging to guide and evaluate repair of congenital heart lesions: A prospective study. J Thorac Cardiovasc Surg 100(2):297, 1990.

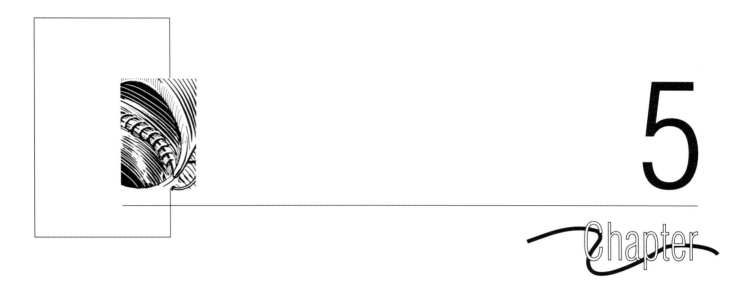

5

Chapter

Perioperative Care

MANAGEMENT OF THE INFANT AND NEONATE WITH CONGENITAL HEART DISEASE

Of the approximately 40,000 children born yearly with congenital heart disease in the United States, nearly half need therapy within the first year of life,[19] and the majority of these will require attention in a critical care setting. As described in previous chapters, the motivation for expanding the scope of reparative operations to the neonate and infant has altered the demographic makeup of intensive care units and has created new challenges for staff in the intensive care unit. During the year ending June 30, 1993, 51% of patients admitted to the Cardiac Intensive Care Unit (CICU) at Children's Hospital in Boston were less than 1 year of age. As shown in Figure 5–1, the number of neonates with heart disease admitted to the 22-bed CICU has steadily risen. Neonates further dominate CICU patient days because of time devoted to preoperative diagnosis and management. Consequently, staff in the CICU must be familiar with the pathophysiology of complex congenital heart defects and also with the special physiology of neonates and young infants, including their responses to anesthesia and surgery.

In general terms, postoperative management of neonates and infants who have undergone either palliative or reparative cardiovascular surgery requires a clear understanding of the cardiac malformation, the extent of dysfunction that existed before the palliation or repair, the operative procedure, all events during the surgery that conceivably could influence the postoperative course, and, finally, the hemodynamics and metabolic conditions that existed immediately after the operation and until the neonate or infant reached the CICU. Optimal management of these critically ill infants can be achieved only when a team of experienced surgeons, cardiologists, anesthesiologists, and nurses work together regularly and harmoniously in the treatment of these patients.

PRACTICAL PHILOSOPHY OF PERIOPERATIVE CARE

Our approach to perioperative management of the neonate and infant is based on a large clinical experience accumulated since the 1970s. It is also influenced by clinical research studies done in our CICU and analysis of factors affecting postoperative morbidity and mortality in these young patients.

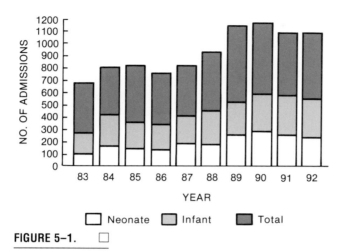

FIGURE 5–1. □

Total number of annual admissions to the cardiac intensive care unit (CICU) between 1983 and 1992. Note the high proportion and increasing number of infants (those less than 1 year old) and neonates.

The philosophy is based on the guiding principle that it is preferable, whenever possible, to repair rather than palliate congenital heart disease and to accomplish this as early as possible in the neonate or young infant. The advantages of a primary corrective operation rather than a staged approach employing initial palliative procedures have been addressed in previous chapters. Inasmuch as reparative procedures usually require cardiopulmonary bypass (CPB), the CICU care of these patients must account for the effects of CPB on the function of multiple organ systems. Increased total body water, transient myocardial dysfunction, elevated pulmonary vascular resistance (PVR), abnormalities of gas exchange, and stress and hormonal responses leading to fluid and electrolyte disturbances must all be considered when proposing a postoperative management plan. These disturbances are transient and are outweighed by the benefit of having a repaired heart and circulation. The philosophy of perioperative care at Children's Hospital in Boston can be summarized as follows:

1. Optimize preoperative function of organ systems by allowing time for resuscitative measures that temporarily restore adequate perfusion.
2. Use extensive postoperative monitoring for assessment of hemodynamics and gas exchange.
3. Prolong the use of anesthesia into the postoperative period to minimize adverse hemodynamic consequences of stress and labile responses to stimuli.
4. Control gas exchange to optimize P_{CO_2} by using mechanical ventilation and muscle relaxants during the early postoperative period.
5. After optimizing preload, use inotropic support to anticipate the predictable decline in cardiac output during the early postoperative period.
6. Use afterload reduction to unburden the neonatal myocardium.

7. Preserve cardiac output with right-to-left atrial level shunts whenever applicable (i.e., after correction of tetralogy of Fallot or the Fontan procedure).
8. Aggressively pursue postoperative diagnosis and therapy of causes for the failing circulation.
9. Develop a team approach to the specialized care of neonates and infants.

The rationale and clinical data supporting this approach are provided in the sections that follow.

CARE OF THE CRITICALLY ILL NEONATE

Care of the critically ill neonate requires an appreciation of the special structural and functional differences of evolving organs.[6] For example, the neonate responds more quickly and extremely to stressful stimuli; this may be expressed by rapid changes in pH, lactate acid, glucose, and temperature.[3] The neonate also has diminished nutrient reserves of fat and carbohydrates. The higher metabolic rate of the newborn, which is manifested by higher oxygen consumption, accounts for the rapid appearance of hypoxia when these patients become dyspneic or apneic and, therefore, deplete alveolar oxygen more quickly. Immaturity of the liver and kidney is associated with reduced protein synthesis and glomerular filtration, thereby affecting drug metabolism. These issues are compounded by the normal increased total body water of the neonate compared with older patients, along with greater capillary permeability,[43] allowing fluid to leak more readily out of the intravascular space. This is especially prominent in the pulmonary vascular bed, which is nearly fully recruited at rest, while lymphatic recruitment, which is required to assist in transporting larger quantities of extravascular pulmonary water, is less available to help decrease mean capillary pressures.[14] Also, in the neonate, systemic blood pressure often does not reliably reflect the adequacy of preload or of oxygen delivery. Because the neonatal myocardium is less compliant, it is less tolerant of increases in afterload and also less responsive to increases in preload.[49, 50, 54] The potential for sustained or labile increases in PVR also exists in neonates, especially those with congenital heart disease, and concern over inciting a pulmonary hypertensive crisis has deterred some from promoting a reparative approach at this early age. Finally, the general and significant stress responses to CPB (see Chapter 4) must also be considered in the overall postoperative management of these young patients.[2]

Clearly, all of these different factors do not preclude performing major cardiac operations in the neonate but simply demand greater vigilance in the care of these children during these early transitional stages of development.[6] Caring for the neonate demands close monitoring of *more* physiologic variables, not fewer, and rapid analysis of events with appropriate and timely therapy. Too often a single abnormality such as hypotension is analyzed in isolation (e.g., without measuring intracardiac oxygen saturations or pressures), and consequently, timely intervention may be delayed. The neonate is unforgiving in this regard and requires informed and rapid decision making.

Whereas neonates may be less tolerant to hemodynamic changes than older children, there is evidence that they are more resilient to ischemic injury. Greater tolerance to hypoxia is characteristic in neonates of many species,[15] as is plasticity of the central nervous system. For example, neonates with obstructive left heart lesions often are seen with hypoxia and profound metabolic acidosis; however, more often than not, after effective resuscitation many remain free of obvious or persistent central nervous system sequelae. There also is increasing evidence that postoperative pulmonary hypertensive crises occur more commonly in a child who has been exposed to high pulmonary pressure and flow beyond the first 4 weeks of life.[8, 24] This has been found to be especially true in lesions such as truncus arteriosus, complete atrioventricular canal defects, and transposition of the great arteries with ventricular septal defects.

Although the technical aspects of repair of complex cardiac malformations on bypass in neonates and young infants seem formidable, surgical advances currently allow routine repair of complex heart disease, even in neonates weighing less than 2500 gm. The survival rate after reparative operations in neonates weighing less than 2500 gm currently exceeds 90% at Children's Hospital in Boston.[7] Table 5–1 shows the results in 100 consecutive neonates admitted to the CICU between January 1987 and March 1991. Sixty-two underwent intervention at a weight of less than 2.5 kg. These interventions included complete repair of truncus arteriosus in a 1490-gm infant and balloon dilatation of critical aortic stenosis in a 1600-gm premature newborn. The survival rate was 81% (50 of 62), and the hospital stay ranged from 4 to 73 days. Twenty-six

patients did not undergo intervention during their initial hospitalization. All were managed medically; survivors were discharged and underwent intervention at a median of 4.3 months. The total survival rate for this group was 69%. The remaining 12 patients had complicating features that precluded intervention; none survived.

RESIDUAL ANATOMIC LESIONS

When either the clinical course or the postoperative hemodynamic or metabolic measurements do not correspond to the expected postoperative recovery, it is prudent to suspect both the accuracy of the preoperative diagnosis and the adequacy of surgical repair. It is ill advised to assume that pre- and intraoperative diagnoses and surgery were optimal and that the patient's heart is failing for some ill-defined reason related to ventricular dysfunction after CPB. Evidence suggests that a residual anatomic lesion is more likely to be the cause of postoperative complications or death than is low cardiac output secondary to myocardial ischemic damage caused by CPB. A review of 257 consecutive patients, including 78 neonates and 67 infants with complex cardiac lesions who were subjected to a single, cold crystalloid cardioplegic strategy, revealed that of the five hospital deaths, only two were due to a low cardiac output (one in an infant with the hypoplastic left heart syndrome and one in an infant with an anomalous left coronary artery arising from the pulmonary artery). No relationship was found between death and the duration of intraoperative myocardial ischemia. Another retrospective review of 32 consecutive neonates and infants who died in the CICU after cardiac surgery revealed that death could be attributed to residual anatomic lesions in 12 of 18 patients who had had reparative operations. Our experience suggests that primary myocardial ischemic damage is seldom the limiting factor in postoperative care. As will be discussed later, low cardiac output does occur in neonates and infants after CPB, but usually it can be anticipated and adequately managed.

Important residual anatomic lesions causing inadequate postoperative performance were also shown to increase length of stay (>28 days) in the CICU. Figure 5–2 shows residual disease as an associated factor linked to prolonged CICU stay in 121 patients drawn from a cohort of 3169 cardiac patients. In patients with an increased length of stay and significant residual anatomic defects, the mortality rate approaches 100% if surgical intervention has been merely palliative. Clearly, patients who linger in the intensive care unit require aggressive

TABLE 5–1. □ SURVIVAL AFTER EARLY INTERVENTION IN 62 OF 100 CONSECUTIVE NEONATES WITH CONGENITAL HEART DISEASE WEIGHING <2.5 KG

	1987	1988	1989	1990
Palliative Operations	4/4 (100%)	6/6 (100%)	6/8 (75%)	2/5 (40%)
Corrective Operations	2/3 (67%)	3/5 (60%)	12/14 (86%)	15/17 (88%)

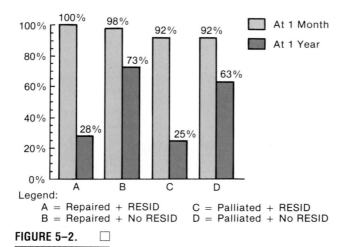

Legend:
A = Repaired + RESID   C = Palliated + RESID
B = Repaired + No RESID   D = Palliated + No RESID

FIGURE 5-2.   □

Survival estimates at 1 year of age for 121 surgical patients with a length of stay >28 days in the CICU between 1985 and 1990. Note that the presence of residual (RESID) disease, whether surgery was palliative or reparative, was a predictor of poor outcome.

diagnostic and therapeutic interventions to identify, and hopefully eliminate, residual anatomic lesions.

MONITORING AND POSTOPERATIVE DATA

Postoperative management in the CICU is based on close monitoring of the patient, including continuous measurement of intracardiac pressures, oxygen saturations, and cardiac output. Routinely measured are left and right atrial pressures, systemic and pulmonary arterial pressures, and also, increasingly, cardiac output using either thermodilution or the Fick method. These measurements allow diagnosis of residual intracardiac or intrapulmonary shunts, obstruction to systemic or pulmonary blood flow, and residual valvar stenosis or regurgitation.

Systemic Arterial Pressure

Continuous monitoring of intra-arterial systemic pressure is very important. Blood pressure measurements obtained by blood pressure cuff in an unstable infant are unreliable. Automated blood pressure cuffs, using Doppler techniques to detect blood flow, offer improved hands-free monitoring but still lack accuracy and reliability during low-flow states and do not offer the beat-to-beat analysis that is so useful in perioperative management. Arterial pressure monitoring can also provide insight into specific hemodynamic abnormalities. Aside from mean arterial pressure, the pulse width and area under the arterial pressure trace are indicators of stroke

volume. A patient with tachycardia, low mean arterial pressure, and a very narrow pulse pressure is likely to have inadequate systemic perfusion. In a patient with a systemic-to-pulmonary artery shunt, the pulse pressure provides some measure of the magnitude of runoff into the pulmonary circulation (i.e., pulmonary blood flow). A narrow pulse pressure and rising atrial pressures may signify impending tamponade.

Pronounced phasic variations in systolic blood pressure induced by positive pressure ventilation in the presence of low atrial pressures are characteristic of a depleted intravascular volume. In a spontaneously breathing patient with diffuse small airway disease, a pulsus paradoxus provides some measure of the work of breathing. Of course, in the spontaneously breathing patient with normal respiratory function and an intact pericardium, pulsus paradoxus generally signifies pericardial effusion or tamponade. Artifacts in arterial pressure tracings must be recognized; otherwise they can complicate management. For example, a small arterial line in the foot of a neonate who has been rewarmed from profound hypothermia may not accurately reflect the perfusion pressure of central organs. The radial artery site is preferred, as it usually provides an adequate trace once the child has warmed. However, the radial artery may also give unreliable blood pressure recordings, particularly in the presence of a Blalock-Taussig shunt or an anomalous origin of the subclavian artery distal to a coarctation. Measurement of blood pressure in both the right arm and the right leg is important in evaluating residual aortic arch obstructions. Again, this examination may be misleading in the presence of an anomalous origin of the subclavian artery, a condition that is not uncommon with an interrupted aortic arch. In such patients, more indirect measures of arch obstruction, such as simultaneous palpation of carotid and femoral artery pulses or Doppler interrogation, must be employed.

Too often, valuable time is lost in resuscitating patients when loss of a blood pressure trace is ascribed to a dampened arterial line. Palpation of either the femoral or carotid arterial pulse is an often forgotten alternative. When in doubt, one or two judicious chest compressions that correlate with restoration of the arterial wave form will confirm the inadequacy of cardiac output, and resuscitative measures must be instituted.

Atrial Pressure

Right and left atrial pressures provide a valuable measure of the preload conditions of the heart and should always be viewed in the context of the patient's underlying disease. They should also be compared with the atrial pressures that were required to achieve successful weaning from CPB. Left atrial pressures are used most commonly to assess intravascular volume requirements. They rarely need to exceed 12 to 14 mm Hg unless there is significant residual abnormality such as a left-to-right shunt, mitral regurgitation or stenosis, or left ventricular dysfunction. Increased left ventricular end-diastolic pressure may be due to depression of systolic or diastolic function, or it may indirectly reflect residual obstruction of the left ventricular outflow tract or valvar regurgitation. Right atrial pressure also provides a reasonably good measure of the patient's intravascular volume and is perhaps most valuable in assessing right ventricular function. A failing right ventricle is more common in neonates and infants than in adults. An elevated right atrial pressure as high as 15 to 18 mm Hg may be seen in the neonate after a right ventriculotomy and is indicative of right ventricular failure. This may be accompanied by pleural or pericardial effusions, hepatomegaly, inability to mobilize peripheral edema, and signs of low cardiac output. Therapy should be directed at improving cardiac output at a lower right atrial pressure.

In neonates, after repair of tetralogy of Fallot, right atrial pressure is invariably higher than left atrial pressure, reflecting the decreased compliance of the hypertrophied neonatal right ventricle, which may receive an additional volume load through a regurgitant pulmonary annulus after a transannular patch repair. If left atrial pressure exceeds right atrial pressure, even with values in the 9 to 12 mm Hg range, the cause of left ventricular dysfunction must be investigated: for example, there may be damage to the anterior descending coronary artery or congenital mitral valve disease.

Pulmonary Artery Pressure

Monitoring of pulmonary artery pressure is useful in diagnosing and assessing therapy for postoperative pulmonary artery hypertension, whether caused by pulmonary venous hypertension (as in mitral stenosis or regurgitation), elevated PVR (as in patients with an atrioventricular canal or previously obstructed total anomalous pulmonary venous connection, older infants with transposition of the great arteries and a ventricular septal defect or truncus arteriosus, or others with more long-standing lesions associated with high pulmonary blood flow), or residual left-to-right shunts.[22, 58] The pulmonary artery line is placed through the right ven-

tricular outflow tract at the time of surgery and can be removed in the CICU by a trained nurse; such removal has a low complication rate. If the catheter is inserted too far, it can reach a wedge position and produce artificially low pulmonary artery pressure and high oxygen saturations. Occasionally the catheter may be inadvertently passed across a ligated, but catheter-patent, ductus arteriosus.

Oxygen saturations in the pulmonary artery that exceed 80% on the first postoperative day may indicate a significant residual left-to-right shunt.[38] This diagnosis must be modified when there is a high PaO_2. For example, a child examined in the CICU after repair of a ventricular septal defect may be ventilated with 30% oxygen and have a PaO_2 of 80 mm Hg and a pulmonary artery oxygen saturation of 78% with the presumption of no significant residual septal defect. However, giving that same child 100% oxygen may produce a PaO_2 of 400 mm Hg, which raises the systemic oxygen content; consequently, the pulmonary artery oxygen saturation increases to 86% without invoking any change in cardiac output, arteriovenous oxygen difference, oxygen consumption, or a left-to-right shunt. Clearly, the physician must be aware of the PaO_2 value; breathing high inspired oxygen adds to the miscalculation of residual shunts. Conversely, pulmonary artery oxygen saturation may be low even in the presence of a large left-to-right shunt if there is a low cardiac output and low, mixed venous oxygen saturation of blood before it reaches the right ventricle and mixes with oxygenated blood from the left ventricle. In this case searching for evidence of low cardiac output will help to identify those patients with normal pulmonary artery oxygen saturation in the presence of residual left-to-right shunts. Note also that one would expect the pulmonary artery pressure to be elevated in the presence of a residual ventricular septal defect that was sufficiently large to produce low cardiac output postoperatively. Even though a "normal" pulmonary artery oxygen saturation can be achieved during low cardiac output states in the presence of a residual shunt, the right atrial oxygen saturation should be critically low and the left atrial pressure should be elevated, reflecting the volume load that a residual ventricular septal defect imparts to the left ventricle. In practice, there rarely is ambiguity about the interpretation of the pulmonary artery oxygen saturation in the presence of a large residual ventricular septal defect. Smaller residual shunts of little hemodynamic importance are more difficult to conclusively demonstrate on the basis of pulmonary artery oxygen saturation. Without a volume load on the left ventricle or a pressure load on the right ventricle, the physician must rely on the difference in oxygen saturation between the right atrium and the pulmonary artery to quantify small shunts. Imprecision in sampling and measuring oxygen saturation and the variability in potential sampling sites from the right atrium (coronary sinus or hepatic veins) make it impossible to interpret 5% to 10% differences in right atrial and pulmonary artery oxygen saturations.

Thermodilution Cardiac Output

The usefulness of pulmonary artery lines for postoperative management can be significantly enhanced by the incorporation of a thermistor for measurement of cardiac output using thermodilution techniques. There are many instances when objective documentation of low or high cardiac output states by thermodilution will confirm tentative diagnoses and facilitate the initiation of an appropriate change in therapy. Measurement of flow is necessary for calculation of resistance. The use of pulmonary artery thermistors has allowed us to document the effects of various agents on PVR, systemic vascular resistance (SVR), and cardiac output during therapeutic trials. In turn, these results have had a significant impact on therapeutic strategies, including ventilatory and other treatment modalities that affect PVR, the use of sedation and anesthesia in the CICU, the use of phosphodiesterase inhibitors, and our current schemes for inotropic support. A No. 3 French catheter with a thermistor and a lumen for monitoring pulmonary artery pressure is placed intraoperatively through the right ventricular outflow tract and secured into position with a pursestring suture. In our initial experience with neonates and infants less than 1 year of age, 134 such catheters were placed. Sixteen of them could not be used in the ICU; four were damaged; three were inadvertently withdrawn, and nine patients had postoperative intracardiac shunts identified on the cardiac output curve (7/9) and confirmed by catheterization, echocardiography, or reoperation. In the remaining 118 patients the median age was 12 days and the mean body surface area was 0.25 m². Diagnoses included transposition of the great arteries (65), ventricular septal defect (26), complete atrioventricular canal (15), truncus arteriosus (6), and other (6). Early in our experience a too-distal position of the catheter was commonly identified by analysis of the contour of the cardiac output curve even though the catheter did not appear to be in a wedge position on the chest radiograph. Catheter reposition was easily accomplished at the bedside. For each of the determinations in 118 patients, analysis was performed to compare consistency of

triplicate determinations, reliability of measurements in neonates compared with those in infants, and determinations made by the physician compared with those made at the bedside by the nurse. Correlation coefficients of reliability were calculated and student paired t tests performed; r values were >0.95 for all three categories, and P values were <.02. There were no major complications related to the catheter. Bleeding was noted in one patient, late bacteremia in one patient, and unsatisfactory pressure wave forms were noted in nine patients. This catheter can provide reliable and reproducible measurements of pulmonary artery pressure and coronary output with low risk in neonates and infants after surgery when used by nurses or physicians. Changes in catheter design may further improve wave forms.

Other Monitoring

Continuous monitoring of the electrocardiogram (ECG) provides essential information regarding the infant's heart rate as well as the respiratory rate, which can be recorded using electrical impedance circuitry with the ECG leads. Adequate monitoring of the ECG is important, not only for heart rate measurement, but also for the rapid detection and description of complex arrhythmias. Alteration of lead selection, simultaneous display of multiple ECG leads, ease of recording from atrial or esophageal pacing wires, and storage and retrieval of wave forms all have become integral aspects of routine bedside monitoring. Some postoperative patient populations (e.g., those who have undergone Fontan procedures) may have an incidence of arrhythmias that exceeds 20%. Adequate monitoring to detect retrograde P waves (producing cannon a waves in the atrial pressure), which elevate mean left atrial pressure, allows changes in therapy, such as slowing the heart rate and atrial pacing, that can have a measurable impact and improve hemodynamics in some critically ill patients.

Continuous measurement of arterial oxygen saturation by pulse oximetry has had a significant impact on critical care and currently is a routine aspect of monitoring for all patients in the CICU where potentially deleterious variations of gas exchange may occur. Rapid analysis of the changes in oxygen saturation produced by therapeutic maneuvers is especially valuable in patients with congenital heart disease in whom oxygenation may also reflect crucial alterations in pulmonary or systemic blood flow or changes in the degree of intracardiac mixing.[20] Despite limitations in accuracy at low oxygen saturations, oxygen saturation monitoring, when combined with end-tidal carbon dioxide sampling, has provided adequate analysis of gas exchange in some chronically ventilated patients in whom arterial access is undesirable or impractical.

Measurement of temperature remains an important general indicator of an infant's well-being in the CICU. Variations in central and peripheral temperatures may herald the onset of infection, alterations in systemic perfusion, or injury to the central nervous system. Fever gives rise to increased oxygen consumption, tachycardia, and increased oxygen demand by the heart and other organs. When cardiac output cannot provide for this increased oxygen demand, mixed venous oxygen saturation decreases as oxygen extraction in the peripheral circulation increases. In patients with right-to-left shunts, the lower mixed venous oxygen saturation is reflected in lower arterial oxygen saturation. This further compromises oxygen delivery and ultimately leads to cellular dysfunction. The central nervous system may be particularly vulnerable to excessive temperatures after an ischemic injury or CPB. Temperature should be monitored postoperatively and hyperthermia treated with surface cooling. Occasionally there is therapeutic value in achieving subnormal temperatures (33°C to 36°C) to minimize oxygen consumption or to treat junctional ectopic tachycardia. Continuous monitoring of rectal or central temperature is needed to avoid excessive hypothermic temperatures, which may precipitate ventricular arrhythmias. When therapeutic cooling is required, cold stress and shivering are generally avoided by maintaining anesthesia and using muscle relaxants.

The importance of monitoring central nervous system activity is becoming increasingly apparent. Abnormal electroencephalograms (EEGs) recorded continuously after surgery in neonates may reflect intraoperative surgical techniques and have some predictive value at the 1-year neurologic examination.[46] Continuous eight-channel EEG recording integrated into the bedside monitor is currently available and may have a role in monitoring certain high-risk patients, especially if sedation, muscle relaxation, and emergence from anesthesia complicate traditional means of neurologic evaluation. Noninvasive measurements of cerebral blood flow with transcranial Doppler echocardiography or near-infrared spectroscopy currently allow monitoring of blood flow to the brain during the perioperative period and assessment of the impact of therapy or altered hemodynamics on the amount of oxygen the brain receives. Whether these monitors of the central nervous system reveal ways in which intervention could be altered or optimized remains unclear.

ANESTHESIA AND VENTILATORY CONTROL

Patients with congenital heart disease who are recovering from surgical reconstruction are especially sensitive to stressful interventions and have marginal organ system reserve and diminished compensatory mechanisms. The postoperative myocardium that has been exposed to CPB, deep hypothermia, or ischemia may be incapable of increasing stroke volume during bradycardia or adjusting to an acute increase in afterload. Myocardial performance is further impaired by ventriculotomy, which is required for repair of a variety of congenital heart diseases.

In healthy infants a painful or stressful stimulus produces tachycardia, hypertension, and a transient decrease in arterial P_{O_2}. In a postoperative cardiac patient the tachycardia may evolve into a hemodynamically compromising, rapid supraventricular arrhythmia, and the hypertension may represent a critical and intolerable increase in ventricular afterload. Hypoxia may be profound and prolonged if the child has cyanotic heart disease or potential right-to-left shunting.

Wakefulness and agitation in mechanically ventilated children increase the work of breathing, exacerbate asynchrony with the ventilator, produce hypercarbia, and increase PVR. Cerebrovascular instability has also been noted.[53] Postoperative pulmonary artery hypertensive crises in infants after thoracic surgery and endotracheal suctioning can be significantly blunted by high doses of narcotics,[27, 28] which also attenuate the impressive increase in stress hormone levels in neonates after CPB.[1]

Sudden death during the first postoperative night after apparently successful and uncomplicated congenital heart surgery is a well-known phenomenon, especially in patients with labile pulmonary artery hypertension and in those with a single ventricle who have undergone palliative surgery; in these latter patients the balance between SVR and PVR plays an important role in hemodynamic stability. These observations have motivated us at Children's Hospital in Boston to extend anesthesia through the first postoperative night, using high-dose continuous infusions of fentanyl (10 to 15 μg/kg/hr) after intraoperative anesthetic doses (50 to 100 μg/kg)[29] in patients with unstable hemodynamics or pulmonary artery hypertension and in most neonates after CPB. Our objective is to minimize hemodynamic lability in unstable patients during the early postoperative hours when cardiac output reaches its nadir and myocardial reserve is diminished. Precise control of P_{CO_2} and pH and, hence, PVR, is more easily achieved in a paralyzed and anesthetized patient. This approach to patient care requires close monitoring of intracardiac, pulmonary, and systemic artery pressures and, in some patients with biventricular repairs, measurement of cardiac output.

Critics of this approach will argue that the use of any anesthetic depresses myocardial function and blunting the endogenous sympathetic response to stimuli lowers vascular tone and invites an increase in the use of inotropic agents. Others argue that controlled ventilation may be hazardous, as inadvertent extubation or other compromise of the airway will leave the patient unable to make a spontaneous compensatory effort. However, two studies from our institution support the notion that high-dose narcotic anesthesia during the first postoperative night can be accomplished in selected patients without additional morbidity and may prove advantageous over conventional analgesic regimens. Neonates undergoing congenital heart surgery were randomized to receive morphine and halothane or high-dose synthetic narcotics for anesthesia and postoperative analgesia; the latter group had decreased levels of stress hormones and a decreased incidence of metabolic acidosis, sepsis, hypotension, and postoperative death, without a longer stay in the ICU.[1]

We prospectively monitored detailed hemodynamic changes and neurologic outcome in the ICU after arterial switch operations in neonates with transposition of the great arteries. One hundred and seventy-one patients with D-transposition who underwent an arterial switch operation were anesthetized with 100 μg/kg of fentanyl (total dose) and received 10 to 15 μg/kg of fentanyl per hour for the first postoperative night. The infusion of fentanyl was continued for patients who were hemodynamically unstable or in whom the chest could not be closed in the operating room. Using this approach, there were no deaths during the first 72 hours postoperatively and only one ICU death in the 171 patients. This low mortality rate was achieved despite a low cardiac index (<2 L/min/m^2) in 24% of the patients and sufficient hemodynamic instability to delay sternal closure or to dictate opening of the chest in 18 patients.

We believe that extending fentanyl anesthesia into the postoperative period for selected infants to minimize the hemodynamic and hormonal stress responses to surgical intervention and perioperative care is of important therapeutic value and has improved clinical outcome.

HEMODYNAMIC SUPPORT
Low Cardiac Output States

Although the principal causes of morbidity and mortality after CPB are attributable to residual or undiagnosed structural lesions (supporting the notion of aggressive diagnostic and postoperative intervention), low cardiac output states do occur and frequently can be predicted.[55, 56] For example, in neonates studied after an arterial switch operation, the cardiac index fell to less than 2 L/min/m^2 in one fourth of the patients during the first postoperative night, while PVR and SVR rose. The addition of afterload reduction and inotropic support opposes this trend. The neonate may also benefit considerably from the use of phosphodiesterase inhibitors, which reduce afterload and increase contractility without causing tachycardia. The beneficial effects of afterload reduction may be especially important for the neonatal myocardium, where increases in afterload may severely compromise left ventricular function. For more refractory but potentially reversible ventricular dysfunction, ventricular assist devices are used when gas exchange appears satisfactory.[47] In selected patients this technique offers potential advantages over extracorporeal membrane oxygenation (ECMO) (see subchapter, "Postcardiotomy Mechanical Ventricular Assistance"), although ECMO is indicated whenever pulmonary function is also significantly impaired.[10, 44] However, we have employed it in fewer than 1% of patients undergoing CPB bypass. With more conventional support of the circulation, most patients can be managed successfully without it.

Intracardiac Shunts

Some children benefit substantially from strategies that allow right-to-left shunting at the atrial level when right ventricular dysfunction occurs postoperatively. A typical example is after early repair of tetralogy of Fallot, when the moderately hypertrophied, noncompliant right ventricle has undergone a ventriculotomy and may be further compromised by an increased volume load from pulmonary regurgitation secondary to a transannular patch on the right ventricular outflow tract. In these children it is very useful to leave the foramen ovale patent, permitting right-to-left shunting of blood and thus preserving cardiac output and oxygen delivery despite the attendant transient cyanosis. If the foramen is not patent or is surgically closed, right ventricular dysfunction can lead to reduced left ventricular filling, low cardiac output, and, ultimately, left ventricular dysfunction. In infants and neonates with repaired truncus arteriosus, the same concerns apply and may even be exaggerated if right ventricular afterload is elevated because of pulmonary artery hypertension. This concept has been extended to older patients with a single ventricle who are at high risk for Fontan operations. If an atrial septal communication or fenestration is left at the time of the Fontan procedure, the resulting right-to-left shunt helps to preserve cardiac output. These children have fewer postoperative complications, as described in Chapter 15.

Infants with tetralogy of Fallot and pulmonary atresia often depend on systemic aortopulmonary collateral vessels for pulmonary flow. After a reparative operation, a residual left-to-right shunt through remaining collateral vessels imposes a diastolic volume load on the left ventricle. Preoperative occlusion of these collateral vessels can be accomplished occasionally by interventional techniques in the cardiac catheterization laboratory, but this may leave the child precariously cyanotic before the operation. In this case, the most effective temporizing therapy consists of reducing oxygen consumption (i.e., with anesthesia and mechanical ventilation) and increasing the systemic perfusion pressure across other remaining systemic-to-pulmonary communications while preparing for surgery.

In patients with tetralogy of Fallot and pulmonary atresia, when the pulmonary arteries are very diminutive and a valved homograft is placed between the right ventricle and pulmonary arteries, the ventricular septal defect (VSD) is left open, and postoperative management of either cyanosis or congestive heart failure is determined by the resistance offered by the pulmonary circuit. The postoperative course of these patients can be variable and demanding of even the most experienced team. After aortopulmonary collateral arteries are occluded and right ventricular–to–diminutive pulmonary artery continuity is established, cyanosis may be intense, and therapy should be aimed at lowering PVR and establishing adequate pulmonary blood flow. However, if the aorta is fully saturated and pulmonary artery oxygen saturation and left atrial pressures are elevated, a left-to-right shunt through the VSD may be developing, producing volume overload of the left ventricle with its consequent hemodynamic effects. This indicates that the VSD should be closed. However, if the patient is not fully saturated systemically but there is evidence of volume overload of the left ventricle with low cardiac output and high left atrial pressure, excessive systemic-to–pulmonary artery collateral flow must be suspected. This often requires early postoperative cardiac catheterization and coil occlusion of residual aortopulmonary collateral vessels.

Assessment of Cardiac Output

Obstruction to blood flow, pulmonary-to-systemic communications, and valvar incompetence consti-

tute abnormalities that result in essentially four pathophysiologic states: systolic pressure overload, diastolic pressure overload, arterial hypoxemia, and pulmonary hypertension. In any of these circumstances, factors influencing cardiac output—end-diastolic volume (preload), systolic wall tension (afterload), myocardial contractility, heart rate, and rhythm—must be assessed and manipulated. Volume therapy (increased preload), followed by judicious use of inotropic agents, is often necessary. Atrial pressure and ventricular response to the changes in atrial pressure must be evaluated. Ventricular response is judged by observing systemic arterial pressure and waveform, heart rate, skin color and peripheral extremity temperature, peripheral pulse magnitude, urine flow, core body temperature, and acid-base balance. As mentioned previously, by measuring cardiac output using a thermodilution technique with a double-lumen pulmonary artery thermistor, diagnostic accuracy is enhanced.

Cardiac Output and Diastolic Function

Occasionally there is an alteration of ventricular relaxation that reduces ventricular compliance. The ventricular cavity size is small, and the stroke volume is decreased. Beta-adrenergic antagonists or calcium channel blockers add little to the treatment of this condition. In fact, the hypotension or myocardial depression produced by these agents frequently outweighs any gain from slowing the heart rate. Instead, a gradual increase in intravascular volume to augment ventricular capacity, in addition to the use of low doses of inotropic agents, has proved to be of modest benefit. Tachycardia must be avoided to optimize diastolic filling time and decrease myocardial oxygen demands. If low cardiac output continues despite the previously described treatment, therapy with vasodilators may be attempted to alter systolic wall tension (afterload) and thus decrease the impediment to ventricular ejection. Although, intuitively, the physician may hesitate to use vasodilators in the presence of a marginal systemic arterial blood pressure, because blood pressure is the product of cardiac output and SVR, a decrease in SVR could increase flow with no undesirable changes in pressure.[16] Because the capacity of the vascular bed increases after vasodilatation, simultaneous volume replacement is indicated. Amrinone may be more useful in these circumstances, as it is a noncatecholamine, nonglycosidic inotropic agent with vasodilating and, perhaps, some lusitropic (improved diastolic state) properties, unlike other inotropic agents.

Cardiac Output and Inotropic Agents

Failure to improve cardiac output after volume and vascular tone adjustments requires the use of an inotropic drug.[4, 12, 23, 64] Table 5–2 lists commonly used vasoactive drugs and their actions. We prefer dopamine in doses of 3 to 10 µg/kg/min; we rarely use more than 15 µg/kg/min because of the known vasoconstrictor and chronotropic properties of dopamine at very high doses. Dobutamine's chronotropic and vasodilatory advantages recognized in adults with coronary artery disease have not always proved equally efficacious in clinical studies in children. In fact, dobutamine has less dopaminergic advantages (or none at all) for the pediatric kidney. This may be an especially important limitation in infants with excess total body water and interstitial edema. The significant chronotropic effect and increased oxygen consumption induced by isoproterenol have also increasingly limited its use in neonates and infants. Epinephrine is useful occasion-

ally for short-term therapy when high systemic pressures are sought, provided the temporary increase in PVR can be tolerated. Occasionally, high doses of epinephrine are necessary to increase pulmonary blood flow across significantly narrowed systemic-to-pulmonary artery shunts when oxygen saturations are low and falling.

In the past, the side effects of inotropic support of the heart with catecholamines seemed less problematic in children than in adults with an ischemic, noncompliant heart. Tachycardia, increased end-diastolic pressure and afterload, and increased myocardial oxygen consumption, in spite of their undesirable side effects, were tolerated by most children in need of inotropic support after CPB. However, with increasing experience in dealing with neonates and young infants, the differences in their response to vasoactive drugs in a CICU setting have become more evident. The less compliant neonatal myocardium, like the ischemic adult heart, may raise its end-diastolic pressure during higher doses of dopa-

TABLE 5–2. ☐ SUMMARY OF SELECTED VASOACTIVE AGENTS

AGENT	DOSES (IV)	PERIPHERAL VASCULAR EFFECT	CARDIAC EFFECT	CONDUCTION SYSTEM EFFECT
Noncatecholamines				
Digoxin (Total digitalizing dose)	20 µg/kg premature 30 µg/kg neonate (0–1 mo) 40 µg/kg infant (<2 yr) 30 µg/kg child (2–5 yr) 20 µg/kg child (>5 yr)	Increases peripheral vascular resistance 1–2 +; acts directly on vascular smooth muscle	Inotropic effect 3–4 +; acts directly	Slows sinus node; decreases AV conduction
Calcium: Chloride Gluconate	10–20 mg/kg/dose (slowly) 30–60 mg/kg/dose (slowly)	Variable; probably depends on serum ionized Ca^{++} level	Inotropic effect 3 +; depends on ionized Ca^{++}	Slows sinus node; decreases AV conduction
Nitroprusside	0.3–5 µg/kg/min	Donates nitric oxide group to relax smooth muscle and dilate pulmonary and systemic vessels	Indirectly increases cardiac output by decreasing afterload	Reflex tachycardia
Amrinone	1–3 mg/kg loading dose 5–20 µg/kg/min maintenance	Systemic and pulmonary vasodilator; platelet and toxic effects not well established in neonates	Increases cardiac output in neonates and infants	Minimal tachycardia

AGENT	DOSE RANGE	PERIPHERAL VASCULAR EFFECT			CARDIAC EFFECT		COMMENT
		Alpha	Beta$_2$	Delta	Beta$_1$	Beta$_2$	
Catecholamines							
Phenylephrine	0.1–0.5 µg/kg/min	4 +	0	0	0	0	Increases systemic resistance, no inotropy; may cause renal ischemia; useful for treatment of TOF spells
Isoproterenol	0.05–0.5 µg/kg/min	0	4 +	0	4 +	4 +	Strong inotropic and chronotropic agent; peripheral vasodilator; reduces preload; pulmonary vasodilator; limited by tachycardia and oxygen consumption
Norepinephrine	0.1–0.5 µg/kg/min	4 +	0	0	2 +	0	Increases systemic resistance; moderately inotropic; may cause renal ischemia
Epinephrine	0.03–0.1 µg/kg/min 0.2–0.5 µg/kg/min	2 + 4 +	1–2 + 0	0 0	2–3 + 4 +	2 + 3 +	Beta$_2$ effect with lower doses; best for blood pressure in anaphylaxis and drug toxicity
Dopamine	2–4 µg/kg/min 4–8 µg/kg/min >10 µg/kg/min	0 0 2–4 +	0 2 + 0	2 + 2 + 0	0 1–2 + 1–2 +	0 1 + 2 +	Splanchnic and renal vasodilator; may be used with isoproterenol; increasing doses produce increasing alpha effect
Dobutamine	2–10 µg/kg/min	1 +	2 +	0	3–4 +	1–2 +	Less chronotropy and arrhythmias at lower doses; effects vary with dose similar to dopamine; chronotropic advantage compared with dopamine may not be apparent in neonates

AV, Atrioventricular; TOF, tetralogy of Fallot.

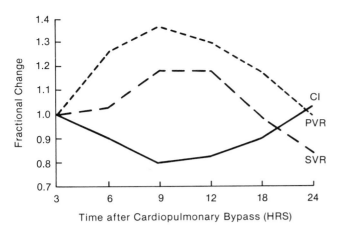

FIGURE 5–3.   □

Fractional change in cardiac index (CI, *solid line*) as a function of time after separation from cardiopulmonary bypass in neonates after an arterial switch operation. The CI fell below 2 L/min/m² in 24% of patients. Changes in systemic and pulmonary vascular resistance (SVR, PVR) are also shown.

mine infusion or develop even more extreme non-compliance. Actual myocardial necrosis caused by high doses of epinephrine infusions has been identified in neonatal animal models after CPB.[5] Although these agents do increase the cardiac output, the concomitant increase in ventricular filling pressure is less well tolerated by the immature myocardium than by that in older children. Similarly, the increases in myocardial oxygen consumption and tachycardia caused by catecholamines have become more significant factors, particularly since coronary transfer procedures have become common. Many of the complex corrective procedures done in neonates and small infants are accompanied by transient postoperative arrhythmias that are either induced or exacerbated by catecholamines; these can have a profound adverse effect on the patient's recovery after surgery. Nevertheless, the predictable, and often significant, decrease in cardiac output documented by numerous investigators after CPB in infants (Fig. 5–3) and older children continues to justify the practice of routinely using inotropic agents to support the heart and circulation while weaning these patients from CPB and during the immediate postoperative period.

Amrinone, a nonglycosidic, noncatecholamine, inotropic agent with additional vasodilatory properties, has emerged as an important inotropic agent for use in neonates and infants after open heart surgery. It has been used extensively in adults for treatment of chronic congestive heart failure but more recently has been introduced to the pediatric practice. The drug appears to exert its principal effect by inhibiting phosphodiesterase, the enzyme that metabolizes cyclic adenosine monophosphate

(cAMP). By increasing intracellular cAMP, calcium transport into the cell is favored, and the increased intracellular calcium stores enhance the contractile state of the myocyte. The drug also appears to work synergistically with low doses of beta-adrenergic agonists, and it has fewer side effects than other catecholamine vasodilators such as isoproterenol. In a controlled trial of amrinone in neonates requiring inotropic support during the first night after an arterial switch operation, we noted a reliable and reproducible increase in cardiac output and decreases in SVR and PVR.[61] This was true when values were compared with baseline hemodynamic values before the administration of amrinone and was even more pronounced when compared with those in neonates randomly picked to receive dopamine therapy alone after an arterial switch operation (Fig. 5–4). From this study, it was concluded that amrinone is safe for use as a potent pulmonary and systemic vasodilator in neonates after open heart surgery. It raises cardiac output without an increase in heart rate provided that preload conditions are maintained with adequate volume replacement. Amrinone is presently the second most commonly employed inotropic agent at Children's Hospital in Boston and is preferred when there is a significant decrease in cardiac output (measured or clinically ascertained) in the presence of a normal or increased afterload. With a 3-mg/kg loading dose over 30 minutes and a continuous infusion of 10 μg/kg/min in an infant weighing 5 kg, the daily drug cost at present is $43. For those weighing more than 5 kg, the cost is directly proportional to body weight and the infusion rate.

When systemic blood pressure is elevated and car-

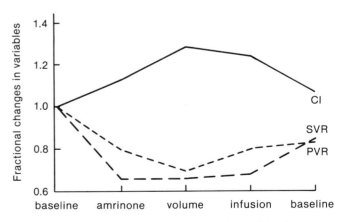

Before, during, and after amrinone infusion

FIGURE 5–4.   □

Increase in cardiac index (CI) shown before and after a loading dose of amrinone, followed by volume replacement restoring left atrial pressure to baseline, continuous infusion of amrinone (30 min), and discontinuation of amrinone with a return toward baseline (30 min). SVR, systemic vascular resistance; PVR, pulmonary vascular resistance.

diac output appears normal, a primary vasodilator, particularly nitroprusside, is indicated to normalize blood pressure and decrease afterload on the left ventricle. Although nitroprusside has no known direct inotropic effects, this potent vasodilator has the advantages of being readily titratable and possessing a short biologic half-life. The use of vasodilators for treatment of pulmonary hypertension has had mixed results because of systemic vasodilating effects that may predominate and limit effectiveness. Tolazaline, prostaglandin E_1, and prostacyclin have all been suggested as useful pharmacologic treatments for this illness.[13, 34, 62]

PULMONARY VASCULAR RESISTANCE AND RIGHT VENTRICULAR FUNCTION

In children, significant increases in PVR after CPB increase right ventricular afterload and may be poorly tolerated if sustained. In the immediate postoperative period, right ventricular function may be transiently impaired by such factors as a right ventriculotomy or prolonged aortic crossclamping. In addition to previously described blood-borne and mechanical factors that may transiently elevate PVR after CPB,[25] the child with congenital heart disease may, by age or diagnosis, be prone to the development of labile pulmonary artery hypertension.[26, 31, 48] For these reasons, the concept of afterload reduction, which has focused primarily on SVR and left ventricular function in the adult cardiac patient, must also be applied to the pulmonary circuit in children.[9, 30, 52, 62]

We have studied many of the factors that influence PVR in children with congenital heart disease and have formulated a clinical management protocol for children after open heart surgery based on some of these findings and on other ongoing investigations (Table 5–3).

Achieving appropriate lung volumes is critical in maintaining functional residual capacity (FRC) and

TABLE 5–3. ☐ FACTORS INFLUENCING PULMONARY VASCULAR RESISTANCE

INCREASED PVR	DECREASED PVR
Lower pH (via acidosis or hypercarbia)	Increased pH (via bicarbonate or hyperventilation)
High airway pressure	Low airway pressure
Atelectasis/pleural effusion capacity	Normal functional residual
Sympathetic stimulation	Blunted sympathetic response (anesthesia)
Alveolar hypoxia	Increased Fio₂*
High hematocrit level	Low hematocrit
Drugs, humoral influence	Drugs, humoral influence
Mechanical obstruction (anatomic, clot)	

*May not be effective immediately after cardiopulmonary bypass; see text.

low PVR.[63] When a normal FRC is reached, PVR is at its lowest. For example, atelectasis, or collapse of the airway, decreases lung volume and compresses the pulmonary microcirculation, which in turn elevates PVR. At the other extreme, hyperinflation produces increased lung volumes, and the capillaries in the alveolar septum become compressed; hence, PVR is also increased. When there are abnormalities of gas exchange and evidence of decreased lung volume or atelectasis on the chest radiograph, positive end-expiratory pressure or an increase in tidal volume (and, hence, mean airway pressure) may actually reduce PVR. These maneuvers may also provide improved ventilation and oxygen supply to other underventilated areas of the lung that had been subjecting the regional pulmonary circulation to the influence of hypoxic pulmonary vasoconstriction, thereby contributing to the elevation of PVR. Newborns have an airway closing capacity that is above the FRC, and therefore some airway closure normally occurs at the end of each normal breath. The addition of even a small amount of positive end-expiratory pressure can prove quite effective in restoring FRC and maintaining gas exchange and a low PVR.[42]

The increased lung water that is characteristic of neonates and infants after CPB can cause significant alterations in lung compliance, including contributions from the chest wall. In this case, the aim is to recruit lung volumes with large tidal volume breaths, accepting the higher associated peak inspiratory pressures. One of the most common causes of a low PaO_2 when the patient arrives in the CICU is an insufficient tidal volume delivered to the lungs, resulting in the inability to recruit all available alveoli. To achieve the desired PCO_2 and avoid increased minute ventilation with excessive respiratory alkalosis from large tidal volume breaths, patients are ventilated with relatively low intermittent mandatory ventilation (IMV) rates of between 12 and 16 breaths per minute.

The effect of hyperventilation with concomitant respiratory alkalosis on PVR has been shown repeatedly in animal models of pulmonary hypertension and in neonates with persistent pulmonary hypertension.[40] In infants after CPB the PVR is very sensitive to changes in pH induced by alterations in PCO_2.[60] Figure 5–5 shows the results in 20 infants less than 1 year old in whom the PCO_2 was manipulated after repair of a VSD or complete atrioventricular canal defect. These patients were hemodynamically stable, received no inotropic support, and had no significant postoperative pulmonary hypertension. They were sedated with morphine (0.1 mg/kg), paralyzed, and mechanically ventilated 4 hours after weaning from CPB. Stepwise changes in PCO_2

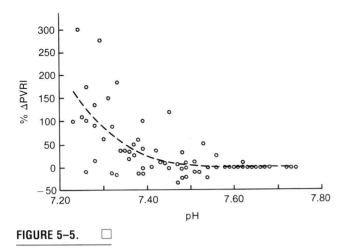

FIGURE 5–5. □

Effect of hyperventilation and respiratory alkalosis on pulmonary vascular resistance in 20 infants after repair of ventricular septal defect or complete atrioventricular (AV) canal. %PVRI, Percentage of change in pulmonary vascular resistance compared with the value at the most alkalotic pH.

were induced by systemic changes in ventilatory rate, allowing the arterial pH to vary according to the P_{CO_2}. The individual patient's percentage of change in PVR compared with the PVR at the most alkalotic setting is shown in Figure 5–5. Notice that as the pH, although still within normal range (7.35 to 7.45), became less alkalotic, the PVR rose, and in several patients it more than doubled. As the pH approached 7.30, our target value, the PVR reached an average value of 9.2 U · m². At this point, pressure in the pulmonary artery reached systemic levels in three of the 20 patients; this was easily and completely reversed by returning to baseline ventilatory settings. Similar results can be obtained by allowing patients to breathe inspired concentrations of carbon dioxide,[45] which makes it unlikely that decreased low lung volumes, secondary to decreased minute ventilation at low IMV rates, could account for the rise in PVR. Moreover, the PaO_2 did not significantly decrease during this maneuver, making alveolar hypoxic pulmonary vasoconstriction an unlikely cause of this effect.

Many mediators of increased pulmonary vascular tone have been suggested, but the role of any single substance remains unclear. It has been suggested that thromboxane and prostacyclin may play an important role in either the genesis of pulmonary artery hypertension (increased thromboxane A_2) or in the reversal of pulmonary hypertension by the mechanical effects of hyperventilation on prostacyclin production. We found that the increase in PVR achieved by increasing P_{CO_2}, which could be eliminated with hyperventilation, was not associated with increased production of either thromboxane or prostacyclin as sampled in the pulmonary artery or

left atrium.[59] However, there are large increases in the endogenous production of epinephrine and norepinephrine as P_{CO_2} rises (Fig. 5–6).[57]

Thus, despite increases in mean airway pressure, moderate hyperventilation tends to decrease PVR postoperatively in the infant who has undergone cardiac surgery. More extreme hyperventilation is not reliably useful in further lowering PVR, even in patients who have persistent pulmonary hypertension postoperatively. Moderate hypercarbia raises PVR, which may profoundly alter hemodynamic stability in selected patients. The net effect on vascular tone induced by changes in pH and P_{CO_2} as a result of changing minute ventilation is significantly more pronounced in the pulmonary vascular bed than in the systemic vascular bed. These findings provide a rationale for our clinical practice of moderate hyperventilation of neonates and infants during the first postoperative hours when PVR may be transiently elevated.

Some have suggested that the effect of respiratory alkalosis on PVR is mediated in part by a direct effect of P_{CO_2} rather than by the hydrogen-ion concentration. However, numerous animal models have demonstrated that the pH itself is the controlling variable and that the level of P_{CO_2} is much less important. Granted, models of pulmonary hypertension using lambs that breathed low concentrations of inspired oxygen may not be relevant to the pulmonary vascular bed of a human infant before or after CPB. The issue is not trivial, as there are justifiable concerns regarding the effects of hyperventilation, including barotrauma, decreased cerebral blood flow, and other potentially adverse effects of CPB on hemodynamics. Therefore, we studied 15

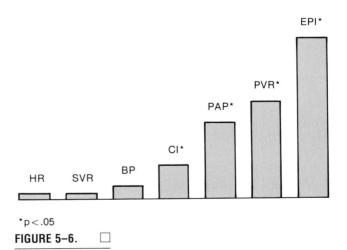

*p < .05

FIGURE 5–6. □

Relative changes in heart rate (HR), systemic vascular resistance (SVR), blood pressure (BP), cardiac index (CI), pulmonary artery pressure (PAP), pulmonary vascular pressure (PVR), and plasma epinephrine levels (EPI) when P_{CO_2} is high (mean, 54 mm Hg) and low (mean, 22 mm Hg).

ventilated infants ages 0.4 to 15.6 months (median, 5.7 months) after corrective cardiac surgery to clarify the role of arterial pH alone on PVR. The study consisted of three stages:

1. Baseline studies were carried out 4 hours after CPB.
2. PVR was increased by decreasing minute ventilation and increasing P_{CO_2}.
3. The pH was raised by an infusion of sodium bicarbonate (4 mEq/kg), with minute ventilation and high P_{CO_2} held constant.

Figure 5–7 shows that with a short trial of hypoventilation to a P_{CO_2} level of 55 mm Hg, the PVR increased. This increase was abolished by infusion of bicarbonate and return of the pH (but not the P_{CO_2}) to baseline. Therefore, increasing the arterial pH with sodium bicarbonate both lowered pulmonary artery pressure and increased the cardiac index, hence decreasing PVR. These effects were observed without changes in P_{CO_2}. Metabolic alkalosis, not hyperventilation-induced respiratory alkalosis exclusively, may be appropriate adjunctive therapy for elevated PVR.

The use of permissive hypercapnia has also been advocated for critically ill children with respiratory failure. The objective is to achieve acceptable end-organ function while inducing less barotrauma and achieving lower mean airway pressures with fewer hemodynamic consequences of high airway pressures. Caution is warranted in applying this principle to children with congenital heart disease after CPB. A relatively mild decrease in pH, which accompanies the increase in P_{CO_2}, may cause a significant increase in PVR and, thus, in afterload on the right ventricle. Patients who suffer from low cardiac output or have less myocardial reserve after a right ventriculotomy may not tolerate a sustained increase in afterload throughout the postoperative period. Infusion of bicarbonate to counterbalance the desired increase in P_{CO_2} may seriously affect the metabolic status of the patient 1 or 2 days after surgery when a contraction alkalosis and diuretic-induced hypochloremic alkalosis combine with bicarbonate therapy to produce a profound persistent metabolic alkalosis that complicates electrolyte balance, digoxin therapy, and management of arrhythmias. Therefore, it remains our preference to use a moderate amount of hyperventilation in the immediate postoperative period, attempting to achieve a pH of 7.45 to 7.48 without much attention to associated P_{CO_2} levels.

Oxygen can be an important pulmonary vasodilator under certain conditions. Alveolar hypoxia has long been recognized as a potent pulmonary vasoconstrictor, and this effect can be reversed by increasing inspired oxygen.[51] In studies of preoperative patients with congenital heart disease, including those with left-to-right shunts, high levels of inspired oxygen have resulted consistently in decreases in PVR of more than 40%. However, both in vitro and in vivo studies have shown that baseline conditions of the lung affect its responsiveness to vasoconstrictors and vasodilators. For example, the effects of CPB and its attendant alteration in the pulmonary circulation may substantially alter the pulmonary bed's responsiveness to high levels of inspired oxygen.

The effect of increasing the inspired oxygen concentration was evaluated in 32 ventilated infants after repair of their congenital heart disease incorporating CPB.[21] When the percentage of inspired oxygen was increased from that in room air to 100%, there was only a trivial decrease in PVR. The lack of pulmonary vasodilating response to oxygen was apparent even in a subgroup of patients with markedly elevated PVR and pulmonary artery hypertension. This lack of responsiveness of the pulmonary vascular bed to oxygen in the immediate postbypass period was in marked contrast to the sensitivity of the pulmonary circuit to changes in pH (Fig. 5–7). The fact that oxygen lost its property as a pulmonary vasodilator in ventilated infants after open heart surgery, even in the presence of moderate alveolar hypoxia and elevated PVR, suggests that CPB may play a significant role in changing the responsiveness of the pulmonary vascular bed to oxygen.

These results may be compared with those from experimental work carried out during the 1980s that suggests an important role of the vascular en-

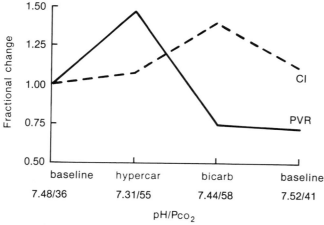

FIGURE 5–7. ☐

Effect of administration of 4 mEq/kg of sodium bicarbonate (bicarb) during mild hypercarbia (hypercar) without change in P_{CO_2}. Note that pulmonary vascular resistance (PVR) falls below the baseline as the pH returns to baseline, even though the P_{CO_2} remains elevated. Thus pH, and not P_{CO_2}, mediates changes in PVR under these conditions.

dothelium in controlling vasomotor tone. The vascular endothelium, in both in vitro and in vivo studies, was found to generate potent diffusible relaxation and contraction factors.[11, 18] Endothelium-derived relaxing factor (EDRF) has been identified as a substance released by the vascular endothelium that results in smooth muscle relaxation of both systemic and pulmonary vessels. Evidence suggests that EDRF may be the free radical nitric oxide, with its precursor being the essential amino acid L-arginine. Moreover, experiments on intact animal lung models suggest that release of EDRF may be responsible for the low PVR in the normal lung and the decreasing PVR in the transitional circulation at birth.

It is possible that the pulmonary vascular endothelium is not sufficiently perfused by its nutrient bronchial circulation during CPB when there is loss of antegrade pulmonary artery flow. Hence, the pulmonary vascular endothelium may suffer an ischemic injury and remain dysfunctional during the first few hours or days after CPB. This hypothesis can be tested by infusing acetylcholine (one of the substances known to release EDRF) into the pulmonary circulation of children before and after CPB. In the presence of endothelial damage, administration of acetylcholine fails to produce vasodilation. Figure 5–8 shows that the potent pulmonary vasodilating properties of acetylcholine administered to patients in the cardiac catheterization laboratory before surgery are altered when the same dose of acetylcholine is infused into the pulmonary artery after CPB. Confirmation that this effect is caused by failure of the endothelium to release nitric oxide (EDRF), not

by the inability of the vascular smooth muscle to relax in response to EDRF, can be verified in patients exposed to inhaled nitric oxide at low concentrations (80 ppm). When inhaled as nitric oxide gas, EDRF may diffuse to pulmonary vascular smooth muscle and cause relaxation.[17] Figure 5–8 also shows the pulmonary vasodilating response to both inhaled nitric oxide and injected acetylcholine in children after CPB. Note the attenuated pulmonary vasodilating response to potent vasodilating doses of acetylcholine. The marked decrease in acetylcholine-induced pulmonary vasodilation after CPB suggests transient pulmonary vascular endothelial dysfunction with consequent failure to release nitric oxide. However, inhaled nitric oxide appears to be a potent pulmonary vasodilator with minimal systemic circulatory side effects because of its unique capacity to avidly bind to hemoglobin once it passes through the smooth muscle endothelial cell barrier to the lumen of the pulmonary blood vessels. Therefore, it becomes inactive when it reaches the systemic circulation. Administration of this agent may have important diagnostic and therapeutic applications in congenital heart disease.

Factors and Actions Influencing Pulmonary Vascular Resistance

The factors and actions affecting PVR can be summarized as follows:

1. *Observation*: Moderate hyperventilation lowers PVR.
   Action: Many repaired postoperative patients benefit from maintenance of Pco_2 at approximately 30 mm Hg. "Permissive hypercapnia" may not be tolerated in these patients if alkaline pH is not maintained. Pulmonary artery pressure may double with Pco_2 at approximately 40 mm Hg.
2. *Observation*: The lowering effect of moderate hypocarbia on PVR is mediated by changes in pH, not Pco_2.
   Action: Metabolic acidosis should be aggressively treated. Metabolic alkalosis with a pH >7.45 minimizes PVR independent of Pco_2.
3. *Observation*: The PVR response to stimuli is intense, but it can be blunted with anesthesia.
   Action: Extend the anesthetic period for labile or fragile patients with continuous infusions of high doses of fentanyl (10 to 20 μg/kg/hr).
4. *Observation*: Appropriate lung volumes are critical in maintaining functional residual capacity and low PVR.
   Action: Recruit alveoli during inspiration with large tidal volume breaths; this reduces hypoxia from ventilation perfusion abnormalities and intrapulmonary shunting.
5. *Observation*: PVR rises with increasing postoperative hematocrit levels, but so does oxygen delivery.
   Action: The optimal hematocrit level may exceed 30%, but a concomitant elevation in PVR may be a limiting factor in the presence of right ventricular dysfunction.
6. *Observation*: PVR tends to increase during the first postoperative night, concurrent with an increase in pulmonary artery pressure and a decrease in cardiac output.

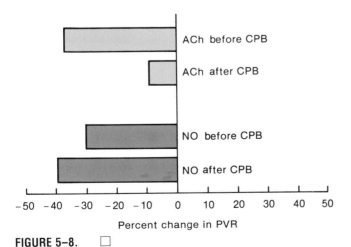

FIGURE 5–8. □

Percentage reduction in pulmonary vascular resistance (PVR) with acetylcholine in preoperative patients is attenuated in postoperative patients despite the retained ability of such patients to vasodilate with inhaled nitric oxide (80 ppm). (From Wessel DL, Adatia I, Giglia TM, Thompson JE, Kulik TJ. Use of inhaled nitric oxide and acetylcholine in the evaluation of pulmonary hypertension and endothelial function after cardiopulmonary bypass. Circulation 88:2128, 1993.)

Action: Inotropic support with afterload reduction is indicated. Amrinone is a frequent second choice of inotropic drug after dopamine, even in neonates.

7. *Observation*: Oxygen is an ineffective pulmonary vasodilator after CPB. pH and P_{CO_2} are important modulators of PVR.

   Action: Prolonged use of high FiO_2 to decrease elevated PVR is discouraged.

8. *Observation*: Pulmonary vascular endothelial dysfunction after CPB is common.

   Action: This may account for the lack of response to FiO_2 and define causes of unexpected or unpredicted pathophysiologic events after CPB. Inhaled nitric oxide (EDRF) is a potent pulmonary vasodilator with minimal systemic effects in selected patients.

PULMONARY VASCULAR RESISTANCE IN THE PATIENT WITH A SINGLE VENTRICLE

Lowering PVR and decreasing right ventricular afterload are useful objectives in patients with repaired, two-ventricle, in-series circulations where pulmonary venous blood is ejected into the systemic circulation and systemic oxygenation depends primarily on the efficiency of gas exchange in the lungs. In contrast, patients with single-ventricle physiology present very different circumstances that require an understanding of oxygenation and the hemodynamics of a circulation arranged in parallel rather than in series. Under certain circumstances, decreasing PVR in these patients may adversely and significantly affect hemodynamics.

Single-ventricle physiology may include many anatomic variants, but all are governed by a common physiologic principle: desaturated systemic venous blood returns to the heart and mixes completely with oxygenated blood returning to the same chamber from the lungs. In the absence of lung disease, the pulmonary venous blood, with oxygen saturations of 95% to 100%, enters the single ventricle and mixes with systemic venous blood having saturations of 55% to 60% or less, depending on the amount of oxygen extraction in the periphery. If pulmonary and systemic blood flows are equal (i.e., QP/QS = 1), the resultant "mixed" systemic oxygen saturation varies from 75% to 80%. As the pulmonary blood flow increases in proportion to systemic flow, the systemic oxygen saturation rises. Consequently, an arterial oxygen saturation of 90% is achieved at the expense of excessive pulmonary blood flow (QP/QS > 3) and, hence, a substantial volume load to the single ventricle, which is required to supply all systemic and pulmonary blood flow (pulmonary flow is three times systemic flow). If both the pulmonary artery and the aorta are anatomically related to the single ventricle and there is

no obstruction, flow to the pulmonary and systemic beds will be partitioned according to the relative resistances of each circuit (i.e., parallel circulations). As the PVR falls below the SVR during the first few hours of life, pulmonary blood flow increases relative to systemic flow, and systemic arterial oxygen saturation increases to more than 80%. Therefore, systemic oxygen saturation becomes a convenient marker of QP/QS. The effects of changes in QP/QS on systemic arterial oxygen saturation for common mixing lesions are shown in Figure 5–9.

The deleterious effects of lungs perfused at high pressure and flows, combined with the adverse effects of volume overload on the neonatal heart (which is less capable of increasing stroke volume in response to increasing preload) lead to hyperdynamic congestive heart failure in which systemic perfusion and oxygen delivery are compromised despite the elevated arterial oxygen saturation. As PVR decreases, the myocardium ultimately fails to provide adequate systemic flow, and more and more of the stroke volume is inefficiently recirculated through the lungs. Therefore, treatment must be aimed at increasing PVR, balancing pulmonary and systemic blood flow ratios, and maintaining adequate systemic blood flow. If there is moderate anatomic obstruction to pulmonary blood flow, the previous scenario does not occur but in cases of extreme pulmonary outflow tract obstruction, QP/QS may become less than 1, with cyanosis progressing as pulmonary blood flow continues to fall. Similarly, high PVR even in the absence of anatomic obstruction will diminish pulmonary blood flow, and as the PVR exceeds SVR, arterial oxygen saturation de-

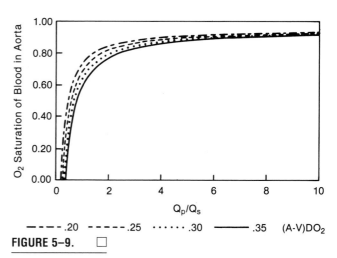

FIGURE 5–9. ☐

Physiology of common mixing (single ventricle) showing an increase in the pulmonary-to-systemic blood flow ratio associated with rising aortic oxygen saturation for any given arteriovenous oxygen gradient (A-V)DO₂.

creases, more profound cyanosis ensues, and systemic oxygen delivery may be inadequate despite improvement in systemic blood flow.

Consequently, the balance between pulmonary and systemic blood flow is the key factor in promoting adequate systemic oxygen delivery. Because PVR must ultimately be low for a patient to qualify for a Fontan procedure, maintaining a high PVR cannot be employed perpetually to achieve the desired balance between PVR and SVR. When pulmonary blood flow is limited in the neonate and young infant, an increase in pulmonary blood flow is most commonly accomplished with a modified Blalock-Taussig shunt. The fixed resistance imposed by the shunt adds to the variability of PVR. Although 3.5- or 4-mm shunts offer considerable resistance to flow when compared with an unobstructed pulmonary artery arising from a single ventricle (or a right ventricle with a large unrestrictive VSD), the origin of pulmonary blood flow from the high-pressure systemic artery permits flow to continue throughout diastole. As PVR falls, shunt flow during systole and diastole may together produce excessive pulmonary blood flow. Consequently, maneuvers to regulate PVR in patients with a systemic-to–pulmonary artery shunt may still prove effective at modifying hemodynamics. This is especially important if the patient has undergone CPB as part of the surgical procedure (e.g., a first-stage operation for hypoplastic left heart syndrome) and ventricular function is transiently depressed or more susceptible to the hemodynamic burden of a volume load, diminished myocardial perfusion pressure, and changes in oxygenation.

Single-ventricle physiology is often characterized by either excessive or diminished pulmonary blood flow. Whenever the pulmonary blood flow is exclusively shunt dependent, the aortic oxygen saturation is directly related to the flow and the perfusion pressure across the shunt and also to the PVR. If the pulmonary blood flow is excessive, the physician must attempt to raise the PVR and lower the SVR or, if necessary, modify the shunt. If pulmonary blood flow is diminished, the PVR must be lowered, the SVR increased, and systemic blood pressure raised. Any mechanical obstruction to pulmonary blood flow either across the shunt or within the mediastinal or intraparenchymal pulmonary arteries must be corrected.

The eventual "reparative" operation for infants with a single ventricle is one of the modifications of the Fontan procedure (see Chapter 15). The benefits from an in-series circuit in these patients include improved systemic oxygenation and a reduction in the obligatory diastolic load borne by any ventricle that is required to fill systemic and pulmonary circuits simultaneously.

Although the subtleties of the "Fontan physiology" are complex and incompletely understood, there are several basic tenets that are accepted in the postoperative management of these patients. The two most important features in the hemodynamics of infants after a Fontan operation are PVR and left atrial pressure, which in turn reflects the diastolic properties of the single ventricle and the function of the systemic atrioventricular (AV) valve. The forces impelling systemic blood from the right atrium through the lungs and the left heart may be counteracted by an elevated end-diastolic pressure; AV valve regurgitation or stenosis; loss of sinus rhythm with retrograde P waves and cannon a waves, which raise left atrial pressure; pulmonary vein stenosis; elevated pulmonary arteriolar resistance; stenotic pulmonary arteries; or cavopulmonary anastomotic narrowing. As might be expected, these children are exquisitely sensitive to changes in PVR and have a very limited ability to compensate for such changes. However, unlike a parallel circuit in which increased PVR results in hypoxemia, a Fontan in-series circuit manifests increased PVR with reduced cardiac output because of limited return to the systemic ventricle. The common causes of increased PVR in the immediate postoperative period include transient and reversible mechanical and blood-borne factors related to CPB, physiologic changes wrought by hypoxia, hypercarbia or acidosis, and the physical changes in the pulmonary artery bed created by excessive positive airway pressure and positive end-expiratory pressure (PEEP) or extrinsic pulmonary compression (e.g., pleural effusion, hemothorax, pneumothorax). Fenestration of the atrial baffle allows for systemic venous decompression while PVR is transiently high. Systemic perfusion is thus preserved. Studies at Children's Hospital in Boston have demonstrated that not only are cardiac output and oxygen delivery improved with fenestration, but also the incidence of pleural effusions has decreased to 9%, and the hospital mortality rate in an increasingly high-risk group of patients has also decreased to less than 5%. The fenestration can be tested with a balloon catheter and closed in the cardiac catheterization laboratory with a clamshell device later in the postoperative period (see Chapter 7).

While pulmonary blood flow is phasic to a certain extent, a substantial proportion of flow occurs during diastole as well. Therefore, the diastolic or relaxation characteristics of the ventricle play an important role in regulating the volume of pulmonary blood flow and, hence, the preload accepted by the ventricle. Consequently, diastolic dysfunction causes low cardiac output. The diastolic properties of the single ventricle are influenced by the preoperative volume and altered ventricular geometry in addition to postoperative events that can aggravate diastolic dysfunction, such as AV valve dysfunction or persistent left-to-right shunts. When the preoperative diastolic load has resulted in ventricular dysfunction (i.e., elevated ventricular end-diastolic pressure), the risks of inadequate ventricular relaxation after a Fontan operation increase substantially. Postoperatively, the output of the single ventricle must meet only the demands of the systemic circuit and thus end-diastolic volume is substantially reduced. As the end-diastolic volume decreases, an alteration in ventricular geometry takes place. In some children, the resulting smaller, hypertrophic ventricle exhibits diastolic dysfunction that was not present at higher end-diastolic volumes. In other instances a subaortic obstruction may appear across a bulboventricular foramen that was unobstructed preoperatively.

Therapeutic manipulations are often not successful in reversing this diastolic dysfunction once it is manifest. In the presence of a low cardiac output, inotropic drugs may not improve hemodynamics and may actually worsen diastolic relaxation, particularly if epinephrine is used in large doses. Similarly, vasodilators reduce ventricular volume. While this is beneficial in diastolic dysfunction, it may exacerbate the problem if there is a small end-diastolic volume. Therefore, intravascular volume must be maintained or augmented to avoid additional reductions in end-diastolic volume. Pharmacologic agents that promote ventricular relaxation (e.g., beta blockers, calcium entry blockers, nitroglycerine) are of theoretic, but as yet limited, clinical benefit in this situation. The potential diastolic benefit of amrinone may prove of greater value.

RESPIRATORY CARE

As previously noted, ventilation and respiratory mechanics exert powerful influences on the hemodynamics of neonates and infants undergoing palliative or reparative operation for congenital heart disease.[33] We seek to remove the uncertainty of gas exchange achieved by spontaneous breathing during the immediate postoperative period and instead use mechanical ventilation, end-expiratory pressure, and manipulation of Pco_2 and pH to influence cardiopulmonary functions.

Intubation of the trachea in the CICU in an awake neonate or infant with congenital heart disease may elicit major hemodynamic and metabolic responses. Therefore, appropriate anesthetic and muscle relaxant techniques should be used to secure the airway. This substantially facilitates the procedure, especially in a fragile postoperative patient who requires reintubation. This maneuver demands an appropriate level of expertise in anesthetic principles and practice on the part of CICU practitioners.

To ensure selected preset mechanical minute ventilation, even through changing pulmonary mechanics, several issues require emphasis. Nasotracheal intubation is preferred, because it provides greater stability of the airway than does orotracheal intubation. A close-fitting endotracheal tube should be selected that permits air to leak at pressures of 25 to 35 cm H_2O. Using this approach we have not had any case of tracheal stenosis requiring tracheostomy in 132 consecutive cardiac patients requiring long-term intubation and staying more than 28 days in the ICU.

Ventilator tubing with an internal diameter of 15 to 25 mm and a wall thickness of 2.4 mm minimizes the compressible volume within the breathing system. Tubing lengths of approximately 40 cm with water traps to remove condensed water vapor (which otherwise collects in the tubing lumen and impedes gas flow) result in a system-compressible volume of 1.1 to 1.5 ml/cm H_2O.

Volume-preset mechanical ventilators are used to achieve mechanical minute ventilation. Warm, filtered, and humidified gas is delivered by the mechanical ventilator. An important consideration in the neonate or young infant is the modification of volume-limited ventilators to allow for continuous flow, which eliminates the work of breathing required to open the inspiratory valve on these machines. This modification requires larger bore tubing to minimize expiratory retard in continuous-flow circuits. Larger bore tubing, in turn, reintroduces the hazards of larger compression volumes that in neonates may approximate or exceed the actual delivered tidal volume. Consequently, sudden changes in lung compliance may result in a significant loss of minute ventilation in the neonate despite the use of volume-preset ventilators. Unlike the older child, the neonate may lose considerable tidal volume when lung compliance changes suddenly and peak inspiratory pressure rises. Equipping the ventilator to sound an alarm when specified peak inspiratory pressures are exceeded is important. It demands that an analysis of the cause be conducted and appropriate action taken.

The mechanical ventilator frequency is set at 12 to 20 breaths/min, the higher values used in neonates. Initially a tidal volume is selected that, by inspection, produces significant movement of the chest wall. The peak inspiratory pressure generated frequently exceeds 25 cm H_2O. Subsequent adjustments, usually in frequency, are guided by the Pa_{CO_2}.

Caution must be used while suctioning the airway in infants during the immediate postoperative period. Increasing airway pressure, diminished motion of the chest wall, visible blood, or blood-tinged or large amounts of normal-appearing secretions in the artificial airway are clear indications to perform this maneuver. Suctioning of the airway is a stressful event that can have a serious adverse effect on hemodynamics. Consequently, we extend the anesthetic period through the first postoperative night in selected patients in an attempt to blunt the pulmonary hypertensive response to this and other external stimuli.

Postoperatively, mechanical ventilation is continued until hemostasis is complete and hemodynamic evaluation reveals a sinus node–initiated or pacemaker-protected heart rate within the 95% confidence limits for age; strong peripheral pulses; capillary refill of <3 seconds; warm distal extremities; an arterial wave form consistent with adequate stroke volume; core temperature <38°C; and no evidence of metabolic acidosis, uncontrolled seizures, or thick, copious secretions. The breath frequency of the mechanical ventilation is decreased until spontaneous breathing begins, noting the patient's respiratory rate and effort along with the hemodynamic effect of weaning. Guided by physical examination, hemodynamic criteria, and arterial blood gas measurements, mechanical ventilatory breath frequency is reduced to <5 breaths/min before the child is extubated. If a patient fails to tolerate spontaneous respiration and weaning from mechanical ventilation using the technique just described, a search for any residual hemodynamic cause must be initiated. Echocardiography serves to identify residual structural abnormalities remaining after surgery or abnormalities that have arisen as a result of the palliation or repair. If echocardiography is inconclusive, the patient is subjected to cardiac catheterization. Noncardiovascular causes of respiratory failure can be broadly grouped into neuromuscular and central nervous system disorders, airway abnormalities proximal to the alveoli, alveolar disease, and compression of lung volume by extrapulmonary factors (e.g., pleural effusion and pneumothorax). Depression of the respiratory center occurs most commonly as a result of the administration of analgesics, sedative hypnotics, or anesthetics. In our experience, ischemic, hypoxic injury to the respiratory center is an unusual cause for disordered respiratory control but occasionally can be a contributing factor.

Diaphragmatic paralysis or paresis caused by injury to the phrenic nerve may precipitate and maintain respiratory failure, particularly in the neonate or young infant, who relies on diaphragmatic function for breathing to a greater extent than do older infants and children, who can recruit accessory and intercostal muscles if diaphragmatic function proves inadequate. A conventional chest radiograph revealing a high hemidiaphragm, especially on the left, should arouse suspicion of diaphragmatic dysfunction. However, this may be masked by positive-pressure ventilation. Ultrasonography or fluoroscopy is useful for identifying diaphragmatic motion or paradoxic excursion. Reversible phrenic nerve injury with recovery of diaphragmatic contraction usually occurs. However, if a patient fails to tolerate repeated extubations, despite maximal cardiovascular and nutritional support, and diaphragmatic dysfunction persists with volume loss in the affected lung, the diaphragm should be surgically plicated. Negative-pressure ventilation has been a useful adjunct in the treatment of these infants and may shorten the period of intubation and positive-pressure ventilation.

Diminished conductance or increased airway resistance arises from several pathologic changes alone or in combination: excessive secretions; swelling of the mucosa as a result of hyperemia or edema, most often resulting from trauma or infection; hyperactive bronchial smooth muscle; or extrinsic compression by neighboring structures. Patients who have secretions from the tracheal aspirate with many visible organisms and polymorphonuclear cells on microscopy, together with fever, an elevated white cell count, or consolidation on the chest radiograph require treatment with appropriate antibiotics. In the presence of mucosal swelling, a nebulized, inhaled alpha agonist promotes vasoconstriction and decreases hyperemia and possibly edema. If bronchospasm is suspected, inhaled or systemically administered bronchodilators may be considered but must be used with caution in light of their tachyarrhythmic potential. If all of these maneuvers fail to improve the patient, the minimum tidal volume and frequency that provide sufficient mechanical minute ventilation to satisfactorily supplement spontaneous ventilation and minimize overinflation of the lungs are determined and used during the recovery phase.

Pulmonary edema, pneumonia, and atelectasis are the most common causes of lower airway and alveolar abnormalities that interfere with gas exchange. If a bacterial pathogen is identified, therapy includes antibiotics; if the cause is pulmonary edema, maintenance of good hemodynamics and, thus, low pulmonary venous pressures is required;

if a cardiogenic basis for increased extrapulmonary water exists, fluid should be restricted and inotropic and diuretic therapy begun. For infants, fluid restriction is frequently incompatible with adequate nutrition, and therefore, an aggressive diuretic regimen is preferable to restriction of caloric intake. Adjustment of end-expiratory pressure and mechanical ventilation serve as supportive therapies until the alveoli and pulmonary interstitium are cleared of the fluid that interferes with gas entry.

Pleural effusions and, less often, ascites may occur in patients after a Fontan operation or tetralogy of Fallot repair. Fluid in the pleural space or peritoneum and intestinal distention compete with intrapulmonary gas for thoracic space. Evacuation of the pleural space or drainage of ascites and decompression of the intestinal lumen allow the intrapulmonary gas volume to increase.

COAGULATION

In the operating room protamine is administered after CPB to reverse the effects of heparin. Continued blood loss in the CICU dictates the need for adequate drainage from the mediastinum to avoid cardiac tamponade while correcting a persistent coagulopathy. Rising atrial pressures, tachycardia, a narrow pulse pressure, hypotension, and poor perfusion are the hallmarks of tamponade. The presence of a draining mediastinal tube does not guarantee protection against this complication. Timely exploration by opening the sternotomy incision in the CICU can provide immediate decompression of the pericardial space and restoration of cardiac output. Transmural pressure and myocardial performance may be optimized in unstable patients by opening the sternum, without significantly increasing the risk of infection. Several risk factors tend to promote persistent hemorrhage, including preoperative cyanosis and polycythemia, reoperation, and multiple suture lines. Both component therapy and fresh whole blood (<24 hours old) are, in most instances, effective in overcoming coagulation disorders. In newborns fresh whole blood ensures that the proper balance of formed and nonformed elements is administered and also avoids the vascular depression that may occur from accumulation of vasodepressant mediators in stored blood.[41] Dilutional and mechanical effects of CPB on platelets may justify the need for platelet transfusion. Additional protamine may be administered to ensure complete reversal of any heparin effect if the partial thromboplastin time (PTT) is elevated. In addition the prothrombin time (PT), thrombin time (TT), fibrinogen levels, platelet counts, bleeding time, and

heparin level can prove useful in discerning the cause of bleeding.[35] Re-exploration of the mediastinum is indicated when there is a persistent or a sudden increase of blood draining from the chest tubes. Evacuation of large amounts of blood or clots is advisable even if the patient remains hemodynamically stable. In our experience, the incidence of reoperation for postoperative bleeding is less than 1%. We prefer to take sufficient time to obtain hemostasis before administering heparin after CPB, and before closing the chest incision.

FLUID, ELECTROLYTES, AND URINE OUTPUT

In general, hourly urine volumes bear a close relation to cardiac output after CPB, provided that the child does not receive diuretics during the immediate postoperative period, when hemodynamics remain uncertain. If urine flow decreases but physical examination and laboratory findings reveal a satisfactory cardiac output, the diminished urine flow is most likely due to hormones whose release is triggered by CPB as well as other interventions. If evidence of good hemodynamic function persists, limited urine flow (1 ml/kg/hr) is acceptable during the first night. Administration of tubular diuretics is not likely to alter the course of vasomotor nephropathy, which may have resulted from diminished perfusion of the kidneys during CPB or subsequent hemodynamic instability, and therefore, diuretics are not indicated solely on the basis of diminished urine flow in the immediate postoperative period. Because of the large water and salt load from crystalloid dilution on CPB, 5% dextrose solutions at half maintenance rates are prescribed during the first postoperative night. However, the large increase in total body water that a neonate can accumulate during CPB can be as high as 600 to 1000 gm. This may be reflected in increased edema of the chest wall, lung, or myocardium, causing decreased total lung compliance and higher cardiac filling pressures. Therefore, diuretics are used after the first night to hasten the elimination of accumulated extravascular water, recognizing that diuretic-induced electrolyte imbalances may occur.[36] If several days of forced diuresis have resulted in a hypochloremic metabolic alkalosis, potassium chloride is supplemented. Intravenous administration of potassium chloride requires precise nursing protocols and an appreciation for the arrythmogenic potential of rapid administration.

When serum chloride levels remain within normal range and alkalosis with high total serum bicarbonate levels persists, treatment with acetazolamide and attempts to decrease the formation of

HCO_3 from carbon dioxide and water should be pursued. There appear to be two potential clinical justifications for this approach. One is for the mechanically ventilated patient who remains alkalotic and in whom a low respiratory rate and minimal respiratory drive persist despite adequate wakefulness and whose Pco_2 is high enough ($Pco_2 > 60$) to affect endogenous catecholamine production and, perhaps, caloric expenditure or unwanted changes in cerebral hemodynamics. Acetazolamide therapy may also be indicated for the ventilator-dependent patient whose total bicarbonate level approaches or exceeds 40 mEq/L with a normal or increased respiratory rate and in whom a trial of extubation is anticipated. These patients typically have increased work of breathing with moderately compensated congestive heart failure on digoxin therapy, a Pco_2 of 60 mm Hg with a normal pH, and serum potassium levels that are periodically low, despite aggressive replacement therapy. If such a patient is then extubated and later observed to have increased respiratory distress and judged to need reintubation and mechanical ventilation, it is important not to hyperventilate the patient once the artificial airway is re-established. It is a common tendency to initially hyperventilate a patient who has just been intubated, thus driving the Pco_2 to the low 30s or high 20s. In such a patient the pH will approach 7.7, the serum potassium will shift into cells, hypotension from positive-pressure ventilation will prompt the administration of calcium, and the cell membrane potential will destabilize. The alkalotic, hypokalemic, hypercalcemic, hypotensive, dilated, digoxin-bound myocardium fibrillates with ease. Treating these patients expectantly with acetazolamide before extubation or avoiding mechanical hyperventilation during reintubation are reasonable options.

NUTRITION

Enteral nutrition is usually begun on the day after cardiac surgery unless bowel dysfunction exists. Ideally, caloric intake should reach 100 to 130 cal/kg/day in infants who weigh <10 kg until they are weaned from mechanical ventilation. Although the enteral route is preferred, parenteral nutrition is necessary in nearly half of neonates after cardiac surgery. Balancing carbohydrate administration with lipids is important, not only for caloric reasons, but also because it permits a respiratory quotient that avoids exclusive carbohydrate metabolism and the associated carbon dioxide production.

THE FUTURE OF CARDIAC INTENSIVE CARE

By 1990, advances in interventional cardiology had eliminated many of the simple short-term surgical admissions to our cardiac intensive care unit. Increasingly, patent ductus arteriosus ligations, closure of atrial septal defects and muscular VSDs, pulmonary and aortic valvotomies, and reoperations for coarctation repairs became management issues for the catheterization laboratory and regular ward, or even outpatient services at Children's Hospital in Boston. Nonetheless, annual admissions to the CICU increased to nearly 1200 during this period. The complexity of cases increased dramatically as the average length of stay rose to 5.5 days. Surgical technique and perioperative diagnosis and management improved measurably as mortality declined from 10% to 4.5% among surgical patients in the CICU, despite the increased proportion of cases such as complex single ventricle, transposition of the great arteries, and difficult aortic arch abnormalities.

We have benefited from a collaborative effort that has emphasized integration of specialized personnel into a cardiovascular program in which the patient with congenital heart disease is the center of attention while traditional departmental or specialty boundaries are much less important. This teamwork philosophy has promoted the development of non-operative interventional techniques, emphasized an expanded role for specialized nursing, and confirmed the value of surgical training and presence on the ICU team. The evolution of cardiovascular intensive care focusing on the neonate and infant requires staff members who are broadly trained in pediatric cardiology, anesthetic principles, and critical care and who are joined by their surgical colleagues to treat all patients in the ICU regardless of their traditional medical or surgical disposition.

The scenario for the sickest patients in the ICU is increasingly driven by technology. The open chest is covered with Silastic, and new, expensive drugs are infused for inotropic support, arrhythmia control, resistance to infections, and total nutrition. Prolonged anesthesia with mechanical ventilation and continuous monitoring of the airway and of multiple vascular pressures are routine activities. Increasingly, advanced forms of atrioventricular sequential pacing are utilized. When the kidneys or liver fail, dialysis or plasmapheresis is employed. Ventricular assist devices or ECMO are used when the heart or lungs fail. In some patients, an organ may even be replaced by another, all at spectacular costs. In fiscal year 1990, 35,000 arterial blood gas analyses were performed on the 1200 cardiac patients admitted to Children's Hospital in Boston. However, this $500,000 expense was dwarfed by costs in personnel and other chargeable items.

In 1986, the total cost of care in ICUs in the United States was estimated at 20% of all inpatient hospital costs, and it amounted to $33.9 billion, an amount approaching 1% of the gross national product. ICU costs vary from two to four times that of a regular ward bed, and in pediatric centers, these costs appear to vary directly with the severity of illness.[37] Use of ICU beds is higher in the United States than in other countries, and the annual growth in the ratio of ICU days to total patient days is steadily increasing.[32] Undoubtedly, necessary attempts at limiting these rising costs will require modification of physician and nurse practice patterns and incorporation of cost awareness into the treatment plan. Educational policies for trainees that address efficiencies in the delivery of health care must also be developed. Education of practitioners with regard to costs associated with the ordering and execution of tests and the use of supplies will increase awareness and help establish a basis for monitoring and accountability of an individual practitioner's use of resources. We must continue to develop safe and effective alternative therapies for congenital heart disease that minimize hospital admissions and the need for critical care beds.[39] Thoracoscopic and transcatheter interventional techniques may offer some hope for cost reduction if patient days in the ICU can be reduced. Some have maintained that the development of less expensive alternatives to intensive care, such as intermediate care (for patients at low risk for mortality who require long-term technical or intensive nursing assistance) is a potentially important cost-savings idea. Certainly we must become more proficient with rigorous institutional reviews of patient outcome and practice patterns. This analysis must provide a rational basis for determining individual patient prognosis among critically ill patients so that resources can be allocated appropriately.

Organization of cost containment and development of financial strategies must be an integral part of critical care planning for the future. The 1990s and early 21st century will demand more responsible and difficult analysis of costs and benefits in the intensive care unit.

REFERENCES

1. Anand KJS, Hansen DD, Hickey PR. Hormonal-metabolic stress response in neonates undergoing cardiac surgery. Anesthesiology 73:661, 1990.
2. Anand KJS, Hickey PR. Halothane-morphine compared with high-dose sufentanil for anesthesia and postoperative analgesia in neonatal cardiac surgery. N Engl J Med 361:1, 1992.
3. Anand KJS, Sippell WG, Aynsley-Green A, et al. Randomized trial of fentanyl anesthesia in preterm neonates undergoing surgery: effects on the stress response. Lancet 1:243, 1987.
4. Bohn DJ, Poirer CS, Demonds JF. Efficacy of dopamine, dobutamine and epinephrine during emergence from cardiopulmonary bypass in children. Crit Care Med 8:367, 1980.
5. Caspi J, Coles JG, Benson LN, et al. Age-related response to epinephrine-induced myocardial stress. A functional and ultrastructural study. Circulation 84(suppl III):III-394, 1991.
6. Castaneda AR, Mayer JE, Jonas RA, et al. The neonate with critical congenital heart disease. Repair—a surgical challenge. J Thorac Cardiovasc Surg 98:869, 1989.
7. Chang AC, Hanley FL, Lock JE, et al. Management and outcome of low birthweight neonates with congenital heart disease. J Pediatr. In press.
8. Clapp S, Perry BL, Farooki ZQ, et al. Down's syndrome, complete atrioventricular canal, and pulmonary vascular obstructive disease. J Thorac Cardiovasc Surg 100:115, 1990.
9. Del Nido PJ, Williams WG, Villamater J, et al. Changes in pericardial surface pressure during pulmonary hypertensive crises after cardiac surgery. Circulation 76(suppl III):III-93, 1987.
10. Delius RE, Bove EL, Meliones JN, et al. Use of extracorporeal life support in patients with congenital heart disease. Crit Care Med 20:1216, 1992.
11. Dinh-Xuan AT, Higenbottam TW, Clelland C, et al. Impairment of endothelium-dependent relaxation in patients with Eisenmenger's syndrome. Br J Pharm 99:9, 1990.
12. Driscoll DJ, Gillette PC, Lewis RM, et al. Comparative hemodynamic effects of isoproterenol, dopamine, and dobutamine in the newborn dog. Pediatr Res 13:1006, 1979.
13. Drummond WH, Gregory GA, Heyman MA, et al. The independent effects of hyperventilation, tolazoline, and dopamine in infants with persistent pulmonary hypertension. J Pediatr 98:603, 1981.
14. Feltes TF, Hansen TN. Effects of an aorticopulmonary shunt on lung fluid balance in the young lamb. Pediatr Res 26:94, 1989.
15. Fisher DJ, Heymann MA, Rudolph AM. Fetal myocardial oxygen and carbohydrate consumption during acutely induced hypoxemia. Am J Physiol 242:H657, 1982.
16. Friedman WF, George BL. Treatment of congestive heart failure by altering loading conditions of the heart. J Pediatr 106:697, 1985.
17. Frostell C, Fratacci MD, Wain JC, et al. Inhaled nitric oxide. A selective pulmonary vasodilator reversing hypoxic pulmonary vasoconstriction. Circulation 83:2038, 1991.
18. Furchgott RF, Zawadzki JV. The obligatory role of endothelial cells in the relaxation of arterial smooth muscle by acetylcholine. Nature 288:373, 1980.
19. Fyler DC. Trends. In Fyler DC (ed). Nadas' Pediatric Cardiology. Philadelphia, Hanley & Belfus, 1992, pp 273–280.
20. Gidding SS. Pulse oximetry in cyanotic congenital heart disease. Am J Cardiol 70:391, 1992.
21. Giglia TM, Wessel DL. Effects of oxygen on pulmonary and systemic hemodynamics in infants after cardiopulmonary bypass. Circulation 82(suppl III):III-78, 1990.
22. Gold JP, Jonas RA, Lang P, et al. Transthoracic intracardiac monitoring lines in pediatric surgical patients: A ten-year experience. Ann Thorac Surg 42:185, 1986.
23. Habib DM, Padbury JF, Anas NG, et al. Dobutamine pharmacokinetics and pharmacodynamics in pediatric intensive care patients. Crit Care Med 20:601, 1992.
24. Hanley FL, Heinemann MK, Jonas RA, et al. Neonatal repair of truncus arteriosus. J Thorac Cardiovasc Surg 105:1047, 1993.
25. Hashimoto K, Miyamoto H, Suzuki K, et al. Evidence of organ damage after cardiopulmonary bypass. The role of elastase and vasoactive mediators. J Thorac Cardiovasc Surg 104:666, 1992.
26. Haworth SG. Pulmonary vascular disease in different types of congenital heart disease. Implications for interpretation of lung biopsy findings in early childhood. Br Heart J 52:557, 1984.
27. Hickey PR, Hansen DD, Wessel DL, et al. Blunting of stress responses in the pulmonary circulation in infants. Anesth Analg 64:1137, 1985.
28. Hickey PR, Hansen DD, Wessel DL, et al. Pulmonary and systemic hemodynamic responses to fentanyl in infants. Anesth Analg 64:483, 1985.
29. Hickey PR, Hansen DD. Fentanyl and sufentanil-oxygen-

pancuronium anesthesia for cardiac surgery in infants. Anesth Analg 63:117, 1984.

30. Hickey PR, Hansen DD. Pulmonary hypertension in infants; postoperative management. In Yacoub M (ed). Annual of Cardiac Surgery. London, Current Science, 1989, pp 16–22.

31. Hoffman JIE, Rudolph AM, Heymann MA. Pulmonary vascular disease with congenital heart lesions: Pathologic features and causes. Circulation 64:873, 1981.

32. Jacobs P, Noseworthy TW. National estimates of intensive care utilization and costs: Canada and the United States. Crit Care Med 18:1282, 1990.

33. Jenkins J, Lynn A, Edmonds J, et al. Effects of mechanical ventilation on cardiopulmonary function in children after open-heart surgery. Crit Care Med 13:77, 1985.

34. Jones ODH, Shore DF, Rigby ML, et al. The use of tolazoline hydrochloride as a pulmonary vasodilator in potentially fatal episodes of pulmonary vasoconstriction after cardiac surgery in children. Circulation 64:134, 1981.

35. Kern FH, Morana NJ, Sears JJ, et al. Coagulation defects in neonates during cardiopulmonary bypass. Ann Thorac Surg 54:541, 1992.

36. Khilnani P. Electrolyte abnormalities in critically ill children. Crit Care Med 20:241, 1992.

37. Klem SA, Pollack MM, Getson PR. Cost, resource utilization, and severity of illness in intensive care. J Pediatr 116:231, 1990.

38. Lang P, Chipman CW, Siden M. Early assessment of hemodynamic status after repair of tetralogy of Fallot: A comparison of 24 hour and one year postoperative data in 98 patients. Am J Cardiol 58:795, 1982.

39. Lawless S, Zaritsky A, Phipps J, et al. Characteristics of pediatric intermediate care units in pediatric training programs. Crit Care Med 19:1004, 1991.

40. Lyrene RK, Welch KA, Godoy G, et al. Alkalosis attenuates hypoxic pulmonary vasoconstriction in neonatal lambs. Pediatr Res 19:1268, 1985.

41. Manno CS, Hedberg KW, Kim HC, et al. Comparison of the hemostatic effects of fresh whole blood, stored whole blood and components after open heart surgery in children. Blood 77:930, 1991.

42. Mansell A, Bryan C, Levinson H. Airway closure in children. J Appl Physiol 33:711, 1972.

43. Mills AN, Haworth SG. Greater permeability of the neonatal lung: Postnatal changes in surface charge and biochemistry of porcine pulmonary capillary endothelium. J Thorac Cardiovasc Surg 101:909, 1991.

44. Moler FW, Custer JR, Bartlett RH, et al. Extracorporeal life support for pediatric respiratory failure. Crit Care Med 20:1112, 1992.

45. Morray JP, Lynn AM, Mansfield PB. Effects of pH and PCO_2 on pulmonary and systemic hemodynamics after surgery in children with congenital heart disease and pulmonary hypertension. J Pediatr 113:474, 1988.

46. Newburger JW, Jonas RA, Wernovsky G, et al. Perioperative neurologic effects of hypothermic arrest during infant heart surgery. The Boston Circulatory Arrest Study. N Engl J Med. In press.

47. Pae WE, Miller CA, Matthews Y, et al. Ventricular assist devices for postcardiotomy cardiogenic shock. A combined registry experience. J Thorac Cardiovasc Surg 104:541, 1992.

48. Rabinovitch R, Haworth SG, Castaneda AR, et al. Lung biopsy in congenital heart disease: A morphometric approach to pulmonary vascular disease. Circulation 58:1107, 1978.

49. Reller MD, Morton MJ, Giraud GD, et al. Severe right ventricular pressure loading in fetal sheep augments global myocardial blood flow to submaximal levels. Circulation 86:581, 1992.

50. Romero TE, Friedman WF. Limited left ventricular response to volume overload in the neonatal period: A comparative study with the adult animal. Pediatr Res 13:910, 1979.

51. Rudolph AM, Yuan S. Response of the pulmonary vasculature to hypoxia and H+ ion concentration changes. J Clin Invest 45:399, 1966.

52. Schranz D, Zepp F, Iversen S, et al. Effects of tolazoline and prostacyclin on pulmonary hypertension in infants after cardiac surgery. Crit Care Med 20:1243, 1992.

53. Shah AR, Kurth CD, Gwiazdowski SG, et al. Fluctuations in cerebral oxygenation and blood volume during endotracheal suctioning in premature infants. J Pediatr 120:769, 1992.

54. Thornburg KL, Morton MJ. Filling and arterial pressure as determinants of RV stroke volume in the sheep fetus. Am J Physiol 244:H656, 1983.

55. Wernovsky G, Giglia TM, Jonas RA, et al. Course in the intensive care unit after preparatory pulmonary artery banding and aortopulmonary shunt placement for transposition of the great arteries with low left ventricular pressure. Circulation 86(suppl II):II-133, 1992.

56. Wernovsky G, Jonas RA, Newburger JW, et al. The Boston Circulatory Arrest Study. Hemodynamics and hospital course after the arterial switch operation. Circulation 86(suppl I):I-237, 1992.

57. Wessel DL, Anand KJS, Hickey PR. Catecholamine and hemodynamic responses to hypercarbia in infants. Anesthesiology 69:A780, 1988.

58. Wessel DL, Elixson EM, Hansen DD, et al. A double lumen transthoracic pulmonary artery catheter for measurement of cardiac output in infants and neonates. Anesthesiology 69:A233, 1988.

59. Wessel DL, Hickey PR, Hansen DD, et al. Prostaglandin metabolism and pulmonary vascular response to changes in PCO_2 in infants. Pediatr Res 21:214A, 1987.

60. Wessel DL, Hickey PR, Hansen DD. Pulmonary and systemic hemodynamic effects of hyperventilation in infants after repair of congenital heart disease. Anesthesiology 67:A526, 1987.

61. Wessel DL, Triedman JK, Wernovsky G, et al. Pulmonary and systemic hemodynamic effects of amrinone in neonates following cardiopulmonary bypass. Circulation 80(suppl II):II-488, 1989.

61a. Wessel DL, Adatia I, Giglia TM, Thompson JE, Kulik TJ. Use of inhaled nitric oxide and acetylcholine in the evaluation of pulmonary hypertension and endothelial function after cardiopulmonary bypass. Circulation 88:2128, 1993.

62. Wheller J, George BL, Mulder DG, et al. Diagnosis and management of postoperative pulmonary hypertensive crisis. Circulation 70:1640, 1979.

63. Witte MK, Galli SA, Chatburn RL, et al. Optimal positive end-expiratory pressure therapy in infants and children with acute respiratory failure. Pediatr Res 24:217, 1988.

64. Zaritsky A, Chernow B. Use of catecholamines in pediatrics. J Pediatr 105:341, 1984.

For the infant with serious congenital heart disease, the perioperative period represents a time of unique physiologic stress. In addition to the hemodynamic burden of the cardiac lesion, patients must also contend with preoperative cardiac catheterization, the surgery itself, general anesthesia, and possible cardiopulmonary bypass with or without hypothermia. Postoperative issues involving fluid imbalance, electrolyte disturbances, and high levels of endogenous/exogenous catecholamines add yet another level of complexity. It is hard to imagine more likely conditions for the occurrence of cardiac rhythm disorders. Fortunately, however, serious perioperative arrhythmias in the infant are uncommon, and most can be managed successfully if detection is prompt and diagnosis is accurate.

The types of rhythm disorders seen in the neonate and infant differ somewhat from those encountered in the older child or adult. Ventricular arrhythmias in general, and ventricular fibrillation in particular, are rather uncommon in very young patients. It is also rare to observe atrial fibrillation in this population, perhaps because the small atrial size cannot support the electrophysiologic requirements for fibrillation. Finally, the incidence of "automatic" tachycardias (i.e., those involving the atrium or atrioventricular junction) is significantly higher in the younger age group. Knowledge of these age-specific features will often assist in the differential diagnosis of complex perioperative arrhythmias.

The key to effective management of arrhythmias in a patient of any age is accurate diagnosis of the underlying electrophysiologic abnormality. The physician must make an effort to understand both the site of origin and the cellular mechanism of the individual disorder so that treatment can be tailored to the specific problem. This is particularly important in the case of automatic tachycardias, which require rather unique therapy. Throughout this section, diagnostic techniques and a deductive approach to the analysis of arrhythmia will be stressed.

DIAGNOSTIC TOOLS

Continuous surveillance of rhythm with a bedside monitor is a fairly standard precaution for any infant with complex heart disease. These devices record one or more surface electrocardiographic leads and can usually be triggered to sound an alarm if bradycardia or tachycardia occurs. Monitors of this type represent the first line of detection for rhythm disorders in the perioperative period. However, when an abnormal rhythm is documented, it is generally not sufficient to depend on the single-lead rhythm strip from the monitor for detailed arrhythmia analysis. Although a simple rhythm strip may occasionally reveal ample clues for accurate diagnosis, a formal 12-lead electrocardiogram should be performed whenever possible. Important details of the P-wave axis and QRS morphology may be seen only when multiple simultaneous electrocardiographic leads are recorded.

At times, even the full 12-lead electrocardiogram is not sufficient for accurate diagnosis. This is primarily true for rapid tachycardias when the P wave is indistinct or obscured by the QRS complex. In this setting, it is necessary to record electrical activity more directly from atrial tissue. Several techniques can be employed for this purpose. In a postoperative patient with temporary epicardial pacing wires in place, atrial activity can be recorded directly from the atrial wires.[19] Using a standard electrocardiographic machine, the leg leads are attached to the patient in the usual fashion to act as ground wires. The two arm leads of the machine are then connected to the temporary atrial wires with a clip or a rubber band (Fig. 5–10). Because lead I of the electrocardiogram reflects the voltage difference between the two arms, a recording of lead I from atrial wires provides a *bipolar* signal containing a large, sharp atrial deflection with very little ventricular activity (Fig. 5–11A). Leads II and III of the electrocardiogram reflect the voltage differences between the right arm and left leg and the left arm and left leg, respectively. Recording of either lead II or III from atrial wires thus provides a *unipolar atrial* signal, which contains a moderately sharp atrial deflection along with a large ventricular component (Fig. 5–11B, C). The resolution of atrial timing with this technique is dramatic and is far superior to that provided by the standard surface electrocardiogram. Examples demonstrating the utility of these recordings will appear throughout this subchapter.

If atrial wires are not available, similar signals can be obtained with the placement of a bipolar transesophageal catheter.[4] Esophageal electrodes are widely available commercially and should be standard equipment in any cardiac unit. The lead can be passed through the mouth or nose and positioned near the mid-esophagus directly behind the left atrium. It is then connected to an electrocardiographic machine or other recording device as previ-

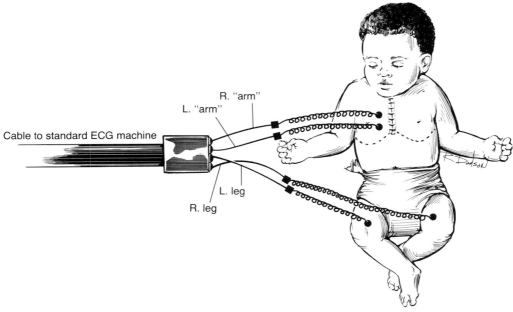

FIGURE 5–10. □

Technique for the recording of electrograms from temporary atrial pacing wires, using a standard electrocardiogram (ECG) device. The leg leads are attached to the patient in the usual fashion, while the arm leads are attached directly to the atrial wires.

ously described. With small manipulations in position, a site can be found which records a sharp atrial signal (Fig. 5–12). For the neonate and infant, optimal signals are typically found at an insertion depth

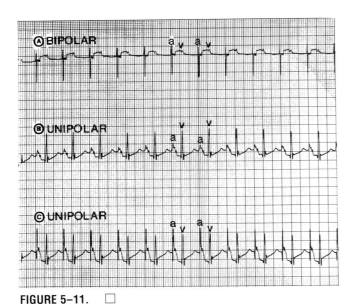

FIGURE 5–11. □

Atrial electrograms recorded during normal sinus rhythm from postoperative atrial pacing wires. *A,* A "bipolar" atrial electrogram made by recording lead I on standard ECG equipment with the arm leads connected to atrial wires. Note the clear, sharp atrial deflection with a small ventricular signal. *B* and *C,* "Unipolar" atrial electrograms made by recording lead II or III on standard equipment with the arm leads attached to atrial wires. Note the clear atrial deflection with a moderate-size ventricular signal.

of 12 to 17 cm (measured from the distal electrode to the nares or mouth).

In addition to their capacity for atrial recording, both atrial wires and the esophageal lead can be used for atrial pacing. This includes support pacing for sinus bradycardia, as well as short bursts of rapid pacing to interrupt re-entry supraventricular tachycardias such as atrial flutter and reciprocating tachycardias from accessory pathways. As will be

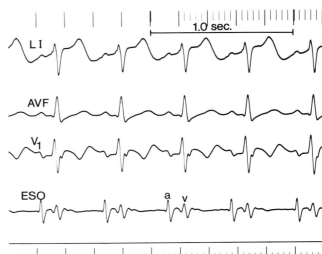

FIGURE 5–12. □

A recording during sinus rhythm of three surface ECG leads along with a simultaneous esophageal electrogram.

discussed later, pacing maneuvers are often preferred over drug therapy for management of these disorders in the compromised infant. Pacing via atrial wires can be accomplished with any standard device; however, transesophageal pacing requires a specialized generator with the capacity for wide pulse widths (approximately 10 milliseconds).

Some complex tachycardias in the infant necessitate more in-depth investigation with formal electrophysiologic study, using intracardiac catheters. Examples include the Wolff-Parkinson-White syndrome or other forms of supraventricular tachycardia caused by accessory pathways, which are not uncommon accompaniments of congenital heart disease. These conditions are usually diagnosed before surgery. Preoperative catheterization can thus include formal mapping of any abnormal pathway location with a view to transcatheter ablation[21] or intraoperative division.[13] It is generally desirable to eliminate these pathways before or during congenital heart surgery whenever possible, even if the patient has not demonstrated supraventricular tachycardia in the preoperative period. Tachycardia can be difficult to manage in the operating room or during recovery from surgery when catecholamines are elevated.

CARDIAC ARRHYTHMIAS IN THE NEONATE AND INFANT

Abnormalities of cardiac rhythm can be separated into the broad classes of tachycardias and bradycardias. As shown in Table 5–4, there are many possible mechanisms for these disorders, each requiring rather specific management. Efforts must be made to narrow the differential diagnosis to the specific mechanism so that therapy can be tailored appropriately.

Pathophysiology of Tachyarrhythmias

There are two general cellular mechanisms for tachycardia. The first involves the familiar concept of "re-entry" or "circus movement" and is by far the most common cause of tachycardia in all age groups.[40] The gross clinical features of re-entry include (1) abrupt onset (usually caused by one or more premature beats), (2) very regular rates, (3) abrupt termination with vagal maneuvers (sometimes successful), and (4) abrupt termination with electrical cardioversion or overdrive burst pacing (virtually always successful). Re-entry is responsible for atrial flutter, atrial fibrillation, accessory pathway tachycardias, atrioventricular nodal re-en-

TABLE 5–4. ☐ CLASSIFICATION OF ARRHYTHMIAS

Bradycardias
  Sinus node dysfunction
  Second degree AV block
    Mobitz I (Wenckebach)
    Mobitz II
  Third degree AV block
Tachycardias
  Disorders of automaticity
    Sinus tachycardia
    Ectopic atrial tachycardia
    Multifocal (chaotic) atrial tachycardia
    Junctional ectopic tachycardia
  Re-entry
    Sinus node re-entry
    Atrial flutter
    Atrial fibrillation
    AV nodal re-entry
    WPW syndrome
      Orthodromic re-entry
      Antidromic re-entry
      Pre-excited atrial flutter/fibrillation
    "Concealed" accessory pathways
      Orthodromic re-entry
  Ventricular tachycardia
    Monomorphic re-entry
    Torsades de pointes

try, and probably most forms of ventricular tachycardia. A second cellular mechanism for tachycardia is "automaticity," a disorder that involves rapid spontaneous depolarization from a single small focus.[1] The gross clinical features for such tachycardias include (1) gradual onset with steady "warm-up" of the rate, (2) a variable rate that changes with manipulation of autonomic tone or body temperature, (3) slight slowing with vagal maneuvers (but never termination), and (4) refractoriness to electrical cardioversion and overdrive pacing maneuvers. Automatic tachycardias can arise from anywhere in the heart, but in the infant, ectopic atrial or junctional foci are the most common source.

Specific Tachycardias

This section will review the more common tachycardias encountered in the infant with congenital heart disease, with emphasis on acute stabilization in the perioperative period. For a more comprehensive discussion of tachycardias and long-term therapy, the reader is referred to several in-depth reviews of this topic.[16, 38, 41]

Sinus Tachycardia

Although sinus tachycardia is not a pathologic rhythm disorder, rapid rates in the infant can sometimes be confused with supraventricular tachycardia. Sinus rates in a stressed infant can exceed 180 beats per minute (bpm) at times, and it is important to recognize the true nature of the rhythm so that inappropriate therapy is not administered. The key features to examine in this setting are the P-wave axis on a 12-lead electrocardiogram and the pattern of rate variation. Sinus tachycardia should generate a normal P-wave axis of $+60$ degrees on the electrocardiogram and should vary slightly in rate over time with changes in sympathetic tone and the respiratory cycle. Sinus tachycardia does not require specific therapy other than elimination of the underlying cause.

Ectopic Atrial Tachycardia

Ectopic atrial tachycardia is an uncommon, but difficult, rhythm disorder caused by abnormal automaticity of a single nonsinus atrial focus.[15] The tachycardia can be either sustained or intermittent and can exhibit a broad range of rates between 100 and 280 bpm. The key diagnostic features include a rapid atrial rate with a P wave that differs in axis or morphology from the P wave in normal sinus rhythm. Because this disorder is caused by abnormal automaticity rather than re-entry, atrial rates tend to vary widely, with "warm-up" at initiation and "cool-down" at termination. There can be intermittent first- and second-degree atrioventricular block (Fig. 5–13), as well as rate-related bundle branch aberration, because of the inability of the normal atrioventricular conduction system to transmit the rapid impulses. However, for the infant with an intact atrioventricular node, the rate of conduction is typically rapid.

Ectopic atrial tachycardia is usually seen as an idiopathic rhythm disorder in patients with a structurally normal heart, but it is also seen occasionally in the infant with congenital heart disease, particularly in the acute postoperative period after surgery at or near the pulmonary veins. Postoperative ectopic atrial tachycardia seems most likely to occur under conditions of high circulating catecholamines and will frequently resolve over a few days as the child recovers and inotropic support is weaned. Rare cases of postoperative ectopic atrial tachycardia may persist beyond the surgical period.

Treatment of this arrhythmia is difficult. Electrical cardioversion and burst overdrive atrial pacing will not interrupt this condition, as it is due to automaticity rather than re-entry. Likewise, drug therapy with agents such as adenosine (which is quite effective in blocking common re-entry supraventricular tachycardia involving the atrioventricular node) has little effect. Thus, acute therapy must involve initial attempts to lower exogenous catecholamines when possible, followed by pharmacologic trials. First-line drugs for this condition include digoxin, which acts primarily by blocking the atrioventricular node and reducing the ventricular response rate, and beta blockers such as intravenous esmolol, which also blocks the atrioventricular node but can frequently slow the ectopic atrial tachycardia focus directly. Intravenous phenytoin (Dilantin) has occasionally been successful in suppressing the ectopic focus. If the rhythm remains refractory to these measures, potent oral medications such as flecainide, propafenone, sotalol, and amiodarone may be tried. For rare cases of persistent ectopic atrial tachycardia that remain refractory to drug therapy, the physician may have to consider electrophysiologic studies with mapping of the focus, followed by attempted surgical or transcatheter ablation of the abnormal atrial site.[39] Fortunately, in most cases of postoperative ectopic atrial tachycardia, it is usually sufficient to maintain rate control by titrating the atrioventricular node response with digoxin and esmolol until the arrhythmia resolves.

Atrial Flutter

Re-entry tachycardia involving atrial muscle is commonly referred to as atrial flutter. The classic electrocardiographic appearance is that of a "sawtooth" atrial rhythm at 300 bpm that is most apparent in leads II, III, and an aVF. However, not all atrial muscle re-entry produces this pattern, particularly in the infant. A wide variety of P-wave morphologies can be observed, and rates can be as slow as 180 bpm or as fast as 400 bpm. The most reliable

FIGURE 5–13. ☐

Ectopic atrial tachycardia recorded on ECG lead II, showing the rapid atrial rate with abnormal P wave morphology, and variable atrioventricular (AV) conduction.

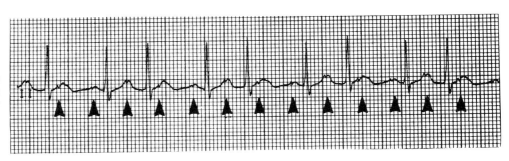

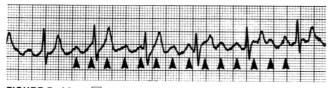

FIGURE 5–14. □

ECG (lead II) recording of classic atrial flutter, showing the rapid, regular, "sawtooth" pattern of atrial depolarization.

electrocardiographic features are a rapid atrial rhythm with abrupt initiation and a strictly regular rate (Fig. 5–14). The ventricular response rate to atrial flutter is quite brisk for the infant, frequently involving a 1:1 conduction ratio, but conduction can vary over time with changes in the autonomic state. Whenever there is confusion regarding the true atrial rate in this condition, an atrial wire recording or an esophageal electrogram can clearly demonstrate the rapid and regular atrial depolarizations (Fig. 5–15).

Atrial muscle re-entry is a fairly common perioperative tachycardia in the neonate and infant. It may occur in conjunction with surgical damage to the sinus node ("tachy-brady" syndrome) but is frequently an isolated abnormality. Congenital heart lesions that cause significant atrial dilatation (e.g., Ebstein's anomaly, Shone's syndrome, atrioventricular canal defects) or extensive atrial surgery (e.g., Fontan, Mustard, or Senning procedures) are associated with the highest incidence of postoperative atrial flutter.

The acute management of atrial flutter is fairly straightforward. Because it is a re-entry tachycardia, both electrical cardioversion and overdrive pacing techniques are highly effective in terminating the condition. Whenever a patient is acutely compromised by this tachycardia, cardioversion or burst pacing should be employed immediately as first-line therapy. Acute drug therapy is not very effective for atrial flutter. In rare cases, intravenous adenosine can terminate the atrial re-entry, but most often it will simply block the atrioventricular node transiently without affecting the underlying atrial tachycardia. Similarly, digoxin and esmolol can slow the rate of atrioventricular conduction over a longer term but do little to terminate the rapid atrial rate. One drug that may occasionally correct the atrial rhythm directly is procainamide; however, this agent can enhance atrioventricular conduction because of vagolytic side effects, and it will often speed up the ventricular rate to undesirable levels. Thus, it is advisable to rely on electrical therapy rather than pharmacology for acute management of this disorder.[6]

Once the primary episode has been terminated, drug therapy can be initiated to prevent recurrence of the flutter. No drug is ideal for this purpose, but as a first-line trial the physician can employ digoxin or a beta blocker, which will at least provide some degree of atrioventricular block to protect against rapid ventricular rates if flutter recurs. For patients with frequent recurrences, intravenous procainamide or oral therapy with quinidine, flecainide, propafenone, sotalol, or amiodarone can be added to digoxin. When flutter occurs in the setting of the sick sinus syndrome, it may be necessary to commence atrial pacing before the use of any potent antiarrhythmic drugs. Pacing at physiologic rates not only protects against further rate slowing from the medications, but also seems to protect against flutter recurrence.

Atrial Fibrillation

Atrial fibrillation is due to the presence of multiple, small, constantly changing re-entry circuits in atrial muscle. It rarely occurs in very young children, perhaps because atrial size is inadequate to support multiple re-entry sites. Nevertheless, it may be seen occasionally in infants with markedly distended atria.

The typical electrocardiographic findings for atrial fibrillation include a pattern of nearly continuous, low-amplitude atrial activity that is irregular and variable. The ventricular response rate also varies in an irregularly irregular fashion (Fig. 5–16). Atrial electrograms from postoperative wires or an esophageal lead will confirm the erratic atrial depolarization if it is unclear on electrocardiographic recordings.

Treatment of atrial fibrillation is similar to that for atrial flutter with the exception that burst overdrive atrial pacing is not effective in terminating the abnormal rhythm. Electrical cardioversion is the usual method of acute conversion and is followed by drug therapy, as outlined for atrial flutter, to prevent recurrence.

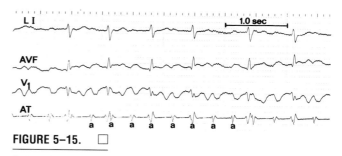

FIGURE 5–15. □

Surface ECG and simultaneous recording made from temporary atrial wires in atrial flutter, showing clear definition of atrial activity.

FIGURE 5–16. □

Surface ECG (lead II) recording of atrial fibrillation.

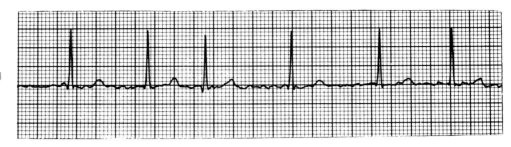

Junctional Ectopic Tachycardia

Junctional ectopic tachycardia is a notoriously difficult form of supraventricular tachycardia. Although rare instances are reported as idiopathic rhythm disorders in otherwise healthy children, junctional ectopic tachycardia is seen almost exclusively as an acute postoperative tachycardia in the infant and young child with congenital heart disease.[12] It appears to be caused by enhanced automaticity of cells in either the atrioventricular node or the proximal His-Purkinje system and is a transient phenomenon lasting only a few hours or days after surgery. If the patient can be supported through this crucial time, the tachycardia will resolve completely, with little risk of recurrence. Unfortunately, this is perhaps the most difficult form of tachycardia to manage in the postoperative period. Before recognition of effective therapy for junctional ectopic tachycardia, high mortality rates (20% to 50%) were associated with this condition. Currently, however, the prognosis is excellent if detection is rapid and appropriate therapy is instituted without delay.

Junctional ectopic tachycardia tends to occur only in young patients (i.e., neonates to infants 2 years of age). It is most common after surgical procedures near the atrioventricular junction (e.g., closure of a ventricular septal defect). However, it can occasionally be seen after surgery that does not involve direct trauma to this area, such as pulmonary artery banding, the Fontan procedure, and others. Its time of onset is variable; it may occur early in the operating room or several hours or as much as 2 days after the procedure.

Because junctional ectopic tachycardia is another of the automatic tachycardias, the rates "warm up" gradually over several hours after initiation. If the peak rate is not too rapid (i.e., less than about 170 bpm), this arrhythmia is fairly well tolerated. However, greatly accelerated rates (ranging from 170 to 290 bpm) can cause severe hemodynamic compromise.

The electrocardiographic findings in junctional ectopic tachycardia are fairly specific. Because the rhythm originates at the atrioventricular junction, there is a rapid ventricular rate with a QRS morphology identical to that of normal sinus beats. However, because the atrium is an "innocent bystander" in this condition, the actual atrial rate is typically slower than that of the ventricle (Fig. 5–17). In some instances of fairly slow junctional ectopic tachycardia, there may be passive 1:1 retrograde conduction to the atrium, but more often there is a retrograde Wenckebach phenomenon or complete retrograde dissociation. This is the only form of supraventricular tachycardia in which the ventricular rate can be faster than the atrial rate. This rate discrepancy is often difficult to appreciate on the surface electrocardiogram, and junctional ec-

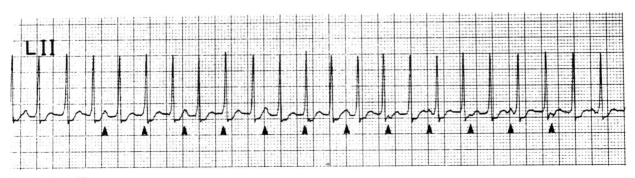

FIGURE 5–17. □

Surface ECG (lead II) recording of rapid junctional ectopic tachycardia that developed in a 14-month-old child after congenital heart surgery for a large ventricular septal defect (VSD). Note the rapid narrow QRS with slower atrial activity (*arrows*).

topic tachycardia is one condition in which an atrial wire recording or esophageal electrogram is almost mandatory for accurate diagnosis (Fig. 5–18). The previously mentioned electrophysiologic features result in two hemodynamic derangements. As in other types of supraventricular tachycardia, the rapid ventricular rates reduce the mean arterial blood pressure and increase atrial pressures because of the short diastolic filling times. However, the presence of dissociated atrial contraction further complicates the situation, as any augmentation of ventricular filling by the "atrial kick" is lost. Thus, the aim in treating junctional ectopic tachycardia is twofold: to restore atrioventricular synchrony and to reduce the junctional rate. Synchrony is the easiest of the two goals to achieve. The atrium can simply be paced at a rate slightly above that of the junctional rhythm, using temporary atrial wires or an esophageal pacing lead. Alternatively, if both atrial and ventricular pacing wires are available, a dual-chamber pacing device can be used to sense the QRS and trigger atrial pacing after a preset interval so that the P wave occurs just before the next QRS is due.[33] Occasionally, restoration of synchrony by either method is the only necessary therapy for junctional

ectopic tachycardia when the rates are not excessive. For greatly accelerated junctional tachycardia, junctional slowing to more physiologic rates must be achieved.

Treatments aimed at slowing automaticity from the atrioventricular junction are varied. Neither electrical cardioversion nor burst overdrive pacing will modify the tachycardia. Some reports have suggested that drugs such as digoxin, beta blockers, and phenytoin are useful in this regard,[17] but in our experience at Children's Hospital in Boston, these agents have rarely been effective. Intravenous propafenone has been used successfully to slow junctional ectopic tachycardia in investigational protocols at some pediatric centers,[14] but the drug is still restricted from general use. Perhaps the most useful advance in treatment for this tachycardia was the observation that mild hypothermia could result in dramatic slowing of the rate.[3] Currently this technique is widely employed. It involves dropping the core body temperature to 34°C using a cooling blanket. When this treatment is instituted, patients must be intubated and paralyzed to prevent shivering, and care must be taken to prevent hypothermia below 33°C to avoid the risk of ventricular fibrillation. Mild hypothermia is well tolerated for periods of hours or a few days when necessary, but the patient should be rewarmed at 8- to 12-hour intervals to determine when junctional ectopic tachycardia has resolved so that therapy can be relaxed. Prolonged hypothermia may interfere with immune function and should not be used longer than necessary. In some cases the tachycardia may not respond to hypothermia, at which point procainamide may be added. Although procainamide has little effect on junctional ectopic tachycardia when used alone at normal body temperature, it can be a potent agent for slowing the junctional rate at a temperature of 34°C.[31]

In rare cases, the above treatment plan may fail to control the junctional rate. A beta blocker can be added to hypothermia along with procainamide, or intravenous amiodarone or propafenone can be tried (if the latter is available under institutional protocols). As a final option, "paired ventricular pacing" could be attempted[37]; this involves attaching both the atrial and ventricular outputs of a dual-chamber pacemaker to ventricular wires, thereby pacing the ventricle with two rapid impulses in succession. If the rate is adjusted appropriately, paired pacing will create one capture beat, which generates systolic contraction, and a closely spaced second beat, which generates electrical depolarization, without mechanical systole. During this brief mechanical pause, the ventricle has time to fill, and the effective rate of ventricular contraction is reduced. The major

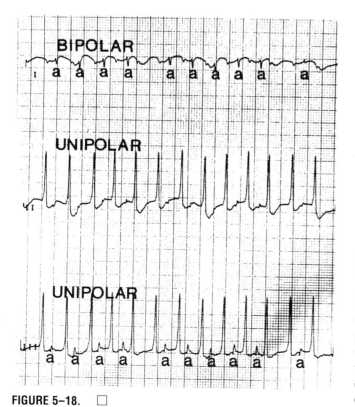

FIGURE 5–18. ☐

Recording made from temporary atrial wires in a patient with junctional ectopic tachycardia, demonstrating a ventricular rate that is faster than the atrial rate. In this case, the atria were activated in a retrograde fashion from the junction, although "retrograde Wenckebach" is present in a 6:5 pattern.

disadvantages of this technique include the fact that atrioventricular synchrony is still absent, and there is the risk of inducing serious ventricular arrhythmias from the rapid stimulation. Paired pacing should be used only when all other measures have failed.

Tachycardias Caused by Accessory Pathways

Accessory atrioventricular conduction pathways are among the most common causes of supraventricular tachycardia in the infant.[25] These pathways can be located anywhere along the tricuspid or mitral valve rings, although right-sided pathways are the more common variety in an infant with congenital heart disease.[7] Anatomic defects with the highest incidence of associated accessory pathways include Ebstein's anomaly, canal defects, and tricuspid atresia.

Accessory pathways can be subdivided on the basis of their conduction patterns. The Wolff-Parkinson-White syndrome, for example, involves a pathway that is capable of bidirectional conduction. During sinus rhythm, anterograde conduction over the pathway depolarizes a small segment of ventricular muscle and is responsible for the short PR interval and delta wave seen on the electrocardiogram. Several varieties of supraventricular tachycardia are possible with this pathway.[29] The most common form of tachycardia involves a circuit that uses the pathway in the retrograde direction followed by anterograde conduction over the normal atrioventricular node (so-called "orthodromic" tachycardia). During orthodromic supraventricular tachycardia, the QRS complex is normal by virtue of the fact that the ventricles are being depolarized over the normal conducting system. Less common forms of Wolff-Parkinson-White tachycardia include the reverse circuit, which uses the pathway in the anterograde direction ("antidromic tachycardia"), as well as atrial flutter or fibrillation. The QRS complex is wide during these latter tachycardias, as the ventricles are being activated over the accessory pathway.

Many accessory pathways are capable of only retrograde conduction[11] and are said to be "concealed." Because there is no anterograde conduction during sinus rhythm, the delta wave and short PR interval are not seen. However, such pathways may still produce orthodromic tachycardia, which can be every bit as difficult as that seen with the Wolff-Parkinson-White syndrome.

Orthodromic re-entry from either type of accessory pathway presents an electrocardiographic picture of a rapid, regular supraventricular tachycardia with a normal QRS complex and a strict 1:1

ratio between the atrium and ventricle. The P waves may be hard to appreciate on a standard electrocardiogram, but when visible, they have a "retrograde" axis of about − 90 degrees and tend to occur 70 milliseconds or more after the QRS (Fig. 5–19). When uncertainty exists, atrial wire recordings or an esophageal electrogram may be helpful in clarifying the atrial depolarization time.

The presence of the Wolff-Parkinson-White syndrome is usually suspected in advance of tachycardic episodes when a routine electrocardiogram is performed as part of the general evaluation of the infant with structural heart disease (Fig. 5–20). As mentioned earlier, such patients should undergo preoperative electrophysiologic studies in the catheterization laboratory so that the pathway can be mapped for catheter ablation or surgical division. Concealed pathways, however, are not detectable on a sinus rhythm electrocardiogram, and they are typically diagnosed only after an episode of tachycardia. Thus, the physician must frequently contend with concealed accessory pathway tachycardia in the postoperative period when the patient is particularly vulnerable.

Acute termination of orthodromic supraventricular tachycardia is relatively easy. Vagal maneuvers (such as application of an ice bag to the face or elicitation of the gag reflex) can be tried and are effective in about 25% of cases. The standard first-line drug for this disorder is adenosine, given by rapid intravenous push. This agent will temporarily block conduction across the atrioventricular node, thereby breaking the re-entry circuit. If adenosine is not successful, the most effective second-line therapy for an infant with postoperative orthodromic tachycardia is probably cardioversion or overdrive atrial pacing. Although digoxin, beta blockers, and verapamil have been used in the past for this form of supraventricular tachycardia, there are serious drawbacks with all three agents. Use of digoxin is hampered by the fact that its onset of action is delayed, and it may also have the undesirable side effect of enhancing conduction across an accessory pathway. Beta blockers are generally not very effective in terminating orthodromic supraventricular tachycardia unless they are used in high doses, which can cause hemodynamic problems from negative inotropic effects. Verapamil should never be used in any infant, because it causes profound myocardial suppression. For acute therapy in the postoperative period, these three agents should probably be avoided.

Unfortunately, orthodromic tachycardia tends to be a recurrent problem, and long-term prevention can be a challenging issue in the postoperative period. The acute measures outlined earlier can be

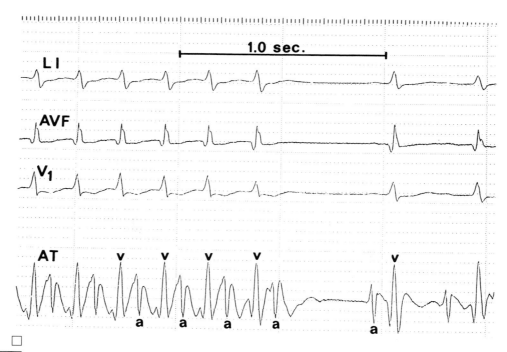

FIGURE 5–19. □

Orthodromic tachycardia in a patient with a concealed accessory pathway, recorded from three surface ECG leads with a simultaneous recording from atrial wires. This tracing shows both supraventricular tachycardia (SVT) and spontaneous conversion to normal sinus rhythm. The P wave during SVT occurs 70 msec or more after the preceding QRS.

repeated as necessary, but it is preferable to find a drug regimen that can minimize the likelihood of recurrence. In our experience at Children's Hospital in Boston, intravenous procainamide, which affects conduction in the accessory pathway directly, is perhaps the most useful drug for this purpose. In difficult cases, a beta blocker can be used in conjunction with procainamide, with careful monitoring of hemodynamics. If tachycardia recurs despite these measures, more potent oral agents such as flecainide, propafenone, sotalol, or amiodarone can be used. Transcatheter ablation of the pathway may be necessary in the postoperative period if medical therapy is not successful.

Re-entry Tachycardia of the Atrioventricular Node

The last variety of supraventricular tachycardia to consider is re-entry within the atrioventricular node. Although this is the most common form of supraventricular tachycardia in the adult,[23] it is extremely rare in young patients. The electrocardiographic appearance is similar to that for orthodromic re-entry from an accessory pathway, except that the "retrograde" P wave occurs nearly simultaneously with the QRS. Recordings from atrial wires or an esophageal lead show an atrial deflection less than 70 milliseconds after ventricular depolarization (Fig. 5–21). Acute therapy is identical to that employed for accessory pathway re-entry.

Ventricular Arrhythmias

Serious ventricular arrhythmias are relatively rare in infants. Although "low-grade" ectopy, such as isolated premature beats or couplets, may be seen in the perioperative period, it is unusual to observe sustained ventricular tachycardia or fibrillation. This contrasts sharply with adult cardiac patients, in whom these disorders are fairly common perioperative issues. Under conditions of acidosis, low cardiac output, and electrolyte disturbance, malignant ventricular arrhythmias may occasionally arise in the infant, requiring aggressive therapy of both the abnormal rhythm and the underlying physiologic derangements.

Two distinct varieties of ventricular tachycardia must be recognized. The first is referred to as "monomorphic" ventricular tachycardia, which is usually due to re-entry within a damaged segment of ventricular muscle.[8] In this case, the electrocardiographic pattern is one of a rapid, wide QRS complex having a constant morphology and regular timing (Fig. 5–22). Slower atrial activity may be completely dissociated from the ventricular complex, but at times there may be passive 1:1 retrograde conduction to the atrium. The absence of atrioventricular dissociation does not rule out ventricular tachycardia. Monomorphic ventricular tachycardia may be difficult to differentiate from some atypical forms of supraventricular tachycardia that involve a wide

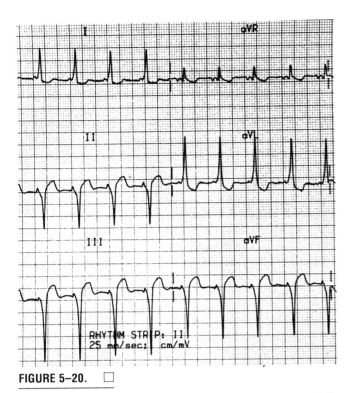

FIGURE 5–20. □

Surface ECG (limb leads) during normal sinus rhythm from an infant with the Wolff-Parkinson-White (WPW) syndrome and an AV canal defect. The short PR interval and delta wave are clearly seen.

QRS complex from bundle branch block, aberration, or accessory pathways. *In the acute setting it is always wise to assume that a wide QRS tachycardia is ventricular tachycardia until enough data have been obtained to definitely prove otherwise.*

The second variety of ventricular tachycardia is the entity referred to as *torsade de pointes*.[20] In this condition, the QRS morphology varies in a distinctive pattern that involves gradual alteration of positive and negative deflections that seem to twist around the isoelectric baseline of the electrocardiogram (Fig. 5–23). Torsade de pointes typically occurs in the setting of abnormal ventricular repolarization with prolongation of the QT interval. Possible causes include electrolyte abnormalities (hypomagnesemia or hypocalcemia), exposure to certain potent antiarrhythmic drugs (e.g., quinidine, procainamide, flecainide), and congenital long QT syndromes.

Sustained ventricular tachycardia must be managed as an emergency. For any compromised patient, basic cardiorespiratory support is initiated, and the tachycardia is treated initially with electrical cardioversion or defibrillation. If the tachycardia is unaffected or recurs, drug therapy must be initiated. For monomorphic disorder ventricular tachycardia, lidocaine is the initial choice, followed by

procainamide if necessary. If the tachycardia remains refractory to these measures, additional drug trials with a beta blocker or bretylium can be attempted. For torsade de pointes, magnesium sulfate and lidocaine, alone or in conjunction with pacing at moderately fast rates, should be employed as initial drug therapy. Procainamide must be avoided in the management of torsade de pointes, as it can further lengthen the QT interval. Above all, the physician must search for reversible underlying causes when treating any malignant ventricular tachycardia in an infant.

Lower grade ventricular arrhythmias in infants rarely require therapy. Most of these minor disorders occur in the setting of hypokalemia or other metabolic disturbance and are best approached by simply correcting the underlying disorder. Indeed, more harm can be caused by unnecessary antiarrhythmic drug administration than would have been caused by the rhythm itself. Isolated ventricular premature beats, even in bigeminy, should generally be observed without treatment. Repetitive ectopy (i.e., couplets and short salvos of nonsustained ventricular tachycardia) in infants should prompt a thorough search for a treatable underlying cause, but it does not require aggressive treatment beyond

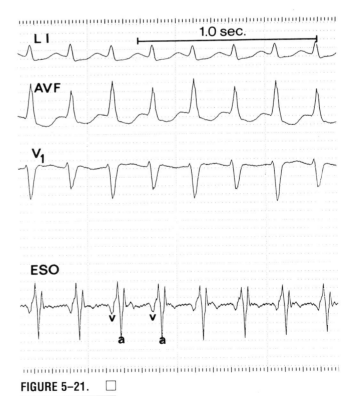

FIGURE 5–21. □

AV nodal reentry tachycardia recorded from three surface ECG leads with a simultaneous recording from an esophageal electrode. The P wave occurs nearly coincident with the QRS complex. This contrasts to the long ventriculoatrial (VA) intervals seen with an accessory pathway (see Fig. 5–20).

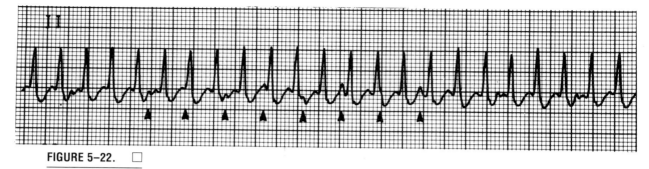

FIGURE 5–22. ☐

Surface ECG recording of monomorphic ventricular tachycardia in a 4-day-old infant. Slower P waves (*arrows*) are dissociated with this rapid QRS.

temporary administration of lidocaine unless there is clear evidence of hemodynamic compromise. If repetitive ectopy persists more than a few days after surgery, more detailed evaluation with Holter monitoring, and possibly formal electrophysiologic testing, may be required to determine the need for chronic suppressive therapy.[22]

Bradycardia Caused by Depressed Function of the Sinus Node

Sinus node dysfunction is an all too common problem after surgery for congenital heart disease. The procedures associated with the highest incidence of this disorder involve extensive atrial baffling (e.g., as in the Mustard, Senning, and Fontan operations). However, damage to the sinus node can occur with any repair, including simple closure of an atrial septal defect. Postoperative sinus bradycardia can be a transient disorder lasting for just a few days after surgery, but more often it represents permanent (and possibly progressive) injury to the sinus node from direct trauma to the node or its arterial supply. In some patients the situation is further complicated by a coexistent re-entry atrial arrhythmia (flutter or fibrillation); this is known as *sick sinus* or *tachy-brady syndrome*.[36]

The electrocardiographic manifestations include inappropriately slow and irregular atrial rates with escape rhythms arising from atrial or junctional foci (Fig. 5–24). Episodic supraventricular tachycardia, as described previously, may also be observed.

Any infant who leaves the operating room with manifestations of sinus node dysfunction should have temporary atrial wires in place. In the early postoperative period, atrial pacing can be used to supply physiologic rates and establish atrioventricular synchrony. If atrial wires are not available, transesophageal atrial pacing can be employed. As an alternative to pacing, isoproterenol can be used on a trial basis to increase the sinus node rate, but

often this results only in acceleration of the junctional escape rhythm and does not necessarily restore synchrony.

After the acute postoperative period, sinus node dysfunction in the infant with a stable escape rhythm is fairly well tolerated and generally does not require immediate pacemaker insertion. However, if supraventricular tachycardia recurs and chronic drug therapy becomes necessary, a pacemaker is frequently placed to protect against further slowing of the escape rhythms. In a patient with intact atrioventricular conduction, a single-chamber atrial unit is sufficient. Specialized atrial pacing devices that are capable of automatic burst pacing to interrupt atrial flutter may be especially attractive for those patients with frequent episodes of supraventricular tachycardia.

Bradycardia Caused by Disorders of Conduction

Atrioventricular conduction disturbances may occur spontaneously or as a result of catheter or surgical trauma. Certain congenital heart defects are associated with developmental abnormalities of the atrioventricular node or the His-Purkinje system (most notably, L-looped ventricles and canal defects) that can result in heart block independent of surgery. In other cases, the conduction system is normal but may be damaged inadvertently during a complex surgical repair (e.g., closure of a ventricular septal defect or the Kono procedure). Improved understanding of the anatomy of the conduction system in abnormal hearts[2] has greatly reduced the incidence of surgical heart block, but at times conduction tissue is so near the region of repair that it cannot be easily avoided.

Acute therapy for atrioventricular block involves support pacing from temporary wires, which are placed in the operating room as a routine precaution for all patients who have undergone an "open" car-

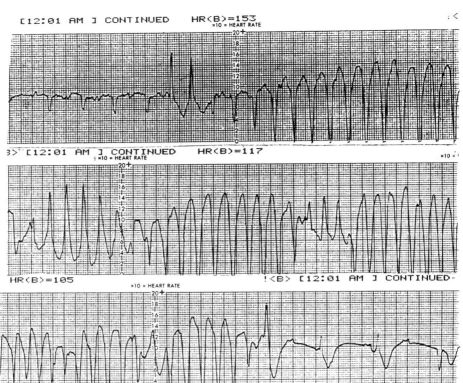

FIGURE 5–23. ☐

Continuous strip Holter monitor ECG recording of torsade de pointes variety of ventricular tachycardia that developed in a patient being treated with quinidine.

diac procedure. Ideally, atrial and ventricular wires should both be available to allow maximum hemodynamic benefit with sequential pacing. Permanent pacing leads can also be inserted in the operating room for future use if the risk of permanent atrioventricular block is considered high. Long-term treatment for these disorders consists of implantation of a permanent pacemaker. Major management decisions thus revolve around (1) when to implant a device and (2) what type of generator/lead system should be used.

The guidelines for implanting a permanent pacemaker in an infant are similar to those for the older child and young adult.[9] Third-degree heart block, related to surgical trauma, that persists more than 10 days after the operation is considered an absolute indication for permanent pacing. This recommendation arose from the observation that the inci-

dence of sudden death approached 50% when pacing was not available for complete atrioventricular block after congenital heart surgery.[18] Likewise, a patient with preoperative third-degree block related to structural heart disease should have a pacemaker implanted at the time of any cardiac surgery, even if the slow rates were well tolerated before operation. Most centers would also recommend pacing for any infant with a Mobitz II second-degree block if the condition persists more than 10 days after surgery. Data are not as clear for patients with Mobitz I second-degree atrioventricular block. If the finding is intermittent and the patient is hemodynamically stable without symptoms, Mobitz I block is often followed conservatively. Electrophysiologic testing during total autonomic blockade[5] may assist in the decision making for such borderline cases. First-degree block, bifascicular block, and isolated bundle

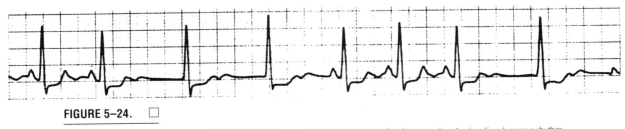

FIGURE 5–24. ☐

Sinus node dysfunction in a young patient after the Fontan operation, showing episodic sinus arrest and a junctional escape rhythm.

branch block are not considered indications for a pacemaker.

The choice of a generator/lead system is influenced by patient size and the severity of underlying heart disease. Although it is technically possible to implant transvenous pacing leads in the infant, small vascular caliber usually limits the system to a single-chamber generator. Additionally, reoperation for lead advancement may become necessary as the child grows. Epicardial implant remains the most common technique for infants at most centers. In fact, epicardial leads are mandatory in many cases, including patients with intracardiac shunting who are at risk for systemic embolization from clot formation on the lead and patients who have undergone (or will undergo) surgery involving cavopulmonary connections.

In small infants with stable hemodynamics, a single-chamber ventricular pacing unit will usually suffice. The system can be upgraded to provide dual-chamber pacing at an elective replacement time when the child has grown. If an infant has poor hemodynamics involving atrioventricular valve regurgitation or high ventricular end-diastolic pressures, dual-chamber pacing should be considered regardless of age. The small size and high reliability of modern pacing devices have drastically reduced the morbidity of permanent pacing in the pediatric population.

ANTIARRHYTHMIC MEDICATIONS

This section will review the basic pharmacology of antiarrhythmic medications in the infant, with emphasis on those agents available in intravenous form for acute stabilization of perioperative arrhythmias. A more comprehensive discussion of these and other antiarrhythmic drugs can be found in several detailed reviews of the topic.[24, 28]

Digoxin

Although digoxin had long been the mainstay of treatment for supraventricular tachycardia in the young, reliance on this drug has decreased as more efficacious and faster acting agents have become available. Nevertheless, digoxin remains a useful option for chronic control of many tachyarrhythmias. In cases of ectopic atrial tachycardia or atrial flutter or fibrillation, digoxin acts mainly as a rate control agent by suppressing rapid conduction in the atrioventricular node. For concealed accessory pathways or atrioventricular nodal re-entry, digoxin may directly prevent the abnormal circuit. Digoxin

should probably be avoided in chronic management of the Wolff-Parkinson-White syndrome because of its potential for enhancing anterograde conduction across the pathway.[30]

Digoxin may be administered intravenously or by mouth. The bioavailability of intravenous digoxin is about 25% greater than that of the orally administered form, so the dose must be reduced accordingly when given by injection. Digoxin dosage for management of arrhythmias is the same as that used for congestive failure (i.e., digitalization over 24 hours, followed by a daily maintenance schedule).[32] Digoxin is cleared exclusively by the kidneys, and it should be used with caution, if at all, in an infant with compromised renal function.

Adenosine

Adenosine is a relatively new and very effective agent for the treatment of the more common forms of supraventricular tachycardia.[26] It is an endogenous nucleoside found in all tissues, but when it is injected as a rapid bolus, it can induce profound slowing of the sinus and atrioventricular nodes. Thus, tachycardias that involve the atrioventricular node as part of their re-entry circuit are promptly terminated when an effective dose reaches the heart. The half-life is extremely short (10 seconds), and much of the drug can be metabolized by blood cells and endothelial cells as it passes through the venous system. Therefore, rapid administration is necessary in a vein as close to the central circulation as possible. In a postoperative patient, a convenient route of injection is a central line or atrial monitoring line. The initial dose for the infant is 0.1 mg per kilogram of body weight, given by rapid intravenous push, followed by a saline flush. If this dose is not effective, a second bolus of 0.2 mg/kg can be tried.

Because of its rapid half-life, adenosine is an extremely safe drug. Several seconds of slow sinus rates and atrioventricular block may follow a dose, but these problems reverse promptly.

Beta Blockers

Beta blockers are effective agents for both primary and secondary treatment of many forms of supraventricular tachycardia and ventricular tachycardia. Unfortunately, because of their negative inotropic effects, these drugs should rarely be used for the sick infant in the postoperative period. Whenever beta blockers are used, it is advisable to choose formulations with the shortest possible half-life so that untoward effects can be corrected quickly if difficulty arises. Esmolol, with a half-life of 10 minutes, is the shortest acting agent available at present. It is a cardioselective beta blocker available only for intravenous use and is an intelligent first choice for a beta blocker in the intensive care setting.

The initial dose is 0.5 mg per kilogram of body weight, given as a rapid bolus. Continuous infusion with 50 to 200 μg/kg/min can then be commenced if the drug is effective. If esmolol is both effective and well tolerated, it can be administered over a long term as a continuous infusion, or the physician can change to a longer acting agent such as propranolol, which has a half-life of about 6 hours.

Propranolol is a nonselective beta blocker that can be administered either intravenously or orally. It can cross-react with noncardiac beta receptors and may aggravate reactive airway disease in susceptible individuals; therefore, it should be avoided in any infant with significant pulmonary disease. The initial intravenous dose is 0.1 mg/kg, given by slow infusion over 10 minutes. The dose can be repeated at 6-hour intervals, or the medication can be changed to oral propranolol, 1 to 4 mg/kg/day in four divided doses.

Lidocaine

Lidocaine is used exclusively for the treatment of ventricular arrhythmias. It is a safe medication with no significant hemodynamic effects at standard doses. Lidocaine is administered as a rapid intravenous bolus at a dose of 1.0 mg per kilogram of body weight, which can be repeated at 10-minute intervals for a total of three doses when necessary. After acute loading, an infusion of 20 to 50 μg/kg/min is used. Serum levels should be checked periodically for patients receiving prolonged therapy.

Procainamide

Procainamide is an extremely useful agent for treatment of acute postoperative tachyarrhythmias. It is effective for a wide range of disorders, including atrial flutter, atrial fibrillation, accessory pathway re-entry, and most forms of ventricular tachycardia. When used in conjunction with hypothermia, it can also assist in the control of refractory junctional ectopic tachycardia. Despite its broad utility, procainamide must be used with caution and only in a closely monitored environment. The side effect of this agent that is of most concern is the small risk of producing new or worsened ventricular arrhythmias[35] related to procainamide's effects on ventricular conduction time and cellular repolarization. Fortunately, this phenomenon of "proarrhythmia" is rare in young patients, but the drug should be administered only with continuous electrocardiographic monitoring and careful attention to the QT interval. Procainamide should be discontinued if the rate-corrected QT interval or the QRS duration is prolonged more than 30% from baseline measurements, particularly if new ventricular ectopy is observed. This drug is usually well tolerated hemodynamically. Because of vasodilation, some decrease in systemic blood pressure may be observed during initial loading, but this effect is easily reversed with administration of fluids.

Intravenous procainamide is administered to the infant as a slow initial loading dose of 5 to 10 mg per kilogram of body weight over 15 to 30 minutes. This can be followed by a constant infusion of 20 to 50 μg/kg/min, with periodic measurements of serum levels. It is not a very useful oral agent in the infant because of difficulties with absorption and the need for frequent dosing. If an oral equivalent to procainamide is required for chronic therapy, quinidine is a reasonable substitute.

Phenytoin

Phenytoin (Dilantin) is useful occasionally for ectopic atrial tachycardia in the postoperative period. It is also indicated for some ventricular arrhythmias, such as those caused by digoxin toxicity. Intravenous Dilantin is administered as an initial slow loading dose of 10 mg per kilogram of body weight over 30 to 60 minutes. Rapid administration can be associated with profound bradycardia and hypotension and must be avoided. The usual maintenance dose for an infant is 5 mg/kg/day in two divided doses, given by the oral route whenever possible.

Magnesium Sulfate

Magnesium sulfate is a useful agent for the control of ventricular tachycardia of the torsades de pointes variety.[34] The dosage range for the infant is not clearly established. At Children's Hospital in Boston, we have found a dose of 25 mg per kilogram of body weight to be safe and fairly effective in anecdotal experience. The rate of administration must be slow (over 15 minutes) to avoid hypotension.

Bretylium

Bretylium has complex electrophysiologic actions that are useful in the management of refractory

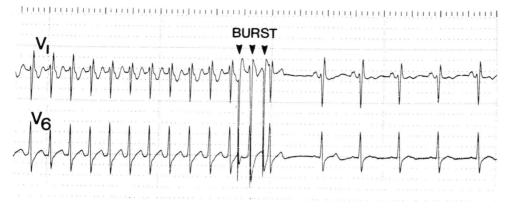

FIGURE 5–25. □

Termination of supraventricular tachycardia with a short burst of atrial pacing (*arrows*).

ventricular tachycardia and ventricular fibrillation.[27] The initial dose for infants is 5 mg per kilogram of body weight, given by rapid intravenous push. This may be repeated after 30 minutes when necessary. If this is effective, an infusion of 15 to 30 µg/kg/min can be started.

There is a biphasic hemodynamic response to this drug. After the initial bolus, bretylium causes a release of norepinephrine from sympathetic nerve terminals, which results in sinus tachycardia and an elevation in blood pressure. After about 1 hour, there is a block at the sympathetic nerve terminals, leading to hypotension that may require volume expansion or catecholamine infusion. Because of these profound cardiovascular effects, bretylium should be restricted to the management of life-threatening ventricular arrhythmias.

Verapamil

Although calcium channel blockers are useful in the treatment of many varieties of supraventricular tachycardia in older patients, *the use of intravenous verapamil is contraindicated in the neonate and infant.* Immature myocytes appear particularly sensitive to calcium channel blockade, resulting in profound hypotension and bradycardia.[10] Given the large number of available alternative therapies, verapamil should be avoided altogether in the acute treatment of arrhythmias for any child younger than 12 months.

ELECTRICAL THERAPY FOR TACHYARRHYTHMIAS

Overdrive burst pacing and direct current cardioversion are useful modalities for the acute treatment of re-entry tachycardias. They are particularly attractive options during the postoperative period,

when side effects from lingering antiarrhythmic drugs need to be avoided.

Overdrive Burst Pacing

Classic re-entry involves circular conduction between two discrete cardiac pathways. If a portion of the circuit can be depolarized at a rate greater than the maximum capacity of one of the pathways, re-entry will be terminated. The technique of overdrive pacing involves brief bursts of electrical stimulation in the atrium (or ventricle) at rates that exceed the conduction potential of the established tachycardia. Arrhythmias that can be treated with this method include atrial flutter, accessory pathway re-entry, atrioventricular node re-entry, and some cases of slow monomorphic ventricular tachycardia. Overdrive pacing is not effective for atrial fibrillation, rapid ventricular tachycardia, or ventricular fibrillation, nor will it terminate automatic focus tachycardia.

For re-entry supraventricular tachycardia, the pacing device is attached to temporary atrial pacing wires (when available) or to a properly positioned esophageal lead. The tachycardia rate is determined, and the generator is set to pace about 10% to 20% faster than the atrium. The physician begins with only three or four beats of burst pacing, and if this is unsuccessful, both the rate and duration of the burst are increased on subsequent attempts (Fig. 5–25). In general, the slower the initial atrial rate, the higher the chance of success with this method. Prolonged pacing at very rapid rates does have the potential to cause atrial fibrillation, and equipment must be on hand for electrical cardioversion in the event this occurs. Overdrive pacing for re-entry ventricular tachycardia should be performed only by individuals experienced with the technique. The pulse generator is attached to temporary ventricular wires, and bursts of ventricular pacing are delivered in the same sequence described for supraventricular tachycardia (Fig. 5–26). Note that direct ventricular pacing is not possible with an esophageal electrode. Acceleration of the ventricular tachycardia rate, or even ventricular fibrillation, can be induced if prolonged rapid pacing is used. Proper precautions for emergency defibrillation need to be available at the bedside.

Direct Current Cardioversion and Defibrillation

Direct current shock is a highly effective method for interrupting re-entrant arrhythmias, including fibrillation. It is a painful procedure, and patients must be fully sedated unless they have already lost consciousness because of hypotension from the arrhythmia. The energy can be delivered either to the thoracic surface with external paddles or directly to the heart with sterile internal paddles if the chest is open. The shock should be synchronized to the QRS complex when used for any supraventricular tachycardia or well-organized ventricular tachycardia, but it must be delivered in an asynchronous fashion for ventricular fibrillation or any rapid polymorphic ventricular tachycardia when there is no suitable QRS to sense. Synchronization ensures that the electrical discharge will occur coincident with the QRS, thereby avoiding a shock during the "vulnerable" period of the T wave, which can precipitate ventricular tachycardia.

For external cardioversion or defibrillation in the infant, the paddles must be positioned to promote a maximum flow of current through the heart muscle. If the paddles are positioned too close together on the anterior part of the chest, much of the current will arc between them, causing poor delivery of energy and possible skin burns. To avoid this, it is preferable to use anteroposterior positioning in small patients, with a flat back paddle between the scapulae and a second paddle along the sternal border at the middle of the chest. The shock energy must be kept to the minimum effective dose to avoid depression of myocardial function. For most supraventricular tachycardias, a starting energy of 0.25 to 0.5 J per kilogram of body weight will usually suffice. If this is unsuccessful, the energy can be doubled and then quadrupled over successive trials. For organized ventricular tachycardia, a starting energy of 1 J/kg is recommended; for ventricular fibrillation, 2 J/kg. The energy required when using internal paddles in direct contact with the heart is much less than that required for the external technique (approximately one tenth of the previously mentioned starting doses).

REFERENCES

1. Akhtar M, Tchou PJ, Jazayeri M. Mechanism of clinical tachycardias. Am J Cardiol 61:9A, 1988.
2. Anderson RH, Ho SY, Becker AE. The surgical anatomy of the conduction tissues. Thorax 38:408, 1983.
3. Bash SE, Shah JJ, Albers WH, et al. Hypothermia for the treatment of postsurgical greatly accelerated junctional ectopic tachycardia. J Am Coll Cardiol 10:1095, 1987.
4. Benson DW, Dunnigan A, Benditt DG, et al. Transesophageal cardiac pacing: History, application, technique. Clin Prog Pacing Electrophysiol 2:2360, 1984.
5. Benson DW, Spach MS, Edwards SB, et al. Heart block in children: Evaluation of subsidiary pacemaker recovery times and ECG tape recordings. Pediatr Cardiol 2:39, 1982.
6. Campbell RM, Dick M, Jenkins JM, et al. Atrial overdrive pacing for conversion of atrial flutter in children. Pediatrics 75:730, 1985.
7. Deal BJ, Keane JF, Gillette PC, et al. Wolff-Parkinson-White syndrome and supraventricular tachycardia during infancy. Management and followup. J Am Coll Cardiol 5:130, 1985.
8. DeBakker JM, Van Capell FJ, Janse MJ, et al. Reentry as a cause of ventricular tachycardia in patients with chronic ischemic heart disease: Electrophysiologic and anatomic correlation. Circulation 77:589, 1988.
9. Dreifus LS, Fisch C, Griffin JC, et al. Guidelines for implantation of cardiac pacemakers and antiarrhythmic devices. J Am Coll Cardiol 18:1, 1991.
10. Epstein ML, Keil EA, Victoria BE. Cardiac decompensation following verapamil therapy in infants with supraventricular tachycardia. Pediatrics 75:737, 1985.
11. Farshidi A, Josephson ME, Horowitz LN. Electrophysiologic characteristics of concealed bypass tracts: Clinical and electrocardiographic correlates. Am J Cardiol 41:1052, 1978.
12. Garson A, Gillette PC. Junctional ectopic tachycardia in children. Electrocardiography, electrophysiology and pharmacologic response. Am J Cardiol 44:298, 1979.
13. Garson A, Moak JP, Friedman RA, et al. Surgical treatment of arrhythmias in children. Cardiol Clin 7:319, 1989.
14. Garson A, Moak JP, Smith RT. Control of postoperative junctional ectopic tachycardia with propafenone. Am J Cardiol 59:1422, 1987.
15. Gillette PC, Garson A. Electrophysiologic and pharmacologic characteristics of automatic ectopic atrial tachycardia. Circulation 56:571, 1977.
16. Gillette PC, Garson A. Pediatric Arrhythmias: Electrophysiology and Pacing. Philadelphia, WB Saunders, 1990.
17. Grant JW, Serwer GA, Armstrong BE, et al. Junctional tachycardia in infants after open heart surgery for congenital heart disease. Am J Cardiol 59:1216, 1987.

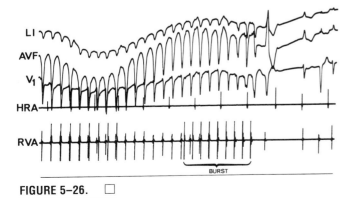

FIGURE 5–26. □

Termination of ventricular tachycardia with a burst of rapid ventricular pacing during a formal electrophysiologic study.

18. Hofschire PJ, Nicoloff DM, Moller JH. Postoperative complete heart block in 64 children treated with and without cardiac pacing. Am J Cardiol 39:559, 1977.

19. Humes RA, Porter CJ, Puga FJ, et al. Utility of temporary atrial epicardial electrodes in postoperative pediatric cardiac patients. Mayo Clin Proc 64:516, 1989.

20. Jackman WM, Friday KJ, Anderson JL, et al. The long QT syndromes: A critical review, new clinical observations and a unifying hypothesis. Prog Cardiovasc Dis 41:115, 1988.

21. Jackman WM, Wang XZ, Friday KJ, et al. Catheter ablation of accessory atrioventricular pathways (Wolff-Parkinson-White syndrome) by radiofrequency current. N Engl J Med 324:1605, 1991.

22. Josephson ME, Horowitz LN. Electrophysiologic approach to therapy of recurrent sustained ventricular tachycardia. Am J Cardiol 43:361, 1979.

23. Josephson ME, Kastor JA. Paroxysmal supraventricular tachycardia. Is the atrium a necessary link? Circulation 54:430, 1976.

24. Klitzner TS, Friedman WF. Cardiac arrhythmias: The role of pharmacologic intervention. Cardiol Clin 7:299, 1989.

25. Ko JK, Deal BJ, Strasburger JF, et al. Supraventricular tachycardia mechanisms and their age distribution in pediatric patients. Am J Cardiol 69:1028, 1992.

26. Lerman BB, Belardinelli L. Clinical electrophysiology of adenosine: Basic and clinical concepts. Circulation 83:1499, 1991.

27. Lucchesi BR. Rationale of therapy in the patient with acute myocardial infarction and life-threatening arrhythmias: A focus on bretylium. Am J Cardiol 54:14A, 1984.

28. Moak JP. Pharmacology and electrophysiology of antiarrhythmic drugs. In Gillette PC, Garson A (eds). Pediatric Arrhythmias: Electrophysiology and Pacing. Philadelphia, WB Saunders, 1990, pp 37–118.

29. Morady F. The spectrum of arrhythmias in preexcitation syndromes. In Benditt DG, Benson DW (eds). Cardiac Preexcitation Syndromes. Boston, Martinus Nijhoff, 1986, pp 119–140.

30. Sellers TD, Bashore TM, Gallagher JJ. Digitalis in the preexcitation syndrome: Analysis during atrial fibrillation. Circulation 56:260, 1975.

31. Sholler GF, Walsh EP, Mayer JE, et al. Evaluation of a staged treatment protocol for rapid junctional tachycardia. Abstract. Circulation 78(suppl II):II-597, 1988.

32. Syoka LF. Pediatric clinical pharmacology of digoxin. Pediatr Clin 28:203, 1981.

33. Till JA, Rowland E, Shinebourne EA, et al. R-wave synchronized pacing in the management of post-surgical His bundle tachycardia. Abstract. Circulation 78(suppl II):II-597, 1988.

34. Tzivoni D, Banai S, Schuger C, et al. Treatment of torsades de pointes with magnesium sulfate. Circulation 77:392, 1988.

35. Velevit V, Podrid P, Lown B, et al. Aggravation and provocation of ventricular arrhythmias by antiarrhythmic drugs. Circulation 65:886, 1982.

36. Vetter VL, Tanner CS, Horowitz LN. Inducible atrial flutter after the Mustard repair of complete transposition of the great arteries. Am J Cardiol 61:428, 1988.

37. Waldo AL, Krongard E, Kupersmith J, et al. Ventricular paired pacing to control rapid ventricular heart rate following open heart surgery. Circulation 53:176, 1976.

38. Walsh EP, Saul JP. Cardiac arrhythmias. In Fyler DC (ed). Nadas' Pediatric Cardiology. Philadelphia, Hanley and Belfus, 1991, p 377.

39. Walsh EP, Saul JP, Hulse JE, et al. Transcatheter ablation of ectopic atrial tachycardia in young patients using radiofrequency current. Circulation 86:1138, 1992.

40. Wit AL, Dillon SM. Anisotropic reentry. In Zipes DP, Jalife J (eds). Cardiac Electrophysiology, From Cell to Bedside. Philadelphia, WB Saunders, 1990, pp 353–363.

41. Zipes DP, Jalife J. Cardiac Electrophysiology, From Cell to Bedside. Philadelphia, WB Saunders, 1990.

POSTCARDIOTOMY MECHANICAL VENTRICULAR ASSISTANCE

Prolonged extracorporeal circulatory support is being applied with increasing frequency to infants and older pediatric cardiac patients with severe cardiopulmonary dysfunction in the hope that survival will be improved. Because of the availability of the technology, early investigators used extracorporeal membrane oxygenation (ECMO) circuits exclusively, and this method continues to be the most common form of postcardiotomy mechanical support.[1, 3, 4, 6, 7, 10] As of April 1991, the National ECMO registry listed 419 neonatal and other pediatric cardiac patients who had been placed on ECMO. In contrast to this significant experience, the use of isolated ventricular assist devices (VADs) in infant and pediatric cardiac patients has been much more limited, with only a few experimental and clinical case reports in the literature.[2, 8, 9] As of the end of 1990, the Clinical Registry of Mechanical Ventricular Assists and Artificial Hearts had listed only five reported uses of VADs in cardiac patients less than 1 year of age.[5] Because of the complexity of its circuitry, including a gas exchange unit and the need for patient anticoagulation, ECMO may not always be the optimal methodology when prolonged circulatory support is required after a cardiotomy.

At Children's Hospital in Boston, beginning in January 1990, we established a program making both ECMO and VADs (i.e., Bio-Medicus, Minneapolis, MN, centrifugal pump) available for infants and other pediatric cardiac patients who require postcardiotomy mechanical ventricular assistance.

RESULTS

All patients admitted to the cardiac intensive care unit between January 1990 and December 1991 (more than 2000) had both ECMO and VAD availability. Most were postoperative patients who had undergone repair or palliation of structural heart defects; a smaller number were patients without structural heart disease who had severe cardiopulmonary compromise secondary to myocarditis or cardiomyopathy. Because of the meager experience with these mechanical assist devices in neonates and infants, specific preliminary criteria based on logic and general experience were established both for the need for mechanical ventricular assistance and for specific indications for the use of either ECMO or VAD. ECMO was used as the support method of choice if there was a component of pulmonary insufficiency or if biventricular dysfunction was present in patients weighing less than 5 kg. An isolated left ventricular assist device (LVAD), an isolated right ventricular assist device (RVAD), or a biventricular assist device (BVAD) was used as the support method of choice if isolated univentricular dysfunction was present in a patient of any size or if biventricular dysfunction was present in a patient weighing more than 5 kg.

In general, patients with cardiopulmonary dysfunction after a cardiotomy were first aggressively evaluated using information from intracardiac lines and from both echocardiography and cardiac catheterization if necessary. If structural heart disease remained, the patient underwent surgical revision. In the absence of reparable residual lesions, aggressive management consisting of inotropic support, afterload reduction, diuretic therapy, sodium bicarbonate supplementation, and open sternotomy was instituted. Often, patients would be transiently maintained on as many as three separate inotropic agents, frequently with epinephrine infusions as high as 0.3 μg/kg/min for as long as 12 to 24 hours before consideration of mechanical assistance. For patients suffering primarily from difficulties with ventilation and gas exchange, aggressive management, including trials of high-frequency jet ventilation, was usually attempted before consideration of the use of extracorporeal mechanical support. Other patients with more profound cardiopulmonary dysfunction who could not be weaned from cardiopulmonary bypass were placed on mechanical support in the operating room.

Using this approach, a total of 21 patients (approximately 1% of all admissions to the cardiac intensive care unit) received prolonged extracorporeal circulatory support between January 1990 and January 1992. Fourteen of these were placed on ECMO, (four preoperatively and 10 postoperatively). A venoarterial system was used in all cases, incorporating the right carotid artery and jugular veins. Of the four preoperative patients, three had transposi-

tion of the great arteries with an intact ventricular septum and were placed on ECMO at 1 day of age after failing to achieve cardiorespiratory stability after birth. All three were profoundly hypoxic; one had suffered a severe pulmonary hemorrhage, and another had primary pulmonary hypertension. Two of these three patients underwent arterial switch operations after 5 and 7 days of ECMO, with one of the two surviving. The third patient suffered a grade IV intraventricular hemorrhage while on ECMO and was not surgically repaired. The fourth preoperative patient was a 1-month-old infant with an unrepaired total anomalous pulmonary venous connection in addition to profound bacterial sepsis. After 1 week on ECMO, which included management of the sepsis, surgical repair was performed; the patient survived. Thus, two of four patients (50%) requiring preoperative ECMO have survived.

The 10 patients placed on ECMO postoperatively ranged in age from 1 month to 2.3 years and weighed from 2.5 to 11.6 kg. Seven of the 10 patients had important pulmonary dysfunction, either parenchymal or pulmonary vascular dysfunction; three had no pulmonary disease but had biventricular dysfunction (body weights: 2.7, 4.4, and 4.5 kg). Seven of the 10 were weaned from ECMO, with five long-term survivors (50%).

Seven patients were placed on VADs, two of them preoperatively. One of these, an 11-month-old patient weighing 6 kg who had profound left ventricular dysfunction from acute viral myocarditis, was placed on an LVAD for 5 days, after which she was successfully removed and became a long-term survivor. The other preoperative patient, a 4-year-old weighing 16 kg who had profound biventricular failure secondary to cardiomyopathy, underwent 4 days of BVAD support as a bridge to transplantation and was successfully transplanted. This patient required RVAD postoperatively for 2 days after the transplantation and was successfully weaned from this as well, but went on to have chronic severe rejection and died 3 months postoperatively.

Of the five patients placed on a VAD postoperatively, one was placed on an LVAD and two on RVADs; two were patients with single ventricle who had had bidirectional cavopulmonary shunts. Four of the five patients were weaned from the assist device, with complete cardiac recovery. Duration of use of the VAD ranged from 18 hours to 8 days. Two patients died late, one from hepatic failure and another from endocarditis and renal failure.

In all VAD patients, Bio-Medicus arterial and venous cannulae were used. For LVAD placement, the ascending aorta and left atrial appendage are cannulated, whereas for RVAD placement, the main pulmonary artery and right atrial appendage are used. Cannulae can be brought through the chest wall either in the suprasternal position or in the left or right parasternal positions after carefully assessing the optimal cannula angle. This allows sternal closure. Flow rates are determined using physiologic principles to maintain a total cardiac output that is adequate for the patient's needs. At the time of weaning, hemodynamic parameters, mixed venous oxygen saturation, acid production, peripheral perfusion, and urine production are carefully monitored as flows are incrementally reduced over a 12- to 24-hour period. Bedside echocardiography is also performed to determine ventricular function. If these parameters remain acceptable for a 4- to 6-hour period at VAD flow rates of 20% or less of predicted cardiac output, the patient is returned to the operating room and decannulated. Generally, activated clotting time is kept between 150 and 170 seconds; however, during weaning it is increased to between 180 and 200 seconds.

In the overall postcardiotomy group, hemorrhagic complications were common among patients on ECMO, significantly altering the outcome or affecting management decisions in six of 10 (60%). Hemorrhage was not clinically important in any of the patients on VADs. All patients on ECMO had significantly positive fluid balances, whereas 83% of those on VADs (five of six) had either even or negative fluid balances.

CURRENT RECOMMENDATIONS

ECMO and VADs are each useful in infant and pediatric patients with severe cardiopulmonary dysfunction. Indications for each device are preliminary and still evolving. At the present time, ECMO is clearly the support method of choice in the pediatric cardiac patient if there is severe pulmonary dysfunction either preoperatively or postoperatively. When single-ventricle dysfunction is present without pulmonary dysfunction, a VAD is the support method of choice, regardless of patient size. When biventricular dysfunction exists without pulmonary dysfunction, a BVAD should be considered. A relative contraindication to the use of a BVAD is patient size, as a BVAD requires four intracardiac cannulae. This can be technically problematic in the patient weighing less than 5 kg.

When isolated cardiac dysfunction is present, especially early after cardiotomy, the hemorrhagic complications that attend the use of ECMO support are overwhelming, severely limiting survival. This has been our experience as well as that of others who have used ECMO in this setting. The isolated VAD—which, unlike ECMO, does not require significant patient anticoagulation and does include a gas exchange unit—offers a great advantage over the ECMO circuit when support is required either intraoperatively or early (first 6 to 12 hours) postoperatively. Generally, activated clotting times have been in the range of 140 to 160 seconds during prolonged VAD use with the Bio-Medicus centrifugal pump. There have been no documented episodes of thrombosis or embolization. In one patient who was kept on extremely low flows (approximately 15% of cardiac output) for more than 12 hours, a very small amount of mural thrombus was detected in both the arterial and the venous cannulae at inspection after removal.

In our experience at Children's Hospital in Boston, the use of a VAD limits both hemorrhagic complications and the ongoing capillary leak that attend total cardiopulmonary bypass and ECMO. Largely because of these hemorrhagic complications, our general experience as well as that of others has been that survival is rare when ECMO is instituted intraoperatively, directly from cardiopulmonary bypass.[1, 3, 4, 6, 7, 10] ECMO is safer (and more appropriate) when the need for support is late after a cardiotomy (i.e., more than 12 hours after cardiopulmonary bypass), when the patient's coagulation system has recovered and extensive suture lines have been relatively well sealed.

It should be emphasized that prolonged extracorporeal circulatory support in infant and older pediatric cardiac patients is an evolving discipline. Although the indications for its use and the criteria for specific device selection cannot yet be formulated with certainty, it seems clear that the exclusive use of ECMO in infants and children with cardiac disease, as advocated by some, does not maximize patient survival. Neither ECMO nor VADs should be considered after a cardiotomy unless residual correctable structural disease has been ruled out.

REFERENCES

1. Anderson HL, Attorri RJ, Custer JR, et al. Extracorporeal membrane oxygenation for pediatric cardiopulmonary failure. J Thorac Cardiovasc Surg 99:1011, 1990.
2. Drinkwater DC, Laks H. Clinical experience with centrifugal pump ventricular support at UCLA Medical Center. Trans Am Soc Artif Intern Organs 34:505, 1988.
3. Kanter KR, Pennington G, Weber TR, et al. Extracorporeal membrane oxygenation for postoperative cardiac support in children. J Thorac Cardiovasc Surg 93:27, 1987.
4. Klein MD, Shaheen KW, Whittlesey GC, et al. Extracorporeal membrane oxygenation for the circulatory support of children after repair of congenital heart disease. J Thorac Cardiovasc Surg 100:498, 1990.
5. Miller CA. Clinical Registry of Mechanical Ventricular Assists and Artificial Hearts. Hershey, PA, Department of Surgery, Hershey Medical Center, 1990.

6. Redmond CR, Graves ED, Falterman KW, et al. Extracorporeal membrane oxygenation for respiratory and cardiac failure in infants and children. J Thorac Cardiovasc Surg 93:1999, 1987.

7. Rogers AJ, Trento A, Siewers RD, et al. Extracorporeal membrane oxygenation for postcardiotomy cardiogenic shock in children. Ann Thorac Surg 47:903, 1989.

8. Taenaka Y, Takano H, Nakatani T, et al. Ventricular assist device (VAD) for children: In vitro and in vivo evaluation. Trans Am Soc Artif Intern Organs 30:606, 1984.

9. Taenaka Y, Takano H, Noda H, et al. Experimental evaluation and clinical application of a pediatric ventricular assist device. Trans Am Soc Artif Intern Organs 35:155, 1989.

10. Weinhaus L, Canter C, Noetzel M, et al. Extracorporeal membrane oxygenation for circulatory support after repair of congenital heart defects. Ann Thorac Surg 48:206, 1989.

6

Conduits: Clinical and Experimental Aspects

An important premise of pediatric cardiac surgery is that any surgical procedure should incorporate growth potential. Although this is readily achieved with the repair of more simple lesions such as atrial or ventricular septal defects, there are many complex lesions for which greater thought must be given to achieving this goal. This is particularly true of lesions in which one of the great vessels is either diminutive or absent. The classic anomaly in which a great vessel must be fabricated in some way is tetralogy of Fallot with pulmonary atresia. Other anomalies often requiring conduit insertion are D- and L-loop transpositions or double-outlet right ventricle with a ventricular septal defect and pulmonary stenosis, as well as truncus arteriosus. Increasing disenchantment with the performance of conduits over the long term has resulted in the elimination of conduits from the repair of anomalies for which they were commonly used in the past, such as in the repair of interrupted aortic arch and in the Fontan procedure.

HISTORY OF THE DEVELOPMENT OF VASCULAR GRAFTS

Allograft Blood Vessels

In the early 1900s, Carrel pioneered the use of transplanted allograft (homograft) arteries and veins as vascular substitutes in an experimental setting, using canine models.[15–17, 37] He developed a number of surgical techniques and instruments that remain in use today. It was not until the development of antibiotics in the 1940s that Carrel's ideas could be applied clinically.

Crafoord, in 1944, was the first to undertake repair of coarctation,[18] followed shortly thereafter by Gross.[34] Gross was concerned that although the elasticity of the aorta would allow resection and direct anastomosis in most cases of coarctation, this was not universally so. He needed a safe arterial substitute and, like Carrel, looked to a nonvalved aortic allograft (Fig. 6–1).[35] In laboratory studies investigating methods of preparation and storage of aortic allografts, Gross found that some methods of storage frequently resulted in catastrophic failure (i.e., death from rupture of the allograft). Nine of 12 dogs that received abdominal aortic allografts that had been frozen to $-72°C$ (CO_2) without a cryoprotective agent died within 2 weeks of surgery when the allograft ruptured. In contrast, none of 25 allografts that had been stored in a balanced salt solution at 4°C ruptured.[33]

During the decade that ensued, many aortic allografts were implanted for coarctation with no widely known reports of failure, although undoubtedly aneurysms, aorto–left bronchial fistulae, and rupture occurred sporadically.[22, 31, 38]

Subsequently, arterial allografts were applied to other peripheral vascular problems such as abdominal aortic aneurysm and iliac and femoral arterial

9

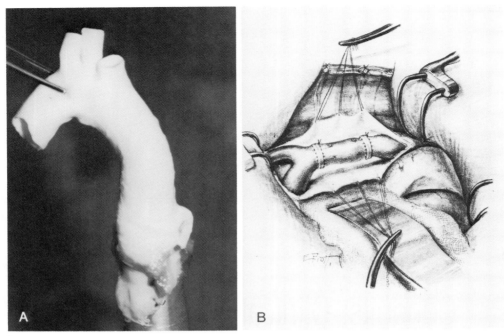

FIGURE 6–1. ☐

The aortic allograft currently is commonly applied as a valve-containing conduit *(A)*, although it was originally used by Gross as a nonvalved conduit for repair of coarctation *(B)*. (From Jonas RA, Mayer JE, Castaneda AR. Unsatisfactory clinical experience with a collagen sealed, knitted Dacron extracardiac conduit. J Cardiac Surg 2:257, 1987.)

occlusive disease. This clinical experience in the early 1950s suggested that there was a higher risk of aneurysm formation or thrombosis with allografts from peripheral muscular arteries such as the femoral artery than there was when proximal, more elastic arteries, such as the ascending aorta, were used.[11, 66] In addition, the logistical and legal problems of collection and storage led to general dissatisfaction with allografts.

Synthetic Vascular Grafts

The explosion of knowledge in the field of plastics technology led to the appearance of numerous durable synthetic fabrics in the late 1940s and early 1950s. These fabrics were soon used by DeBakey and others to construct synthetic tube grafts or conduits. Dacron (polyethylene terephthalate) was recognized as more stable and resistant to degradation when in a biologic milieu than some of its polymer cousins such as nylon and Ivalon.[21, 26, 80, 87]

Edwards emphasized in an early report[25] that the porosity of fabric tubes gave them an advantage over nonporous alternatives. A totally impervious conduit, such as a Silastic tube, showed progressive accumulation of pseudointima, forming an inert capsule (both inner and outer) with no adhesion of that capsule to the prosthesis, much like the thick

nonadherent capsule surrounding a pacemaker generator.[3]

Wesolowksi and coworkers pursued the relationship between synthetic conduit porosity and healing with a wide range of laboratory studies.[88, 90] In 1961 they concluded that optimal healing occurred with a water porosity of 5000 ml/cm^2/min at a pressure of 120 mm Hg. Most of the higher porosity, knitted Dacron grafts currently in use have a porosity of approximately 2000 ml/cm^2/min. In the nonheparinized patient undergoing peripheral vascular surgery, this high porosity can be controlled at the time of implantation by preclotting the graft with the patient's own blood. This is not adequate for the fully heparinized patient undergoing cardiac surgery. Numerous attempts have been made since the 1960s to achieve temporary porosity control with biologic sealants other than the patient's own fibrin clot. However, early investigators had persistent problems with cracking and separation of sealant materials.[6, 42, 51] An alternative approach was simply to use less porous fabric. This led to the introduction of woven fabric tubes with a baseline porosity of 100 to 250 ml/cm^2/min, such as the Cooley Veri-Soft graft (Meadox Medical; Newark, NJ). Because acceptable blood loss in the heparinized patient requires a porosity of less than 50 ml/cm^2/min, even these grafts require preclotting. Another technique that has become popular has been to bake these

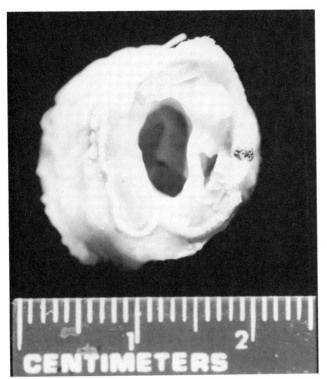

FIGURE 6–2.   □

Low-porosity Dacron conduit can rapidly accumulate a thick pseudointima ("peel"). This 14-mm Dacron conduit needed replacement within 15 months of implantation. (From Jonas RA, Schoen FJ, Ziemer G, et al. Biological sealants and knitted Dacron conduits: Comparison of collagen and fibrin glue pretreatments in circulatory models. Ann Thorac Surg 44:283, 1987.)

work of the prosthesis. These loops are said to encourage fibrous and vascular ingrowth and thus anchor the pseudointima.[41, 67, 79] At the same time, they decrease the porosity of the fabric, but only to a limited degree. Therefore, the search has continued for a suitable technique of incorporating a biologically degradable component within the graft.

Biologic Sealants for Synthetic Grafts

Wesolowski studied the "sealant" concept with a number of materials, including aldehyde cross-linked collagen.[89] He determined from this study that delayed resorption of the absorbable component (such as strongly cross-linked collagen) actually accelerated pseudointima formation and graft occlusion. He concluded that the absorbable component should be cleared at the rate of autologous fibrin.

A knitted Dacron graft, sealed with human albumin, was released briefly in the early 1980s but was subsequently withdrawn from the U.S. market because of manufacturing and packaging difficulties.[24, 36] Another graft, the Tascon knitted graft, was presealed with a thin, luminal coating of glutaraldehyde cross-linked collagen. Laboratory studies at Children's Hospital in Boston revealed that resorption of the collagen was very slow, and because the coating was on the luminal surface, there was poor adhesion of pseudointima to the graft (Fig. 6–3).[47, 48]

moderate-porosity, woven tube grafts after soaking them in heparinized blood or albumin. To avoid the need for any graft preparation, very tightly woven, very low porosity grafts, such as the Cooley Lo-Por graft (Meadox Medical; Newark, NJ), were introduced. Such grafts have a baseline porosity of approximately 50 ml/cm[2]/min. They are difficult to handle because of their rigidity and difficulty with needle penetration. In addition, Edwards' and Wesolowski's predictions about the healing of such grafts proved to be correct.[25, 88] These grafts accumulate a poorly adherent, thick pseudointima with areas of hemorrhagic dissection between the luminal surface of the graft and the pseudointima. Although this may not be of clinical significance in a large-diameter (greater than 20 mm), straight tube graft (e.g., one used for replacement of an abdominal aortic aneurysm), it is certainly significant in smaller grafts, particularly when placed in growing children (Fig. 6–2).

Another approach, such as that popularized by Sauvage et al., has been to introduce velour internally, externally, or both. The velour fibers form loops that project above or below the basic frame-

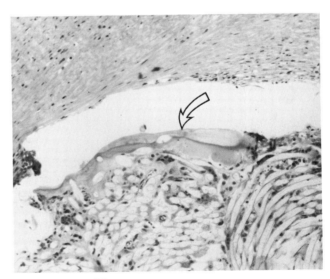

FIGURE 6–3.   □

Photomicrograph of a knitted Dacron conduit with a lining of glutaraldehyde-treated collagen on its luminal surface (Tascon conduit). Failure of the collagen lining to resorb *(arrow)*, even after several months of implantation, resulted in poor adhesion of pseudointima, repeated dissection deep to the pseudointima, and rapid accumulation of thick pseudointima. (From Jonas RA, Mayer JE, Castaneda AR. Unsatisfactory clinical experience with a collagen sealed, knitted Dacron extracardiac conduit. J Cardiac Surg 2:257, 1987.)

In a small clinical trial, it was confirmed that the graft failed early in a number of cases because of rapid accumulation of pseudointima (Fig. 6–4).[46] Collagen can be less strongly cross-linked by using formaldehyde rather than glutaraldehyde. This is the basis of the Hemashield process (Meadox Medical; Newark, NJ) that currently is commercially available in the United States. Laboratory studies using subcutaneous implants of treated Dacron in rats, as well as circulatory implants in sheep, have suggested that this material has little effect on the normal healing process of the Dacron graft. Studies have confirmed excellent porosity control to less than 10 ml/cm^2/min.[47, 48]

Another approach currently undergoing scrutiny by the U.S. Food and Drug Administration is to use the tropocollagen subunits of collagen as found in gelatin (Vascutek; Inchinnan, Scotland). This material is highly water soluble and has been used as a plasma expander for many years. The collagen subunits are weakly cross-linked using aldehyde. The degree of cross-linking can be controlled by chemically converting some of the amino groups that take part in the cross-link to carboxyl groups. Laboratory studies undertaken at Children's Hospital in Boston suggest that this approach also does not significantly impede the normal healing process of knitted Dacron grafts (Fig. 6–5).[50]

Fibrin glue is a human fibrinogen–bovine thrombin, two-component material that can be applied to porous vascular prostheses.[39] Although appropriate resorption is likely, the material has the potential for viral transmission, as well as the disadvantage of a tedious dissolving, mixing, and application process.

A number of researchers continue to pursue the concept of a composite fabric in which one of the yarns incorporated in the weave is bioresorbable.[9, 29, 86] Careful assessment must be made of the rate of decay of fabric strength; the fabric must have sufficient long-term strength to resist aneurysm formation.

Small-Diameter Arterial Prostheses

Microporous expanded polytetrafluoroethylene (PTFE) is a form of Teflon in which the polymer is arranged as a lattice of nodes interconnected by filaments. During its development in the early 1970s, many variations of internodal spacing (pore size) were tested, with the conclusion that a pore size of 20 to 30 μm was optimal for healing.[13] Early clinical implants had a tendency toward aneurysmal dilatation; this has been overcome by the addition of an external PTFE wrap or by increasing the thickness of the graft wall. In its current commercial form, this material (known as Gore-Tex or Impra) has proved to be considerably more successful than Dacron as a small (< 7 mm in internal diameter) arterial prosthesis. Important disadvantages of PTFE are persistent needle-hole bleeding (which is only partially overcome by the use of PTFE suture in the fully heparinized patient) and the difficulty of conforming this material in larger sizes to the irregular course sometimes required for cardiac reconstructive purposes.

Endothelial Lining of Synthetic Prostheses

An important area of contemporary research is the seeding of endothelial cells onto Dacron or PTFE grafts.[40] Such cells can be mechanically or enzymatically debrided from a suitable dispensable autologous vessel and are then suspended in the patient's blood, which is used to preclot the prosthesis. Cell culture techniques can be used to increase the number of cells.[84] Despite promising early results, these techniques present logistic difficulties. In addition, there is emerging doubt that even if endothelial cells remain viable when bonded directly to synthetic material, many important functions such as their antithrombogenic properties, including the synthesis of prostacyclin, may not be preserved in this setting. Attention is currently being directed at the role of the basement membrane in facilitating normal endothelial cell function.

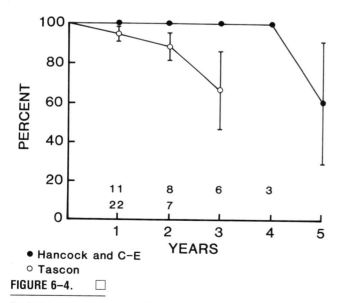

● Hancock and C–E
○ Tascon
FIGURE 6–4. ☐

The Tascon conduit performed significantly worse than the Hancock and Carpentier-Edwards (C-E) conduits in a small clinical trial, as illustrated by the percentage of patients who were free from conduit replacement plotted against the duration of implantation. (From Jonas RA, Ziemer G, Schoen FJ, et al. A new sealant for knitted Dacron prostheses: Minimally cross-linked gelatin. J Vasc Surg 7:414, 1988.)

FIGURE 6–5. □

Photomicrographs of unimplanted grafts showing current methods of temporarily decreasing the high porosity of knitted Dacron conduits. *A,* Graft presealed with albumin. *B,* Graft presealed with gelatin. In each case the sealant material is indicated by a star. (hematoxylin and eosin stain)

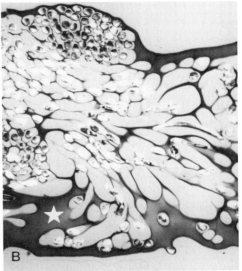

Biologic Grafts Other Than Arterial Allografts

A number of vascular xenografts have been described since Carrel first reported the use of frozen and formalin-preserved arterial xenografts as arterial substitutes.[16] Rosenberg and associates[75] described the treatment of bovine carotid arteries with ficin, to remove the antigenicity of the smooth muscle, followed by collagen cross-linking with dialdehyde starch. Although this graft is useful as a subcutaneous arteriovenous fistula for hemodialysis, its susceptibility to thrombosis and aneurysm formation has limited its application for other vascular reconstructive purposes.

Human umbilical vein treated with glutaraldehyde and incorporated within a mesh of Dacron has functioned as well as saphenous vein for above-knee, femoropopliteal bypass, although there is an increasing risk of aneurysmal degeneration, thrombosis, and false aneurysm formation at the sites of anastomoses over time.[20]

VASCULAR PROSTHESES FOR RECONSTRUCTIVE CARDIAC SURGERY

Aortic Allograft Conduits

The first conduits used in a cardiac reconstructive procedure were constructed from the patients' own pericardium. These grafts were interposed between the right ventricle and pulmonary artery for tetralogy of Fallot with pulmonary atresia.[59, 74] Because adequate pericardium often is not available in these patients and because of the hemodynamic advantages of incorporating a valve in the conduit, Ross

and Somerville introduced the concept of a valved, aortic allograft conduit in Britain (see Fig. 6–1).[76] Unlike Gross's allograft conduits for coarctation, Ross included the aortic valve with the aortic root and ascending aorta, thus re-creating the valved right ventricular outflow tract. Ross's allografts were collected from cadavers, generally within 24 to 48 hours of death. After dissection, the allografts were treated with an antibiotic solution for a few days and were then stored in either a balanced salt solution or in tissue culture medium at 4°C for up to 4 weeks. When allografts were introduced in the United States, at least two important changes to Ross's original method were made. First, instead of a weak antibiotic solution to "sterilize" the allografts, high-power irradiation was employed. Instead of being stored in a balanced salt solution, with or without tissue culture medium at 4°C, many allografts were freeze dried. These techniques, particularly in combination, led to death of cells and severe damage to the collagen within the valve leaflets. Although Ross had observed calcification in the wall of this conduit, valve leaflet calcification had been extremely rare.[76, 78] In contrast, stenosis rapidly developed in the valve of the irradiated, freeze-dried allograft, and therefore, allografts fell into general disrepute in the United States.[64]

Bioprosthetic Conduits: Glutaraldehyde-Treated, Porcine-Valved Dacron Conduits

In the early 1970s, very low porosity, woven Dacron conduits became available.[10] Such conduits were combined with the glutaraldehyde-treated pig valve as pioneered by Carpentier et al.[14] The immense logistic advantages of such conduits, which could be stocked in a complete range of sizes, proved attractive, and during the ensuing decade many thousands of these Hancock and Carpentier-Edwards conduits were implanted.

Within just 5 years, reports of the unsatisfactory performance of these conduits appeared (Fig. 6–6).[1, 5, 67] As could have been predicted from Wesolowski's studies in 1963, a thick pseudointima frequently accumulated rapidly. In addition, others noted that glutaraldehyde tanning of pig valves resulted in rapid calcification in children.[30, 91] Thus, a combination of pseudointima formation and valve stenosis resulted in a less than 50% freedom from conduit replacement within 9 years of implantation.[45] In their favor, however, it should be noted that the mode of failure of these conduits was only very rarely catastrophic. Simple monitoring of the systolic murmur and right ventricular hypertrophy on the electrocardiogram allowed for elective replacement of these conduits, which easily shelled out of their covering of pseudoadventitia, at very low risk.

Addition of a valve to the conduit appeared to accelerate pseudointima formation,[27] and thus one response to the problem was a more liberal use of nonvalved conduits. However, by this time the outstanding long-term results of Ross and others using allografts[23, 55] became widely appreciated, and in the mid-1980s the allograft once again became the conduit of first choice for cardiac reconstruction in the United States.

CURRENT METHODS OF ALLOGRAFT PREPARATION

Allografts stored at 4°C gradually lose cellular viability and tissue integrity and are discarded within 4 to 6 weeks of collection. This presents a major logistic problem, particularly in the management of smaller children, where the number of appropriate-size donors is limited. Major advances in cryopreservation technology currently allow the preservation of many cells, such as sperm and red cells, and even complete embryos, which can be preserved possibly indefinitely. Whereas Gross used an uncontrolled rate of freezing to the temperature of dry ice (−72°C), current practice involves a controlled rate of freezing to the temperature of liquid nitrogen (−196°C). In addition, a cryoprotectant such as dimethyl sulfoxide (DMSO) also helps to prevent the formation of intracellular ice crystals during the freezing process. The specific antibiotics employed can also influence the long-term performance of allografts. Studies by Armiger and associates[4] suggested that a combination of cefoxitin, lincomycin,

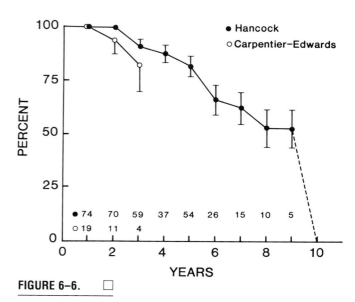

FIGURE 6–6. ☐

Actuarial freedom from replacement of porcine valves containing woven Dacron conduits.

polymyxin B, vancomycin, and amphotericin (CLPVA) was optimal for facilitating ongrowth and ingrowth of recipient cells into the leaflets of the allograft valve. More recent studies have resulted in modification of this antibiotic mixture in an attempt to maximize cellular viability,[12] although this may increase the risk of persistent bacterial contamination, necessitating discarding of the allograft.

The organization of regional organ and tissue banks has facilitated the collection of allografts. Most donors in the United States have been brain-dead (but heart-beating) multiple-organ donors. The collection has been undertaken in the sterile setting of an operating room. To supply the rapidly increasing demand for a wide range of allograft sizes, it will be important in the coming years to expand collection to cadavers, as has been the practice in Britain, New Zealand, and other countries since the 1960s.[52]

CELLULAR VIABILITY AND LONG-TERM ALLOGRAFT PERFORMANCE

A long-standing controversy has centered on the importance of continuing viability of donor cells in the maintenance of allograft durability. The point of view espoused by Barratt-Boyes for many years has been that the allograft is primarily a collagenous skeleton and that donor cellular viability is unimportant. Preservation of the mucopolysaccharide ground substance, as well as the ultrastructure of collagen and elastin during preparation, is considered important. Appropriate preparation is also important to encourage both ongrowth and ingrowth of recipient cells onto the valve leaflets.[4] This lappet of tissue at the critical hinge area of the valve is important for leaflet durability. The usual mechanism of failure of allografts is rupture of the leaflets, resulting in valvar regurgitation. In the case of aortic allografts, the conduit wall almost always becomes heavily calcified, so it is unlikely that viability of cells could influence the durability of conduit function. In the case of pulmonary allografts, calcification of the arterial wall is much less common and, when present, much less pronounced relative to aortic allografts.[2] This may be related to (1) the fact that the arterial wall of the pulmonary allograft is thinner (60% of aortic allograft thickness) and (2) the elastin concentration, as elastin tends to be the nidus for calcification. At least three laboratory studies[2, 53, 68] have suggested that pulmonary allografts harvested from immature animals and implanted into growing animals can increase in size with time (Fig. 6–7). Whether this represents growth secondary to viable cells or to simple dilatation is as yet unknown.

An alternative to the collagenous skeleton theory is the theory supported by O'Brien et al. for many years.[72, 73] O'Brien and coworkers believe that continuing viability of donor fibroblasts is important for the maintenance and continuing synthesis of collagen. In an anecdotal case in which a valve was retrieved 10 years after implantation, they were able to demonstrate by chromosome studies that donor cells were viable. Others have argued that this does not confirm a functional role for any remaining viable donor cells.[2] There is little disagreement that the majority of endothelial cells become necrotic during the collection, preparation, and storage procedures. Yankah and associates[92, 93] quantitated the percentage of viable endothelial cells in a rat model and found that all endothelial cells were dead within 5 days of harvesting.

If the importance of cellular viability is accepted, then modifications must be made to the harvesting, preparation, and storage methods to guarantee maximal cell viability. This has been the stimulus for recent modification of the antibiotic solution used by CryoLife, Inc., to sterilize the valve before cryopreservation. Cryopreservation itself must be carefully controlled to maximize cellular viability. When this is done properly, long-term viability will be much enhanced relative to that with simple storage at 4°C.

Failure of allografts implanted in children as conduits is primarily a result of outgrowth of the conduit. Neopulmonary valvar regurgitation is generally well tolerated; and therefore, it is unlikely that the question of the importance of cell viability in

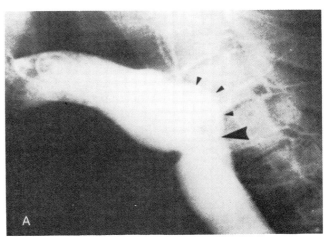

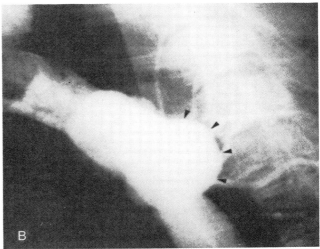

FIGURE 6–7. □

A laboratory study of pulmonary allografts implanted at systemic pressure in sheep demonstrated progressive aneurysmal dilation. *A,* Angiogram 3 months after implantation showing mild allograft dilation. *B,* Angiogram 5 months after implantation shows aneurysmal dilation of the allograft.

determining the durability of allografts will be solved in this setting. Implantation of aortic allografts as orthotopic aortic valve replacements is a much more demanding application than the use of allografts as conduits. Apart from O'Brien et al.'s series of 192 cryopreserved, aortic allograft valve replacements with a 10-year freedom from failure,[72] there are no published long-term series using potentially viable allografts as valve replacements. Cryopreserved allografts have been implanted in large numbers in the United States only since the late 1980s, so it is likely to be many years before this issue is resolved.

Role of Rejection in Determining Allograft Durability

Until the widespread application of cryopreserved allografts in the mid-1980s, most allografts used clinically were nonviable, so immune reactions to cellular elements were irrelevant. Collagen is a ubiquitous protein that does not stimulate an immune response per se, and fibroblasts, in contrast to endothelial cells, do not express class II antigens, which are important in the rejection response. After the introduction of cryopreserved "viable" allografts, attention was directed at the potential role of immune mechanisms in damaging allograft durability. In a series of elegant experiments, Yankah and co-workers[93] demonstrated that implantation of a viable aortic allograft in the abdominal aorta of inbred species of rats resulted in accelerated rejection of skin grafts from the same donor species. This has led some centers to use short-term immunosuppression in patients after allograft valve insertion. However, this does not seem to be justified until a more formal clinical study has conclusively demonstrated significant benefits of such an approach.

FAILURE OF ALLOGRAFT CONDUITS

Catastrophic failure of allograft conduits used for cardiac reconstruction has not yet been reported. However, based on the clinical experience of vascular surgeons during the 1950s,[22, 31, 38] it seems likely that with more widespread application of this biologic material, there will be failure by allograft rupture or the formation of pseudoaneurysms or conduit-to-bronchus fistulae. More recently, enthusiasm has developed for the use of pulmonary allografts to maximize the pool of available allograft sizes. When applied in a situation where it will be exposed to pressure equal to or greater than systemic pressure, a pulmonary allograft conduit can show rapid dilatation.[2, 53, 68] Because the pulmonary valve itself lacks a fibrous annulus, there is a significant risk of pseudoaneurysm formation at the proximal anastomosis. In fact, such pseudoaneurysms necessitated two reoperations among the first 100 pulmonary allografts inserted at Children's Hospital in Boston between 1985 and 1989.[54] Also, there was rupture of a pulmonary allograft exposed to systemic pressure as part of the reconstruction for a neonate with hypoplastic left heart syndrome.[54] Therefore, it would seem prudent to limit the use of pulmonary allografts to sites where the predicted intra-allograft pressure will be substantially subsystemic. In addition, any child receiving an allograft conduit must be carefully followed for life for early detection of the potential complications described.

THE FUTURE: AUTOGRAFTS AND THE "LIVING BLOOD VESSEL EQUIVALENT"

The growth potential of tubular segments of arterial autograft in children has been confirmed over many years by experience with renovascular reconstruction using segments of iliac artery.[57, 71] Furthermore, the potential for a relatively narrow strip of autologous tissue to provide appropriate growth when incorporated as a small part of the circumference of an otherwise nongrowing tube has been observed in a number of reconstructive cardiac procedures, including the Mustard and Norwood procedures. These observations led us to incorporate a strip of free arterial autograft as part of a conduit, the rest of which is constructed of pericardium. Appropriate growth was confirmed in 10 1-month-old lambs over 12 months (Fig. 6–8). To date, a single clinical implant, consisting of a longitudinal strip of free aortic autograft on an aortic allograft, has been inserted and has also demonstrated satisfactory growth.[81]

The "living skin equivalent" has been an important advance in the treatment of extensive skin loss caused by burns. Using cell culture methods, the layers of the dermis are built up, resulting in skin that is histologically and functionally similar to normal skin.[7] Concerted efforts are currently under way to fabricate a living blood vessel equivalent employing the same technology. Vessels are grown on glass mandrels with an intima, media, and adventitia being reproduced. If such a vessel could be imbued with appropriate growth potential, it would present a tremendous advance for the child with great vessel atresia who undergoes reconstructive cardiac surgery in early life.

CLINICAL INDICATIONS FOR CONDUIT INSERTION

The classic indications for conduit insertion have been tetralogy of Fallot with long-segment pulmonary atresia (pulmonary atresia with ventricular septal defect [VSD]), the so-called Rastelli procedure for D-transposition with a VSD and pulmonary stenosis,[74] and the repair of truncus arteriosus. Double-outlet right ventricle with a subpulmonary ventricular defect represents part of the spectrum between tetralogy of Fallot and transposition and is a rarer indication for conduit placement. L-loop transposition (corrected transposition with a VSD and pulmonary stenosis) requires conduit placement because of the course of the right coronary artery across the right-sided left ventricular outflow tract.

In the early years of ready availability of the por-

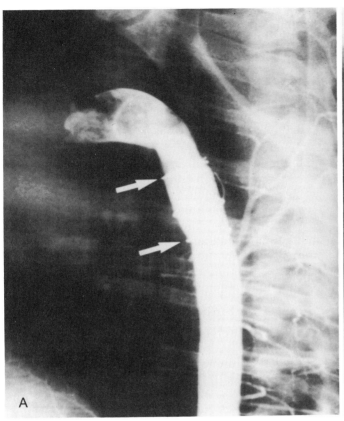

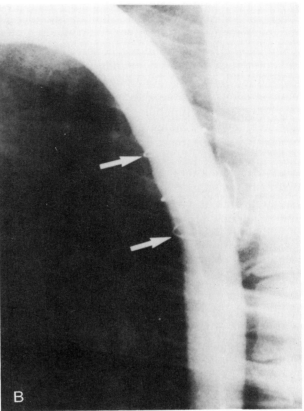

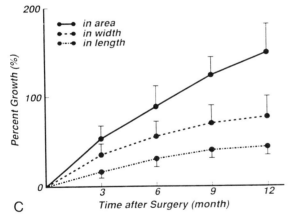

FIGURE 6–8. □

A laboratory study of a composite conduit containing a longitudinal strip of arterial autograft confirmed its growth potential. *A,* Postoperative aortogram 7 days after operation. *B,* Aortogram 12 months after operation. The white arrows indicate composite aortic conduit. *C,* Growth of the autologous aortic strip in length, width, and area with time. (From Sawatari K, Kawata H, Armiger LC, Jonas RA. Growth of composite conduits utilizing longitudinal arterial autograft in growing lambs. J Thorac Cardiovasc Surg 103:47–51, 1992.)

cine-valved Dacron conduit, before its high rate of failure was suspected, conduits were applied to a number of reconstructive problems where they easily can be avoided. For example, children with moderately severe hypoplasia of the main pulmonary artery as part of simple tetralogy had conduits placed for the perceived benefit of a competent valve in the right ventricular outflow tract.

Availability of the Hancock conduit also coincided with the introduction of the Fontan procedure for children with a single functional ventricle. These children demonstrated within a short time that the gradient resulting from pseudointima accumulation and stenosis of the porcine valve was a major hemodynamic disadvantage. Accordingly, innovative techniques were devised by Kreutzer and coworkers,[61] Bjork et al.,[8] and others to eliminate the need for a conduit as part of the Fontan procedure. A more recent modification described independently by Jonas and Castaneda,[44] Puga et al.[64] and de Leval et al.[23] has been the double cavopulmonary anastomosis. An intra-atrial baffle is placed to create a lateral cavopulmonary pathway to direct inferior vena caval blood to the cavopulmonary anastomosis.

Other operations that have fallen into disrepute

with the recognition of the unsatisfactory long-term performance of conduits include the Damus-Stansel-Kaye procedure for transposition and the left ventricular–apical aortic conduit. Damus,[19] Stansel,[85] and Kaye[56] described an operation for D-transposition with an intact ventricular septum based on the premise that it was desirable to use the left ventricle as the systemic ventricle, making a more physiologic correction of transposition than was achieved by atrial inversion procedures such as the Mustard or Senning operations. The main pulmonary artery was divided and the proximal end anastomosed to the side of the aorta. A conduit was then placed between the right ventricle and distal end of the main pulmonary artery. Not only did this carry the late complication of a high reoperation rate for conduit obstruction, but also the early mortality was high. Although the concept of an anastomosis between the pulmonary artery and the aorta has been preserved (for the bypass of subaortic obstruction with a single ventricle), the Damus-Stansel-Kaye operation has otherwise become of little more than historical interest.

Long, severe, tunnel subaortic stenosis or left ventricular outflow tract obstruction continues to be a major surgical challenge. After a brief period of enthusiasm for the placement of a valved conduit from the left ventricular apex to the descending thoracic aorta,[70] it soon became clear that this was not a satisfactory long-term solution. Frequently, it was difficult to achieve an unobstructed proximal anastomosis in the diminutive cavity of the very hypertrophied left ventricle. Stents only partially solved this problem and were highly susceptible themselves to pseudointima accumulation. Probably the most compelling reason surgeons have largely abandoned this procedure was the great difficulty in reoperating and replacing such conduits, in contrast to the relative ease of replacing a right ventricle-to-pulmonary artery conduit. Currently, extended aortic root replacement with an allograft[82] or various procedures for enlarging the left ventricular outflow tract, such as the Konno operation,[60] have replaced the apical aortic conduit.

Not only have conduits been used less frequently for the Fontan procedure and left ventricular outflow tract obstruction, but, in addition, a concerted effort has been made to minimize their use in the more traditional setting of tetralogy of Fallot with pulmonary atresia and D-transposition with a VSD and pulmonary stenosis. If there is some development of the main pulmonary artery, wide mobilization of the pulmonary artery branches allows the proximal part of the main pulmonary artery to be anastomosed directly to an infundibular incision in the right ventricle. The anterior wall of the pulmo-

nary artery and the ventriculotomy can be supplemented with an autologous pericardial patch. The appreciation of the elasticity and consequent mobility of the pulmonary arteries has developed in part from the widespread application of Lecompte's anterior pulmonary artery translocation procedure, performed as part of the arterial switch procedure for D-transposition of the great arteries.[63] Lecompte and associates also described translocation of the pulmonary arteries anterior to the aorta as part of the REV procedure for transposition of the great arteries with a VSD and pulmonary stenosis.[77] Another technique described by Jacobs and colleagues[43] involves the use of the left atrial appendage as a source of autologous tissue with growth potential. The reconstructed right ventricular outflow tract is roofed anteriorly with autologous pericardium.

GENERAL TECHNIQUE OF ALLOGRAFT CONDUIT INSERTION

The cryopreserved allograft must be thawed for approximately 10 minutes in a water bath at 37°C. The dimethyl sulfoxide is rinsed out by serial dilution. A small segment must be sent for bacteriologic culture. The walls and valve tissue are carefully examined, and the coronary arteries are suture ligated. The allograft is cut to length. The distal anastomosis is fashioned with a continuous Prolene suture. The allograft should be oriented so that the anterior leaflet of the mitral valve (which should be left attached to the allograft aortic valve during the dissection) lies mainly posteriorly and slightly rightward. In the case of tetralogy with pulmonary atresia, for example, this allows the natural curve of the allograft to lie appropriately. It also avoids the bar of ventricular septal muscle lying in the line of the right ventricular outflow. A direct anastomosis is fashioned between the anterior mitral leaflet of the allograft and the superior half of the incision in the right ventricle. The anastomosis is completed with a hood or roof of autologous pericardium treated with 0.6% glutaraldehyde for 30 minutes. Particularly in the case of the pulmonary allograft, it is important that this suture line catch the collagenous vessel wall and not be limited to the muscle below the allograft valve.

A pulmonary artery monitoring line should be placed through a mattress suture just inferior to the anastomosis in the right ventricular free wall; it should be directed into the distal part of the pulmonary artery under direct vision. This allows monitoring of pulmonary artery pressure in the early postoperative period and also shows any pullback gradient between the distal pulmonary artery and the right ventricle across both anastomoses when it is withdrawn, generally on the day after surgery.[32] As discussed previously, it is probably not wise to use pulmonary artery allografts when they will be exposed to full systemic pressure, particularly in children beyond infancy.

RESULTS OF SURGERY

Rigid prosthetic conduits containing a porcine valve, when used in the 1970s and early 1980s, carried a high early mortality rate. Undoubtedly this reflects in part the complex underlying anatomy and physiology of many of these children. However, there also was technical difficulty in suturing rigid low-porosity, woven Dacron to thin, friable, small pulmonary arteries. The rigid metal valve stent often lay over the left main coronary artery and could cause coronary compression and ischemia. Thus, in Jonas et al.'s analysis, published in 1985,[45] of 12 years of experience with prosthetic conduits, there was a 22% early mortality rate among 201 patients. Long-term actuarial survival of hospital survivors was 83% at 9 years. No patient was free of the need for conduit replacement by 10 years from the time of surgery (see Fig. 6–6). Postoperative catheterization frequently revealed a significant gradient between the right ventricle and the pulmonary artery. An early study at Children's Hospital in Boston[69] revealed that of 19 patients with Hancock conduits catheterized a mean of 1.6 years after surgery, five had gradients greater than 75 mm, and only four had gradients less than 20 mm. Repeated cardiac catheterizations revealed rapid progression of these high early gradients (Fig. 6–9). At the time of replacement surgery, the cause of obstruction was found to be a combination of valve calcification and accumulation of pseudointima peel in most patients.

There have been many reports over the years documenting superior performance of antibiotic-treated, nonfrozen aortic allografts stored at 4°C.[23, 28, 55, 83] To date, there is only early data with respect to cryopreserved allografts.[58, 62, 65] However, laboratory data suggest that there is unlikely to be a significant difference from the long-term performance of frozen aortic allografts and those stored at 4°C.[49] At Children's Hospital in Boston, 178 aortic and 138 pulmonary allografts were placed between 1985 and 1989. Significant early gradients greater than 20 mm rarely have been seen, whereas with the prosthetic conduits they were the rule. Four of the 138 children with pulmonary allografts (2.9%) developed aneurysms, two true and two false, necessitating

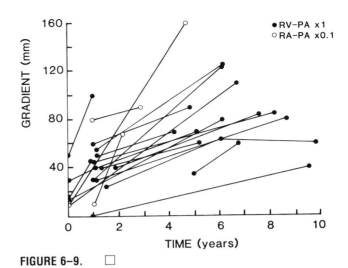

FIGURE 6–9. □

Serial transconduit gradients for right ventricular (RV)–pulmonary arterial (PA) (× 1) and right atrial (RA)–PA (× 0.1) low-porosity Dacron conduits. Note the high early postoperative gradients and the rapid progression of gradients. (From Jonas RA, Freed MD, Mayer JE, et al. Long-term followup of patients with synthetic right heart conduits. Circulation 72[suppl II]:77, 1985.)

reoperation. One child with hypoplastic left heart syndrome died after rupture of an 11-mm pulmonary allograft. In every case, the pulmonary allograft was exposed to at least systemic pressure. Three of the 178 children who had an aortic allograft inserted (1.7%) developed a false or true aneurysm, although most aortic allografts showed evidence of heavy calcification of the conduit wall within 6 to 12 months of insertion. True calcification of the valve leaflet has been rare in 7 years of followup, although more recent experience has suggested that leaflet calcification may be more common in very small allografts (<10 mm internal diameter) inserted in young infants and neonates.

INDICATIONS FOR CONDUIT REPLACEMENT

Right ventricular hypertension is frequently well tolerated for many years. However, review of experience with simple tetralogy of Fallot suggests that patients with right ventricular hypertension and a right ventricular scar have a definite risk of ventricular ectopy and sudden death. At Children's Hospital in Boston, our policy has been to undertake conduit replacement if right ventricular pressure approaches systemic pressure or if there are symptoms or signs of right ventricular failure. Balloon dilatation of conduit obstruction has rarely been of benefit other than over the very short term.

With the current widespread application of allografts, it is important once again to note that, as with any biologic material, there is likely to be an incidence of tissue failure. This is likely to result in the formation of false aneurysms, true aneurysms, or fistulae between the conduit and the bronchus. Unlike the failure mode of synthetic conduits, which is progressive but predictable, allowing timely elective replacement, it seems likely that at least some late allograft failure will prove more catastrophic unless careful follow-up has occurred. In spite of this hopefully very small, late risk, allografts appear to be an important advance over prosthetic alternatives, with a lower risk of early mortality, a markedly decreased incidence of early transconduit gradients, and a probable decreased incidence of need for conduit replacement.

REFERENCES

1. Alfieri O, Blackstone EH, Kirklin JW, et al. Surgical treatment of tetralogy of Fallot with pulmonary atresia. J Thorac Cardiovasc Surg 76:321, 1978.
2. Allen MD, Shoji Y, Fujimura Y, et al. Growth and cell viability of aortic versus pulmonic homografts in the systemic circulation. Circulation 84 (suppl III):94, 1991.
3. Andrade JD. Interfacial phenomena and biomaterials. Med Instrum 7:110, 1973.
4. Armiger LC, Gabin JB, Barratt-Boyes HG. Histological assessment of orthotopic aortic valve leaflet allografts: Its role in selecting graft pretreatment. Pathology 15:67, 1983.
5. Bailey WW, Kirklin JW, Bargeron LM, et al. Late results with synthetic valved external conduits from venous ventricle to pulmonary arteries. Circulation 56(suppl II):73, 1976.
6. Bascom JU. Gelatin sealing to prevent blood loss from knitted arterial grafts. Surgery 50:504, 1961.
7. Bell E, Ehrlich HP, Buttle DJ, et al. Living tissue formed in vitro and accepted as skin equivalent tissue of full thickness. Science 211:1052, 1981.
8. Bjork VO, Olin CL, Bjarke BB, et al. Right atrial-right ventricular anastomosis for correction of tricuspid atresia. J Thorac Cardiovasc Surg 77:452, 1979.
9. Bowald S, Busch C, Eriksson I. Absorbable material in vascular prostheses. A new device. Acta Chir Scand 146:391, 1980.
10. Bowman FO, Hancock WD, Malm JR. A valve containing Dacron prosthesis. Arch Surg 107:724, 1973.
11. Brock L. Long-term degenerative changes in aortic segment homografts, with particular reference to calcification. Thorax 23:249, 1968.
12. Brockbank K. Personal communication, June, 1991.
13. Campbell CD, Goldfarb D, Detton DD, et al. Expanded polytetrafluroethylene as a small artery substitute. Trans Am Soc Artif Intern Organs 20:86, 1974.
14. Carpentier A, Lemaigre G, Robert L, et al. Biological factors affecting long-term results of valvular heterografts. J Thorac Cardiovasc Surg 58:467, 1969.
15. Carrel A. Heterotransplantation of blood vessels preserved in cold storage. J Exp Med 9:226, 1907.
16. Carrel A. Results of the transplantation of blood vessels, organs, and limbs. JAMA 51:1662, 1908.
17. Carrel A. Ultimate results of aortic transplantations. J Exp Med 15:389, 1912.
18. Crafoord C, Nylon G. Congenital coarctation of the aorta and its surgical treatment. J Thorac Surg 14:347, 1945.
19. Damus PS. A proposed operation for transposition of the great vessels. Correspondence. Ann Thorac Surg 20:724, 1975.
20. Dardik H, Dardik I. Successful arterial substitution with modified human umbilical vein. Ann Surg 183:252, 1976.
21. Deterling RA, Bhonslay SB. An evaluation of synthetic materials and fabrics suitable for blood vessel replacement. Surgery 38:71, 1955.
22. DeWeese MS, Fry WJ. Small-bowel erosion following aortic resection. JAMA 179:142, 1962.
23. de Leval MR, et al. Total cavopulmonary connection: A logical alternative to atriopulmonary connection for complex Fontan operations. J Thorac Cardiovasc Surg 96:682–695, 1988.
24. Dumurado D, Guidoin R, Marois M, et al. Albuminated Dacron prostheses as improved blood vessel substitutes. J Bioeng 2:79, 1978.
25. Edwards WS. The effect of porosity in solid plastic artery grafts. Surg Forum 8:446, 1957.
26. Edwards WS, Tapp JS. Chemically treated nylon tubes as arterial grafts. Surgery 38:61, 1955.
27. Fiore AC, Peigh PS, Robison RJ, et al. Valved and nonvalved right ventricular pulmonary arterial extracardiac conduits. J Thorac Cardiovasc Surg 86:490, 1983.
28. Fontan F, Choussat A, Deville C, et al. Aortic valve homografts in the surgical treatment of complex cardiac malformations. J Thorac Cardiovasc Surg 87:649, 1984.
29. Galletti PM, Ip TK, Chiu TH, et al. Extending the functional life of bioresorbable yarns for vascular grafts. Trans Am Soc Artif Intern Organs 30:399, 1984.
30. Geha AS, Laks H, Stansel HC, et al. Late failure of porcine valve heterografts in children. J Thorac Cardiovasc Surg 78:351, 1979.
31. Gerber A, Rubaum N. Gastrointestinal hemorrhage due to rupture of an aortic homograft. Calif Med 105:377, 1966.
32. Gold JP, Jonas RA, Lang P, et al. Transcutaneous intracardiac monitoring lines in pediatric surgical patients: A 10 year experience. Ann Thorac Surg 42:185, 1986.
33. Gross RE, Bill AH, Peirce EC. Methods for preservation and transplantation of arterial grafts. Surg Gynecol Obstet 88:689, 1949.
34. Gross RE, Hufnagel CA. Coarctation of the aorta: Experimental studies regarding its surgical correction. N Engl J Med 233:287, 1945.
35. Gross RE, Hurwitt ES, Bill AH. Preliminary observations on the use of human arterial grafts in the treatment of certain cardiovascular defects. N Engl J Med 239:578, 1948.
36. Guidoin R, Snyder R, Martin L, et al. Albumin coating of a knitted polyester arterial prosthesis: An alternative to preclotting. Ann Thorac Surg 37:547, 1984.
37. Guthrie CC. Survival of engrafted tissues. III. Blood vessels. Heart 2:115, 1910.
38. Hagland LA, Sweetman WR, Wise RA. Rupture of an abdominal aortic homograft with ileal fistula. Am J Surg 98:746, 1959.
39. Haverich A, Walterbusch G, Borst HG. The use of fibrin glue for sealing vascular prostheses of high porosity. Thorac Cardiovasc Surg 29:252, 1981.
40. Herring M, Glover JL (eds). Endothelial Seeding in Vascular Surgery. Orlando, FL, Grune & Stratton, 1987.
41. Holub DA, Trono R, Klima T, et al. Macroscopic, microscopic, and mechanical analyses of prototype double velour vascular grafts. Bull Tex Heart Inst 5:365, 1978.
42. Humphries AW, Hawk WA, Cuthbertson AM. Arterial prosthesis of collagen impregnated Dacron tulle. Surgery 50:947, 1961.
43. Jacobs ML, Baffa JM, Murphy JD, et al. Autologous flaps for right ventricular outflow tract construction in infants. Circulation 84(suppl II):240, 1991.
44. Jonas RA, Castaneda AR. Modified Fontan procedure: Atrial baffle and systemic venous to pulmonary artery anastomotic techniques. J Cardiac Surg 3:91, 1988.
45. Jonas RA, Freed MD, Mayer JE, et al. Long-term followup of patients with synthetic right heart conduits. Circulation 72(suppl II):77, 1985.
46. Jonas RA, Mayer JE, Castaneda AR. Unsatisfactory clinical experience with a collagen sealed, knitted Dacron extracardiac conduit. J Cardiac Surg 2:257, 1987.
47. Jonas RA, Schoen FJ, Levy RJ, et al. Biological sealants and knitted Dacron: Porosity and histological comparisons of vas-

cular graft materials with and without collagen and fibrin glue pretreatments. Ann Thorac Surg 41:657, 1986.

48. Jonas RA, Schoen FJ, Ziemer G, et al. Biological sealants and knitted Dacron conduits: Comparison of collagen and fibrin glue pretreatments in circulatory models. Ann Thorac Surg 44:283, 1987.

49. Jonas RA, Ziemer G, Britton L, et al. Cryopreserved and fresh antibiotic sterilized valved aortic homograft conduits in a longterm sheep model. J Thorac Cardiovasc Surg 96:746, 1988.

50. Jonas RA, Ziemer G, Schoen FJ, et al. A new sealant for knitted Dacron prostheses: Minimally cross-linked gelatin. J Vasc Surg 7:414, 1988.

51. Jordan GL, Stump MM, Allen J, et al. Gelatin impregnated prosthesis implanted into porcine thoracic aorta. Surgery 53:45, 1963.

52. Kadoba K, Armiger L, Sawatari K, et al. The influence of time from donor death to graft harvest on conduit function of cryopreserved aortic allografts in lambs. Circulation 84(suppl III):100, 1991.

53. Kadoba K, Armiger LC, Sawatari K, et al. Mechanical durability of pulmonary allograft conduits at systemic pressure: Angiographic and histological study in lambs. J Thorac Cardiovasc Surg. 105:132–141, 1993.

54. Kadoba K, Sawatari K, Jonas RA. Mechanical failure of pulmonary homografts at systemic pressure. J Am Coll Cardiol 15:78A, 1990.

55. Kay PH, Ross DN. Fifteen years' experience with the aortic homograft: The conduit of choice for right ventricular outflow tract reconstruction. Ann Thorac Surg 40:360, 1985.

56. Kaye MP. Anatomic correction of transposition of the great arteries. Mayo Clin Proc 50:638, 1975.

57. Kent KC, Salvatierra O, Reilly LM, et al. Evolving strategies for the repair of complex renovascular lesions. Ann Surg 206:272, 1987.

58. Kirklin JW, Blackstone EH, Maehara T, et al. Intermediate term fate of cryopreserved allograft and xenograft valved conduits. Ann Thorac Surg 44:598, 1987.

59. Klinner W. Indikationsstellung und operative technik fur die korrketur der Fallotschen tetralogie. Langenbecks Arch Klin Chirurgie 308:40, 1964.

60. Konno S, Imai Y, Iida Y, et al. A new method for prosthetic valve replacement in congenital aortic stenosis with hypoplasia of the aortic valve ring. J Thorac Cardiovasc Surg 70:909, 1975.

61. Kreutzer G, Galindez E, Bono H, et al. An operation for the correction of tricuspid atresia. J Thorac Cardiovasc Surg 66:613, 1973.

62. Lamberti JJ, Angell WW, Waldman JD, et al. The cryopreserved homograft valve in the pulmonary position: Early results and technical considerations. J Cardiac Surg 3:247, 1988.

63. Lecompte Y, Zannini L, Hazan E. Anatomic correction of transposition of the great arteries: New technique without use of a prosthetic conduit. J Thorac Cardiovasc Surg 82:629, 1981.

64. Puga FJ, Chiavarelli M, Hagler DJ, et al. Modification of the Fontan operation applicable to patients with left atrioventricular valve atresia or single A-V valve. Circulation 76:III55, 1987.

65. McGrath LB, Gonzalez-Lavin L, Graf D. Pulmonary homograft implantation for ventricular outflow tract reconstruction: Early phase results. Ann Thorac Surg 45:273, 1988.

66. Meade JW, Linton RR, Darling RC, et al. Arterial homografts. Arch Surg 93:392, 1966.

67. Mitchell RS, Miller CD, Bilingham ME, et al. Comprehensive assessment of the safety, durability, clinical performance, and healing characteristics of a double velour knitted Dacron arterial prosthesis. Vasc Surg 14:197, 1980.

68. Molina JE, Edwards J, Bianco R, et al. Growth of fresh-frozen pulmonary allograft conduit in growing lambs. Circulation 80:183, 1980.

69. Norwood WI, Freed MD, Rocchini AP, et al. Experience with valved conduits for repair of congenital cardiac lesions. Ann Thorac Surg 24:223, 1977.

70. Norwood WI, Lang P, Castaneda AR, et al. Management of infants with left ventricular outflow obstruction by conduit interposition between the ventricular apex and thoracic aorta. J Thorac Cardiovasc Surg 86:771, 1983.

71. Novick AC, Stewart BH, Straffon RA. Autogenous arterial grafts in the treatment of renal artery stenosis. J Urol 118:919, 1977.

72. O'Brien MF, Stafford EG, Gardner MAH, et al. A comparison of aortic valve replacement with viable cryopreserved and fresh allograft valves, with a note on chromosomal studies. J Thorac Cardiovasc Surg 94:912, 1987.

73. O'Brien MF, Stafford G, Gardner M, et al. The viable cryopreserved allograft aortic valve. J Cardiac Surg 2(suppl):153, 1987.

74. Rastelli GC, Ongley PA, Davis GD, et al. Surgical repair for pulmonary valve atresia with coronary-pulmonary artery fistula: Report of case. Mayo Clin Proc 40:521, 1965.

75. Rosenberg N, Gaughran ERL, Henderson J. The use of segmental arterial implants prepared by enzymatic modification of heterologous blood vessels. Surg Forum 6:242, 1956.

76. Ross DN, Somerville J. Correction of pulmonary atresia with a homograft aortic valve. Lancet 2:1446, 1966.

77. Rubay J, Lecompte Y, Batisse A, et al. Anatomic repair of anomalies of ventriculo-arterial connection (REV): Results of a new technique in cases associated with pulmonary outflow tract obstruction. Eur J Cardiothorac Surg 2:305, 1988.

78. Saravalli OA, Somerville J, Jefferson KE. Calcification of aortic homografts used for reconstruction of the right ventricular outflow tract. J Thorac Cardiovasc Surg 80:809, 1980.

79. Sauvage LR, Berger K, Woos SJ, et al. An external velour surface for porous arterial prostheses. Surgery 70:940, 1971.

80. Sauvage LR, Wesolowski SA. The healing and fate of arterial grafts. Surgery 38:1090, 1955.

81. Sawatari K, Kawata H, Armiger LC, et al. Growth of composite conduits utilizing longitudinal arterial autograft in growing lambs. J Thorac Cardiovasc Surg 103:47–51, 1992.

82. Schaffer MS, Campbell DN, Clarke DR, et al. Aortoventriculoplasty in children. J Thorac Cardiovasc Surg 92:391, 1986.

83. Shabbo FP, Wain WH, Ross DN. Right ventricular outflow reconstruction with aortic homograft conduit: Analysis of the long-term results. Thorac Cardiovasc Surg 28:21, 1980.

84. Shindo S, Takagi A, Whittemore AD. Improved patency of collagen-impregnated grafts after in vitro autogenous endothelial cell seeding. J Vasc Surg 6:325, 1987.

85. Stansel HC. A new operation for D-loop transposition of the great arteries. Ann Thorac Surg 19:565, 1975.

86. van der Lei B, Darius H, Schror K, et al. Arterial wall regeneration in small caliber vascular grafts in rats. J Thorac Cardiovasc Surg 90:378, 1985.

87. Vorheese AB, Jaretzki A, Blakemore AH. The use of tubes constructed from Vinyon "N" cloth in bridging arterial defects: A preliminary report. Ann Surg 135:332, 1952.

88. Wesolowski SA. The healing of vascular prostheses. Surgery 57:319, 1965.

89. Wesolowski SA, Fries CC, Domingo RT, et al. The compound prosthetic vascular graft: A pathologic survey. Surgery 53:19, 1963.

90. Wesolowski SA, Fries CC, Karlson KE, et al. Porosity: Primary determinants of ultimate fate of synthetic vascular grafts. Surgery 50:91, 1961.

91. Williams DB, Danielson GK, McGoon DC, et al. Porcine heterograft valve replacement in children. J Thorac Cardiovasc Surg 84:446, 1982.

92. Yankah AC, Hetzer R. Procurement and viability of cardiac valve allografts. In Yankah AC, Hetzer R, Miller DC, et al (eds). Cardiac Valve Allografts 1962–1987. New York, Springer-Verlag, 1988, p 23.

93. Yankah AC, Wottge HU, Muller-Rucholtz W. Prognostic importance of viability and a study of a second set allograft valve: An experimental study. J Cardiac Surg 3:263, 1988.

7
Chapter

Interventional Cardiology

EXPERIMENTAL BASIS FOR INTERVENTIONAL TECHNIQUES

Although interventional cardiology has its roots in the early 1950s[41] and 1960s,[34] progress in the field was initially hampered by the lack of experimental data. There are few naturally occurring models of congenital heart disease in animals, and those available have limited applicability to human disease. Early studies by Dotter and Judkins[5] and Gruntzig and Hopff[10] of dilating atherosclerotic lesions emphasized the importance of the soft nature of the plaque: as the vessel was dilated, the plaque was thought to be redistributed within the vessel wall, allowing for improved flow. Such lesions do not occur in children with congenital heart disease. Creation of valvar stenoses or septal defects has been very difficult. Placing an animal on bypass, making its circulation worse by adding a shunt or an obstruction, and then weaning the animal from support carries very high mortality and morbidity rates. Closed heart procedures to accomplish the same goals can mimic the physiology of congenital lesions, but rarely that of the anatomic substrate. Nonetheless, important information has been derived from animal studies, permitting the introduction of novel techniques with low early morbidity and high initial success rates.

Vessel Dilatation

The basic experimental models for dilatation of congenitally narrowed vessels have relied heavily on earlier experimental surgical studies. Resection of a large fraction of the vascular lumen, with wrapping of the site by absorbable suture, produces a significant lesion that remains stenotic as the animal grows.[23, 24] The result is a vessel whose outside diameter is smaller than normal and whose inside diameter is further compromised by intimal hyperplasia. Gradients of 30 to 40 mm Hg are attainable across both experimental aortic coarctations and stenoses of the pulmonary artery branches, although greater degrees of obstruction produce severe, acute ventricular dysfunction and often result in early death.

In the absence of a soft vascular wall, dilatation of a postoperative experimental lesion succeeds by tearing the intima and part of the media; the vessel then heals in an open position. Tears do not occur with small degrees of vascular stretch; both stenosed and normal vessels stretch at moderate dilatation diameters and then recoil to their original diameter once the balloon is removed. The degree of stretch necessary to produce intimal and medial disruption varies with the nature of the native vessel and the lesion. Balloon-to-vessel diameter ratios of

1.4 to 1.6 mm will disrupt aortic arches; larger ratios are needed for pulmonary artery branches (2.0 to 3.0), pulmonary veins (3.0 to 4.0), or systemic veins (3.0 to 4.0). Thus, veins are much more compliant than either systemic or pulmonary arteries and require larger balloons for effective dilatation.

Compliance is not only vessel dependent, but also lesion dependent. When experimental lesions are made in an identical fashion,[23, 24] pulmonary arterial stenoses are more compliant than aortic coarctations; however, when nonabsorbable suture is used to wrap the vessels, both lesions become much less compliant and require small balloons inflated to high pressure for dilatation. Thus, the optimum balloon size for a given experimental lesion is only partly predictable. The same uncertainty applies to clinical lesions.

The absence of intimal and medial disruption at small dilatation diameters does not mean that the vessel is unaffected. Blood flow in the vascular wall via the vasa vasorum increases within minutes of a sustained vascular stretch[4] and remains elevated for hours. Pretreatment with indomethacin abolishes most of the hyperemia. The role that this response plays in the healing of a dilated vessel is unclear.

As noted previously, successful dilatation of a nonatheromatous lesion implies intimal and medial disruption; we have never observed long-term gradient relief in animals without a documented vascular tear. As a result, vessels that were dilated soon after surgery (less than 1 month) suffered rupture of the suture lines. Reconstitution of the adventitial scar tissue seems to be necessary for successful postoperative dilatations, a process that (in animals) was functionally complete after 2 months. The medial fibers of the aortic or pulmonary arterial wall separate in layers, with hemorrhage into both the media and the interstitium. Especially in pulmonary arteries, the tear can extend throughout the media, stopping only at the adventitia. Such transmedial tears are associated with (but not entirely caused by) large balloon sizes and are conceivably the cause of late aneurysm formation after dilatation in some animals.

Immediately after the dilatation of experimental lesions, the vessel wall becomes very fragile and can be disrupted with standard catheter manipulation.[23, 24] Healing occurs by the layering of platelets over the lesion within a few days, followed by refashioning of the intima by fibroblast proliferation within the media. On gross inspection, healing appears to be complete at about 6 weeks after dilatation. In some animals who underwent dilatation of aortic coarctation, medial thinning was accompanied by the late formation of aneurysms. Healing

results in a fibrotic medial layer and may also be accompanied by intimal "bridges" that span the vascular lumen, with shallow, false passages under the intimal bridges. Whereas aortic aneurysms appear to be progressive, at least in some animals, intimal bridges seem to have no functional consequences.

Stents

At present, few stents have been used in the management of infants with congenital heart disease. Beekman and Mullins and their coworkers[2, 28] have adapted similar forms of experimental vascular stenoses to assess the effects of stent placement in pulmonary arteries and aortae. These studies have demonstrated several advantages of intravascular stents over standard balloon dilatation techniques. The initial vascular stretch in response to dilatation is not lost with stent placement, enabling smaller balloons to give adequate relief from the stenosis. Vascular endothelialization of stents in pulmonary arteries and aortas appears to be good as long as the stent is in close apposition to the vessel wall after expansion; those parts of the stent that are free in the vessel lumen or overlie side branch orifices do not become endothelialized as readily,[2, 28] although microscopic endothelialization may occur nonetheless.

Intermediate follow-up after stent placement demonstrates that intimal proliferation may significantly reduce the luminal diameter, especially in smaller vessels. Although stents do not grow along with an experimental animal, preliminary data suggest that a stent in the pulmonary arteries may be redilated to a larger diameter weeks to months after the first implantation.[28]

Valve Dilatation

In the absence of septal defects, inflation of an occlusive balloon across a cardiac valve will interrupt cardiac output and eventually produce cardiac standstill. The earliest experiences in open heart surgery[47] seemed to indicate that venous inflow occlusion was much better tolerated than ventricular outflow occlusion, and thus inflow occlusion became the method of choice for short (1- to 3-minute), direct-vision procedures to open the pulmonary valve.[26] However, the precise limits of tolerance for each form of occlusion in closed-chested animals were unclear, as was the importance of ventricular decompression during occlusion. Balloon occlusion of the pulmonary valve in an intact animal produces progressive bradycardia and hypotension that become severe after 60 to 80 seconds and irreversible after 90 to 120 seconds. The development of a double-balloon, caval occlusion catheter resulted in the ability to mimic inflow occlusion in the catheterization laboratory. This resulted in marked hypotension, but much less bradycardia, and electrocardiographic changes suggestive of ischemia (Fig. 7–1). Subsequent development of large-bore balloon catheters that could be reliably inflated and deflated within 10 to 12 seconds made inflow occlusion techniques unnecessary.

Like arteries and veins, valves and valve rings are also compliant to various degrees; a valve dilated with a 20-mm balloon will not result in a valve area of 3.14 cm². Pulmonary valves are more compliant than aortic valves, and the pulmonary annulus can be dilated with a balloon 50% larger than the annulus without producing major intracardiac damage.[37] In contrast, the aortic annulus is relatively rigid: balloons only 20% larger than the annulus can seriously damage the normal outflow tract, producing cusp avulsions, hemorrhage into the anterior leaflet of the mitral valve, and even aortic rupture.[11]

In addition to issues related to balloon diameter, dilatation balloons have length, and cardiac structures are often curved. When the balloons are inflated to the atmospheres necessary to split valve leaflets (three to five atmospheres), the balloons straighten and force the heart to deform around this rigid balloon. In the pulmonary outflow tract, such

damage could be significant, producing myocardial hemorrhage (Fig. 7–2).

Closure Techniques

Coils

Gianturco coils were first developed for the obliteration of small peripheral arteries, but subsequently they have become invaluable in the closure of unwanted intrathoracic vessels. In vitro studies have demonstrated that coils 50% to 100% larger than the vessel to be closed will adopt a linear configuration and provide little obstruction to flow. Coils that are nearly the same size as the artery to be occluded will reform into a circle aligned along the axis of flow and will only minimally impede flow. In contrast, coils 20% to 30% larger than the vessel will form a dense knot that effectively obstructs flow (Fig. 7–3).

Umbrellas

Rashkind[33] first demonstrated the feasibility of transcatheter closure of cardiac defects with an umbrella-like device. The creation of an animal model of a patent ductus arteriosus (PDA)[20] allowed testing of the original Rashkind PDA umbrella. The development of endocarditis was observed in the early postimplant period in deliberately infected an-

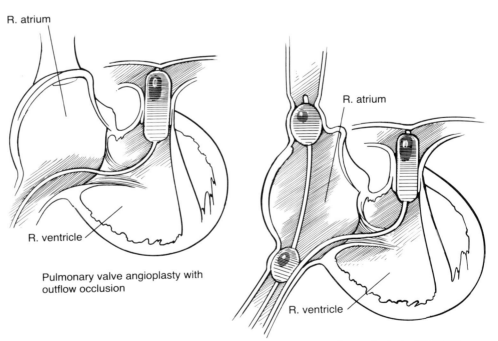

FIGURE 7–1. □

Occlusion of the right ventricular outflow tract *(left panel)* produces hypotension, bradycardia, and ectopy and is irreversible after 60 to 90 seconds in experimental animals. Combined inflow and outflow occlusion produces hypotension and tachycardia and is tolerated for 90 to 120 seconds.

R. atrium

R. ventricle

Pulmonary valve angioplasty with outflow occlusion

R. atrium

R. ventricle

Pulmonary valve angioplasty with inflow occlusion

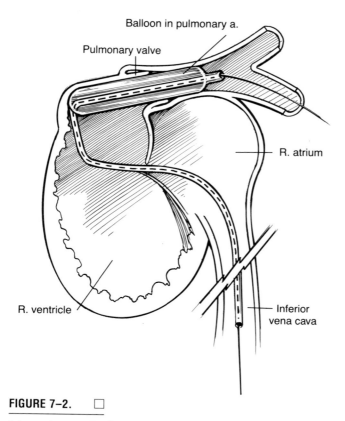

FIGURE 7–2. ☐

A long, pulmonary valve dilatation balloon will straighten the normally curved right ventricular outflow tract in infant lambs, producing hemorrhage in the anterior right ventricular free wall.

preparation has been used to evaluate the button device for the closure of atrial septal defects.[45]

Although neither late arrhythmias nor neurologic complications were noted in these animals, their absence must be verified after use of umbrellas in children. Also, atrial septal defects in lambs are not identical to those in children. The ovine atrial septum is small and tunnel-like and therefore has ideal circumferential borders for umbrella attachment, making ovine atrial septa easier to close than human septa. These differences serve to emphasize the tentative nature of preliminary animal studies. Similarly, although there are animal models of ventricular septal defects, such defects are either close to valvar structures or are held open with mechanical tunnels,[48] and thus, they cannot be used to evaluate occlusive devices for children.

CLINICAL TRANSCATHETER ENLARGEMENT OF STENOTIC VESSELS

Balloon Dilatation

Native Infant Coarctations

Unrepaired aortic coarctations were among the first congenital lesions to be dilated with angio-

imals, and damage to right heart valvar structures occurred if the device was forcefully retrieved from the pulmonary artery to the vena cava without being folded up. Similar animal studies with hooked umbrellas were unsatisfactory: the hooks attached to the first place that the device contacted within the heart, which determined the ultimate position of the device.

Therefore, we first experimented with the hinged, double-umbrella device, which later was further modified to allow the umbrella to fold back on itself (the so-called "clamshell" design). In early animal trials,[25] several important observations were made:

1. Atrial septal defects expand in size after implantation of an occlusive device, and the extent of expansion is probably related to the compliance of the defect.
2. The compliance of a defect can be assessed by balloon sizing.
3. Umbrellas that accidentally detach during insertion tumble to a branch of the pulmonary artery or the aorta, but then align along the vascular axis so that they do not occlude flow.
4. Correctly implanted umbrellas are first covered with a glistening coat of fibrin and then become endothelialized within 6 to 12 weeks (Fig. 7–4). A similar animal

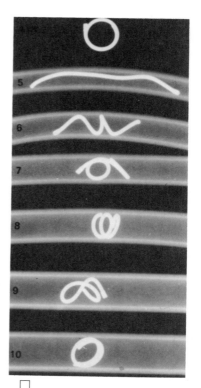

FIGURE 7–3. ☐

A 10-mm coil has been extruded in tubes from 5 to 20 mm in diameter. The coil is nonocclusive in both small and large tubes.

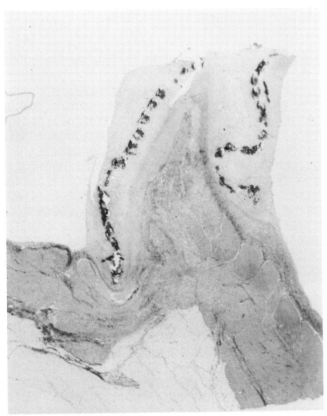

FIGURE 7–4. □

Ovine atrial septum after catheter closure with a clamshell umbrella. The atrial myocardium is covered by Dacron fabric *(dark spots)* and also by densely adherent endocardium.

plasty balloons. In the initial series[18] there was a low morbidity rate in neonates undergoing dilatation, with good immediate gradient reduction, but a very high rate (more than 50%) of restenosis within the first 6 months. This early experience has subsequently been reconfirmed,[27] supporting our current policy of reserving dilatation of neonatal coarctation for the rare infant who is not a candidate for surgery.

Dilatation of native coarctation in older infants and in children remains controversial. Although at this time we still prefer surgical coarctectomy, there is a nationwide trend toward dilatation of primary coarctations in older children. The arguments in favor of dilatation may be summarized as follows:

1. Dilatation of native coarctation is a safe procedure, with mortality rates of less than 1% and major morbidity rates of less than 3% to 4%.[15, 32, 49] Specifically, postoperative infections, damage to the recurrent laryngeal nerve, and spinal cord injury have not been reported.
2. Dilatation is largely successful, reducing the measured postoperative gradient to less than 20 mm Hg in at least 80% of patients.[15, 32, 49] Restenosis is rare.

3. In several series dilatation appeared as safe as surgery and just as successful.[15, 32, 49]
4. The disadvantages of dilatation are either relatively minor (e.g., injury to the femoral artery) or rare (e.g., aneurysm formation).

At the Children's Hospital in Boston, we continue to favor surgery as the initial form of management for most infants for the following reasons:

1. Mortality and morbidity rates from coarctation surgery have decreased significantly.
2. Resection and end-to end anastomosis of the coarctation produce a more consistent and greater gradient reduction than that produced by dilatation angioplasty; normally, there is a reverse gradient between the arms and legs,[17] with systolic pressure in the legs being higher because of pulse amplification. Even a 10–to 15–mm Hg gradient between arm and leg pressures at rest may represent a significant obstruction. These "mild" residual gradients may become high with exercise, predisposing the adolescent and adult with partially "repaired" coarctation to the risks of late hypertensive complications.
3. Repairing mild residual obstructions after partially successful dilatation may pose special risks, as collateral formation may be inadequate to protect the spinal column during crossclamping.
4. It is likely that the recurrence of a coarctation gradient, and thus the nidus for late bacterial endocarditis, is related to turbulent flow across the narrowed segment. Resection with end-to-end anastomosis provides a more favorable flow profile within the aortic arch.

Until a large, prospective trial comparing optimum dilatation techniques with optimum surgical techniques is performed, resolution of this issue will be difficult.

Recurrent Coarctations

Indications and the technique for dilatation of recurrent coarctation are much less controversial. We favor balloon dilatation for correction of nearly all residual or recurrent stenoses. Percutaneous access is obtained through the femoral artery, the precise anatomy of the obstruction is defined angiographically, and a balloon about three times the diameter of the obstruction is chosen, provided that the balloon is not more than 50% larger than the normal vessel proximal or distal to the coarcted segment. For rigid obstructions, this balloon size will suffice (or will even be too large in some older children). For compliant obstructions, the balloon will expand to its full size at low pressure (two atmospheres), and a larger balloon will be required. In general, when a subtle waist is seen at low pressures, dilatation will result in inadequate gradient improvement; when a striking waist is seen (and then eliminated at high pressure), dilatation will produce excellent gradient reduction but increase the risk of aneurysm. It may prove necessary to change the balloon several times to achieve a postdilatation gradient of 10 to 15 mm Hg without producing an aneurysm.

The timing of dilatation for recurrent coarctations depends on the date of the original operation and the age of the child. As noted previously, 2 to 3 months should be allowed after surgery to permit the vessel to heal and form an adventitial scar. We almost never dilate less than 2 months after surgery and will shorten the postoperative wait (to perhaps 6 weeks) only if the patient requires vigorous medical management (e.g., assisted ventilation) because of recurrent coarctation. Long-lasting hypertension seems to be more likely if native coarctations are left unrepaired for more than 2 to 5 years. At the Children's Hospital in Boston we have used the same timing for recurrent coarctation. In symptomatic patients, recurrent coarctations are dilated at the time of diagnosis; in asymptomatic patients, significant lesions are usually dilated within 2 years after the initial diagnosis.

The degree of obstruction that warrants intervention has been determined with few supporting data. We have arbitrarily chosen a resting gradient of more than 25 mm Hg. At present, little information is available to indicate that the resting gradient is the best way to assess coarctation obstruction or the late effects of relatively low residual gradients acquired early in life. The decision to intervene at relatively low gradients is influenced by the low morbidity and mortality rates associated with dilating recurrent coarctations.

Between 1984 and early 1992, 40 infants less than 1 year of age with recurrent aortic coarctation underwent dilatation at Children's Hospital in Boston; preliminary results of the first 27 patients were reported in 1987.[43] There was one death (in a sick infant), caused by occult bleeding at the vascular entry site. In 33 procedures (82%) there was a postdilatation gradient of less than 25 mm Hg, or less than half the predilatation gradient. Late restenosis did occur, but was rare (four patients). Minor complications were relatively common (pulse loss without injury to the leg and blood loss requiring transfusion). Angiographic results ranged from excellent, with a smooth lumen and little evidence of aneurysm formation, to tortuous paths with considerable vascular irregularity. In general, the angiographic appearance improves over time with ingrowth of intimal tissue. There is little late angiographic follow-up of these patients. Thus far, no late aneurysm formation has been seen, but the number of patients followed extensively is limited.

Stenotic Pulmonary Arteries in Infants

Balloon dilatation of hypoplastic or stenosed pulmonary arteries is among the most important interventional techniques in congenital heart diseases. Surgical alternatives are frequently inadequate, and relief of these stenoses plays a central role in the long-term outcome of surgical repairs. As noted previously, even stenotic pulmonary arteries are compliant, stretching passively but reversibly to two or three times their functional diameter. Parenthetically, these observations underscore the shortcomings of using dilators intraoperatively to assess pulmonary artery size: a vessel that may accommodate a 10-mm dilator will frequently recoil to 5 to 6 mm despite elevated perfusing pressures. In addition, balloon dilatation has provided important information about the nature of obstructed pulmonary arteries. Many pulmonary arteries appear diffusely "hypoplastic," in that the vessels are small centrally but do not taper normally. With rare exceptions, the so-called "hypoplastic" pulmonary artery is, in fact, a vessel with two or three serial obstructions with "normal" vessel intervening (Fig. 7–5). Interventional cardiologists successfully enlarge such vessels by dilating each significant segmental stenosis.

As with coarctation, dilatation of narrowed pulmonary arteries works by tearing the intima and part of the media.[22, 40] Very large balloons (on average, 4.3 times the size of the narrowed artery) are needed to accomplish this. Precise angiographic def-

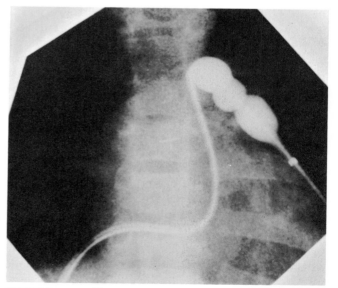

FIGURE 7–5.   ☐

A so-called hypoplastic (3-mm) pulmonary artery after inflation of a 12-mm balloon to 6 atmospheres. A vessel that appeared to be uniformly small is seen to have several discrete lesions.

inition of arterial anatomy in two planes will demonstrate not only narrowed areas, often involving more than one lobe, but also the anatomy of adjacent vessels. To deliver the dilating balloon to a distal, narrowed pulmonary artery, a robust guide wire should be advanced to the distal part of the lung, following the path of the largest distal pulmonary arterial vessel. If a large dilating balloon is inflated in small but normal distal branches, a saccular aneurysm will result (Fig. 7–6). Such aneurysms, although apparently benign,[40] undoubtedly interfere with blood flow and gas exchange within the lung.

Because of the risk of catheter perforation in a recently damaged vessel, at Children's Hospital in Boston we originally avoided multiple dilatations in the same procedure.[22] However, the availability of extremely soft, torque-controlled wires has made it safe to cross even freshly dilated vessels, allowing several vessels to be dilated at the same time.

Initial reports of dilating peripheral pulmonary arteries indicated an overall success rate of only 60%.[22, 40] Failure was due primarily to rigid lesions that could not be torn, even at seven to eight atmospheres of inflating pressure. Newer high-pressure polyethylene balloons can withstand much higher (18 to 20) atmospheres of pressure. Although these relatively rigid, large-bore balloon catheters are difficult to manipulate through small hearts, their use has significantly increased success rates.[8] Rarely, dilatation fails because of marked vessel compliance; usually such failure is due to kinking or folding of the vascular channel, in which case enlargement of these vessels requires the use of endo-

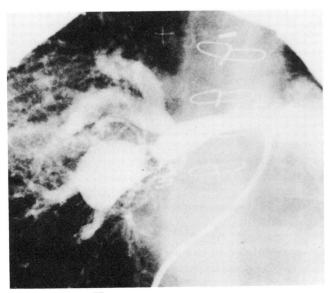

FIGURE 7–6. □

Aneurysm of the anterior segment of the right middle lobe 1 year after "successful" dilatation. This lesion was seen immediately after dilatation and has not gotten larger.

vascular stents. Stents have been rarely used in infants, because they do not grow as the patient grows.

Although the safety of catheter dilatation of pulmonary arteries has improved with experience, morbidity persists, and rare deaths continue to occur.[1, 40] Therefore, the indications for this procedure are limited to the following clinical conditions that have demonstrable long-term adverse effects:

1. Pulmonary artery stenoses producing right ventricular pressures near or higher than systemic levels.
2. Pulmonary artery stenoses contributing to symptomatic right heart failure or persistent cyanosis in patients with septal defects.
3. Unilateral pulmonary artery stenoses that contribute to significant pulmonary hypertension in the unaffected lung.
4. Unilateral pulmonary artery stenoses that markedly reduce flow to the affected lung. For example, if total flow to the left lung (normally 45% of cardiac output) is less than 20% of cardiac output, that lung will begin to function as an area of ventilatory dead space: oxygen exchange will be preserved, but carbon dioxide delivery to the lung (and hence removal) will be impaired. Because the actual flow disturbance required to produce symptoms or long-term disability is unclear, intervention for this indication remains somewhat arbitrary.

Between 1984 and 1992 at Children's Hospital in Boston, pulmonary arteries were dilated in 34 infants, many on more than one occasion. The early results, reported in 1989, which included 135 patients, only 7 of them infants,[40] indicated aneurysm formation in 5% and unilateral pulmonary edema[8] in 3%, with an overall mortality rate of 1.5%. In that series, 56% of procedures succeeded (>50% gain in diameter and >30% decrease in right ventricular pressure); restenosis occurred in 12%.

More recently, the use of high-pressure balloons was successful in another 60%[8] of patients in whom standard dilatation techniques failed. Thus, the overall success rate of the procedure is currently 88%, with a mortality rate of 1% to 2% and a morbidity rate of about 4%.

Systemic and Pulmonary Veins

Congenital narrowings of systemic or pulmonary veins in infants are rare. In fact, they are more commonly seen after surgical repair of complex lesions (e.g., the atrial inversion operation for transposition of the great arteries, use of atriopulmonary baffles in the modified Fontan operation, and repair of a total anomalous pulmonary venous connection). Although the techniques for dilating systemic and pulmonary veins are similar, the results are quite different.

Veins are the most compliant of vessels. Unlike

arteries, they have a very thin medial layer, so the amount of vessel that can be "safely" torn in an angioplasty procedure is limited. As such, native venous stenoses presumably have little capacity to be dilated, whereas postoperative stenoses should have a better potential for successful dilatation.

Being compliant, veins can be dilated only with very large balloons (six to ten times the narrowest spot), although dilating pressures higher than four to six atmospheres are rarely required. The earliest reports of dilating pulmonary veins were discouraging,[6] and even subsequent reports using very large balloons[19] indicated that restenosis occurred within 1 year in essentially every case. Presumably, early restenosis was caused by plastic, reversible deformation of the veins without a medial tear, and this was the basis for our early use of stents to treat pulmonary vein stenosis.

Results were better after balloon dilatation of systemic venous stenoses that followed Mustard or Senning operations for transposition of the great arteries,[19] although these procedures are rarely needed in infants. Presumably, this enhanced success was due to a different mechanism of venous stenosis: caval obstructions after a Mustard procedure generally occur within the heart, where the baffle passes over the old atrial septum. Dilatation of these strictures produces tears in atrial tissue that can then heal in an open position. To date, there are few, if any, reports of successful balloon dilatation of extracardiac venous narrowings.

Dilatation of stenotic venous baffles is safe unless attempted in the early postoperative period. The number of patients who have been followed for more than several years is small, and thus the incidence of restenosis is not known but is probably significant.

Intravascular Stents in Congenital Heart Disease

Originally designed to treat atherosclerotic iliac arteries, the possibilities of using expandable metal stents in congenital heart disease was first explored in animals by several investigators.[2, 28] By 1989 enough data were available to begin clinical trials in Boston and Houston.[29] To date, stents have been used to enlarge pulmonary arteries, pulmonary veins, systemic venous baffles, and, in rare cases, dynamic obstructions within the right and left ventricles. However, stents have been used only 10 times in infants, all in the Boston series. Thus, our experience is limited.

Stent Enlargement of Pulmonary Arteries

During the process of balloon dilatation, most pulmonary arteries enlarge before the intima and media begin to tear. Stents may take advantage of this natural elasticity by preventing recoil, effecting permanent vessel enlargement. Even considering that the thickness of the stent itself (0.5 mm for the Palmaz iliac stent) reduces net vessel dilatation, prevention of recoil allows stents to dilate pulmonary artery branches more effectively than does balloon dilatation alone.

This advantage is countered by several limitations:

1. Stents may promote intimal hyperplasia in pulmonary arteries, causing late restenosis.
2. Stents do not grow as the child grows, and thus may limit ultimate vascular size.
3. Stents require large delivery systems.
4. Stents are difficult to position accurately in a vascular tree with short-segment vessels and many branches.

Nonetheless, stents have proved invaluable in infants and children with peripheral pulmonary artery stenosis who failed standard balloon dilatation techniques.

To remain in position, stents must be dilated to a size somewhat larger than the diameter to which the vessel can be easily stretched. Pulmonary arteries are dilated first using standard balloon dilatation techniques. If the vessel stretches by twofold or more and cannot be permanently enlarged by a vascular tear, stent placement should be considered.

To date, our indications for stent enlargement of pulmonary artery branches at Children's Hospital in Boston have been much stricter than those for balloon dilatation alone.[29] Postoperative lesions producing suprasystemic right ventricular pressures, significant pulmonary hypertension, or clinical right heart failure have been the major indications. Smaller coronary or renal stents (with a maximum diameter of 5 to 9 mm) have been placed in infants only for life-threatening lesions.

Despite these limited indications, we have implanted five stents in the pulmonary arteries of three infants. On average, they have more than doubled pulmonary artery diameter, with little restenosis at early follow-up. Stents have been especially helpful in enlarging central pulmonary arteries obstructed by kinks or vascular compression (Fig. 7–7). No patient has died. One stent became dislodged during passage through the right ventricle and was left unexpanded in the right pulmonary artery. Angiography 9 months later revealed no stenosis.

Stent Enlargement of Pulmonary Veins

Although stent enlargement of pulmonary veins has the same theoretical advantages seen with sys-

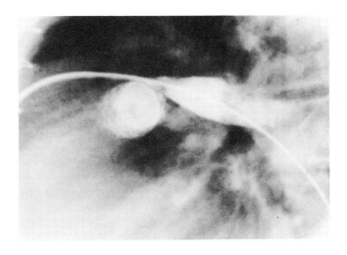

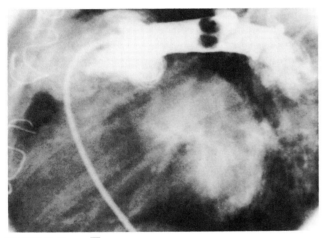

FIGURE 7–7. □

"Folded" or kinked proximal left pulmonary artery before *(upper panel)* and after *(lower panel)* successful dilatation and stent placement. When a large, 15-mm balloon was inflated at this site, no waist was seen in the balloon, even at low pressures *(lower panel).*

temic veins, the results are very different. Stent enlargement for narrowed pulmonary veins, whether congenital or postoperative, has proved successful immediately, with marked increases in vessel diameter and flow. Unfortunately, most cases of pulmonary vein stenosis appear to be due to a diffuse intrapulmonary and extrapulmonary process. Often, in addition to a focal narrowing at the venous entry to the left atrium, the veins within the lung are also small,[12] despite being subjected to very high pressures. After the proximal stenosis is relieved, the veins tend to rapidly decrease in size, and in nearly every case they progressively restenose either within the lung upstream from the stent or within the stent because of progressive proliferation of intimal tissue.

Of 12 attempts at stent placement in pulmonary

veins (in eight patients), 10 were successful. Two stents in infants were malpositioned: one dislodged into the descending aorta, and one remained attached to the atrial septum. Each of the 10 patients showed dramatic early improvement. However, five of seven patients followed more than 6 months had substantial restenosis, usually about 3 to 5 months after the procedure. Angiography revealed progressive pulmonary venous encroachment from the parenchymal end of the stent. Redilation of stents in pulmonary veins has successfully enlarged the stent itself, but failed to enlarge the narrowed intrapulmonary vein.

Clinical experience with stents in pulmonary veins seems to support the notion that congenital or late postoperative pulmonary vein stenosis is a diffuse, progressive disease, first localized to the pulmonary vein but later tending to extend throughout the proximal pulmonary veins. To date, all attempts to relieve these stenoses (i.e., surgery, balloon dilatation, stent enlargement) have failed.

TRANSCATHETER RELIEF OF STENOTIC VALVES

Stenotic Pulmonary Valves

Pulmonary valve dilatation was the first catheter technique to achieve widespread clinical use.[13] Techniques have been refined and improved such that, at Children's Hospital in Boston, nearly every case of isolated pulmonary stenosis, regardless of the patient's age, is managed safely and successfully without surgery. It is the procedure of choice.

In neonates, pulmonary valves are thickened, the pulmonary annulus is frequently small, and right ventricular dysfunction is common. Nonetheless, nearly all neonates are significantly improved after dilatation. Avoiding open heart surgery in these patients seems to improve clinical outcome.[53]

Dilatation of neonatal valves is a technically demanding procedure. There is little antegrade flow in patients who are PDA-dependent, making balloon flotation catheters useless for crossing the valve. The right ventricular cavity is small and hypertrophied, reducing the space for catheter manipulation. The neonatal myocardium is delicate and can be perforated with the softest catheters, and in severe cases the valvar opening has a diameter less than 1 mm. Once the valve is crossed successfully, a balloon larger than the valve orifice must be negotiated through this tiny, muscle-bound right ventricle. Although improvements in technique have helped, patience, persistence, and multiple approaches are required to confidently dilate every neonatal pulmonary valve.

All neonates whose pulmonary stenosis is severe enough to produce cyanosis, heart failure, or signs of low cardiac output should undergo balloon valvotomy within a day or two of diagnosis. Even asymptomatic neonates who are estimated to have supra-systemic right ventricular pressure should undergo early elective dilatation. Valvar stenoses do not spontaneously regress, and gradients may increase (and cardiac output decrease) as the ductus and foramen ovale close. Indeed, the procedure may be safer in neonates than in older patients, as cardiac output and oxygenation can be maintained during temporary valve occlusion.

The results of neonatal pulmonary valve dilatation have been good. Since 1985, 61 neonates have undergone attempted dilatation, without a death. The valve was crossed in 59 (97%), with adequate clinical relief in 57. Two neonates had very small (4 mm) annuli and thickened valves; the gradient fell marginally, and surgical patching of the pulmonary outflow tract was repaired 2 days later. All other patients left the catheterization laboratory with subsystemic right ventricular pressures. Five neonates required late intervention: in three balloon valvotomy was repeated for recurrent valvar stenosis, and two required surgical outflow patching for persistent, severe subpulmonary stenosis.

Aortic Stenosis

The first reports of balloon aortic valvotomy[16] followed those of pulmonary valvotomy by several years. This reluctance was based on several concerns: blunt surgical aortic valvotomies had not produced good clinical results, the aortic regurgitation likely to follow balloon dilatation might be poorly tolerated, and the large-bore catheters required for retrograde balloon dilatation posed considerable risks to small femoral arteries. Nevertheless, balloon aortic valvotomy has proved to be a reasonable therapy for congenital aortic stenosis, with risks and benefits comparable to those of open surgical valvotomies.[44]

Like neonatal pulmonary valvotomy, balloon aortic valvotomy of the neonate is a technically demanding procedure, with safe vascular access and catheter manipulation across the valve posing particular difficulties. However, unlike in valvar pulmonary stenosis, balloon size brings additional risks to the dilatation of neonatal aortic stenosis. A small balloon may produce no gradient relief, whereas slightly larger balloons can cause severe aortic regurgitation. Multiple balloon catheter changes

lengthen the procedure in a sick neonate. After a difficult initial learning curve (producing two deaths in the first five cases) we can currently dilate neonatal aortic valves with adequate degrees of safety.

Despite what appeared to be technically satisfactory gradient relief, some neonates have continued to fare poorly after balloon dilatation. It was eventually learned that clinical results in neonatal aortic stenosis depend not only on the valvotomy, but also on the other anatomic left heart structures. A retrospective multivariate analysis by Rhodes and associates[36] revealed that the combined measurements of left ventricular volume and the diameters of the aortic and mitral valve annuli and the aortic arch are important determinants of outcome. In all neonates who died after balloon valvuloplasty, two of these four measurements were more than two standard deviations below the mean.

Any neonate with critical aortic stenosis who has heart failure or cardiogenic shock requires prompt valvotomy. A predilatation period of prostaglandin therapy will help almost any infant with aortic stenosis and an atrial septal defect. A left-to-right shunt at the atrial level and a right-to-left shunt at the ductal level will bypass the distressed left heart and maintain cardiac output. Neonates with virtually intact atrial septa derive little, if any, benefit from prostaglandin therapy and require urgent anatomic relief.

Most likely, balloon dilatation of congenital aortic stenosis is little different from surgical valvotomy under direct vision. Both are palliative procedures with limited therapeutic goals, seeking to incompletely open fused commissures that are malformed or even absent. These dysmorphic, immature valves do not lend themselves to precise splitting of commisures, even under direct vision. However, the extent to which a commisural incision is necessary or tolerated cannot be determined with the heart opened. In contrast, balloon valvotomies permit gradual valvotomies to be performed (e.g., with an 8-mm balloon, then a 9-mm balloon, then a 10-mm balloon). Immediate assessment of postdilatation gradients allows the physician to stop as soon as satisfactory results are achieved. In addition, without anesthesia and surgery, which may or may not include cardiopulmonary bypass, the neonate seems to have a better chance to survive suboptimal anatomic results such as moderate residual aortic stenosis and aortic regurgitation. Finally, balloon valvotomy maintains an undistorted operative field for the patient's ultimate anatomic management: valve replacement.

The technical problems associated with dilating aortic valves in infants are similar to those in neonates, but less onerous.

The indications used for balloon aortic valvotomy in infants are the same as those used for surgical valvotomies: symptoms, strain evidenced on the electrocardiogram, or transvalvar gradients >60 mm Hg. The wisdom of this policy has yet to be documented by late follow-up studies.

Between 1984 and 1991, 83 neonates and infants with congenital aortic stenosis have undergone balloon dilatation at Children's Hospital in Boston; 41 were neonates less than 1 month of age. The five deaths in neonates (12%) were due to small left heart structures, balloon-induced aortic regurgitation, or endocarditis. Only one death occurred in infants more than 1 month of age (2%); this 7-week-old infant was in shock. Restenosis occurred in four of the neonates (10%); each was successfully redilated. To date, there have been no late deaths. The average gradient reduction (62%) was somewhat better (75%) in infants more than 4 months of age, supporting the notion that valve morphology is not favorable in neonates but perhaps is more favorable in older infants because of continued postnatal maturation.

Congenital Mitral Stenosis

Congenital mitral stenosis, a very rare condition, may be due to a parachute subvalvar apparatus, leaflet thickening and fusion, shortened and fused chordal attachments, "supravalvar" rings, or any combination of these. Because pure leaflet thickening is a relatively minor part of this pathology, one would have anticipated little gradient relief from balloon valvotomy. However, the results have been better than expected,[46] with about 50% of patients enjoying significant gradient relief. At Children's Hospital in Boston, we currently attempt palliation in all infants and young children with symptomatic mitral stenosis in the catheterization laboratory.

Although the methods used for dilating valves in infants with mitral stenosis differ little from those used in older children, the procedure is much more demanding. There is little room between the stenosed valve and the ventricular apex, making centering of balloons across the valve difficult. Currently available balloons larger than 12 mm are long, have a large profile, and do not fit in the femoral veins or left ventricles of infants weighing less than 6 kg. These large-bore catheters commonly produce occlusion of the iliac vein. Because catheter access to dilate an infant's mitral valve can really be achieved only by way of the femoral vein, bilateral iliac vein occlusion effectively prevents subsequent mitral valve dilatations. Despite these technical limita-

tions, dilatation has proved useful in delaying the need for early valve replacement.

The results of balloon dilatation for congenital mitral stenosis are clearly worse than those for stenosis caused by rheumatic fever, and indications for its use in infants are correspondingly stricter (i.e., heart failure producing failure to thrive, systemic or higher pulmonary artery pressures, or frequent hospitalizations).

Of 10 infants who underwent dilatation of a congenitally stenosed mitral valve at the Children's Hospital in Boston, five had leaflet fusion with shortened chords, four had a parachute valve, and one had primarily a supravalvar ring fused to the leaflets. Six had significant (>50%) gradient reduction, although unfortunately, restenosis within 12 months was common. It is suspected that patients in whom restenosis occurs early after dilatation never had splitting of fused commissures, but perhaps had only "plastic deformation" of valvar and subvalvar structures. Mild-to-moderate mitral regurgitation (two of 10 patients) is not common, but is perhaps not unwanted. Over the course of months, mitral regurgitation may increase left atrial and left ventricular size and "improve" left ventricular diastolic compliance, making ultimate mitral valve replacement an easier procedure.

Tricuspid Stenosis

We have attempted dilatation in only three patients with tricuspid valve stenosis, all associated with pulmonary atresia and an intact ventricular septum. In one patient with severe annular hypoplasia (a 6-mm annulus in a 3-year-old child), the procedure was unsuccessful. In the other two patients, using techniques similar to those described for congenital mitral stenosis, balloon dilatation produced significant gradient relief (Fig. 7–8).

TRANSCATHETER CLOSURE OF UNWANTED VESSELS

Many vascular closure techniques were first developed by interventional radiologists; however, transcatheter closure of abnormal vessels within the thorax is managed primarily by interventional cardiologists at the time of cardiac catheterization. Although vascular "glues," "spiders," and detachable balloons are available for transcatheter closure of abnormal vessels, we prefer to use Gianturco coils.[7] These simple devices are versatile and flexible, can be delivered through a multitude of delivery catheters as small as No. 3 French, and can be reli-

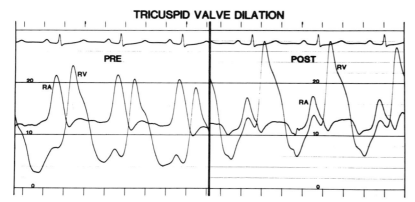

TRICUSPID VALVE DILATION

FIGURE 7–8. ☐

Simultaneous right atrial and right ventricular tracings before (pre) and after (post) balloon dilatation of congenital tricuspid stenosis in a patient who had "repaired" pulmonary atresia with an intact ventricular septum.

ably retrieved after inadvertent embolization. If stable at the time of discharge from the catheterization laboratory, coils do not migrate.

Aortopulmonary Collaterals

Abnormal (non-PDA) vessels that arise from the thoracic aorta or its branches may improve oxygenation in unrepaired patients with cyanotic congenital heart disease but can cause adverse effects before, during, and after repair. They reduce systemic perfusion and may obscure the operative field during cardiopulmonary bypass, add a volume load to the left ventricle, and compete with effective sources of pulmonary blood for space in the pulmonary vascular tree. Clearly, all "significant" aortopulmonary collaterals that can be safely closed should be closed, preferably before repair. As confidence in the use of coils has increased, smaller and smaller vessels are being considered significant. In circulations in which pulmonary blood is, by definition, tenuous (e.g., after the Fontan procedure) or left heart function is impaired, relatively small vessels can cause significant clinical disability.

Not all systemic arteries providing blood to the lungs require closure. However, estimating the quantity of collateral blood flow is problematic. There is no chamber for this blood to mix adequately with systemic venous return, and the anastomosis of aortopulmonary collaterals with pulmonary vessels may occur too far distally in the lung to permit catheters to sample oxygen saturation. Thus, qualitative features of the vessels are generally used, rather than measured volume flow, to estimate significance.

Obviously, vessels as large as a surgically created Blalock-Taussig shunt (3 to 4 mm in infants and toddlers) can carry an entire cardiac output to the lungs and must be considered significant. Even smaller vessels that opacify pulmonary veins after passage through the lungs may pose problems in

tenuous clinical circumstances. It is now suspected that relatively small aortopulmonary collaterals arising from the head and neck vessels may predispose patients to develop neurologic complications after cardiopulmonary bypass.[52] Even 2-mm vessels arising from the base of the vertebral artery may require closure before open heart surgery.

As with all transcatheter closure techniques, coils rely on clot formation to completely seal off vessels. To promote clot formation, the coils are soaked in topical thrombin.

The ideal vessel for coil embolization has a long, straight segment distal to any normal branches and a distal stenosis to prevent embolization into the lung. However, with diligence and care, almost all aortopulmonary collaterals, even arteries with a proximal stenosis close to the aortic lumen, can be closed with coils.

Factors that would argue against preoperative closure include (1) a large collateral in a cyanotic patient such that closure would reduce aortic oxygen saturation below 70%, (2) a collateral that is the sole source of blood supply to a significant part of the lung (i.e., a lobe or several segments), and (3) collaterals that are easy to close in the operating room before starting cardiopulmonary bypass or arteries that need to be connected to the pulmonary arteries (unifocalization).

Although originally used in older children, coils can now be safely delivered through No. 3 to 4 French catheters, extending their use to infants. The more aggressive approach to rehabilitation of diminutive pulmonary arteries in younger children[39] has furthered the use of coils in infants. In one infant an errant coil traveled to the lungs. Six errant coils were retrieved from older patients using standard snare techniques. In two other cases, the coils were left in situ within intraparenchymal pulmonary arteries. At angiography 1 to 3 years later, these dislodged coils had narrowed but had not occluded 2- to 3-mm sublobar pulmonary arteries.

The most common "complication" of coil embolization is a low-grade fever 12 to 24 hours after the procedure. Although we have not observed infection, atelectasis, or pleural effusions in any of these patients, such fever can interfere with the timing of previously planned operative repairs.

Surgical Shunts

Surgical takedown of previously placed aortopulmonary shunts can lengthen or complicate cardiac repairs. Although the classic or modified right Blalock-Taussig shunt (with a left arch) poses few, if any, problems, closure of posterior left-sided shunts or Potts anastomoses can require a tedious dissection through old scar tissue and may place adjacent structures, such as the phrenic nerve, at risk. The decision of whether to close shunts preoperatively or intraoperatively is made jointly between the surgeon and cardiologist and is usually added to the end of a preoperative diagnostic catheterization. "Repair" of pulmonary atresia with an intact ventricular septum currently can be accomplished at cardiac catheterization, with closure of the atrial septal defect and shunt using coils and umbrellas.[9]

Although detachable balloons have been successfully used in rare cases, we prefer coils for closing surgical shunts. These are more difficult to close than most aortopulmonary collaterals: the catheter takes an acute turn at the subclavian artery, there is rarely distal stenosis, and very high flow can dislodge even properly placed coils. Thus, the initial closure rates were less than 80%, and coil dislodgement to the lungs was relatively common.[31] The procedure was simplified by adopting the technique of distal balloon occlusion. An appropriate-size balloon, inflated in the pulmonary artery under the shunt, stabilizes the first coil and allows multiple coils to be delivered to densely occlude the shunt before balloon release (usually 5 to 10 minutes). Since adopting that technique, we have successfully closed nearly all Blalock-Taussig shunts without complication (Fig. 7–9).

A Potts shunt can be closed in larger patients using a double umbrella delivered via the descending aorta. However, this procedure has not been performed in infants.

Pulmonary Arteriovenous Malformations

Pulmonary arteriovenous malformations, which are extremely rare in infancy, may be isolated, may be associated with the Osler-Weber-Rendu syndrome, or may form after a Glenn anastomosis. Coil embolization of vascular malformations has not led

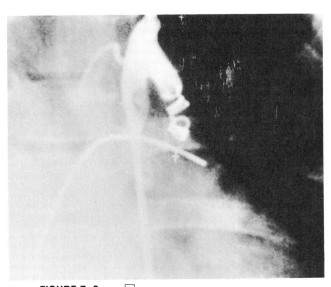

FIGURE 7–9. ☐

Multiple coils used to completely occlude a Blalock-Taussig shunt.

to systemic thrombotic or embolic events and has become the treatment of choice for these lesions.

TRANSCATHETER CLOSURE OF CARDIAC DEFECTS

Patent Ductus Arteriosus

The Rashkind double umbrella[35] has allowed extension of the use of transcatheter closure to the infant with a patent ductus arteriosus. Neonatal patent ductus, especially in a premature infant, does not have a ductus diverticulum on the aortic side to allow anchoring of any devices currently available; thus, for the foreseeable future, surgical ligation will continue to be needed for closure of a patent ductus in a premature neonate.

The techniques for catheter closure (Fig. 7–10) have been described previously.[30, 51] In general, at least a year is allowed for the duct to close spontaneously; infants less than 1 year of age who undergo catheter closure of a PDA usually have heart failure, growth failure, pulmonary hypertension, or other medical problems that make closure advisable. This is rare. Of the 100 patients who underwent catheter closure of a patent ductus at Children's Hospital in Boston between 1988 and 1991, only nine were less than 1 year of age; all had clinically successful closures.

Atrial Septal Defects

Transcatheter umbrella closure of atrial septal defects, first performed in 1976,[14] has been success-

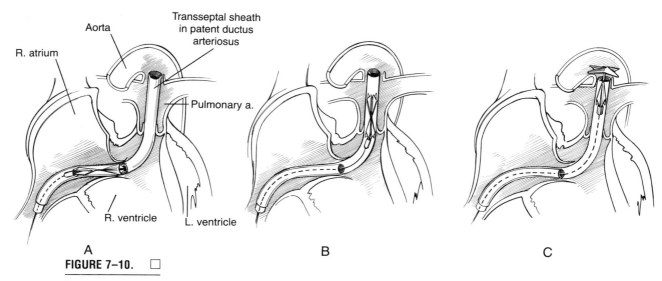

FIGURE 7–10. ☐

Transcatheter closure of a patent ductus arteriosus allows the catheter to approach the duct via a long sheath advanced from the femoral vein.

fully completed in more than 400 patients. Recent observations that stainless steel arms may fracture in situ (without apparent morbidity) after fixation have prompted a design change in the most widely used device, the Bard clamshell occluder.[38] Nonetheless, the high success rate (more than 90%) and minimal morbidity, even in high-risk cases, indicate that catheter closure of atrial septal defects, and of other atrial defects, will continue to play an expanding role in the management of congenital heart disease.

As with PDA, atrial septal defects rarely require closure in the first year of life; most such closures are performed surgically (and incidentally) at the time of surgical management of more complex lesions. Rarely, they are closed in the catheterization laboratory, usually in infants who are ill and have residual atrial level shunts. Catheter closure of these defects is relatively straightforward: percutaneous access is obtained from the femoral vein, a catheter and guide wire traverse the atrial defect to the left atrium, and a No. 10 French long sheath is advanced to the mid–left atrium (Fig. 7–11A). One set of umbrella arms is opened in the left atrium, the whole system is withdrawn until the umbrella encounters the atrial septum, and the sheath is withdrawn until the right atrial arms expand, allowing the umbrella to straddle the septum. Once the position appears appropriate, the device is released (Fig. 7–11B).

Thus far, only four infants have undergone atrial septal defect closure in the catheterization laboratory at Children's Hospital in Boston; three had right-to-left shunts through the foramen ovale, but one had a left-to-right shunt and was at increased

risk for open heart surgery. Each procedure was successful in that the shunt was abolished or became clinically insignificant. No infant has had evidence of cardiac arrhythmias or trauma; none has had a stroke.

Ventricular Septal Defects

Initially, transcatheter closure of ventricular septal defects was accomplished in older children and adults,[21] but the methodology was rapidly adapted to infants.[3] This is a technically difficult procedure

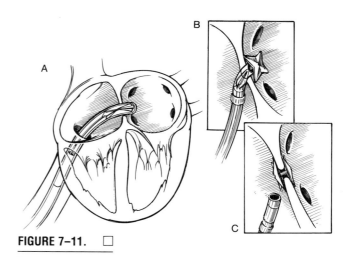

FIGURE 7–11. ☐

During umbrella closure of an atrial septal defect, the umbrella is advanced from the inferior vena cava to the atrium via a long sheath, the distal arms are opened in the left atrium (A and B), and then the entire system is withdrawn until the distal arms engage the septum, allowing the proximal arms to be deployed before release of the device (C).

in infants, but the preliminary results have been encouraging.

Atrioventricular canal, paramembranous, malalignment, and posterior muscular ventricular septal defects are all located close to the atrioventricular or semilunar valves. Umbrellas anchored in any of these defects would place the function of those valves at risk. Thus, more than 90% of ventricular septal defects are not suitable for catheter closure. Although single, midmuscular, or isolated anterior septal defects can be closed with double umbrellas, they are successfully closed surgically through the tricuspid or pulmonary valve, without a ventriculotomy. Therefore, transcatheter closure is primarily indicated for complex apical or anterior muscular ventricular septal defects or multiple "Swiss cheese" defects (Fig. 7–12). Of 80 ventricular septal defects

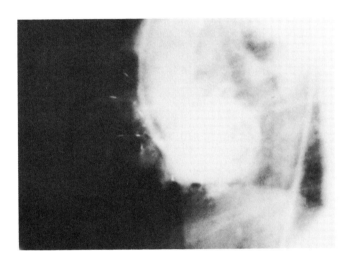

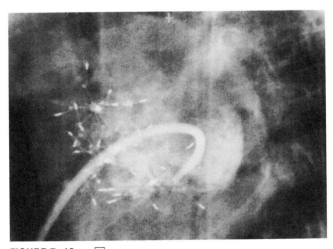

FIGURE 7–12. □

Left anterior caudal view of multiple ventricular septal defects *(upper panel)* closed using four separate clamshell umbrellas arranged along the circumference of the apical ventricular septum *(lower panel).*

closed at our catheterization laboratory, seven have been in infants. Access to the defect usually is obtained via a Brockenbrough approach to the left atrium and ventricle, and a balloon catheter is floated over a preformed wire across the defect. Once this catheter reaches the pulmonary artery, a second venous catheter (from the jugular vein for apical defects; from the femoral vein for anterior defects) is advanced to the pulmonary artery. A long guide wire is snared in the pulmonary artery and retrieved via the second venous sheath, creating a through-and-through wire course (e.g., from the femoral vein to the right atrium, left atrium, left ventricle, ventricular septal defect, right ventricle, right atrium, and, finally, to the jugular vein), which is used to deliver the No. 8 or No. 10 French sheath to the defect via the straightest, most direct course.

Once catheter access traverses the ventricular septal defect, balloon sizing and precise angiography are needed to choose the most appropriate umbrella and location. Umbrella delivery follows the same procedure as described for atrial septal defects.

Despite the complex nature of septal defects closed with transcatheter techniques, the results in these seven infants have been encouraging. Placement was successful in all seven patients, with no mortality, strokes, persistent arrhythmias, or cardiac damage. Adequacy of closure is difficult to assess in many patients; associated paramembranous ventricular septal defects or other lesions have required later open repair. Nonetheless, at late catheterization, pulmonary-to-systemic flow ratios were less than 1.5:1 in all but two infants. Both of these infants had significant residual ventricular septal defects that were closed successfully at postoperative catheterization.

Clearly, further advances in umbrella design and closure techniques will expand the role of catheter closure of complex muscular ventricular septal defects.

FUTURE DIRECTIONS

Two forms of catheter-directed therapy, currently only rare in infants, are likely to assume major importance in the future. The advent of a reliable and relatively safe form of catheter-delivered cytopathic energy (i.e., radiofrequency electricity) has revolutionized the treatment of several forms of childhood arrhythmias, not only the Wolf-Parkinson-White syndrome,[42] but also ectopic atrial tachycardias[50] and atrioventricular nodal re-entry tachycardias. Improved understanding of catheter design, short- and long-term effects of catheter-delivered energy, and the genesis of neonatal and postoperative arrhythmias will undoubtedly increase the use of this promising technique.

In addition, gene therapy is also making rapid advances in cardiovascular medicine. At present, physical techniques are generally used to introduce genes into target cardiovascular organs. Catheter-directed therapy will be used to assist in that effort. These and other new applications of catheter-directed therapy in infants will help ensure an ever-increasing role for interventional cardiology.

REFERENCES

1. Arnold LW, Keane JF, Kan JS, et al. Transient unilateral pulmonary edema following successful balloon dilation of peripheral pulmonary artery stenosis. Am J Cardiol 62:327, 1988.
2. Beekman RH, Moller DW, Lupinetti FM, et al. Balloon expandable stent repair of experimental coarctation in dogs. Circulation 84(suppl II):513, 1991.
3. Bridges ND, Perry SB, Keane JF, et al. Preoperative transcatheter closure of congenital muscular ventricular septal defects. N Engl J Med 324:1312, 1991.
4. Cragg AH, Einzig S, Rysavy JA, et al. The vasa vasorum and angioplasty. Radiology 148:75, 1983.
5. Dotter CT, Judkins MP. Transluminal treatment of arteriosclerotic obstruction. Circulation 30:654, 1964.
6. Driscoll DJ, Hesslien PS, Mullins CE. Congenital stenosis of individual pulmonary veins: Clinical spectrum and unsuccessful treatment by transvenous balloon dilation. Am J Cardiol 49:1767, 1982.
7. Fuhrman BP, Bass JL, Castaneda-Zuniga W, et al. Coil embolization of congenital vascular anomalies in infants and children. Circulation 70:285, 1984.
8. Gentles T, Lock JE, Perry SB. High-pressure balloon dilation of pulmonary arteries. J Am Coll Cardiol 22:867, 1993.
9. Giglia TM, Mandell VS, Connor AR, et al. Diagnosis and management of right ventricular dependent coronary circulation in pulmonary atresia with intact ventricular septum. Circulation 86:1516, 1992.
10. Gruntzig A, Hopff H. Perkutane Rekanalisation chronischer arterieller verschlusse mit einem neuen diltationskatheter: Modification der Dotter-Technik. Dtsch Med Wochenschr 99:2502, 1974.
11. Helgason H, Keane JF, Fellows KE, et al. Balloon dilation of the aortic valve: Studies in normal lambs and in children with aortic stenosis. J Am Coll Cardiol 9:816, 1987.
12. Jenkins KJ, Sanders SP, Orav EJ, et al. Individual pulmonary vein size and survival in infants with totally anomalous pulmonary venous connection. J Am Coll Cardiol 22:201–206, 1993.
13. Kan JS, White RJ, Mitchell SE, et al. Percutaneous balloon valvuloplasty: A new method for treating congenital pulmonary valve stenosis. N Engl J Med 307:540, 1982.
14. King TD, Mills NL. Secundum atrial septal defects: Nonoperative closure during cardiac catheterization. JAMA 235:2506, 1976.
15. Lababidi Z, Daskalopoulos DA, Stoeckle H Jr. Transluminal balloon coarctation angioplasty: Experience with 27 patients. Am J Cardiol 54:1288, 1984.
16. Lababidi Z, Wu J, Walls JT. Percutaneous balloon aortic valvuloplasty: Results in 23 patients. Am J Cardiol 53:194, 1984.
17. Leandro J, Smallhorn JF, Benson L, et al. Ambulatory blood pressure monitoring and left ventricular mass and function after successful surgical repair of coarctation of the aorta. J Am Coll Cardiol 20:197, 1992.
18. Lock JE, Bass JL, Amplatz K, et al. Balloon dilation angioplasty of coarctations in infants and children. Circulation 68:109, 1983.
19. Lock JE, Bass JL, Castaneda-Zuniga W, et al. Dilation angioplasty of congenital or operative narrowings of venous channels. Circulation 70:457, 1984.
20. Lock JE, Bass JL, Lund G, et al. Transcatheter closure of patent ductus arteriosus in piglets. Am J Cardiol 55:826, 1985.
21. Lock JE, Block PC, McKay RG, et al. Transcatheter closure of ventricular septal defects. Circulation 78:361, 1988.
22. Lock JE, Castaneda-Zuniga WF, Fuhrman BF, et al. Balloon dilation angioplasty of hypoplastic and stenotic pulmonary arteries. Circulation 67:962, 1983.
23. Lock JE, Niemi BA, Burke BA, et al. Transcutaneous angioplasty of experimental aortic coarctation. Circulation 66:1280, 1982.
24. Lock JE, Niemi T, Einzig S, et al. Transvenous angioplasty of experimental branch pulmonary artery stenosis in newborn lambs. Circulation 64:886, 1981.
25. Lock JE, Rome JJ, Davis R, et al. Transcatheter closure of atrial septal defects: Experimental studies. Circulation 79:1091, 1989.
26. Mistrot J, Neal W, Lyons G, et al. Pulmonary valvulotomy under inflow stasis for isolated pulmonary stenosis. Ann Thorac Surg 21:30, 1976.
27. Morrow WP, Vick GW, Nihill MR, et al. Balloon dilation of unoperated coarctation of the aorta: Short and intermediate term results. J Am Coll Cardiol II:133, 1988.
28. Mullins CE, O'Laughlin MP, Vick GW III, et al. Implantation of balloon expandable intravascular grafts by catheterization in pulmonary arteries and systemic veins. Circulation 77:188, 1988.
29. O'Laughlin MP, Perry SB, Lock JE, et al. Use of endovascular stents in congenital heart disease. Circulation 83:1923, 1991.
30. Perry SB, Lock JE. Frontloading of double umbrellas: Improved delivery of umbrella devices. Am J Cardiol 70:917–920, 1992.
31. Perry SB, Radtke W, Fellows KE, et al. Coil embolization of aortopulmonary collaterals and shunts in patients with congenital heart disease. J Am Coll Cardiol 12:100, 1989.
32. Rao PS, Najjar HN, Mardini MK, et al. Balloon angioplasty for coarctation of the aorta: Immediate and long-term results. Am Heart J 115:657, 1988.
33. Rashkind WJ. Transcatheter treatment of congenital heart disease. Circulation 67:711, 1983.
34. Rashkind WJ, Miller WW. Creation of an atrial septal defect without thoracotomy: A palliative approach to complete transposition of the great arteries. JAMA 196:991, 1966.
35. Rashkind WJ, Mullins CE, Hellenbrand WE, et al. Nonsurgical closure of patent ductus arteriosus: Clinical application of the Rashkind PDA occluder system. Circulation 75:583, 1987.
36. Rhodes LA, Colan SD, Perry SB, et al. Predictors of survival in neonates with critical aortic stenosis. Circulation 84:2325, 1991.
37. Ring JC, Kulik TJ, Burke BA, et al. Morphologic changes induced by dilation of the pulmonary valve annulus with overlarge balloons in normal newborn lambs. Am J Cardiol 55:210, 1985.
38. Rome JJ, Keane JF, Perry SB, et al. Double umbrella closure of atrial septal defects: Initial clinical applications. Circulation 82:751, 1990.
39. Rome JJ, Mayer JE, Castaneda AR, et al. Tetralogy of Fallot with pulmonary atresia: Rehabilitation of diminutive pulmonary arteries. Circulation 88:1691, 1993.
40. Rothman A, Perry SB, Keane JF, et al. Early results and follow up of balloon angioplasty for branch pulmonary artery stenosis. J Am Coll Cardiol 15:1109, 1990.
41. Rubio-Alvarez V, Limon RL, Soni J. Valvulotomias intracardiacas por medio de un cateter. Arch Inst Cardiol Mexico 23:183, 1953.
42. Saul JP, Hulse JE, De W, et al. Catheter ablation of accessory atrioventricular pathways in young patients: Use of long

vascular sheaths, the transseptal approach, and a retrograde left posterior parallel approach. J Am Coll Cardiol 21:571–583, 1993.

43. Saul JP, Keane JF, Fellows KE, et al. Balloon dilation angioplasty of postoperative aortic obstructions. Am J Cardiol 59:943, 1987.
44. Sholler GF, Keane JF, Perry SB, et al. Balloon dilation of congenital aortic stenosis: Results and influence of technical and morphologic features on outcome. Circulation 78:351, 1988.
45. Sideris EB, Sideris SE, Fowlkes JP, et al. Transvenous atrial septal defect occlusion with a "buttoned" double-disk device. Circulation 81:312, 1990.
46. Spevak PJ, Ball JL, Ben-Shachar G, et al. Balloon angioplasty for non rheumatic mitral stenosis in children. Am J Cardiol 66:472, 1990.
47. Swan H, Zeavin L, Blount SG Jr, et al. Surgery by direct vision in the open heart during hypothermia. JAMA 153:1081, 1953.
48. Synhorst DP, Lauer RM, Doty DB. Hemodynamic effects of vasodilator agents in dogs with experimental ventricular septal defects. Circulation 54:472, 1976.
49. Tynan M, Finley JP, Fontes V, et al. Balloon angioplasty for the treatment of native coarctation: Results of valvuloplasty and angioplasty of congenital anomalies registry. Am J Cardiol 65:790, 1990.
50. Walsh EP, Saul JP, Hulse JE, et al. Transcatheter ablation of ectopic atrial tachycardia in young patients using radiofrequency current. Circulation 86:1138, 1992.
51. Wessel DL, Keane JF, Parness I, et al. Outpatient closure of the patent ductus arteriosus. Circulation 77:1068, 1988.
52. Wong PC, Barlow CF, Hickey PR, et al. Factors associated with choreoathetosis following cardiopulmonary bypass in children with congenital heart disease. Circulation 86II:118, 1992.
53. Zeevi B, Keane JF, Fellows KE, et al. Balloon dilation of critical pulmonary stenosis in the first week of life. J Am Coll Cardiol II:821, 1988.

2

Part

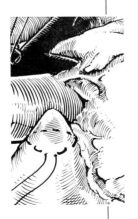

Congenital Heart Defects
and Procedures

8

Chapter

Atrial Septal Defect

An atrial septal defect is broadly defined as a communication between the left and right atria that allows abnormal shunting of blood between the two chambers. Of the four anatomic types of communication, only one represents a true defect in the interatrial septum: the ostium secundum atrial septal defect. The sinus venosus defect and the coronary sinus septal defect represent abnormalities in the remnants of the right and left horns of the embryologic sinus venosus, whereas the ostium primum defect represents an abnormality in the septum of the atrioventricular canal. In these three defects the true atrial septum, made up of the septum primum and septum secundum, is normal. Despite their various origins, all four of these lesions are considered to be atrial septal defects because the pathophysiologic changes induced by them are generally similar. Ostium secundum, sinus venosus, and coronary sinus septal defects will be discussed in this chapter; however, the ostium primum defect, because it is part of the spectrum of the atrioventricular canal defect, will be covered in Chapter 10.

In general, isolated atrial septal defects do not cause significant symptoms in infancy, and therefore, the surgeon is not usually involved in their management in patients in this age group. However, in a small percentage of infants significant symptoms do occur, and the surgeon's judgment and skills are required. The major focus of this chapter will be on the management of infants who have atrial septal defects that cause symptoms.

ANATOMY

Developmental Considerations

The atrial septum forms from a composite of embryologic structures.[21] The thick, muscular upper aspect of the atrial septum (septum secundum) is formed from the invaginated roof of the embryologic atria. Its inferior border is marked by the limbus, the oval-shaped free edge of the septum secundum. The lower aspect of the atrial septum is formed by the thin, mobile septum primum tissue, which fuses with endocardial cushion tissue during development. The free edge of the septum primum extends superiorly and posteriorly to overlap the free edge of the limbus on its left atrial aspect, defining the foramen ovale. Throughout fetal life right atrial pressure is slightly higher than left atrial pressure, and the septum primum bulges into the left atrium, providing a pathway for a relatively large volume of blood (most of it highly oxygenated umbilical blood) to pass from the inferior vena cava to the left atrium. This communication closes after birth, when left atrial pressure rises above right atrial pressure, allowing the mobile septum primum to abut against the limbus.

Morphologic Features

The anatomic landmarks of the right atrium are important, because atrial septal defects are almost exclusively exposed surgically through a right atrial incision. The normal structures of the right atrium are shown in Figure 8–1.

An ostium secundum defect is one that is confined within the fossa ovalis. If the limbus is normal and the septum primum does not appear deficient, such a lesion is called a *patent foramen ovale.* Deficiency of the septum primum is the most common cause of a true ostium secundum atrial septal defect. The deficiency in the septum primum may vary from a few small fenestrations to complete absence, in which case the inferior border of the septal defect becomes confluent with the posterior wall of the inferior vena cava. In these cases the eustachian valve of the inferior vena cava may be mistaken for the lower border of the defect by the inexperienced observer. Surgical closure undertaken with this misperception will result in drainage of the inferior vena cava to the left atrium. An ostium secundum defect may also result from a normal septum primum and deficient limbus tissue, in which case the defect will be relatively high in the septum. Insufficient septum secundum and limbus are thought to

be extremely unusual in situs solitus hearts, although this has not been rigorously studied.

The sinus venosus defect can occur in any position along the remnant of the right horn of the sinus venosus, which extends from the orifice of the superior vena cava to the orifice of the inferior vena cava along the most posterior aspect of the right atrium, overlying the connection of the right pulmonary veins to the left atrium. The most common position for a sinus venosus defect is at the superior sinoatrial junction. The defect is superior to the limbus. Its lower edge is a rim of tissue that borders on the most superior extent of the septum secundum, while the upper aspect of the defect becomes confluent with the back wall of the superior vena cava. This defect is frequently (>90% of cases) associated with partial anomalous connection of the right pulmonary veins.[13] Most commonly the veins in the right upper and middle lobes drain to the superior vena cava or sinoatrial junction; however, the venous drainage of the entire right lung may be anomalous, or there may be no anomalous drainage.

Rarely, sinus venosus defect may occur in other

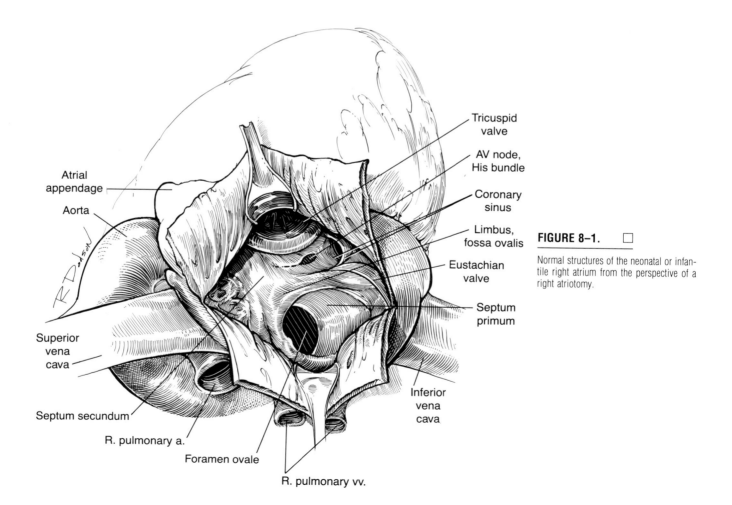

Atrial appendage

Aorta

Superior vena cava

Septum secundum

R. pulmonary a.

Foramen ovale

R. pulmonary vv.

Tricuspid valve

AV node, His bundle

Coronary sinus

Limbus, fossa ovalis

Eustachian valve

Septum primum

Inferior vena cava

FIGURE 8–1. ☐

Normal structures of the neonatal or infantile right atrium from the perspective of a right atriotomy.

positions. It may be directly posterior to the fossa ovalis, not bordering on the orifice of the superior or inferior vena cava. In this case the right pulmonary veins may appear to enter the atria ambiguously when viewed from inside the heart, but appear normally related to the venae cavae and the heart when viewed from outside. A sinus venosus defect may also appear inferiorly at the inferior vena cava–sinoatrium junction. In this case the lower aspect of the defect becomes confluent with the inferior vena cava. Anomalous venous drainage from the right lung to the inferior vena cava may or may not accompany this defect. Partial anomalous venous drainage of any of the pulmonary veins may occur occasionally in isolation—without a sinus venosus atrial defect—either with a completely intact atrial septum or with a patent foramen ovale or secundum atrial septal defect.

Coronary sinus septal defects result from deficiencies in the remnant of the left horn of the sinus venosus, which extends along the length of the coronary sinus to the level of the coronary sinus orifice, including the thebesian valve. A number of associated lesions can exist with this condition; these constitute the spectrum of the unroofed coronary sinus syndrome.[11, 18] The opening of the coronary sinus is always present in its usual position; however, the wall between the coronary sinus and the left atrium is variably deficient. This wall may be fenestrated in various locations along its length, or it may be completely absent. Such a defect in the wall between the coronary sinus and the left atrium allows an abnormal communication between the left and right atria via the otherwise normal coronary sinus orifice. In this syndrome, a left superior vena cava commonly (but not invariably) exists, connecting to the base of the left atrial appendage. When a left superior vena cava is present, there is no connecting vein between the right and left superior venae cavae in approximately 90% of cases. The unroofed coronary sinus syndrome can occur in otherwise normal hearts; however, it is frequently found in cases of heterotaxia.

Ostium secundum defects account for 7% to 10% of all cardiac anomalies and more than 80% of all atrial defects.[5] Sinus venosus defects account for approximately 5% to 10% of atrial septal defects. Coronary sinus defects are rare. The remainder of atrial septal defects are of the atrioventricular canal type. Combinations of these different types can occur together.

PATHOPHYSIOLOGY AND NATURAL HISTORY

Very small atrial septal defects may provide enough resistance to restrict flow; however, essen-

tially all clinically significant atrial septal defects behave as nonrestrictive defects, and the amount of shunting is determined by the relative compliances of the left and right ventricles during diastole. In the neonatal and early infancy periods, the left and right ventricles have similar thicknesses and, therefore, similar compliance characteristics, resulting in very little left-to-right shunting. As a result it is unusual for isolated atrial septal defects to cause symptoms in early infancy. As the right ventricular compliance increases in response to the reduced afterload of the pulmonary circulation, the left-to-right shunt increases. In spite of increasing shunts, however, most infants remain asymptomatic. The natural history of atrial septal defects after infancy is well established and provides strong evidence that these lesions should be corrected. This pathophysiology will not be reviewed here.

Important exceptions to the typically benign natural history of atrial septal defects in infancy do occur. In a small but significant fraction of patients with isolated defects (5%), congestive heart failure or failure to thrive develops during infancy.[4, 8, 15] In our experience, about half of the infants in this small group fail solely on the basis of hemodynamics, and the other half have significant compromise to other major organ systems that, along with the septal defect, contributes to failure. The natural history in these infants has been shown to result in a mortality rate of as much as 10% if surgical correction is not undertaken.[12] Pulmonary hypertension has also been reported in infants and children, although the incidence is extremely low, and causality cannot be assigned with confidence.[3] The reason congestive heart failure occurs during infancy in some patients with atrial septal defects is not clear. Cardiac catheterization in these patients does not reveal obvious differences in shunt size between them and the larger group of patients who are asymptomatic.[15, 20] In our pathologic collection, several specimens of isolated secundum atrial defects exist in which the clinical history was that of a patient who died from congestive heart failure in infancy. In these cases the septum primum was essentially completely absent. Notably, in these cases the left atrium and ventricle were mildly but significantly hypoplastic, with well-formed left atrial and ventricular structures. It could be speculated that intrauterine limitations to inflow through the foramen ovale, induced by the absent septum primum, may have caused subtle size and compliance deficiencies in the development of the left side of the heart. These deficiencies, associated with the atrial septal defect, may then contribute to congestive heart failure in infants.[22] It must be emphasized that clinical physiologic data supporting this intriguing contention are not readily available.

Unlike ventricular septal defects, most atrial septal defects do not close spontaneously. When closure does occur, it is usually in the first year of life, and the defects are relatively small. There have been a number of reports of spontaneous closures in infants, with closure rates reported as high as 39%.[4, 6, 15] It must be recognized that concepts regarding the natural history of small and moderate-size atrial septal defects are changing because of the increasing ability to identify such lesions with the more widespread use of echocardiography.

DIAGNOSIS AND INDICATIONS FOR SURGERY

Because most atrial septal defects do not cause symptoms early in life, the diagnosis is often first suspected when a murmur is heard on routine examination. When present early in life, symptoms are typically related to the size of the left-to-right shunt; however, intermittent cyanosis and paradoxic embolism may occur also. Chest radiograph and electrocardiographic findings will support the diagnosis when the shunt is large. Echocardiography is routinely performed. Two-dimensional echocardiographic and color Doppler studies will show the size and position of the defect and document left-to-right flow. In addition, right ventricular volume overload can be confirmed, indicating the physiologic significance of the lesion. In sinus venosus defects, the echocardiographic assessment of the pulmonary venous connections can often be difficult.

In the older child, if the echocardiographic study and physical examination clearly demonstrate an atrial septal defect associated with evidence of a right-sided volume overload, elective intervention to close the defect is pursued without catheterization. However, in infants cardiac catheterization is usually performed to confirm the diagnosis, clarify the hemodynamics, or rule out associated lesions.

The main indication for surgical closure in infants is the presence of an atrial septal defect that causes symptoms. A less clear indication is the presence of an asymptomatic septal defect with echocardiographic evidence of a right ventricular volume overload or catheterization evidence of a QP/QS > 1.5.

The timing of closure in the asymptomatic infant deserves further comment. For the typical asymptomatic or minimally symptomatic patient, elective repair at 4 to 5 years of age is widely recommended. This practice has apparently been based on the consideration that this is a convenient time for elective repair, with little harm done to the patient by waiting until this age. In the early years of cardiac surgery the considerations of technical ease and safety probably also influenced the belief that this age was the ideal one for repair. Because very few atrial septal defects close spontaneously after the first year, the hope that the defect will close without intervention should not be a major impetus for delaying surgery.

Although there no longer appear to be technical or safety reasons to delay surgery until the age of 4 to 5 years, there are also no compelling reasons to proceed earlier in the asymptomatic patient other than to avoid the small risk of a paradoxic embolus. Thus, because there is no good reason to wait until 4 to 5 years of age, it is not unreasonable to electively close large atrial septal defects late in infancy. If symptoms are present or if there are important psychosocial or other considerations, intervention should be pursued at any age without hesitation.

Currently, in a small number of institutions (including Children's Hospital in Boston) closure of ostium secundum atrial septal defects that have certain anatomic characteristics can be achieved in the cardiac catheterization laboratory using permanent occluders introduced through a percutaneous, transluminal vascular approach. This subject is discussed in detail in Chapter 7. This technique represents an important option for the patient with a secundum defect of small to moderate size. Larger or more complex defects cannot be closed at present using this method.

Our experience with atrial septal defects in infants during the 1980s and early 1990s has molded our current approach to this set of lesions. During this time at Children's Hospital in Boston, a total of 195 patients with isolated ostium secundum atrial defects have had surgery. Of these, 35 were atypical in that they had symptoms possibly attributable to the defect within the first 24 months of life. The age range of these patients was 5 months to 24 months.

Nineteen of these 35 patients were failing to thrive (mean weight < fifth percentile) and had clinical and echocardiographic evidence of a large left-to-right shunt. Two were infants, and 17 were between 1 and 2 years of age. These 19 patients had no other defects or medical problems.

In the remaining 16 of these 35 patients, other complex, noncardiac congenital anomalies were present (typically gastrointestinal, neurologic, or pulmonary). Eight of these were infants, and eight were between 1 and 2 years of age. Typically, these patients had only moderate left-to-right shunts (mean QP/QS of 2.7; range, 1.6 to 4) at cardiac catheterization. The contribution of the cardiac lesion to the overall failure to thrive in this group was difficult to quantify because of multisystem problems. The failure to thrive had persisted in spite of maximal management of all noncardiac problems (mean weight < third percentile).

Since the early 1980s, a total of 85 sinus venosus defects have been surgically repaired at Children's Hospital in Boston. Fifteen of these 85 patients underwent surgery before the age of 2 years: seven were infants, and eight were between 1 and 2 years of age. The indication for surgery in these 15 patients was failure to thrive.

During the same period a total of 32 coronary sinus septal defects were repaired. In nine of these the coronary sinus septal defect was isolated, whereas the other 23 defects were associated with complex, intracardiac structural lesions. In two of the nine patients with isolated defects, surgical correction was performed before 1 year of age. The indication for surgery in these two patients was failure to thrive with marked delay in growth.

SURGICAL MANAGEMENT

Historical Perspective

Because of their anatomic simplicity, atrial septal defects were the subject of some of the earliest attempts at surgical repair of intracardiac defects. Several ingenious closed methods for closure, such as the atrioseptopexy method of Bailey et al.[1] and the closed suture technique of Sondergaard,[19] were applied in the late 1940s and early 1950s. Open repair, using the atrial well technique, was performed at Children's Hospital in Boston by Gross and coworkers in 1952,[9] and repair under direct vision using moderate hypothermia and inflow occlusion was performed in 1953 by Lewis and Taufic.[14] In 1954, Gibbons introduced cardiopulmonary bypass for closing an atrial septal defect.[7] In the present era cardiopulmonary bypass is used almost exclusively for surgical closure of atrial septal defects. Repair in an infant was first reported by Hastreiter et al. in 1962,[10] and since then a number of closures in infants have been reported.[2, 3, 8, 15–17, 20]

Surgical Technique

Ostium Secundum Atrial Septal Defect

A standard median sternotomy approach is used. Because of the relative simplicity of the operation, cosmetic considerations may justify keeping the upper aspect of the incision well below the sternomanubrial junction. The sternum itself is usually completely split. In patients who weigh more than 6 kg,

cardiopulmonary bypass is routinely conducted at 32°C core temperature with bicaval cannulation, aortic crossclamping, and cardioplegic protection. An alternative to aortic crossclamping with cardioplegia is to induce electrical ventricular fibrillation during the intracardiac portion of the repair. Continuous electrical stimulation of the ventricles with the fibrillator is mandatory, as spontaneous conversion to an organized rhythm may occur at these warm temperatures. The disadvantages of this approach are that (1) coronary sinus blood flow continues, potentially obscuring the intracardiac anatomic landmarks, and (2) spontaneous defibrillation may occur with the potential for air embolism if the defibrillator is accidentally dislodged. Short periods (5 to 15 minutes) of ventricular fibrillation at relatively warm core temperatures (32°C) in the nonhypertrophied heart with normal coronary arteries are otherwise well tolerated. Attention should be given to maintaining adequate aortic perfusion pressure if this technique is used. In the infant weighing less than 5 kg, cardiopulmonary bypass with deep hypothermic circulatory arrest may be considered. We have used this in the past, but currently we reserve it for small infants with more complex lesions such as sinus venosus defects or the unroofed coronary sinus syndrome.

The details of the repair itself are generally straightforward (Fig. 8–2). An oblique incision is made, beginning in the right atrial appendage and extending well anterior to the sinoatrial area toward the inferior vena cava. The positions of the coronary sinus and all systemic and pulmonary veins should be identified and the rim of the defect completely visualized. The septum primum is further inspected to determine the presence of other fenestrations. If the septum primum is markedly deficient, the inferior rim will be absent, and the defect will be confluent with the back wall of the inferior vena cava. In this case the eustachian valve should be clearly identified to avoid mistaking it for the lower rim of the defect. An assessment is made as to whether primary closure or patch closure will be performed. This decision is based on the size and shape of the defect and on the integrity and pliability of the defect edges. The guiding principle is that significant tension should be avoided. Clearly, a patch is not necessary for most infants. With either patch or primary closure, a running suture of polypropylene is used, beginning at the inferior rim of the defect. If the limbus is deficient anteriorly, care should be taken to avoid injury to the coronary sinus and the atrioventricular node. Before completing the suture line at the superior aspect of the defect, the left atrium is filled with cold saline to

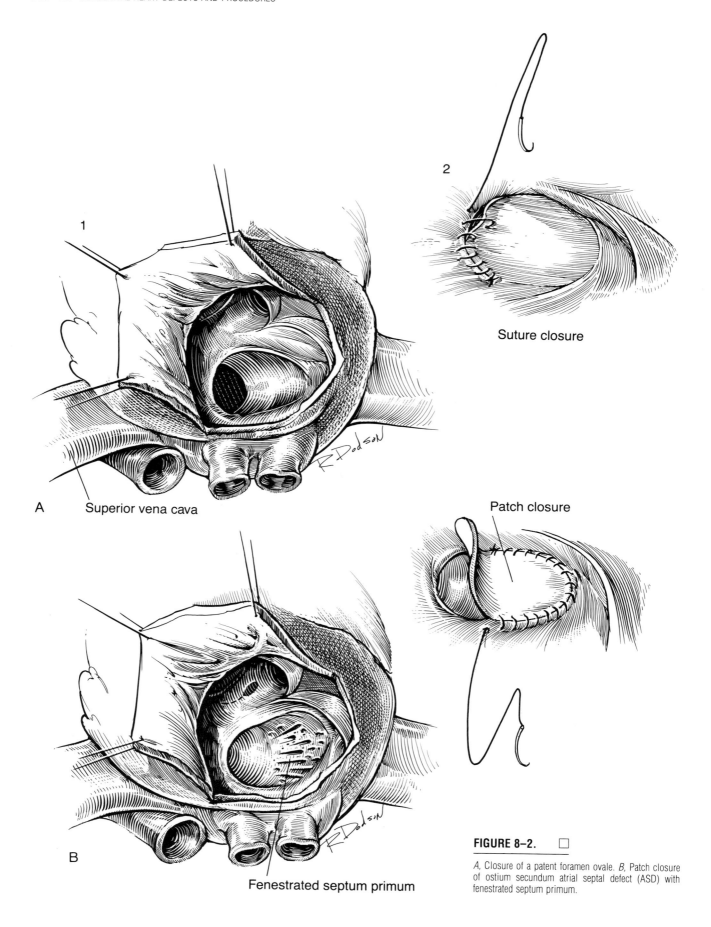

2

Suture closure

A   Superior vena cava

Patch closure

B   Fenestrated septum primum

FIGURE 8–2.   □

A, Closure of a patent foramen ovale. *B,* Patch closure of ostium secundum atrial septal defect (ASD) with fenestrated septum primum.

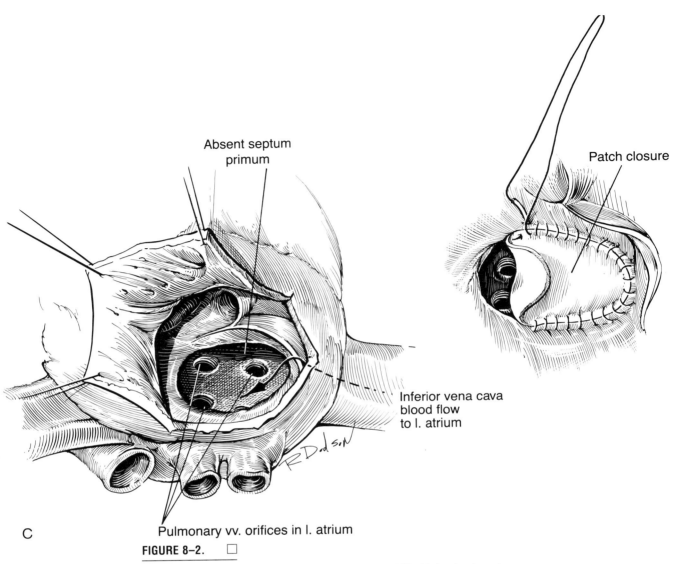

Absent septum
primum

Patch closure

Inferior vena cava
blood flow
to l. atrium

Pulmonary vv. orifices in l. atrium

C

FIGURE 8–2. □

Continued. C, Morphology and patch closure of ostium secundum ASD with absent septum primum.

remove air. The suture line is then completely inspected and the right atriotomy closed with a running polypropylene suture.

Cardiopulmonary bypass techniques and precautions after structural repair are routine. The choice of patch material, if one is used, does not appear to be important in most instances. However, if regurgitation of the atrioventricular valve is present, pericardium is recommended to reduce the risk of hemolysis induced by contact of the regurgitant jet with the prosthetic material.

Sinus Venosus Defect

The cardiopulmonary bypass technique is similar to the technique used for repair of the ostium secundum atrial septal defect, except that the upper venous cannula is placed high in the superior vena cava or the innominate vein if continuous cardiopulmonary bypass is to be used (Fig. 8–3). The best technique for repairing the lesion will depend on the degree of anomalous pulmonary venous drainage and the size of the defect.

At one end of the morphologic spectrum, the defect is large and the pulmonary veins drain either normally or ambiguously at the sinoatrial junction. In this case the entire lesion, including the pulmonary veins and the defect, is accessible through an incision in the right atrial appendage. Repair is accomplished with a fresh autologous pericardial patch and running polypropylene suture, making sure that the anomalous pulmonary veins drain unobstructed under the patch, through the defect, and to the left atrium. If the defect is small and

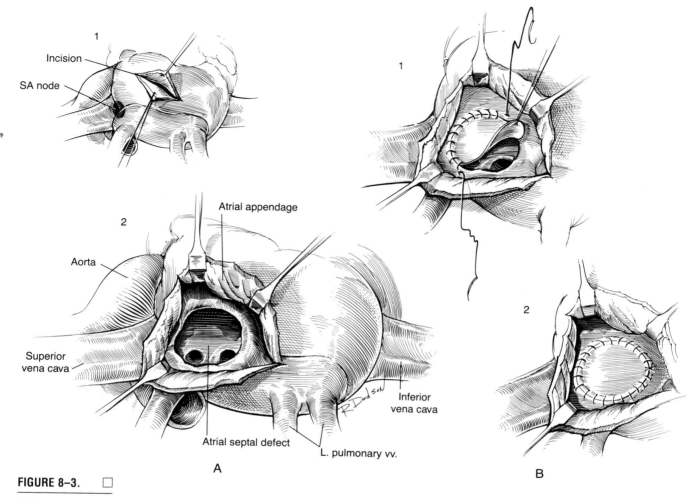

FIGURE 8–3. ☐

A, Sinus venosus defect at the superior cavoatrial junction from the perspective of a right atriotomy. *B,* Patch closure of a superior cavoatrial sinus venous defect via a right atriotomy.

there is concern that its orifice may be restrictive to drainage of the anomalous pulmonary veins, the defect can be enlarged by a radial incision at its antero-inferior margin.

For anomalous pulmonary veins that enter the superior vena cava cephalad to the sinoatrial junction, several different approaches have been utilized, as access to the anomalous veins through a right atrial incision is inadequate.

One approach is to incise the posterolateral aspect of the superior vena cava longitudinally, just in front of the entrance of the anomalous veins into the superior vena cava. The incision is then extended across the sinoatrial junction, well posterior to the sinoatrial node. Before making this incision, the area is carefully inspected to avoid injury to any identifiable arterial supply to the sinoatrial node. A piece of fresh pericardium is then carefully tailored to fit as a baffle inside the superior vena cava so that it will encompass all of the anomalous pulmo-

nary veins as well as the defect, allowing unobstructed flow from the pulmonary veins into the left atrium under the baffle. At the same time the baffle cannot be so redundant that flow from the superior vena cava to the right atrium is compromised. The basic goal of the baffle construction is to allow unobstructed pulmonary venous blood flow under the baffle and unobstructed systemic venous blood flow around the baffle within the superior vena cava. The baffle suture line must be extremely precise and is performed with running 6-0 or 7-0 polypropylene suture. In this repair, the choice of baffle material may be critical. Mobile, viable, fresh pericardium easily responds to small pressure differences between the systemic and pulmonary venous beds, adjusting to the most optimal position within the superior vena cava to allow unobstructed flow of both systemic and pulmonary venous drainage. If there is concern over patency between the superior vena cava and the right atrium after placement of

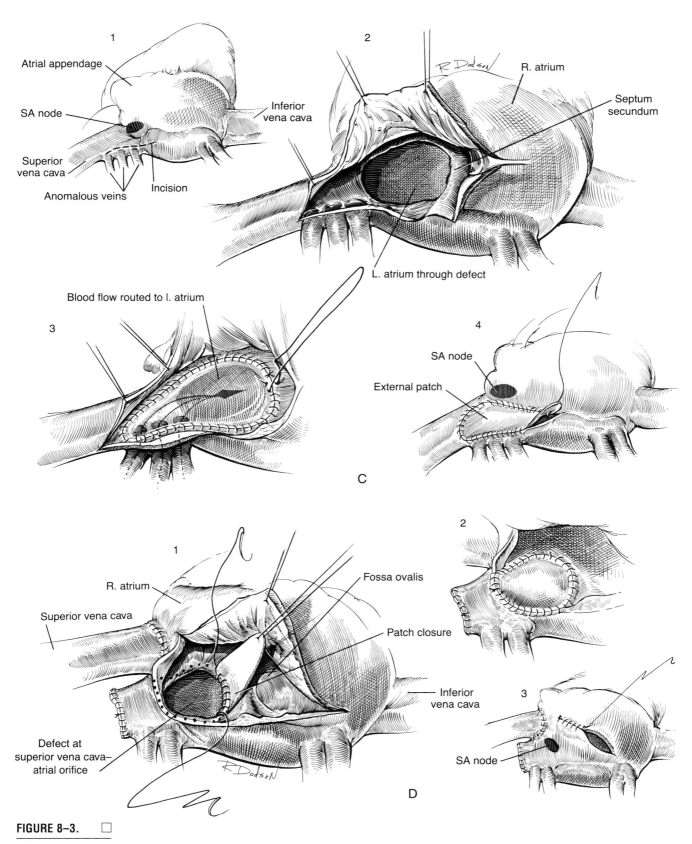

FIGURE 8–3. □

Continued. C, Exposure and incision for repair of a sinus venosus defect at the superior cavoatrial junction with anomalous drainage of the right upper lobe pulmonary veins using a posterolateral cavoatrial incision. *D,* Repair of the same defect using superior caval transection and implantation into the right atrial appendage.

Illustration continued on following page

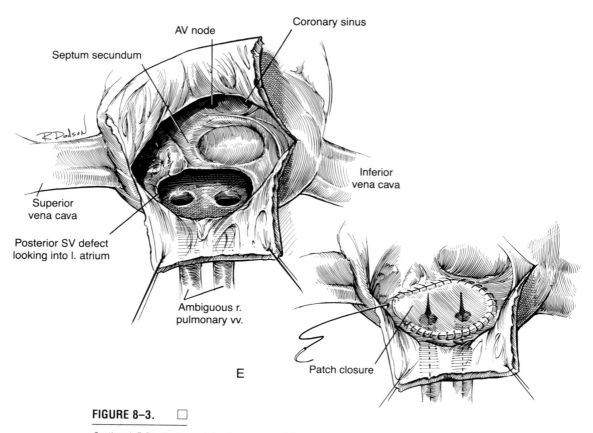

Septum secundum

AV node

Coronary sinus

Superior
vena cava

Inferior
vena cava

Posterior SV defect
looking into l. atrium

Ambiguous r.
pulmonary vv.

E

Patch closure

R Dodson

FIGURE 8–3. ☐

Continued. E, Repair of a posterior sinus venosus defect with ambiguously draining right pulmonary veins.

the baffle, a second patch made of pericardium or Gore-Tex may be used to augment the original longitudinal superior vena caval incision, rather than primarily closing it. A similar technique can be used to repair a sinus venosus defect adjacent to the inferior vena cava or to repair some forms of the scimitar syndrome. In this syndrome, if the atrial septal defect is small or absent, the septum primum can be completely removed to enlarge or to create a septal defect before the baffle is placed.

If the anomalous pulmonary veins drain so cephalad into the superior vena cava that an extremely long baffle would be required, it may be best to allow a small anomalous vein that enters the superior vena cava in a very cephalic position to be left to drain on the systemic side. If these high anomalous veins are too large to ignore, an alternative reconstruction is possible. An incision is made in the right atrial appendage, and the right atrial orifice of the superior vena cava is closed with a pericardial patch and running suture so that the entire superior vena cava and anomalous pulmonary veins drain across the defect into the left atrium. The superior vena cava is then transected just above the highest anomalous pulmonary vein, and the cardiac end of the cava is oversewn, allowing this part of

the superior vena cava to act as a conduit for drainage of the anomalous veins into the left atrium. The cephalic end of the cava is then anastomosed end to end to a large incision in the superior aspect of the right atrial appendage. This technique is also a good option if the arterial supply to the sinoatrial node is likely to be injured by the use of the pericardial baffle reconstruction.

Many other complex techniques have been described for reconstructing the sinus venosus defect, including the use of U-shaped patches and autologous atrial flaps; however, we have not found a compelling reason to employ these methods.

Coronary Sinus Septal Defect

Cardiopulmonary bypass considerations for coronary sinus septal defects (Fig. 8–4) are the same as those for secundum atrial septal defects. In the presence of a left superior vena cava, a third venous cannula may be necessary if no communicating vein exists between the right and left superior venae cavae and continuous cardiopulmonary bypass is to be employed. Alternatively, in very small infants in whom three venous cannulae would be cumbersome, moderate hypothermia (25°C) and temporary liga-

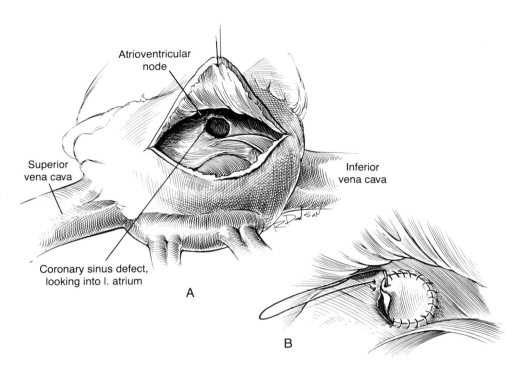

FIGURE 8–4. ☐

Exposure and repair of a coronary sinus septal defect via a right atriotomy.

(labels in figure:)
Atrioventricular node
Superior vena cava
Inferior vena cava
Coronary sinus defect, looking into l. atrium
A
B

tion of the left superior vena cava can be considered. If a coronary sinus septal defect exists in isolation, either as a completely unroofed coronary sinus or as a large coronary sinus fenestration to the left atrium, simple pericardial patch closure of the coronary sinus orifice is performed. In the case of a coronary sinus fenestration, the fenestration itself must be clearly identified, and the surgeon must be satisfied that it will not restrict coronary sinus drainage to the left atrium after closure of the coronary sinus orifice. This can occur if the fenestration is situated very close to the coronary sinus orifice and is distorted at the time of the patch placement. In all cases the anterosuperior rim of the patch on the coronary sinus orifice must be precisely applied to avoid atrioventricular nodal injury.

Unroofed Coronary Sinus

When a left superior vena cava exists with an unroofed coronary sinus, a more complex repair may be required (Fig. 8–5). In this situation the left superior vena cava enters the left atrium just superior to the left upper pulmonary vein orifices. When no connecting innominate vein is present between the two superior venae cavae, as is commonly the case, the defect is repaired by excision of as much native atrial septum as possible; this is followed by placement of a complex pericardial patch, using a running suture technique, so that all of the pulmonary veins drain under the patch to the mitral valve orifice. The orifices of the inferior vena cava, right su-

perior vena cava, and left superior vena cava all drain on the right atrial side of the patch to the tricuspid valve. When excising the native atrial septum, the atrioventricular node must be carefully identified. The three-dimensional relationships among the systemic veins, pulmonary veins, and mitral orifice must be given careful consideration when tailoring the patch.

An alternative approach to the problem of an unroofed coronary sinus with a left superior vena cava and no connecting vein is to construct a pericardial tunnel from the orifice of the left superior vena cava in the left atrium to the right atrium, followed by closure of the coronary sinus orifice. This technique may be less advisable in small infants.

When a connecting vein is present between the two superior vena cavae, the repair proceeds more simply by ligating the left superior vena cava below the connecting vein and patching the orifice of the coronary sinus as described previously. The left superior vena cava must also be ligated at the cardiac side of a hemiazygos vein, if one is present. This approach is generally not recommended in the presence of an absent or inadequate connecting vein.

RESULTS

Of the 35 patients in whom ostium secundum atrial septal defects were repaired before 24 months of age, 19 had large shunts and failure to thrive but no other anomalies. There were no deaths in this

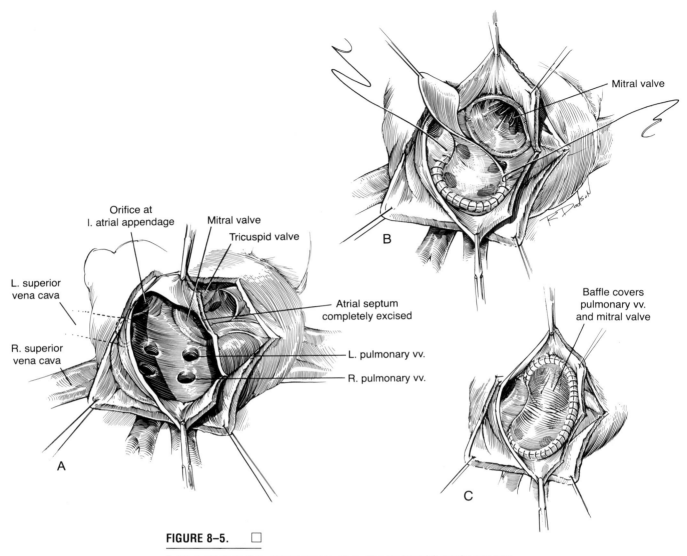

FIGURE 8–5.   ☐

Exposure and repair of an unroofed coronary sinus with a persistent left superior vena cava.

group, and the hospital stay averaged 4.7 days (range, 3 to 8 days). Deep hypothermic circulatory arrest was used for two patients and continuous cardiopulmonary bypass for 17. Six defects were patched, and 11 were closed primarily.

In the 16 other patients with smaller shunts (mean QP/QS = 2.7); failure to thrive; and multiple, chronic noncardiac problems, repair was also accomplished with no deaths; however, the hospital stay was somewhat longer (mean, 8.7 days; range, 3 to 30 days). Deep hypothermic circulatory arrest was used in six patients and continuous cardiopulmonary bypass in 10. Three patients were repaired with patches, and 13 underwent primary closure.

Fifteen sinus venosus defects were repaired in infants. There was no mortality. No patients manifested pulmonary or systemic venous obstruction in the postoperative period, and all patients were discharged from the hospital in normal sinus rhythm.

Nine coronary sinus septal defects were repaired in infants. Only two of these were isolated defects, and each had an accompanying left superior vena cava. Repair was performed using deep hypothermic circulatory arrest and a complex atrial baffle. Neither patient has shown evidence of baffle obstruction or leak during short-term follow-up.

SUMMARY

These results indicate that atrial septal defects of all types can be effectively and safely repaired in small infants. Deep hypothermic circulatory arrest or continuous cardiopulmonary bypass may be used as appropriate. In infants, ostium secundum defects can often be closed primarily without the risk of recurrence; however, this decision must be made on an individual basis.

The technical approach to sinus venosus and coronary sinus septal defects must be carefully planned because of subtle but critical variations in the anatomy of these defects. It is important that the surgeon remain flexible in the reconstructive approach to these lesions.

The difficult clinical problem of how to manage the failing infant with a small to moderate atrial septal defect associated with significant, chronic, noncardiac disease involving the pulmonary, neurologic, or gastrointestinal systems has been addressed. If failure to thrive persists after optimized management of the noncardiac problems, surgical closure of the atrial defect can be performed without undue mortality or morbidity in an attempt to optimize overall patient care. In mid- to long-term follow-up in seven of these patients, symptomatic improvement and improved growth were noted in all. One other child died several years after surgery from complications related to a noncardiac anomaly.

The question of optimal timing of surgery for the asymptomatic, isolated atrial septal defect may need re-evaluation. Large ostium secundum, sinus venosus, and coronary sinus septal defects are highly unlikely to close spontaneously, especially after the first year of life. Elective surgery at age 4 to 5 years provides no important technical advantage for the surgeon and no psychological advantage for the patient or the patient's family. There appears to be no compelling reason why elective repair should not be undertaken at the end of the first year of life.

REFERENCES

1. Bailey CP, Nichols HT, Bolton HE, et al. Surgical treatment of forty-six interatrial septal defects by atrio-septo-pexy. Ann Surg 140:805, 1954.
2. Bull C, Deanfield J, de Leval M, et al. Correction of isolated secundum atrial septal defect in infancy. Arch Dis Child 56:784, 1981.
3. Cabezuelo-Huerta G, Vazquez-Perez J, Frontera-Izquierdo P. Atrial septal defect with pulmonary hypertension in infancy. An Esp Pediatr 12:105, 1979.
4. Cockerham JT, Martin TC, Guitierrez FR, et al. Spontaneous closure of secundum atrial septal defect in infants and young children. Am J Cardiol 52:1267, 1983.
5. Feldt RH, Avasthey P, Yoshimasu F, et al. Incidence of congenital heart disease in children born to residents of Olmsted County, Minnesota, 1950–1969. Mayo Clin Proc 46:794, 1971.
6. Ghisla RP, Hannon DW, Meyer RA, et al. Spontaneous closure of isolated secundum atrial septal defects in infants: an echocardiographic study. Am Heart J 109:1327, 1985.
7. Gibbons JH. Application of a mechanical heart-lung apparatus to cardiac surgery. Minn Med, p 171, 1954.
8. Gordovilla-Zurdo G, Cabo-Salvador J, Moreno-Granados F, et al. Surgery of symptomatic interauricular communication in the first year of life. An Esp Pediatr 29:94, 1988.
9. Gross RE, Pomeranz AA, Watkis E Jr, et al. Surgical closure of defects of the interauricular septum by use of an atrial well. N Engl J Med 247:455, 1952.
10. Hastreiter AR, Wennemark JT, Miller RA, et al. Secundum atrial septal defects with congestive heart failure during infancy and early childhood. Am Heart J 64:467, 1962.
11. Helseth HK, Peterson CR. Atrial septal defect with termination of left superior vena cava in the left atrium and absence of the coronary sinus. Ann Thorac Surg 17:186, 1974.
12. Hunt CE, Lucas RV Jr. Symptomatic atrial septal defect in infancy. Circulation 47:1042, 1973.
13. Lewis FJ. High defects of the atrial septum. J Thorac Cardiovasc Surg 36:1, 1958.
14. Lewis FJ, Taufic M. Closure of atrial septal defects with the aid of hypothermia: Experimental accomplishments and the report of the one successful case. Surgery 33:52, 1953.
15. Navajas A, Pastor E, La Fuente P, et al. Symptomatic atrial septal defect in infancy. An Esp Pediatr 14:25, 1981.
16. Ohkita Y, Miki S, Kusuhara KM, et al. Two cases of secundum atrial septal defect corrected in infancy. Nippon Kyobu Geka Gakkai Zasshi 34:892, 1986.
17. Phillips SJ, Okies JE, Henken D, et al. Complex of secundum atrial septal defect and congestive heart failure in infants. J Thorac Cardiovasc Surg 70:696, 1975.
18. Raghib G, Ruttenberg HD, Anderson RC, et al. Termination of left superior vena cava in left atrium, atrial septal defect, and absence of coronary sinus. Circulation 31:906, 1965.
19. Sondergaard T. Closure of atrial septal defects: Report of three cases. Acta Chir Scand 107:492, 1954.
20. Spangler JG, Feldt RH, Danielson GK. Secundum atrial septal defect encountered in infancy. J Thorac Cardiovasc Surg 71:398, 1976.
21. Van Mierop LHS. Embryology of the atrioventricular canal region and pathogenesis of endocardial cushion defects. In Feldt RH, McGoon DC, Ongley PA, et al. (eds). Atrioventricular Canal Defects. Philadelphia, WB Saunders, 1976, p 1.

Anomalies of the Pulmonary Veins

Total anomalous pulmonary venous connection (TAPVC) encompasses a wide spectrum of congenital heart anomalies, both anatomically and physiologically. Management of TAPVC varies from a low-risk, relatively elective, technically simple procedure (such as that for TAPVC to the coronary sinus) to the most urgent of neonatal cardiac surgical emergencies, carrying a significant risk of early or late death (such as that for obstructed infradiaphragmatic TAPVC).

Unique to this anomaly is the absence of definitive means of medical palliation; therefore, severely obstructed TAPVC represents almost the only true surgical emergency across the entire spectrum of congenital heart surgery. The heterogeneous nature of this anomaly can be explained by its embryologic origin.

PATHOLOGIC ANATOMY

Embryology

The lungs develop as an outpouching from the foregut. They carry with them a plexus of veins derived from the splanchnic (systemic) venous plexus, which drains to the heart through the cardinal and umbilicovitelline veins (Fig. 9–1). TAPVC occurs when the pulmonary vein evagination from the posterior surface of the left atrium fails to fuse with the pulmonary venous plexus surrounding the lung buds. In place of the usual connection to the left atrium, at least one connection of the pulmonary plexus to the splanchnic plexus persists. Accordingly, the pulmonary veins drain to the heart through a systemic vein.[23]

Anatomy

Persistent splanchnic venous connections can occur at almost any point in the central cardinal or umbilicovitelline venous systems. In one classification described by Darling and coworkers,[7] TAPVC is described as *supracardiac* when the anomalous connection is to an ascending vertical vein, usually on the left and connected to the left innominate vein; as *cardiac* when the pulmonary veins connect directly to the right atrium or to the coronary sinus; and as *infracardiac* when the connection is to intra-abdominal veins. In a large series of autopsies from Children's Hospital in Boston, approximately 45% of the cases of TAPVC were supracardiac, 25% were cardiac, and 25% were infracardiac.[8] In 5% of the patients, pulmonary venous connection was *mixed*, with at least one of the main lobar pulmonary veins connecting to a different systemic vein relative to the remaining veins.

Pulmonary venous obstruction can occur at any point in the anomalous pathway, but it is most commonly seen with an infracardiac connection, where it is almost always present to some degree. When

157

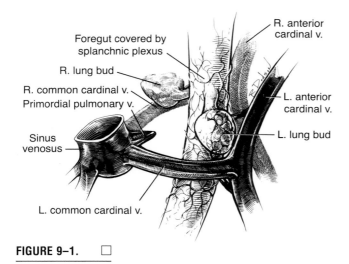

FIGURE 9–1. □

Total anomalous pulmonary venous connection (TAPVC) results when the primordial pulmonary vein fails to unite with the plexus of veins that surround the lung buds and is derived from the splanchnic venous plexus, including the cardinal veins and umbilicovitelline veins.

pulmonary venous obstruction is present, there are usually morphologic changes in pulmonary arterioles with an increase in arterial muscularity and extension of muscle into smaller and more peripheral arteries.[12]

Associated Anomalies

Although most patients with TAPVC have no associated major cardiac defects, many different associated anomalies have been reported, including tetralogy of Fallot and double-outlet right ventricle.[8] Associated anomalies, particularly a single functional ventricle, are much more likely to occur with heterotaxia syndrome.[3]

In patients with TAPVC, the left atrial volume is small, and left ventricular volume is often at the lower limit of normal. This may be related to the leftward deviation of the ventricular septum that is present with right ventricular hypertension.[11, 34] It may also be partially related to absence of pulmonary venous return directly to the left atrium during fetal development. Endocardial fibroelastosis of the left ventricle has also been reported.[19] The relative hypoplasia of the left ventricle is consistent with the low cardiac indices often seen in these patients postoperatively.[27]

Pathophysiology

Because both pulmonary and systemic venous blood returns to the right atrium in all forms of

TAPVC, survival of the child is dependent on the presence of a right-to-left intracardiac shunt. This almost always occurs through a patent foramen ovale that is rarely restrictive (i.e., there is no pressure gradient between the right and left atria).[9] Mixing of systemic and pulmonary venous return results in at least some degree of cyanosis in all patients. The degree of cyanosis is determined by the amount of pulmonary blood flow relative to systemic blood flow, and this, in turn, is determined largely by the presence or absence of pulmonary venous obstruction. Pulmonary venous obstruction is almost always accompanied by pulmonary arterial and right ventricular hypertension. In fact, significant pulmonary venous obstruction is unlikely in the child with right ventricular pressure that is less than 85% of systemic pressure (Fig. 9–2).[16] When no pulmonary venous obstruction is present, pulmonary blood flow is often increased, as pulmonary venous blood is returning to the compliant right heart. This increase in pulmonary blood flow may result in pulmonary hypertension with pressure as high as systemic pressure. However, suprasystemic right ventricular pressure is unlikely in the absence of pulmonary venous obstruction. The observed muscularity of pulmonary arterioles is reflected in a tendency for the patient to have labile pulmonary vascular resistance postoperatively, resulting in so-called "pulmonary hypertensive crises."

Both pulmonary venous obstruction and in-

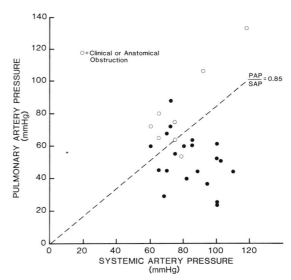

FIGURE 9–2. □

Pulmonary venous obstruction, demonstrated either at surgical correction or at postmortem examination, is likely to occur in patients with TAPVC to the coronary sinus when right ventricular pressure is greater than 85% of systemic pressure at cardiac catheterization. (From Jonas RA, Smolinsky A, Mayer JE, Castaneda AR. Obstructed pulmonary venous drainage with total anomalous pulmonary venous connection to the coronary sinus. Am J Cardiol 59:431–435, 1987.)

creased pulmonary blood flow are likely to cause an increase in extravascular lung water, which may be largely interstitial, although in severe cases of pulmonary venous obstruction, this can progress to frank pulmonary edema, with fluid extravasation into the alveoli.

An interesting feedback loop can occur in some cases of supracardiac TAPVC. The anomalous vertical vein carrying the entire pulmonary venous return may pass between the left main bronchus and left pulmonary artery. Some degree of pulmonary venous obstruction will result in increased pressure within the left pulmonary artery, which further exacerbates the compression of venous return between the bronchus and the left pulmonary artery. Ultimately, a severe degree of obstruction may ensue.[5]

CLINICAL FEATURES

The presenting features of the child with TAPVC are determined by the degree of pulmonary venous obstruction. If obstruction is severe, the child may be profoundly cyanosed and in respiratory distress within hours of birth. Such a child will be tachycardic and hypotensive.

In children without serious pulmonary venous obstruction, clinical status is determined by the level of pulmonary blood flow and the degree of pulmonary hypertension. The child with significant pulmonary hypertension and greatly increased pulmonary blood flow will fail to thrive and may have tachypnea and diaphoresis, particularly when feeding. The degree of cyanosis will be mild. If pulmonary artery pressure is only minimally elevated, the child may progress well for years with only a mild degree of cyanosis.

PREOPERATIVE EVALUATION

Diagnostic Studies

In the child with serious obstruction, analysis of arterial blood gas reveals severe hypoxia (e.g., Po_2 less than 20 mm Hg), often with associated metabolic acidosis. The chest radiograph shows a normal heart size with generalized pulmonary edema. The electrocardiogram demonstrates right ventricular hypertrophy, but this is to be expected in the neonate. Two-dimensional echocardiography is very reliable in establishing the diagnosis of TAPVC. Ventricular septal position and Doppler assessment of any tricuspid regurgitant jet will give a useful estimate of right ventricular pressure. Avoidance of cardiac catheterization in the desperately ill neonate

with obstructed TAPVC has been an important advance in the preoperative management of this condition.[29] The osmotic load induced by angiography in the past often exacerbated the degree of pulmonary edema.

In older children, cardiac catheterization may be indicated. The important hemodynamic data to be collected include right ventricular and pulmonary artery pressures, as well as a measure of the degree of pulmonary venous obstruction as determined by the gradient between the pulmonary artery wedge pressure and right atrial pressure. Generally there is minimal or no gradient across the foramen ovale, and therefore, balloon or blade septostomy is not recommended. (Some centers do recommend balloon septostomy as a palliative procedure, although we prefer to proceed to early repair.) The point at which a step-up in oxygen saturation is observed within the systemic venous systems helps to localize the site of the pulmonary venous connection. Pulmonary arteriography demonstrates the anomalous pulmonary venous pathway during the levophase (which may be significantly delayed if obstruction is present).

MEDICAL MANAGEMENT

Obstructed TAPVC

Since the discovery of prostaglandin, obstructed TAPVC remains perhaps the only true surgical emergency within the field of congenital heart disease. Other than intubation and positive-pressure ventilation with 100% oxygen, along with correction of metabolic acidosis, no medical measures have been demonstrated to adequately palliate this problem, although one report has suggested that maintenance of ductal patency with prostaglandin E_1 may be useful.[36] Certainly this should provide some increase in cardiac output by allowing a right-to-left shunt through the ductus. However, in the child who is already profoundly hypoxic because of inadequate pulmonary blood flow, the increase in systemic cardiac output is achieved only at the expense of a further decrease in pulmonary blood flow. Nevertheless, if mixed venous saturation increases as the cardiac index increases, it is conceivable that there could be a net improvement in arterial saturation.

Nonobstructed TAPVC

As pulmonary vascular resistance decreases, there is a progressive increase in the volume load for the right heart. The child should be treated with standard decongestive measures. Optimally surgery should be undertaken early in infancy to minimize the secondary deleterious effects of the long-standing volume load on the heart and lungs, as well as the effects of long-standing cyanosis.[4, 24, 28, 32]

SURGICAL MANAGEMENT

History

TAPVC was first described by Wilson in 1798.[35] In 1951, Muller achieved surgical palliation by anastomosing the anomalous common pulmonary venous trunk to the left atrial appendage.[21] TAPVC was first corrected by Lewis et al. in 1956, using hypothermia and inflow occlusion.[20] Correction using cardiopulmonary bypass was described in the same year by Burroughs and Kirklin.[6] The application of deep hypothermic circulatory arrest, as popularized by Barratt-Boyes and coworkers,[1] resulted in a marked improvement in surgical mortality among infants, including neonates in extremis because of obstructed TAPVC.

Indications for and Timing of Surgery

Because there is no possibility of spontaneous resolution of TAPVC, the diagnosis alone is an indication for surgery. The timing of surgery should be determined by the presence or absence of pulmonary venous obstruction.

Obstructed TAPVC

Because there is no effective means of medical palliation of obstructed TAPVC, the neonate with severe hypoxia and acidosis should be taken immediately to the operating room after echocardiographic diagnosis. Although the use of extracorporeal membrane oxygenation has been described as a preoperative intervention,[18] there would seem to be little to be gained by this, as standard cardiopulmonary bypass can be established just as quickly and allows immediate repair of the pulmonary venous obstruction. If necessary, ECMO can be applied postoperatively.[18, 33]

Nonobstructed TAPVC

Surgical correction should be undertaken at a convenient time, early in infancy, before the deleterious pathologic changes secondary to cyanosis and a long-standing volume load on the heart and lungs have a chance to develop.[4, 24, 28, 32]

Technical Considerations

Anesthesia for Obstructed TAPVC

The hypoxic, acidotic neonate with obstructed TAPVC requires meticulous anesthetic management. Pulmonary resistance should be minimized by hyperventilation with 100% oxygen. Anesthesia is induced with a high dose of fentanyl, which will decrease pulmonary vasoreactivity.[13] If an inotropic agent is required, isoproterenol is preferred as long as the patient does not become unduly tachycardic. In view of the mildly hypoplastic nature of the left heart, however, a rapid heart rate of up to 200 beats per minute may, in fact, be necessary to maintain adequate cardiac output. Metabolic acidosis should be aggressively treated with bicarbonate or tris(hydroxymethyl) aminomethane (THAM). There may be a large calcium requirement, and blood glucose may be labile. Occasionally, there is associated sepsis and renal failure. Digoxin is probably not useful, and it also lowers the threshold for ventricular fibrillation.

Emergency Surgical Management of Obstructed Infracardiac TAPVC

Adequate venous access and an arterial monitoring line, preferably in an umbilical artery, are essential. A pulse oximeter also provides extremely useful information. It is best to avoid surface cooling, because these desperately ill children may fibrillate at a relatively high core temperature (greater than 30°C), particularly if large doses of digoxin have been given at the referral center. The chest is opened by a median sternotomy, and at least one lobe of the thymus, usually the left, is excised. A patch of anterior pericardium is harvested. This can be treated with 0.6% glutaraldehyde for 30 minutes, which considerably improves ease of handling. It is essential that there be minimal disturbance of the myocardium after the pericardium is opened. Even the slightest retraction of the ventricular myocardium can result in ventricular fibrillation.

After systemic heparinization, bypass is commenced with an arterial cannula in the ascending aorta and venous return via a single cannula inserted into the right atrial appendage. Immediately after bypass is begun, the ductus arteriosus is dissected free and ligated. This should be done in all cases, irrespective of whether ductal patency has been demonstrated. After at least 5 minutes of cooling so that myocardial temperature is less than 25°C, and with perfusion continuing, the heart is gently retracted out of the chest to allow dissection of the anomalous descending vertical vein. Retraction should not be excessive; otherwise it will cause kinking of the coronary arteries and interfere with myocardial perfusion. A heavy ligature is tied around the vertical vein at the point where it pierces the diaphragm. The vertical vein is divided and filletted proximally to the level of the superior pulmonary veins. The heart is then replaced in the pericardium. By the time the rectal temperature is less than 18°C, the esophageal temperature will be 13°C or 14°C, and tympanic temperature will be approximately 15°C. The ascending aorta is clamped, and cardioplegic solution is infused into the root of the aorta. Bypass is ceased, and blood is drained from the child. The venous cannula is removed.

A transverse incision is made from the right atrial appendage and is carried posteriorly through the foramen ovale into the left atrium. Because the right pulmonary veins do not anchor the left atrium, excellent exposure of the previously dissected vertical vein is obtained. The incision in the posterior wall of the left atrium is carried inferiorly parallel to the vertical vein (Fig. 9–3). It may also be ex-

tended superiorly into the base of the left atrial appendage. The common pulmonary vein to left atrium anastomosis is performed using continuous 6–0 absorbable polydioxanone suture. Excellent exposure is obtained by the approach described, and there is no possibility of kinking or malalignment, as may be the case with the alternative technique of performing the anastomosis with the heart everted from the chest. The foramen ovale and the more posterior part of the right atriotomy can be closed with a pericardial patch. Direct suture closure of the foramen ovale has a tendency to narrow the anastomosis and should be avoided. Before the atrial septal defect is closed, the left heart should be filled with saline, and air can be vented through the cardioplegia site in the ascending aorta. After closure of the right atriotomy, the left heart is filled with saline, the venous cannula is reinserted, and bypass is recommenced. The aortic crossclamp is released with the cardioplegic site bleeding freely. During rewarming a pulmonary artery monitoring line is inserted through a horizontal mattress suture in the

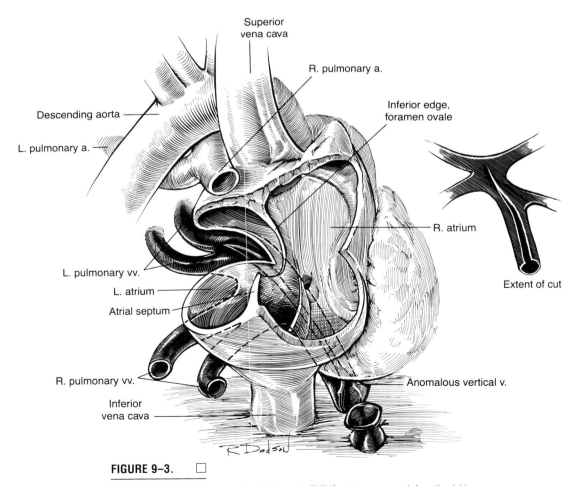

FIGURE 9–3. □

Operative exposure obtained with infradiaphragmatic TAPVC, using an approach from the right.

infundibulum of the right ventricle.[10] Insertion of a left atrial monitoring line through a pulmonary vein should be avoided because of the small size of the pulmonary veins. However, it is possible to insert a left atrial line through the left atrial appendage.

On occasion some of us prefer the approach of everting the apex of the heart from the chest. The pulmonary confluence to left atrial anastomosis is constructed by an external rather than an internal approach.

Weaning from Cardiopulmonary Bypass

Once rewarming to a rectal temperature of at least 35°C is completed, the patient can be weaned from cardiopulmonary bypass. Although this should be uneventful in any patient after elective surgery, it can be a critical phase in the management of a patient who is acutely ill and has had a previous obstruction. Such patients tend to have markedly labile pulmonary vascular resistance. Their response to cardiopulmonary bypass is often a substantial, although brief, temporary increase in pulmonary resistance. Therefore, it is useful to monitor pulmonary artery pressure, in addition to aortic and left atrial pressure, at the time of weaning from bypass. Is it not uncommon for pulmonary pressure to be close to systemic levels for the first 10 to 15 minutes after weaning from bypass. During this time, ventilatory management is critical. Once again, the patient should be maintained on 100% oxygen, and the P_{CO_2} should be lowered to at least 30 mm Hg. Isoproterenol is frequently useful as an inotropic agent in further lowering pulmonary resistance. Because of the mildly hypoplastic nature of the left ventricle and the left atrium, it may be necessary to maintain relatively high left atrial pressures, perhaps as high as 15 to 20 mm Hg. In the presence of a widely open anastomosis, pulmonary pressure should fall to less than two thirds to one half of systemic pressure within 15 to 30 minutes of weaning from bypass. If pulmonary pressure remains elevated, an obstructed anastomosis should be suspected. Intraoperative two-dimensional echocardiography can give excellent visualization of this area.

Elective Surgical Management of Nonobstructed Supracardiac TAPVC

The general operative approach to nonobstructed supracardiac TAPVC is similar to that for infracardiac TAPVC. Deep hypothermic circulatory arrest in the infant provides optimal exposure and, therefore,

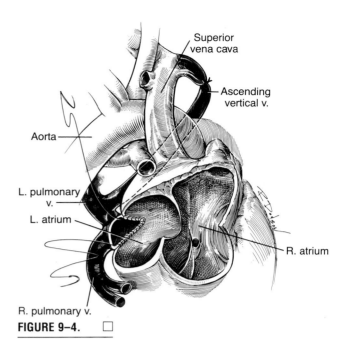

FIGURE 9–4. ☐

Excellent exposure of the horizontal pulmonary venous confluence is obtained by a single atrial incision extended through the foramen ovale into the left atrium for supracardiac TAPVC. Autologous pericardium is used to close the foramen ovale, supplement the anastomosis, and enlarge the left atrium in supracardiac TAPVC.

the most consistently wide open anastomosis. The horizontal pulmonary venous confluence is dissected free during the cooling period. In this case, after cessation of cardiopulmonary bypass and removal of the venous cannula, the right atrial transverse incision is carried across the atrial septum at the level of the foramen ovale into the left atrium. It is then continued transversely, extending into the base of the left atrial appendage. A longitudinal incision, parallel to the posterior wall of the left atrial incision, is made in the horizontal pulmonary venous confluence. A direct anastomosis is fashioned between the left atrium and the pulmonary venous confluence, using continuous 6–0 polydioxanone suture (Fig. 9–4). The anastomosis is begun at the most leftward point, using a continuous suture technique and working toward the right. Once again, it is best to close the foramen ovale with a patch of autologous pericardium. This avoids any narrowing of the anastomosis and also helps to supplement the size of the small left atrium. The anomalous ascending vertical vein is always ligated. Pulmonary hypertension is rare after elective cases in which pulmonary artery pressure has usually been only mildly elevated before surgery.

Elective Surgical Management of TAPVC to the Coronary Sinus

It was previously thought that obstruction of TAPVC to the coronary sinus was extremely rare, but a review of TAPVC at the Children's Hospital in Boston revealed a surprisingly high incidence of 22% of such cases.[16] Therefore, two-dimensional echocardiography should carefully assess the point of junction between the pulmonary veins and the coronary sinus, which was the most common point of obstruction in this series. If there is any doubt about this area, cardiac catheterization should be performed. In the absence of obstruction, a simple unroofing procedure of the coronary sinus will suffice. The tissue between the foramen ovale and coronary sinus is incised (Fig. 9–5A), and the incision in the roof of the coronary sinus is carried to the posterior wall of the heart. The resulting atrial septal defect is closed with an autologous pericardial patch (Fig. 9–5B).

In an attempt to decrease the incidence of bradyarrythmias after this procedure, Van Praagh and colleagues suggested the "fenestration" procedure, which includes unroofing of the coronary sinus toward the left atrium and closure of the coronary sinus stoma within the right atrium.[30] This technique allowed for preservation of the tissue between the coronary sinus and the foramen ovale, where it was thought that important internodal conduction pathways may have existed. Experience with this operation at Children's Hospital in Boston between 1972 and 1980 demonstrated that in the 10 patients in whom this procedure was used, there was no decrease in the incidence of bradyarrhythmias when compared with the more traditional procedure. Although no cases of restriction at the point of fenestration were observed at this hospital, there have been cases reported by others.[34]

If two-dimensional echocardiography reveals a potential site of obstruction at the junction of the coronary sinus with the horizontal confluence (Fig. 9–6), an operation similar to that for supracardiac TAPVC should be performed. The horizontal confluence should be filletted and a parallel incision made in the posterior wall of the left atrium, extending into the left atrial appendage. A direct anastomosis can be fashioned using continuous absorbable polydioxanone suture.

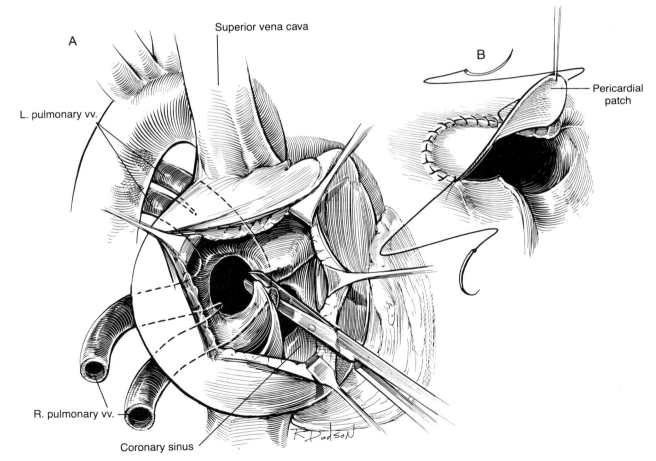

FIGURE 9–5. □

A, Unobstructed TAPVC to the coronary sinus is treated by incision of the tissue between the coronary sinus ostium and the foramen ovale, with complete unroofing of the coronary sinus. *B,* Autologous pericardium is used to close the resultant atrial septal defect in TAPVC to the coronary sinus.

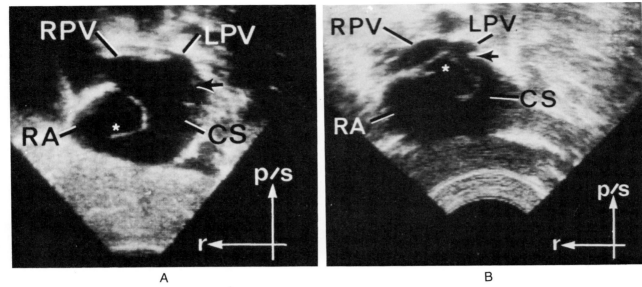

A

B

FIGURE 9–6. ☐

A, Preoperative two-dimensional echocardiogram from a patient with unobstructed total anomalous pulmonary venous connection. The subxiphoid long-axis cut shows a wide connection *(arrow)* between the pulmonary venous confluence and the dilated coronary sinus (CS). *B,* Preoperative two-dimensional echocardiogram of a patient with obstructed total anomalous pulmonary venous connection. The subxiphoid long-axis cut shows a narrowed connection *(arrow)* between the pulmonary venous confluence and the mildly dilated coronary sinus. *, Eustachian valve; LPV, left pulmonary vein; p/s, posterior and superior; r, rightward; RA, right atrium; RPV, right pulmonary vein. (From Jonas RA, Smolinsky A, Mayer JE, Castaneda AR. Obstructed pulmonary venous drainage with total anomalous pulmonary venous connection to the coronary sinus. Am J Cardiol 59:431–435, 1987.)

Elective Surgical Management of TAPVC to the Right Atrium

Using deep hypothermic circulatory arrest, as described for the previous procedures, an autologous pericardial baffle can be used to direct the anomalous veins through the atrial septal defect, which may be surgically enlarged, into the left atrium.

Failure to Wean from Cardiopulmonary Bypass

If the right ventricle appears to be incapable of generating the high pressures required in the early period after weaning from bypass, it may be useful to consider applying extracorporeal membrane oxygenation (ECMO) for a period of several days to allow a gradual decrease in pulmonary vascular resistance.[18, 33] This principle has been successfully applied for the high pulmonary resistance encountered in neonates with diaphragmatic hernias. Although this procedure has not been applied at Children's Hospital in Boston for obstructed TAPVC, there are undoubtedly some children who would benefit from ECMO. Although cannulation can be performed as recommended for diaphragmatic hernia, with arterial cannulation of the carotid artery and venous return via a multifenestrated tube inserted into the right atrium through the internal jugular vein,[17] we prefer aortic and atrial cannula-

tion. The cannulae are brought through stab incisions in the neck, and the sternum is closed.

Intensive Care Management

The heavily muscularized pulmonary arterioles of the child with obstructed TAPVC remain particularly labile for up to several days after corrective surgery. During this period, pulmonary resistance should be minimized by appropriate ventilatory management. The stress response of pulmonary vasoconstriction should be minimized by maintaining a constant state of anesthesia, using a fentanyl infusion supplemented with hourly boluses of pancuronium, 0.1 mg per kilogram of body weight. Arterial P_{CO_2} should be maintained at approximately 30 mm Hg, and the inspired oxygen concentration should be titrated so as to achieve a pulmonary pressure (as measured by the indwelling pulmonary artery line) that is less than two thirds of systemic pressure. A low-dose isoproterenol infusion of up to 0.1 µg per kilogram of body weight per minute may also be continued for 24 to 48 hours for its pulmonary vasodilatory effects. After 24 to 48 hours of hemodynamic stability, the level of anesthesia may be lightened, with careful observation for pulmonary hypertensive crises. These are particularly likely to occur in response to the stress of endotracheal tube suctioning, which should be performed carefully after hyperventilation. Experience with inhaled nitric oxide suggests that this may be a useful selective pulmonary vasodilator that can be applied successfully in this setting.

RESULTS OF SURGERY AT THE CHILDREN'S HOSPITAL IN BOSTON

Early Results

Surgical results have improved dramatically since the 1960s. Before 1970, repair of TAPVC in infancy generally carried a mortality rate greater than 50%.[2, 22] Between 1970 and 1980, many centers reported mortality rates of between 10% and 20%.[25, 34] More recent reports have described an early mortality rate of less than 10%.[16, 29]

During the 10-year period between 1977 and 1986, 67 infants and older children underwent repair for TAPVC at Children's Hospital in Boston. This total excludes children with complex multiple anomalies that included TAPVC, usually as part of the heterotaxia syndrome. Table 9–1 illustrates the distribution of the various anatomic forms of TAPVC.[15] It can be seen that the most common form was supracardiac TAPVC, which made up 42% of cases. There was no early mortality among the 20 patients with TAPVC to the coronary sinus of the right atrium. There was a 7% mortality rate among patients with supracardiac TAPVC. The highest mortality rate was seen with infracardiac TAPVC, in which three of 16 patients died early.

More recently, between 1983 and 1989, 27 infants underwent surgery at Children's Hospital in Boston, as reported by vanderVelde and associates,[31] with no early deaths.

Late Results and Complications

Despite an initial satisfactory course, pulmonary venous obstruction develops in between 5% and 10% of children after surgery for TAPVC, often within 3 to 6 months.[29, 31] Most commonly this takes the form of an obliterative intimal fibrous hyperplasia affecting the pulmonary veins close to their junction with the original common pulmonary vein and, therefore, somewhat remote from the actual line of anastomosis with the original true left atrium. This entity is particularly difficult to deal with surgically and is also unresponsive to balloon dilatation. Attempts at repair using a pericardial patch have generally been unsuccessful. Patching techniques using flaps of atrial tissue may be more successful in relatively mild cases.[26]

Anastomotic obstruction owing to inadequate growth of suture lines can occur in spite of the use of absorbable sutures or interrupted suture techniques. This form of obstruction can usually be managed by additional surgery. Generally, there is dilatation of a secondary chamber behind the anastomosis. Simple incisions connecting the two chambers, followed by endocardial approximation, generally suffice to deal with this problem.

Table 9–1 illustrates the late deaths that occurred among the 67 infants and children who underwent repair at the Children's Hospital in Boston between 1977 and 1986. Late death was usually related to the development of pulmonary venous obstruction.

In the more recent series of 27 infants, seven showed postoperative echocardiographic evidence of pulmonary venous obstruction.[31] In two patients this was found to be at the pulmonary vein–to–left atrial anastomosis (one with an infradiaphragmatic and one with a mixed connection). In three patients, obstruction of individual pulmonary veins developed, and two patients were found to have obstruction at the junction of the pulmonary venous confluence with a left vertical vein that had previously drained to the coronary sinus, which had been unroofed as part of the operative procedure. Five of the seven patients in whom pulmonary venous obstruction developed died postoperatively.

Jenkins et al.[14] reviewed the size of the individual pulmonary veins and related this to outcome in infants less than 4 months old at presentation. They found that the sum of the diameters of the individual pulmonary veins indexed for body surface area was significantly larger ($P = .01$) in unobstructed survivors (72.0 ± 16.3) than in patients who died without surgery (43.4 ± 11.3) or those in whom obstruction developed or who died late (52.1 ± 11.6 mm/m^2). They concluded that the size of the pulmonary veins is an important determinant of outcome in patients with TAPVC.

TABLE 9–1. □ DISTRIBUTION OF TAPVC

CONNECTION	NO. OF CASES	EARLY DEATHS	LATE DEATHS
Supracardiac	28	2	0
Infracardiac	16	3	1
Coronary sinus	17	0	2
Right atrium	3	0	0
Mixed	3	1	1
Total	67	6	4

REFERENCES

1. Barratt-Boyes BG, Simpson M, Neutze JM. Intracardiac surgery in neonates and infants using deep hypothermia with

surface cooling and limited cardiopulmonary bypass. Circulation 43,44(suppl I):25, 1971.
2. Behrendt DM, Aberdeen E, Waterson DJ, et al. Total anomalous pulmonary venous drainage in infants. I. Clinical and hemodynamic findings, methods, and results of operation in 37 cases. Circulation 46:347, 1972.
3. Bharati S, Lev M. Congenital anomalies of the pulmonary veins. Cardiovasc Clin 5:23, 1973.
4. Borow KM, Green LH, Castaneda AR, et al. Left ventricular function after repair of tetralogy of Fallot and its relationship to age at surgery. Circulation 61:1150, 1980.
5. Burroughs JT, Edwards JE. Total anomalous pulmonary venous connection. Am Heart J 59:913, 1960.
6. Burroughs JT, Kirklin JW. Complete surgical correction of total anomalous pulmonary venous connection. Report of three cases. Proc Staff Meet Mayo Clin 31:182, 1956.
7. Darling RC, Rothney WB, Craig JM. Total pulmonary venous drainage into the right side of the heart. Lab Invest 6:44, 1957.
8. Delisle G, Ando M, Calder AL, et al. Total anomalous pulmonary venous connection: Report of 92 autopsied cases with emphasis on diagnostic and surgical considerations. Am Heart J 91:99, 1976.
9. Gathman GE, Nadas AS. Total anomalous pulmonary venous connection: Clinical and physiologic observations of 75 pediatric patients. Circulation 42:143, 1970.
10. Gold JP, Jonas RA, Lang P, et al. Transcutaneous intracardiac monitoring lines in pediatric surgical patients: A 10-year experience. Ann Thorac Surg 42:185, 1986.
11. Hammon JW, Bender HW, Graham TP, et al. Total anomalous pulmonary venous connection in infancy: Ten years' experience, including studies of postoperative ventricular function. J Thorac Cardiovasc Surg 80:544, 1980.
12. Haworth SG, Reid L. Structural study of pulmonary circulation and of the heart in total anomalous pulmonary venous return in early infancy. Br Heart J 39:80, 1977.
13. Hickey PR, Hansen DD, Wessel DL, et al. Blunting of stress responses in the pulmonary circulation of infants by Fentanyl. Anesth Analg 64:1137, 1985.
14. Jenkins KJ, Sanders SP, Coleman L, et al. Pulmonary vein size and outcome in infants with totally anomalous pulmonary venous connection. Circulation 84(suppl II):351, 1991.
15. Jonas RA, Castaneda AR. Total anomalous pulmonary venous connection: Surgical aspects. In Nelson N (ed). Current Therapy in Neontal/Perinatal Medicine. Philadelphia, BC Decker, 1990, p 374.
16. Jonas RA, Smolinksy A, Mayer JE, et al. Obstructed pulmonary venous drainage with total anomalous pulmonary venous connection to the coronary sinus. Am J Cardiol 59:431, 1987.
17. Karl TS, Iyer KS, Sano S, et al. Infant ECMO cannulation technique allowing preservation of carotid and jugular vessels. Ann Thorac Surg 50:488, 1990.
18. Klein MD, Shaheen KW, Whittlesey GC, et al. Extracorporeal membrane oxygenation for the circulation support of children after repair of congenital heart disease. J Thorac Cardiovasc Surg 100:498, 1990.

19. Leblanc JG, Patterson MW, Taylor GP, et al. Total anomalous pulmonary venous connection. J Thorac Cardiovasc Surg 95:540, 1988.
20. Lewis FJ, Varco RL, Taufic M, et al. Direct vision repair of triatrial heart and total anomalous pulmonary venous drainage. Surg Gynecol Obstet 102:713, 1956.
21. Muller WH. The surgical treatment of transposition of the pulmonary veins. Ann Surg 134:683, 1951.
22. Mustard WT, Keon WJ, Trusler GA. Transposition of the lesser veins (total anomalous pulmonary venous drainage). Prog Cardiovasc Dis 11:145, 1968.
23. Neill CA. Development of the pulmonary veins: With reference to the embryology of pulmonary venous return. Pediatrics 18:880, 1956.
24. Newburger JW, Silbert AR, Buckley LP, et al. Cognitive function and duration of hypoxemia in children with transposition of the great arteries. N Engl J Med 31:1495, 1984.
25. Norwood WI, Hougen TJ, Castaneda AR. Total anomalous pulmonary venous connection: Surgical considerations. Cardiovasc Clin 11:353, 1981.
26. Pacifico AD, Mandke NV, McGrath LB, et al. Repair of congenital pulmonary venous drainage to the coronary sinus. J Thorac Cardiovasc Surg 64:132, 1972.
27. Parr GV, Kirklin JW, Pacifico AD, et al. Cardiac performance in infancy after repair of total anomalous pulmonary venous connection. Ann Thorac Surg 17:561, 1974.
28. Rabinovitch M, Herrera-deLeon V, Castaneda AR, et al. Growth and development of the pulmonary vascular bed in patients with tetralogy of Fallot with or without pulmonary atresia. Circulation 64:1234, 1981.
29. Sano S, Brawn WJ, Mee RBB. Total anomalous pulmonary venous drainage. J Thorac Cardiovasc Surg 97:886, 1989.
30. Van Praagh R, Harken AH, Delisle G, et al. Total anomalous pulmonary venous drainage to the coronary sinus. J Thorac Cardiovasc Surg 64:132, 1972.
31. vanderVelde M, Parness IA, Colan SD, et al. Two dimensional echocardiography in the pre- and post-operative management of total anomalous pulmonary venous connection. J Am Coll Cardiol 18:1746, 1991.
32. Walsh EP, Rockenmacher S, Keane JF, et al. Late results in patients with tetralogy of Fallot repaired during infancy. Circulation 5:1062, 1988.
33. Weinhaus L, Canter C, Noetzel M, et al. Extracorporeal membrane oxygenation for circulatory support after repair of congenital heart defects. Ann Thorac Surg 48:206, 1989.
34. Whight CM, Barratt-Boyes BG, Calder AL, et al. Total anomalous pulmonary venous connection. Long-term results following repair in infancy. J Thorac Cardiovasc Surg 75:52, 1978.
35. Wilson J. A description of a very unusual formation of the human heart. Philos Trans R Soc Lond 88:346, 1798.
36. Yee ES, Turley K, Hsieh WR, et al. Infant total anomalous pulmonary venous connection: Factors influencing timing of presentation and operative outcome. Circulation 76(suppl III) 83:1987.

10

Chapter

Atrioventricular Canal Defect

Atrioventricular canal defects encompass a spectrum of lesions that are caused by maldevelopment of the endocardial cushions. Abnormalities of atrioventricular valve form and function and of interatrial and interventricular communications may result.

This chapter will be concerned primarily with atrioventricular canal defects that require surgical reconstruction and in which there is the potential for a biventricular heart. Variations that have severe straddling, stenosis, or atresia of either the left or right component of the atrioventricular valve, or forms that have one severely hypoplastic ventricle, will not be considered in detail. It must be kept in mind, however, that these "unbalanced" defects also fall along a spectrum that at one end merges with defects that do have the potential for biventricular reconstruction.

The atrioventricular canal defect may be isolated or may be one component of a more complex lesion. Associated cardiovascular lesions will be discussed in this chapter. However, cases in which the defect is part of the heterotaxia syndrome will not be discussed, as the atrioventricular canal defect is usually not considered the primary pathophysiologic problem, and repair of the atrioventricular canal defect in this syndrome is often not considered.

The intracardiac, morphologic complexity and variability of this defect rival those of any other congenital heart defect; nevertheless, surgical re-

construction can be performed with outstanding results, even in small infants.

ANATOMY

Developmental Considerations

To completely understand this lesion, it must be appreciated that the normal atrioventricular canal is a three-dimensional structure, not only encompassing the two dimensions of the plane of the atrioventricular valves, but also possessing depth, with the atrial and ventricular components of the canal septum extending above and below the plane of the atrioventricular valve annuli. The atrial portion of the atrioventricular canal septum extends posteriorly from the plane of the valve annuli and merges with the true atrial septum, while the ventricular portion of the atrioventricular canal septum extends anteriorly from the valve annuli and merges with the true ventricular septum. The atrial and ventricular portions of the atrioventricular canal septum also converge with each other between and at the level of the atrioventricular valve annuli, thereby separating the common atrioventricular valve into the mitral and tricuspid components. A normal atrioventricular canal septum, including both the atrial and ventricular components, appears to be necessary for normal formation of the two atrioventricular valves.[35]

Development of the normal atrioventricular canal is accomplished by the proliferation of endocardial cushion tissue. The superior and inferior cushions grow across the common orifice to divide it into the mitral and tricuspid orifices. Growth of tissue from the superior and inferior cushions also closes the ostium primum in the atrial septum, and growth of tissue from the inferior cushion contributes to the closure of the secondary interventricular foramen in the ventricular septum. Growth and development of the superior and inferior cushions, along with the lateral dextrodorsal conus cushion, contribute to formation of the normal leaflets of the mitral and tricuspid valves. Contribution to the valvar and subvalvar apparatus is also made by excavation and attenuation of ventricular muscle just beneath the valve annuli.[35]

When this embryologic process fails, one of the various forms of the atrioventricular canal defect occurs. It is important to emphasize that all forms of this defect, whether mild or severe, have morphologic abnormalities of all three aspects of the atrioventricular canal: the atrial and ventricular portions of the atrioventricular canal septum and the atrioventricular valves themselves.

Morphologic Variations

Varying degrees of abnormality in the development of the endocardial cushions result in the spectrum of atrioventricular canal lesions. In spite of the variations, all forms of this lesion have the following common morphologic features:

1. Deficiency of the atrioventricular canal septum
2. Abnormal formation of the atrioventricular valves
3. A "scooped out" ventricular septum with a shortened dimension of the inlet-to-apex ventricular septal distance
4. An "unwedged" aortic valve with a "gooseneck" deformity of the left ventricular outflow tract and increased dimension of the apex-to-outlet ventricular septal distance
5. Inferior displacement of the coronary sinus, atrioventricular node, and proximal conduction system at the ventricles.

The deficiency in the atrioventricular canal septum causes the "scooped out" appearance of the crest of the ventricular septum. This causes the atrioventricular valves to be positioned closer to the apex of the heart than normal. The aortic valve cannot become wedged between the mitral and tricuspid annuli, as in the normal heart, because of maldevelopment of the superior and inferior cushions. As a result, the left ventricular outflow tract is lengthened and narrowed, creating the "gooseneck"

deformity of the left ventricular outflow tract. The abnormality of the atrioventricular valves themselves may be quite variable. Even when two well-developed atrioventricular valve annuli form, morphologic abnormalities of the leaflets of the left-sided and right-sided valves (especially the anterior leaflet of the left-sided valve) are almost always present.

Each of these morphologic abnormalities may range from mild to severe in any individual case; however, because all of the various morphologic abnormalities are interrelated, the degree of severity of one abnormality (for example, abnormality of the atrioventricular valves) generally is similar to that of most of the other abnormalities, although some variation in the degree of these associations does exist.

The degree of severity of the morphologic abnormality at each of these levels often carries physiologic implications. In the most severe (complete) form of the defect, the atrial, ventricular, and valvar components are "in common," resulting in a physiologic interatrial communication; a physiologic interventricular communication; and a single, or common, atrioventricular valve (Fig. 10–1).[36]

In less severe forms, only one or two of these three components are "in common" in the physiologic sense, although all three components are still morphologically abnormal. As a result, there may be no physiologic interatrial communication or no physiologic interventricular communication. At the atrioventricular valve level there may be a common valve annulus, two well-formed annuli, or a condition somewhere between these two morphologic extremes. These less severe forms of the atrioventricular canal defect have been called by various names and subcategories, following the concepts first put forth by Wakai and Edwards.[38] This practice, al-

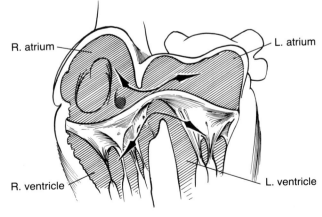

FIGURE 10–1. ☐

Schematic four-chamber view of complete atrioventricular (AV) canal defect, showing common valve and atrial and ventricular communications.

though sometimes helpful, is too simplistic and may detract from complete understanding of the lesion by de-emphasizing the continuous morphologic spectrum of all atrioventricular canal defects.

Within this spectrum the mildest form of the defect is one in which two atrioventricular valve annuli form, and a "cleft" in the anterior leaflet of the left valve is present. The subvalvar aspect of the valve annuli and chordal structures adheres along the top of the only mildly "scooped out" ventricular septum (resulting in the atrioventricular valves being slightly closer to the apex, thus preventing an interventricular communication); the supravalvar aspect adheres to the atrial septum (preventing an interatrial communication); and the aortic valve is partially wedged between the relatively well formed atrioventricular valves (minimizing the gooseneck deformity). In this lesion there is no potential for intracardiac shunting even though deficiencies of the atrial and ventricular aspects of the atrioventricular canal septum are present. The only potential for pathophysiology is regurgitation through the cleft in the anterior leaflet of the left-sided atrioventricular valve. This is a relatively rare form of the atrioventricular canal defect.

In terms of increasing physiologic (and morphologic) complexity, the next form of the defect is also one in which two atrioventricular valve annuli form, but the deficiency in the atrial aspect of the atrioventricular canal septum results in development of an ostium primum defect. At the atrioventricular valve level, this lesion is not "in common," as there are two separate valve annuli. However, the valves are abnormal, with the anterior leaflet of the left-sided valve typically having a cleft. At the ventricular level the lesion is also not "in common," as atrioventricular valve tissue has become adherent to the ventricular septal crest, eliminating the potential for an interventricular communication. Nevertheless, the ventricular septum is abnormal, exhibiting the typical "scooped out" appearance. This form of the atrioventricular canal defect occurs frequently. The apical position of the atrioventricular valves and the gooseneck deformity can often be identified in this lesion.

Various other more complex forms also occur, but with less frequency. These forms have frequently, and with some confusion, been referred to as transitional atrioventricular canal defects.[5] In these forms an ostium primum interatrial communication is usually present. An interventricular communication may be present, because the atrioventricular valve tissue has not become completely adherent to the crest of the "scooped out" ventricular septum. The size of the interventricular communication may vary from moderate to almost nonexistent. Occa-

sionally an interventricular defect is present without an interatrial defect.

Two separate atrioventricular valve annuli may exist in this form; however, the development of the valve annuli may vary from being well established, to tenuously established, to common. When the atrioventricular valves are tenuously separated, a thin fibrous bridge of tissue may connect the superior and inferior common atrioventricular valve leaflets above the crest of the ventricular septum. A deep cleft between the left-sided superior and inferior leaflets is, by necessity, present, and the subvalvar aspect of this "annulus" may be relatively tightly adherent to the crest of the ventricular septum, or it may be suspended above the ventricular septum with a substantial interventricular communication beneath it. By definition, an ostium primum defect is always present with this particular variation. A common atrioventricular valve annulus occurs when the superior and inferior leaflets do not physically connect above the crest of the ventricular septum. In some variations the superior and inferior common atrioventricular valve leaflets may approach each other but not physically touch. These two leaflets are usually densely adherent to the crest of the ventricular septum. In this form of the atrioventricular canal defect an ostium primum defect is usually present, a common atrioventricular valve orifice is present by definition, and a small interventricular communication may be present where the superior and inferior atrioventricular valve leaflets do not completely adhere to the crest of the ventricular septum. It becomes somewhat a matter of definition as to whether an interventricular communication is truly present when the superior and inferior leaflets are both completely adherent to the crest of the ventricular septum, with the only potential for interventricular communication being the small bare area of the mid-portion of the ventricular septal crest, where the superior and inferior leaflets approach each other but do not touch.

These gradations emphasize that it is best to consider all forms of the atrioventricular canal defect as a continuous spectrum of lesions involving the atrial, ventricular, and valvar portions of the canal. Each particular form should be described by its unique anatomic and physiologic features, not by an artificial categorization. Nevertheless, it is important to be familiar with the various published classification systems, as they are frequently used.[5, 27, 38] The physician should be aware, however, that at the present time at least six separate definitions of the "intermediate" form of the atrioventricular canal defect exist in the literature.

The most severe (complete) forms of the atrioventricular canal defect exist when a common atrioventricular valve is present and the superior and inferior valve leaflets are not adherent to the crest of the ventricular septum. In these cases large, nonrestrictive interventricular communications are present, along with an ostium primum interatrial defect. These complete forms of this defect are frequently encountered. The number and configuration of common atrioventricular valve leaflets can be variable, and it is often difficult to clearly distinguish the classic leaflet configuration referred to in most texts. Chordal structures from individual valve leaflets situated above the septal crest may attach to the crest itself, straddle into both ventricles, or attach all on one side of the ventricular septal crest. Commissures may overlie the ventricular septal crest, or they may not, resulting in leaflets that "bridge" or "straddle" the septal crest. In our experience Rastelli's classic leaflet designations are somewhat simplistic and of little clinical value.[27] Historically, much attention has been given to these leaflet and chordal details. In our view these details are not nearly as important as understanding some of the other relationships already discussed and others that will be discussed later.

Variations in the degree of severity of the other morphologic abnormalities of the atrioventricular canal defect can also have important surgical significance. Recognition of the abnormal position of the conduction tissue is critical to avoid heart block. Because of the deficiency of the atrioventricular canal septum, the conduction system is displaced in all forms of the defect.[6] The orifice of the coronary sinus and the atrioventricular node are both more inferior than usual when visualized through the right atrium. The node is situated in the right atrial tissue close to the inferior edge of the interatrial defect, between the orifice of the coronary sinus and the crux of the heart, where the inferior aspect of the crest of the interventricular septum joins the atrioventricular groove. This has been called the *nodal triangle* to distinguish it from the triangle of Koch, which can still be identified in the atrioventricular canal defect but does not harbor the node. The bundle of His penetrates the atrioventricular junction at the crux and travels along the crest of the ventricular septum, giving off the left-sided bundles. About midway along the ventricular septal crest, moving in an inferior-to-superior direction, the bundle branches move off the crest of the septum, leaving the superior aspect of the crest of the ventricular septum free of conduction tissue.

Severe forms of the gooseneck deformity can cause tunnel-like, subvalvar obstruction of the left ventricular outflow tract; however, this is unusual. Additionally, membranes, abnormal chordal and papillary structures of the atrioventricular valve, and accessory endocardial cushion tissue can also obstruct the left ventricular outflow tract.[26, 32]

The position of the papillary muscles of the left-sided atrioventricular valve structures must be carefully evaluated, as two very closely spaced papillary muscles or a solitary papillary muscle may result in a parachute mitral valve after closure of the cleft between the left superior and inferior leaflets.[12]

Attention must also be given to the amount and quality of atrioventricular valve tissue. Surgical manipulation of the leaflet tissue, by necessity, sequesters a certain amount of the surface area of the leaflets. Proper coaptation of the reconstructed atrioventricular valves may not be possible if insufficiency of the leaflet surface area is severe. Deficiency of atrioventricular valve tissue and obstruction of the left ventricular inflow and outflow tracts appear to be more common when atrioventricular canal defects occur in patients without the trisomy 21 chromosomal abnormality.[13]

Another important consideration, first emphasized by Bharati and Lev,[5] relates to how well the common atrioventricular valve is centered over the ventricular septum. When it is positioned equally over both ventricles, usually both are of normal size and a repair resulting in two functioning atrioventricular valves and ventricles is possible. However, the common atrioventricular valve may be centered primarily over one ventricle or the other. The ventricle associated with the smaller portion of the atrioventricular valve orifice is often correspondingly hypoplastic. In severe cases it is clear that a single-ventricle reconstruction is all that can be accomplished. In less severe cases the decision to attempt a two-ventricle repair can be extremely difficult. This decision is based on clinical judgment, which in turn is based on a number of factors, including (1) which ventricle is hypoplastic, (2) the quality of the atrioventricular valve tissue itself, (3) an assessment of ventricular cavity size and ventricular outflow tracts, (4) the status of the pulmonary vasculature, and (5) an assessment of the risks of the alternative single-ventricle repair. Although careful consideration of these factors can be helpful in deciding whether to attempt a two-ventricle repair, unfortunately, specific guidelines for making this decision have not been formulated.

Associated Cardiovascular Lesions

Attention must be given to associated anatomic cardiovascular abnormalities that are not intrinsically related to the atrioventricular canal defect itself. These abnormalities include a left superior vena cava, anomalous pulmonary venous connection, secundum atrial septal defect, additional ventricular septal defects (usually posterior muscular), patent ductus arteriosus, accessory orifice of the left atrioventricular valve, aortic arch abnormalities, and conotruncal defects, including tetralogy of Fallot, double-outlet right ventricle, and transposition of the great vessels. The specific anatomic and physiologic points of importance associated with these lesions will be discussed in the section, "Surgical Technique."

A particular complex that we have encountered on a number of occasions, and that has been described by others,[13, 24] is the existence of a partial atrioventricular canal defect consisting of an ostium primum interatrial defect and a cleft mitral valve associated with a single left ventricular papillary muscle, aortic coarctation, or a hypoplastic aortic arch.

As mentioned, the atrioventricular canal defect frequently is also one component of the complex heart disease associated with the heterotaxia syndromes. In many heterotaxia cases (especially patients with asplenia), two-ventricle reconstructions are not possible. Still, occasionally a patient with polysplenia will have two well-balanced ventricles and can therefore be considered for a two-ventricle repair.

PATHOPHYSIOLOGY AND NATURAL HISTORY

The pathophysiology of the various forms of atrioventricular canal defect depends on the degree of each of three main hemodynamic abnormalities: interatrial shunting, interventricular shunting, and atrioventricular valve regurgitation. In addition, associated cardiovascular abnormalities may predictably modify the pathophysiology. The most prominent finding in the complete form of this defect is usually a large left-to-right ventricular level shunt. The pathophysiology is basically similar to that of a large, isolated ventricular septal defect. The details and implications of a large left-to-right ventricular level shunt are reviewed in Chapter 11 and will not be discussed here. The pathophysiologic changes may be somewhat more accelerated in the complete form of atrioventricular canal defect than in the isolated ventricular septal defect[25] because of the addition of the atrial level shunt and the potential for further ventricular volume overload from atrioventricular valve regurgitation; also, in patients with trisomy 21, there is a potential for intrinsic pulmonary parenchymal and vascular deficiencies. As a result the patient with the complete form of this

defect usually develops symptoms of heart failure early in infancy.

If the defect is accompanied by trisomy 21, pulmonary vascular obstructive disease seems to develop more quickly than in defects without trisomy 21. Some studies confirm this contention,[9, 11, 19, 34] whereas others fail to show any clear difference in the degree of histologic pulmonary vascular disease between patients with and those without trisomy 21.[17, 25] Upper airway obstruction, sleep apnea, and hypoventilation are definitely more common with trisomy 21, as is the tendency for the development of pulmonary infections.[11] These factors may play a role in the findings of higher calculated pulmonary vascular resistance during cardiac catheterization and in the accelerated development of pulmonary vascular obstructive disease that may occur in trisomy 21 patients. Setting aside the issue of trisomy 21, there appears to be no question that pulmonary vascular obstructive disease develops more rapidly in patients with complete atrioventricular canal defects than in patients with an isolated ventricular septal defect, with the great majority having advanced Heath-Edwards changes by 1 year of age.

Predictably, clinically important congestive heart failure develops during infancy in patients with the complete form of atrioventricular canal defect. Without medical or surgical management, life expectancy is less than 6 months in half of the patients and less than 2 years in 80%.[4] The cause of death within the first several years of life is congestive heart failure or infectious pulmonary complications. After this period obstructive pulmonary vascular disease and decompensation of the atrioventricular valve increasingly affect survival.[4] In our experience, mild atrioventricular valve incompetence is present in about 35% of patients in the first year of life; however, severe incompetence is rare, occurring in only 4%.[16]

In forms of the atrioventricular canal defect without a large interventricular communication, the predominant pathophysiologic lesion is usually a large atrial level shunt. If the atrioventricular valve functions normally, the patient's signs and symptoms are similar to those of any other patient with a large atrial septal defect (see Chapter 8). If the atrioventricular valve is incompetent, however, the volume load caused by this lesion will accelerate congestive heart failure.

If obstruction of the left ventricular outflow tract is associated with the defect, congestive heart failure is also accelerated. Associated cardiac lesions such as tetralogy of Fallot, double-outlet right ventricle, transposition of the great arteries, aortic arch abnormalities, left-sided obstructive lesions, and patent ductus arteriosus also affect the patient's physiology and symptomatology in ways expected for these lesions. For example, moderate obstruction of the right ventricular outflow tract from associated tetralogy of Fallot may cause some degree of cyanosis; however, it also may significantly delay the onset of congestive heart failure by restricting pulmonary blood flow.

DIAGNOSIS AND INDICATIONS FOR SURGERY

The diagnosis is suggested by the typical physical findings of atrial or ventricular level left-to-right shunting, possibly associated with the auscultatory findings of atrioventricular valve regurgitation. Chest radiographic findings are typical of a large left-to-right shunt but are nonspecific. Electrocardiographic findings are more specific. These basic aspects of the diagnosis have been well described in many standard texts.[1]

Echocardiography is probably the most useful diagnostic modality for defining the morphologic details of the atrioventricular canal defect. The specific anatomic details regarding the atrial and ventricular communications, the atrioventricular valve abnormality, the left ventricular outflow tract, the degree of ventricular balance, the status of the papillary muscles, and the associated lesions can usually be clearly delineated. Physiologic parameters can also be estimated, but not with the accuracy of anatomic details. The direction of shunting, degree of shunting, and degree and specific cause of atrioventricular valve regurgitation can all be estimated.

In more recent years, cardiac catheterization has not been routinely performed unless specific information regarding the size of the shunt and the amount of pulmonary vascular resistance is required. This is almost never necessary in infants less than 6 months old. After this age, however, careful delineation of the physiology of the pulmonary vasculature becomes more important. Occasionally cardiac catheterization is required even when there are no pulmonary vascular concerns to confirm anatomic detail when echocardiographic examination is not definitive.

Indications for surgery depend on the form of the atrioventricular canal defect, but if symptoms of congestive heart failure are present, corrective surgery should be undertaken as soon as possible, regardless of the type of defect. For the complete form, this may be as early as the first few weeks of life. Complete repair is the procedure of choice, with the patient's age and size having no bearing on this decision. Only in extremely unusual circumstances would a pulmonary artery band be considered. Such circumstances would include uncontrollable heart failure in the presence of an active respiratory infectious problem that precludes cardiopulmonary bypass, uncorrectable associated lesions such as multiple muscular ventricular septal defects, or uncertainty over the degree of ventricular imbalance.

In the asymptomatic patient with the complete form of atrioventricular canal defect, elective repair is undertaken by 6 months of age. The timing of elective repair is based on several lines of reasoning. First, irreversible pulmonary vascular obstructive disease can develop within the first year. Second, there are no increased risks of technical problems related to complete repair at this time.[16] Finally, at Children's Hospital in Boston our results suggest that the mortality rate is lower for repair in the first 6 months of life than for repair in the second 6 months.[16]

In forms of the atrioventricular canal defect that are less complete, patients may remain asymptomatic longer. In cases characterized by the ostium primum defect only and without an interventricular defect or atrioventricular valve regurgitation, symptomatology may not appear for a number of years, as is true of patients with simple atrial septal defects. These patients should undergo elective corrective surgery, preferably at or before 1 year of age (see Chapter 8). An important consideration in this regard is the functional status of the left atrioventricular valve. Once regurgitation develops, cleft edges tend to thicken. Although in certain cases this can be beneficial in that it allows more secure closure of the cleft, distortion and foreshortening of the valve leaflets can also occur. This makes valve repair (i.e., closure of the cleft) less likely to achieve complete valve competence. Therefore, repair should be performed at the first sign of left atrioventricular valve regurgitation, regardless of age and absence of symptoms.

When associated cardiovascular anomalies that are surgically correctable accompany the atrioventricular canal defect, complete repair of the associated lesion is also undertaken at the time of the canal repair. Such lesions include a persistent left superior vena cava, anomalous pulmonary venous connection, patent ductus arteriosus, secundum atrial septal defect, muscular ventricular septal defect, aortic arch obstruction, and conotruncal defects.

SURGICAL MANAGEMENT

Historical Perspective

The first repair of a complete atrioventricular canal defect was performed by Lillehei and associates in 1954 using cross circulation,[22] and the first reports of successful repair of the isolated ostium primum defect appeared in 1955.[18, 39] This success was achieved in spite of the fact that the complex anatomy of the atrioventricular canal defect was poorly understood at that time. Generally, subsequent surgical management of this lesion carried a high mortality rate because of this lack of anatomic understanding.[21] During the ensuing decade many contributions were made that provided important insight into the complexity of this lesion, resulting in improved outcome. In 1958, Lev described the conduction system in the atrioventricular canal defect, thereby allowing avoidance of complete heart block.[20] Other major contributions to our understanding of the anatomy were made by Bharati and coworkers[5, 6] and Rastelli and associates.[27]

Various surgical techniques, using either one or two patches for the reconstruction and emphasizing the management of the atrioventricular valve tissue, naturally followed.[23, 29, 30] As outcome improved through the 1960s, attempts at repair earlier in life were made. Rastelli and associates[28] reported their results in 1968, with some of the repairs having been performed in infants, and Barratt-Boyes reported infant repair using deep hypothermic circulatory arrest in 1973.[2] Frequent reports of repair of complete atrioventricular canal defects in infants have appeared subsequently, with the best results generally suggesting about a 10% mortality rate.[3, 14] Complete repair during infancy has been recommended at Children's Hospital in Boston since the 1970s.[8, 10]

Currently, reports by some groups still recommend routine surgical palliation for infants, using pulmonary artery banding.[15, 31, 33, 40] Our present approach is to perform pulmonary artery banding only in extremely unusual circumstances.

In 1978, Carpentier suggested that the left atrioventricular valve be constructed as a "trifoliate" valve without closure of the cleft.[7] We disagree with this as a routine approach both on an anatomic basis (i.e., the cleft does not have the characteristics of a normal commissure in that the chords from each side of the cleft do not converge to a common papillary muscle) and on a functional basis (i.e., our experience is that open clefts can behave unpredictably in the postoperative period, with the potential for the development of severe regurgitation at the left atrioventricular valve). This is an area of disagreement, and successful results have been reported with both approaches. New insights into subtle variations in atrioventricular valve morphology may help to resolve this controversy.

Surgical Technique

The approach to cardiopulmonary bypass is standard. A median sternotomy is performed, the thymus gland is mobilized or subtotally resected, and a large patch of pericardium is removed and fixed in glutaraldehyde. Continuous cardiopulmonary bypass with bicaval cannulation is used for patients weighing more than 8 kg, and deep hypothermic circulatory arrest may be considered for those weighing less than 4 kg. If continuous cardiopulmonary bypass is to be used, the inferior venous cannula must be introduced low, essentially into the inferior vena cava itself, to provide adequate exposure for the lower end of the repair. During the initial phases of cardiopulmonary bypass, the ligamentum arteriosum (or patent ductus) is routinely clipped or ligated.

Cleft Mitral Valve

In the rare form of the atrioventricular canal defect consisting of only an incompetent cleft mitral valve (Fig. 10–2), surgical exposure is accomplished through an interatrial groove incision. Alternatively, a right atrial incision, followed by an atrial septal incision, can be performed. After the mitral valve is exposed, the left ventricle is filled with cold saline, and the valve is observed for leaflet coaptation, cleft coaptation, and leaflet prolapse. In the majority of cases of cleft mitral valve, the incompetence is through the cleft, although there may be some degree of central incompetence as well. The repair proceeds by precise placement of simple polypropylene sutures in the cleft, beginning at its base and moving centrally. Absolute alignment of the cleft in all its dimensions is of critical importance. The surgeon must avoid the tendency to "unroll" the cleft edges, and instead place the sutures where the edges naturally coapt. If the leaflet tissue is extremely delicate, judgment must be exercised regarding the security of the simple sutures. It may be necessary to use pledgetted mattress sutures instead; however, these increase the likelihood of distortion and sequestration of the valve tissue.

Sutures are placed along the cleft, moving centrally until the first set of chordal attachments are approached. The valve is then tested again with saline. If central coaptation is adequate, the repair is complete. If central regurgitation is present and is not due to a poorly aligned cleft repair, pledgetted mattress sutures are placed in the annulus at the bases of both valve commissures to reduce the circumference of the annulus and thereby correct the central incompetence. If leaflet prolapse is present,

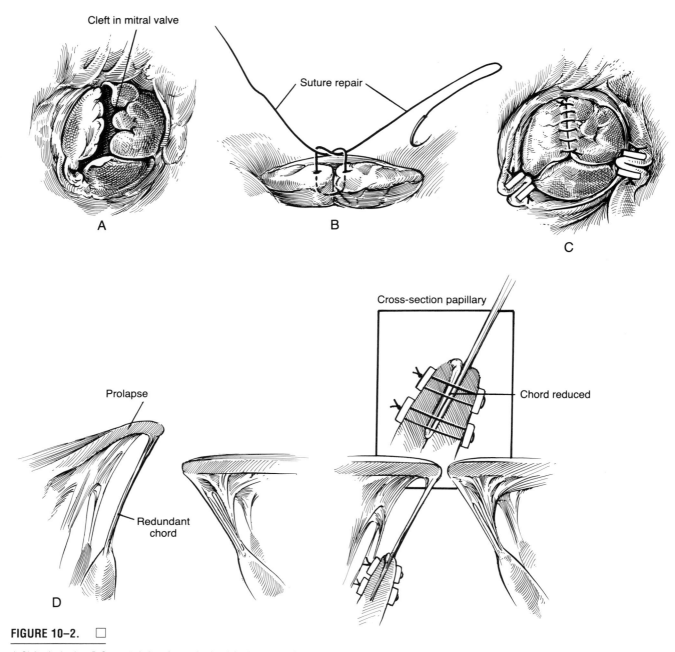

FIGURE 10-2. ☐

A, Cleft mitral valve. *B,* Suture technique for repair of a cleft mitral valve. *C,* Annuloplasty repair for central mitral regurgitation. *D,* Repair of a prolapsed segment of the mitral valve.

the responsible chords are appropriately foreshortened. We have not encountered an isolated cleft mitral valve with regurgitation in infants; however, the principles of cleft repair can be generalized to the more complex lesions discussed below.

Ostium Primum Defect with a Cleft Mitral Valve

When an ostium primum interatrial defect is present with a cleft mitral valve (Fig. 10-3), the approach is exclusively through a right atrial incision. The mitral valve is addressed first, looking through the atrial defect. Repair of the mitral valve cleft proceeds as described for the isolated cleft mitral valve. The interatrial communication is then closed with a patch of glutaraldehyde-treated autologous pericardium (Fig. 10-4). It is important to avoid synthetic patch materials, which can cause hemolysis if residual regurgitation of the left-sided atrioventricular valve is present.

The patch is placed with a running suture technique using 5-0 polypropylene suture, beginning at

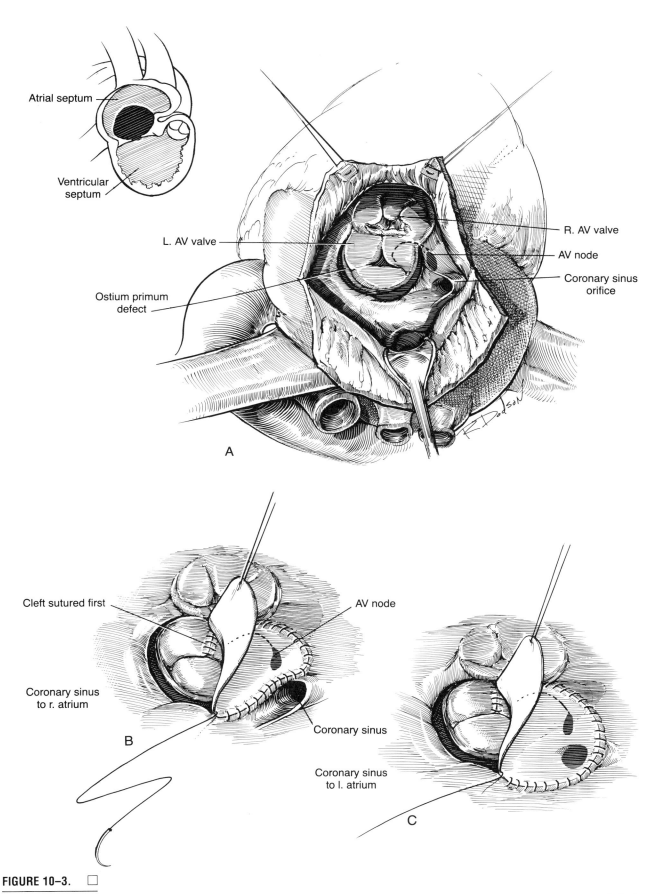

Atrial septum

Ventricular septum

L. AV valve

Ostium primum defect

R. AV valve

AV node

Coronary sinus orifice

A

Cleft sutured first

Coronary sinus to r. atrium

B

AV node

Coronary sinus

Coronary sinus to l. atrium

C

FIGURE 10–3. ☐

A, Partial forms of AV canal defect with ostium primum defect and cleft in the left-sided AV valve as seen from the surgeon's perspective via a right atriotomy. *B,* Patch repair allowing the coronary sinus to drain to the right atrium. *C,* Patch repair allowing the coronary sinus to drain to the left atrium.

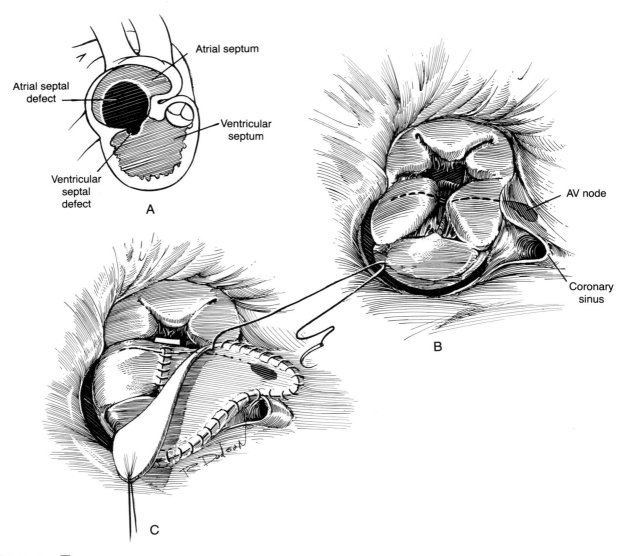

FIGURE 10–4. □

A, Morphology of partial AV canal defects with small ventricular communication. *B,* Surgeon's view via a right atriotomy. *C,* Repair using pledgetted suture to close a ventricular septal defect, cleft closure, and pericardial patch closure of ostium primum defect.

the base of the mitral cleft. The suture line continues to the surgeon's right, where the critical area of
the conduction system and the coronary sinus are
located. The edge of the patch is sutured superficially to the mitral valve tissue that is adherent to
the underlying ventricular septal crest. Suture
depth is critical, as the proximal conduction bundles
travel along the underlying crest of the ventricular
septum at this level. As the suture line approaches
the inferiormost extent of the ventricular septal
crest, it should be directed well to the right ventricular side of the crest, using the available tissue from
the right-sided atrioventricular valve inferior leaflet. As the annulus is approached, the suture line
undergoes transition from the atrioventricular valve

tissue to the atrial free wall. Then, working with
the atrial free wall and septum, the suture line progresses sequentially anterior, inferior, and finally
posterior to the coronary sinus and atrioventricular
node, essentially surrounding these structures.
Thus, the coronary sinus drains under the patch to
the left atrium.

The suture line then approaches the posteroinferior free edge of the ostium primum defect. Attention is then returned to the area of the base of the
cleft mitral valve, where the other end of the suture
line is placed in the mitral valve tissue along the
superior aspect of the crest of the ventricular septum. This suturing proceeds until the transition
from the atrioventricular valve tissue to the atrial

wall is completed at the annulus, and the superior free edge of the ostium primum defect is approached. The two ends of the suture line then approach each other along the rim of the ostium primum defect. If an ostium secundum defect is also present, this may be incorporated under the single patch.

If a left superior vena cava is present, several options exist. If a large connecting innominate vein is present, the left superior vena cava may simply be ligated as it enters the heart, thus avoiding the large right-to-left shunt that would occur because the coronary sinus is draining to the left atrium. If no connecting vein is present, it is not advisable to ligate the left superior vena cava, although this certainly does not consistently result in complications as a result of venous obstruction. In this situation the patch is placed so that the coronary sinus drains to the right atrium. To accomplish this, after the initial suture line of the patch surrounds the nodal triangle, instead of passing posterior to the coronary sinus to approach the edge of the ostium primum defect, the suture line is directed between the node and the coronary sinus, placing it just inside the orifice of the dilated coronary sinus ostium, along its anterosuperior aspect, to approach the edge of the ostium primum defect. This suture line is not preferred by some in the absence of a left superior vena cava because of the theoretical increased risk of nodal injury and the increased difficulty of working close to the rim of the smaller coronary sinus; however, others routinely place the coronary sinus in the right atrium.

Partial Form With Interventricular Communication

Occasionally, in the presence of an ostium primum defect with two separate atrioventricular valves, the subvalvar aspect of the atrioventricular valve will not completely adhere to the crest of the ventricular septum. If the resulting interventricular communication is of no hemodynamic significance, it may be ignored, and the repair can proceed as previously described. However, if the defect, or the combined effect of several such defects, is physiologically significant, it must be surgically addressed. If there is one or several discrete communications between fibrous attachments of the valve or valve chords to the crest, it may be possible to primarily close the defects directly by approximating the adjacent subvalvar fibrous attachments with simple or mattress sutures. Occasionally, multiple defects are present along the entire length of the ventricular septal crest, and a different approach is required. If the interventricular communication is relatively large, the approach is essentially the same as that

described later for repair of the complete form of atrioventricular canal defect. If multiple short chordae are attached along the crest of the ventricular septum, as is often the case with this variant, the interventricular communications can be closed by placing multiple interrupted mattress sutures along the right ventricular side of the crest of the septum and then through leaflet tissue to pull the leaflet down to the septum, thereby obliterating the interventricular communication. This technique is most applicable when the communications exist under the superior bridging leaflet. Pressure on the conduction tissue traveling along the crest of the ventricular septum can occur if this method is used for communications under the inferior leaflets.

Partial Form With Common Atrioventricular Valve Annulus

In the partial atrioventricular canal defect in which two separate atrioventricular valve annuli do not form but the left superior and inferior leaflets are densely adherent to the ventricular septal crest, the repair basically proceeds as in the case of an ostium primum defect with a cleft atrioventricular valve (see Fig. 10–4). The only addition to the procedure is that one or two pledgetted sutures may be required in the mid-portion of the crest of the ventricular septum to connect the tips of the left superior and inferior leaflet, thereby creating the base of the "cleft" and simultaneously closing the potentially small interventricular communication.

Complete Forms

In the complete form of the atrioventricular canal defect (Fig. 10–5), in addition to a common atrioventricular valve and ostium primum defect, there is a large interventricular communication under both the superior and inferior atrioventricular valve leaflets. Chordal attachments from the valve leaflets vary. They may attach to the crest of the ventricular septum or to the ipsilateral or contralateral ventricular cavities. The valve leaflet morphology also varies with regard to number, positioning, and degree of development of commissures. A single patch of autologous, glutaraldehyde-treated pericardium is preferable. The positions of the chordal attachments and commissures of the common atrioventricular valve do not change patch placement; however, these anatomic details may require that certain chordal attachments be severed and some leaflets incised to accurately place the patch. After the right atrium is opened, the leaflets are assessed by filling the ventricles with saline. The details of the coaptation of the superior and inferior leaflets overlying

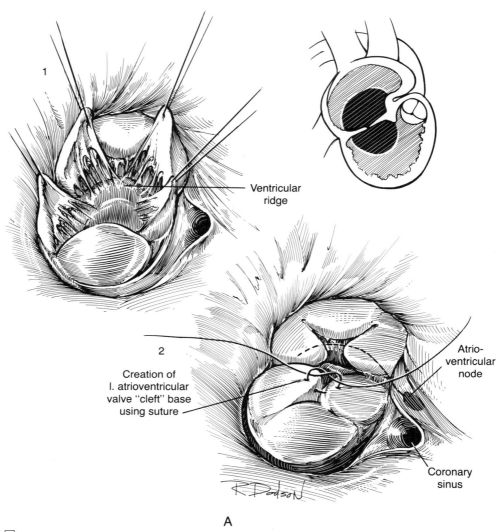

FIGURE 10–5. ☐

A, Morphology of the complete form of AV canal defect from several perspectives. This is the surgeon's view through a right atriotomy. Naturally occurring commissures overlie the ventricular septal crest. (1) Superior and inferior leaflets under tension to show crest of ventricular septum. (2) Leaflets in natural position with initial mitral "cleft" suture in place.

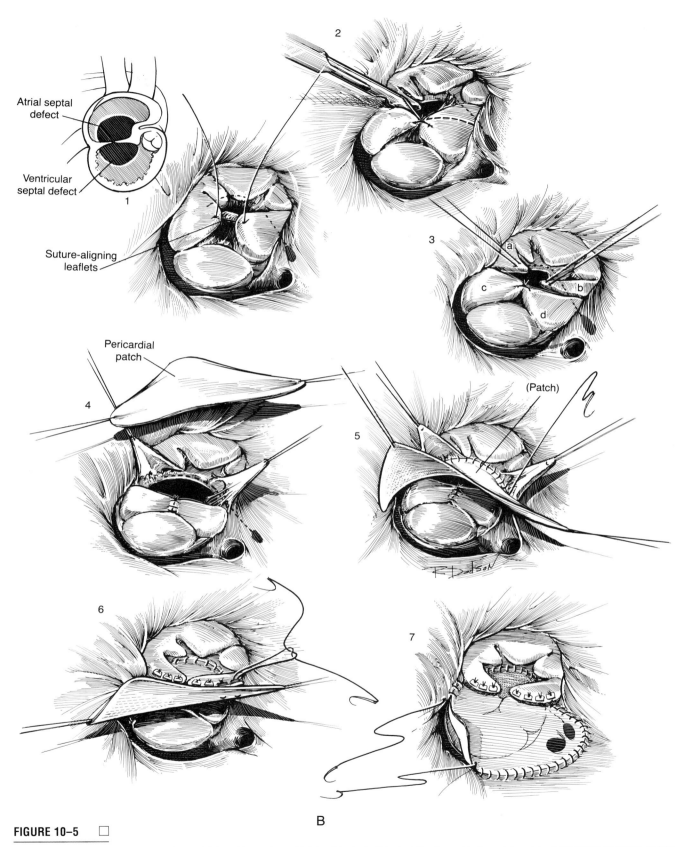

FIGURE 10–5 ☐

Continued. B, Morphology of a complete AV canal defect with superior and inferior AV valve leaflets straddling the ventricular septal crest. Leaflet incisions are shown, and the technique of single patch repair with closure of cleft is demonstrated. (1) Superior and inferior leaflets in natural position with suture placed to align cleft and leaflets. (2) Incisions in bridging leaflets. (3) Incised leaflets (a) right superior, (b) right inferior, (c) left superior, and (d) left inferior. (4) Exposure of ventricular septum. (5) Patch placed along crest of ventricular septum. (6) Attachment of leaflets to patch. (7) Completion of patch suture line in atrium.

the ventricular septal crest are studied, and a marking suture is placed to identify the point of creation of the base of the left atrioventricular valve "cleft," directly above the ventricular septal crest. This marking suture is critical, because it determines the point of partition of the common atrioventricular valve into left-sided and right-sided valves, and it also determines the alignment of the cleft.

At this point in the operation the "width" of the canal is measured precisely between the two points on opposite sides of the annulus where the ventricular septal crest approaches the atrioventricular groove. This measurement determines the width of the patch at the annular level. The patch width at this point is extremely important (Fig. 10–6). If it is too wide, there will be patch redundancy, essentially increasing the left atrioventricular valve annulus and potentially causing insufficient left atrioventricular valve tissue for the surface area of the orifice. This would promote regurgitation at the left atrioventricular valve. Conversely, if the left atrioventricular valve tissue is judged to be truly insufficient, then the patch width can be made more narrow, essentially accomplishing an annuloplasty. Caution must be exercised, however, because this can be overdone, causing tension on the patch and thereby increasing the likelihood of patch dehiscence. The positions of the valve commissures are also noted in relation to the crest of the ventricular septum. If superior and inferior commissures overlie the septal crest, leaflet incisions can be avoided. If valve leaflets bridge the crest, they must be incised

in a line parallel to and overlying the crest, with the incision extending to the annular level.

After these incisions are made, the crest of the interventricular septum is examined. If there is adequate exposure for placing the patch, all chordal attachments are preserved. If chordal attachments obscure the right side of the ventricular septal crest, the minimum number of chords necessary to adequately expose the septum are incised. Resuspension of the leaflets to the patch, performed later in the procedure, will provide the valve with the stability lost from these chordal transections; however, the general approach should be that every chord that is transected will potentially add to valve instability. The papillary muscle configuration of the left ventricle is also noted, primarily to identify the variant in which either a single papillary or two closely spaced papillary muscles are present.

The patch is first attached to the ventricular aspect of the defect just to the right side of the crest, beginning in the mid-portion of the ventricular septum just beneath the marking suture placed to create the base of the left-sided valve "cleft." The inferior and superior running suture lines continue along the septal crest until the annulus of the atrioventricular valve is reached. Some then reinforce the suture line with selectively placed, pledgetted interrupted sutures. The running sutures are then set aside under slight tension, while the leaflets are suspended from the patch. If no leaflet tissue has been cut, the patch can be sandwiched between naturally occurring commissures; the leaflet edges on

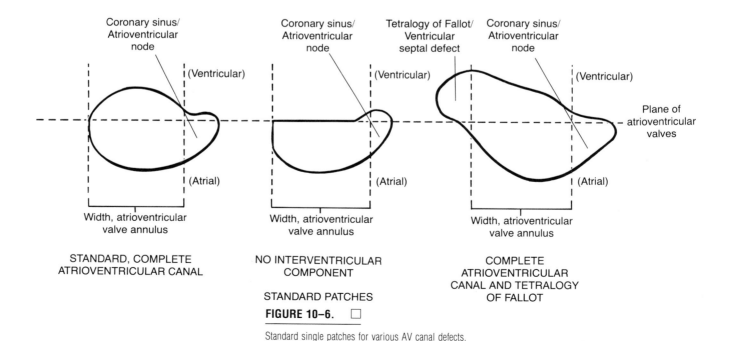

FIGURE 10–6. □

Standard single patches for various AV canal defects.

the left and right sides of the patch are then attached to the patch with interrupted plegetted sutures. If bridging leaflet tissue has been cut, the patch is situated between the cut leaflet edges, and the cut edges on both the left and right sides of the patch are attached to the patch. The leaflets must be attached to the patch at an appropriate patch depth so that valve competence is preserved. This depth can be judged by observing the leaflet level when chordal structures are under slight tension.

The left atrioventricular valve "cleft," which has been created by this leaflet reconstruction, is then closed as previously described. If a single left-sided papillary muscle or two closely spaced papillary muscles are present, the valve must be carefully assessed for the possibility of causing mitral stenosis with cleft closure.[12] The left atrioventricular valve is then tested by filling the left ventricle with saline, and any additional incompetence is managed as described previously for the cleft mitral valve. An incompetent valve after repair may be related to insufficient valve tissue, but this is not common. This view is supported by our experience, which indicates that valve insufficiency after repair is not associated with preoperative insufficiency.[16] In the great majority of cases, postrepair insufficiency occurs in patients whose atrioventricular valves were competent before repair. The appearance of "inadequate" valve tissue is usually related to (1) excessively rightward attachment of the patch in the right ventricle, (2) a patch that is too wide (redundant) or (3) failure to divide the superior or inferior leaflets sufficiently to the right ventricular side. The resultant central incompetence can be prevented or improved by the use of annuloplasty. When the rare patient with truly insufficient atrioventricular valve tissue is encountered, the only option may be placement of a left atrioventricular valve prosthesis.

The atrial aspect of the patch is then sutured as previously described for the ostium primum defect, with similar attention given to the coronary sinus and atrioventricular node. This is accomplished by continuing the running polypropylene sutures previously used to attach the patch in the ventricle.

Associated Lesions

Surgical management of associated cardiac defects, such as patent ductus arteriosus, aortic arch obstruction, secundum atrial septal defects, and muscular ventricular septal defects, is carried out as described in the chapters dealing with these lesions. Secundum atrial septal defects—and, occasionally, muscular ventricular septal defects—that are close to the main interventricular communication may be incorporated within the primary patch.

If the muscular ventricular septal defect is more anterior or apical, it must be addressed separately.

Obstruction of the left ventricular outflow tract associated with the atrioventricular canal defect is unusual, in spite of the narrowed and elongated left ventricular outflow tract that naturally occurs as part of this lesion. Left ventricular outflow tract obstruction with this defect can be caused by a number of lesions. Discrete subaortic membranes and excrescences of endocardial cushion tissue can be easily removed surgically. More problematic lesions include obstruction from functional atrioventricular valve tissue (leaflets, chords, or papillary muscle) and from tunnel-like stenosis. Obstruction from functional atrioventricular valve tissue may require excision and prosthetic replacement of the left atrioventricular valve. Tunnel stenosis is best addressed by performing an aortoventriculoplasty sparing the aortic valve, if possible. In the atrioventricular canal defect, this procedure does not run the risk of conduction injury. Single-ventricle reconstructions should be given due consideration in the most severe forms of these complex cases.

Occasionally, an accessory orifice of the left-sided atrioventricular valve is encountered. This lesion covers a wide morphologic spectrum. It may be small and insignificant, in which case it is of no consequence and should be left alone. More significant second orifices may be associated with a papillary muscle arrangement such that one papillary muscle is committed to each orifice, essentially causing a parachute of the primary orifice. The bridge of tissue between the two orifices should never be cut, as this results in unsupported valve tissue and regurgitation. If a single papillary muscle supports the primary orifice, the cleft should be carefully assessed. Complete closure of the cleft has the potential to produce stenosis.

Management of various associated conotruncal lesions may complicate the technique of repair.[37] In tetralogy of Fallot associated with the complete form of the atrioventricular canal defect, the shape of the single pericardial patch is somewhat modified compared with the patch used for the isolated defect (see Fig. 10–6). With this association the ostium primum defect may be small or adherent to the atrioventricular valve tissue, compromising exposure to the left side of the atrioventricular valve. A posterior incision in the atrial septum, extending into the ostium primum defect, is often helpful in improving exposure to the left-sided structures. The atrial aspect of the patch may need to be modified to account for this. The anterosuperior margin of the ventricular aspect of the patch must also be enlarged to account for the anterior extension of the interventricular defect and the malalignment of the conal septum. This part of the patch is sutured in place in continuity with the rest of the patch, allowing enough redundancy at the anterosuperior end of the ventricular portion of the patch so that flow from the left ventricle to the aorta is uncompromised. Most often in this condition the superior atrioventricular leaflet bridges the septal crest, and this leaflet must be incised. Incision of this leaflet should be carefully modified by making the incision to the tricuspid side of the usual incision to account for the deviation of the conoventricular septum. This will help avoid left ventricular outflow obstruction after placement of the patch. The entire rim of the subaortic extension of the interventricular communication (i.e., the tetralogy–ventricular septal defect component) may not be readily visible through the usual right atrial approach. This part of the ventricular suture line may be completed when the obstructive component of the defect in the right ventricular outflow tract is addressed through the typical longitudinal, infundibular, right ventricular outflow tract incision. The inferior aspect of the ventricular portion of the patch must also be given careful consideration. In this lesion the interventricular communication is often largely obliterated under the inferior atrioventricular valve leaflet, and therefore this part of the patch should be made quite shallow.

Surgical management of the right ventricular outflow tract obstruction is handled as described in Chapter 13 for isolated tetralogy of Fallot. However, the surgeon's judgment should lean significantly toward providing pulmonary valve competence, because in tetralogy of Fallot with an atrioventricular canal defect the tricuspid valve is already abnormal. Free pulmonary regurgitation may not be as well tolerated as it is in isolated tetralogy of Fallot. Residual right ventricular outflow obstruction, however, is also not acceptable. For the moderately to severely deformed right ventricular outflow tract, employing a valved conduit—preferably a cryopreserved allograft—should be given serious consideration.

Transposition of the great vessels associated with a well-balanced atrioventricular canal defect, although rare, is managed in the same manner used for isolated transposition of the great vessels. An arterial switch operation is performed when possible. Appropriate attention must be given to the anatomic details of the transposition, however, as described in Chapter 26 for isolated transposition of the great vessels.

Just as in isolated double-outlet right ventricle, the anatomic variability of double-outlet right ventricle associated with a well-balanced atrioventricular canal defect causes the decision-making process

for treatment of this lesion to be complex. (It should be noted, however, that the great majority of cases of double-outlet right ventricle and transposition of the great arteries are associated with unbalanced canal defects).[36] Double-outlet right ventricle with a subaortic ventricular septal defect is managed similarly to tetralogy of Fallot, whereas double-outlet right ventricle with morphologic features similar to transposition of the great vessels may be managed by an arterial switch operation. More intermediate forms of double-outlet right ventricle must be managed on an individual basis. The important consideration, however, is to determine by preoperative echocardiography and cardiac catheterization with angiography, and by inspection at surgery, whether the left ventricle can eject unobstructed to a normal-sized semilunar valve after the atrioventricular canal reconstruction is completed. If this is the case, the physician may consider a two-ventricle repair by taking one of several approaches: The approach may be similar to that for tetralogy of Fallot, except that more extensive modification of the patch is required so that the left ventricle is baffled to the aorta. It may involve an arterial switch operation with baffling of the left ventricle to the pulmonary artery, or it may involve an anastomosis from the main pulmonary artery to the aorta (as in the Damus-Kaye-Stansel procedure) with patch baffling of the left ventricle to the pulmonary valve or to both semilunar valves, with the addition of a conduit from the right ventricle to the pulmonary artery. Even with these complex conotruncal defects, the option of single-ventricle management is taken only if the canal defect is unbalanced or the left ventricle cannot be reliably aligned with either semilunar valve. Because the interventricular communication is frequently noncommitted in relation to both semilunar valves or because important chordal attachments are in the way, a Fontan operation may be necessary.

Postoperative Care

In general, postoperative management of atrioventricular canal defects follows the principles outlined for all surgically corrected cardiac defects in infants. Even in the best of circumstances, however, the atrioventricular valves in the repaired canal defects are not normal. During the first 24 hours postoperatively, cardiac function may be somewhat depressed, as it is in all cardiotomy patients. After repair of atrioventricular canal defects, it is important to treat patients aggressively with inotropic support in an attempt to avoid the elevated atrial filling pressures that occur with volume resuscita-

TABLE 10-1. ☐ ATRIOVENTRICULAR CANAL DEFECT REPAIRS NOT INVOLVING A VENTRICULAR COMPONENT (N = 258)

AGE (mo)	NUMBER*	1972–1976	1977–1981	1982–1986	1987–1991
0–12	36 (8)	5 (2)	6 (1)	12 (4)	13 (1)
13–24	25 (0)	1 (0)	3 (0)	13 (0)	8 (0)
>24	197 (2)				

*Numbers refer to cases; numbers in parentheses refer to deaths.

tion. Reliance on volume resuscitation may result in annular dilatation and atrioventricular valve regurgitation. Ideally, atrial filling pressures in the first 24 hours should be kept in the range of 5 to 10 mm Hg, with additional resuscitative efforts given in the form of inotropic support. Afterload reduction may also be particularly helpful in these patients.

Patients with associated trisomy 21 have a tendency to develop transient, relatively slow nodal rhythms postoperatively. This is usually a junctional escape rhythm secondary to sinus bradycardia. Atrioventricular conduction is not affected, and atrial level external pacing, using temporary wires, will capture the ventricles without difficulty. In the early postoperative course the nodal rhythm may be well tolerated; however, if augmentation of cardiac output is necessary, atrial pacing can accomplish this effectively by increasing the heart rate and adding effective atrial contraction.

RESULTS

During the period from 1972 to 1991, 719 patients with various forms of the atrioventricular canal defect have undergone surgical repair at Children's Hospital in Boston. This number includes only patients in whom two-ventricle reconstructions were performed.

As mentioned, from the perspective of morphology and surgical reconstruction, it is most instructive to view all atrioventricular canal defects along a continuous spectrum. For analysis of surgical outcome, however, patients were assigned to one of two large groups based on whether a ventricular septal defect was surgically addressed. In 258 of these patients there was either no interventricular communication or the existing one was considered so small that it was not surgically addressed. The other 461 patients had closure of an interventricular communication as a component of the repair. This categorical distinction is justified, because the pathophysiology, natural history, and optimal timing of surgery can all be dichotomized by the presence of a significant interventricular communication.

Forms Without Interventricular Communications

In the first group of 258 patients in which the interventricular septum was not surgically addressed, 197 were repaired after 2 years of age, reflecting the later presentation of patients with atrial septal defect physiology. Of the remaining 61 patients, 36 were repaired in infancy (0 to 12 months of life) and 25 between the ages of 1 and 2 years. Table 10–1 gives the short-term outcome (30 days or in hospital) of the 61 patients younger than 24 months of age at operation. Patients were categorized by age and date of surgery. There were two deaths among the 197 patients more than 2 years of age (1%). One patient had a significantly hypoplastic left ventricle; both patients had significant mitral regurgitation postoperatively that contributed to their death.

Of the patients who underwent surgery within the first year of life, either significant preoperative mitral regurgitation or associated lesions such as subaortic stenosis or aortic coarctation were present in a high percentage. Postoperative mitral valve insufficiency was an important factor in all of the deaths in this group, with reoperation for valve replacement or plasty a frequent occurrence among the patients who died. The outcome for infants with this complex defect has improved during the most recent 5-year period, as indicated in Table 10–1. Patients between 1 and 2 years of age at the time of surgery had less preoperative mitral regurgitation and fewer associated anomalies, as reflected in their later presentation and their better outcome.

A particularly high-risk lesion is the combination of a partial atrioventricular canal defect (no interventricular communication) associated with a hypoplastic aortic arch and coarctation, and a mildly hypoplastic left ventricle with either two closely spaced papillary muscles or a single papillary muscle. We have encountered this syndrome in six patients, five during infancy and one just over 2 years of age. Three of these patients have died, one has required multiple operations, and one has persistent significant mitral regurgitation because the cleft in the mitral valve could not be closed owing to a single left-sided papillary muscle. Long-term follow-up in the entire group of 258 patients has identified an additional three late deaths.

Forms With Interventricular Communications

During this 20-year period, of the 461 patients with atrioventricular canal defects who underwent operations that included closure of an interventric-

TABLE 10–2. ☐ REPAIR OF ATRIOVENTRICULAR CANAL DEFECT INVOLVING A VENTRICULAR COMPONENT* (N = 461)

AGE (mo)	1972–1976	1977–1981	1982–1986	1987–1991
0–6	6 (4)	26 (7)	48 (8)	70 (1)
7–12	7 (6)	37 (11)	59 (5)	66 (3)
13–24	3 (3)	10 (1)	22 (3)	4 (0)
>24	9 (3)	32 (1)	31 (1)	31 (5)

*Numbers refer to cases; numbers in parentheses refer to deaths.

ular communication, there were 62 early deaths (13.4%). A breakdown of these cases, however, as shown in Table 10–2, gives important insight into the changes in surgical approach and the improved results over time. The number of infant repairs has risen dramatically in successive 5-year intervals, while the mortality rate has decreased by an order of magnitude (from 25% to 2.9%) when the period before 1976 is compared with the period after 1987. For the interval from 1987 to 1991, the mortality rate in infants less than 6 months old was one in 70 (1.4%) and in infants between 7 and 12 months old, three in 66 (4.5%).

Table 10–3 shows other trends over the 20-year period that may have affected the improved outcome. The number of complex associated lesions has increased over time, reflecting an increasingly complex patient population; patent ductus arteriosus, patent foramen ovale, and secundum atrial septal defect, all of which occurred frequently, are excluded from these percentages. Table 10–4 shows the associated lesions addressed in this population. In spite of this trend toward more complex lesions, the percentage of primary repairs has increased and the need for reoperation has decreased over time. The indications for reoperation have primarily consisted of left atrioventricular valve insufficiency, residual ventricular septal defects, and complete heart block (pacemaker implantation). In more recent years, reoperation for residual ventricular septal defect and for pacemaker insertion has been essentially eliminated.[16] The reoperation rate for residual left atrioventricular valve regurgitation has also shown a decreasing trend; however, it has remained at about 7% in more recent years. Analysis of our results in infants indicates that the presence of double-orifice

left atrioventricular valve and significant perioperative residual regurgitation at the left atrioventricular valve are the only variables (of 46 variables examined) that are associated with perioperative death.[16] The use of pledgets to support delicate tissue, the selective use of left atrioventricular valve annuloplasty and of closure of the left atrioventricular valve cleft, and careful intraoperative assessment of the valve repair for residual regurgitation under direct vision have unquestionably contributed to these improved results. The remaining incidence of significant residual regurgitation at the left atrioventricular valve, although low, contributes substantially to the existing mortality. Further conceptual understanding of the structural and functional variations of the atrioventricular valve as they pertain to this lesion may be necessary before residual regurgitation at the left atrioventricular valve can be reduced to the very low incidence currently seen for other residual lesions. Improved understanding promises to allow continued refinement in the selection of various reconstructive techniques, such as varying the patch width to modify the size of the annulus, the use of annuloplasty, and management of the cleft in the left-sided atrioventricular valve.

Palliative procedures such as pulmonary artery banding or systemic-to-pulmonary artery shunting were performed only in highly selected patients with complex associated lesions (multiple ventricular septal defects, borderline hypoplastic ventricle, or uncorrectable conotruncal anomalies) or other complex problems at the time of presentation (e.g., sepsis with associated tracheoesophageal fistula). In addition, in more recent years, many of the patients with palliative procedures had undergone initial palliation at other institutions.

In the most recent 5-year period, the majority of patients with complex associated lesions underwent

TABLE 10–3. ☐ ATRIOVENTRICULAR CANAL DEFECT REQUIRING INTERVENTRICULAR REPAIR: TIME-RELATED TRENDS*

	1972–1976	1977–1981	1982–1986	1987–1991
Associated lesions	16%	22%	22%	39%
Primary complete repair	56%	81%	87%	88%
Reoperations	36%	21%	16%	9%

*Percentiles refer to percentage of all procedures performed during the specified time periods.

TABLE 10–4. ☐ ANOMALIES ASSOCIATED WITH ATRIOVENTRICULAR CANAL DEFECTS REQUIRING INTERVENTRICULAR REPAIR (N = 461)

LESION	NO.	%
Tetralogy of Fallot	36	8
Left superior vena cava	26	6
Ventricular septal defect	23	5
Polysplenia complex	11	2
Coarctation	9	2
Hypoplastic left ventricle	6	1
Hypoplastic right ventricle	5	1
Anomalous pulmonary venous return	5	1
Subaortic stenosis	3	1
Double-outlet right ventricle	3	1
D-transposition	3	1
Double-outlet mitral valve	3	1
L-transposition	2	<1
Interrupted aortic arch	1	<1

primary total repair. Of the 136 infants operated on in this time period, 41 (30%) had associated anomalies; however, only six (4%) underwent a pulmonary artery band or a systemic-to-pulmonary artery shunt. During the same period five patients with associated coarctation of the aorta underwent staged primary repair in which the coarctation repair was followed within a short period (i.e., several days) by the repair of the atrioventricular canal defect.

In our series of complete atrioventricular canals, we have encountered five patients who had prominent, double-orifice left atrioventricular valves. Three of these five patients died perioperatively, although none of them had left atrioventricular valve insufficiency or hemodynamics suggestive of severe stenosis. It may be that these patients had unrecognized associated left heart deficiencies that could have contributed to their demise, although this is only speculative.

Long-term follow-up was available in 217 of the 394 patients who were discharged from the hospital. There were seven (3.2%) late deaths in this group.

SUMMARY

The atrioventricular canal defect can occur in many forms. In the forms without a significant interventricular communication, elective repair should be performed within the first year of life. When mitral insufficiency or associated cardiovascular lesions cause symptoms early in life in this group, repair should be performed at the time of presentation. This symptomatic subgroup of infants with partial atrioventricular canal defects represents a high-risk population, as reflected in the relatively high mortality rates (see Table 10–1). An aggressive and committed approach to primary repair early in infancy has been taken in these cases, and the improved results from 1987 to 1991 support the validity of this approach. The mitral valve appears to be the critical issue in these cases. Preoperative mitral regurgitation or stenosis usually indicates a significant valve problem in these partial forms of the atrioventricular canal defect, and aggressive surgical management of the valve is critical to success. When preoperative mitral valve regurgitation is present, delaying the repair runs the risk of further degeneration of the valve, precluding acceptable valve reconstruction. The fact that medication can prevent serious congestive heart failure should not be used as an argument in favor of delaying reconstruction. When stenosis is present, careful management of the mitral cleft is critical.

Forms of the atrioventricular canal defect that include an interventricular communication should be electively repaired by 6 months of age, or as soon as significant symptoms develop. Management of left-sided atrioventricular valve tissue is critical to the outcome. The improvement in our most recent results is related to the elimination of residual defects (e.g., ventricular septal defects and heart block) and to improved left atrioventricular valve function in the postoperative period. Our most recent 5-year experience suggests that repair within the first 6 months of life may carry an added benefit when compared with repair between 6 months and 1 year (see Table 10–2). Palliative surgery should be reserved for the rare cases in which it is not clear whether a two-ventricle repair will be possible or in which cardiopulmonary bypass is temporarily contraindicated because of sepsis or associated medical problems.

Two areas remain in which further conceptual understanding of this defect will produce improved clinical outcome. First, the ongoing controversy over the best method of reconstruction of the left atrioventricular valve reflects a poor understanding of subtle variations in valve morphology. Both the cleft closure approach and the trifoliate approach clearly work in specific cases; they also fail in certain cases, reflecting poor selection of the reconstructive approach. In some patients who have deficient tissue, either method may fail. It is quite likely that most of the failures using either technique would have been avoided if a more appropriate reconstructive approach, based on appreciation of subtle morphologic criteria, had been taken. Until these factors are appreciated, our experience suggests that closure of the cleft is most likely to produce the least amount of morbidity. In the rare patient with truly dysplastic and deficient atrioventricular valve tissue, left-sided valve replacement should be undertaken primarily.

The second area involves an understanding of ventricular balance. Well-balanced defects and highly unbalanced defects present no problem; however, in more intermediate cases there are few proven guidelines for deciding between univentricular and biventricular reconstruction.

REFERENCES

1. Adams FH, Emmanouildes GC, Riemenschneider TA (eds). Moss' Heart Disease in Infants, Children, and Adolescents. 4th ed. Baltimore, Williams & Wilkins, 1990.
2. Barratt-Boyes BG. Correction of atrioventricular canal defects in infancy using profound hypothermia. In Barratt-Boyes BG, Neutze JM, Harris EA (eds). Heart Disease in Infancy: Diagnosis and Surgical Treatment. Edinburgh, Churchill Livingstone, 1973, p 110.
3. Bender HW Jr, Hammon JW JR, Hubbard SG, et al. Repair

of atrioventricular canal malformation in the first year of life. J Thorac Cardiovasc Surg 84:515, 1982.

4. Berger TJ, Blackstone EH, Kirklin JW, et al. Survival and probability of cure without and with operation in complete atrioventricular canal. Ann Thorac Surg 27:104, 1979.

5. Bharati S, Lev M. The spectrum of common atrioventricular orifice (canal). Am Heart J 86:533, 1973.

6. Bharati S, Lev M, McAllister HA Jr, et al. Surgical anatomy of the atrioventricular valve in the intermediate type of common atrioventricular orifice. J Thorac Cardiovasc Surg 79:884, 1980.

7. Carpentier A. Surgical anatomy and management of the mitral component of atrioventricular canal defects. In Anderson RH, Shinebourne EA (eds). Pediatric Cardiology. London, Churchill Livingstone, 1980, pp 477–490.

8. Castaneda AR, Mayer JE Jr, Jonas RA. Repair of complete atrioventricular canal in infancy. World J Surg 9:590, 1985.

9. Chi TL, Krovetz JL. The pulmonary vascular bed in children with Down's syndrome. J Pediatr 86:533, 1975.

10. Chin AJ, Keane JF, Norwood WI, et al. Repair of complete common atrioventricular canal in infancy. J Thorac Cardiovasc Surg 84:437, 1982.

11. Clapp S, Perry BL, Farooki ZQ, et al. Down's syndrome, complete atrioventricular canal, and pulmonary vascular obstructive disease. J Thorac Cardiovasc Surg 100:115, 1990.

12. David I, Castaneda AR, Van Praagh R. Potentially parachute mitral valve in common atrioventricular canal: Pathologic anatomy and surgical importance. J Thorac Cardiovasc Surg 84:178, 1982.

13. De Biase L, Di Ciommo V, Ballerini L, et al. Prevalence of left-sided obstructive lesions in patients with atrioventricular canal without Down's syndrome. J Thorac Cardiovasc Surg 91:467, 1986.

14. Fox LS. Optimal management of patients with complete atrioventricular septal defect. Clin Cardiol 12:145, 1989.

15. Frid C, Thoren C, Book K, et al. Repair of complete atrioventricular canal: 15 years experience. Scand J Thorac Cardiovasc Surg 25:101, 1991.

16. Hanley FL, Fenton K, Mayer JE, et al. Repair of atrioventricular canal defects in infancy: Twenty year trends. J Thorac Cardiovasc Surg 106:387, 1993.

17. Haworth SG. Pulmonary vascular bed in children with complete atrioventricular septal defect: Relation between structural and hemodynamic abnormalities. Am J Cardiol 57:833, 1986.

18. Kirklin JW, Daugherty GW, Burchell HB, et al. Repair of the partial form of persistent common atrioventricular canal: Ventricular communication. Ann Surg 142:858, 1955.

19. Laursen HB. Congenital heart disease in Down's syndrome. Br Heart J 8:32, 1976.

20. Lev M. The architecture of the conduction system in congenital heart disease. I. Common atrioventricular orifice. Arch Pathol 65:174, 1958.

21. Levy MJ, Cuello L, Tuna N, et al. Atrioventricularis communis. Clinical aspects and surgical treatment. Am J Cardiol 14:587, 1964.

22. Lillehei CW, Cohen M, Warden HE, et al. The direct vision intracardiac correction of congenital anomalies by controlled cross circulation: Results in thirty-two patients with ventricular septal defects, tetralogy of Fallot, and atrioventricularis communis defects. Surgery 38:11, 1955.

23. Maloney JV Jr, Marable SA, Mulder DG. The surgical treatment of common atrioventricular canal. J Thorac Cardiovasc Surg 43:84, 1962.

24. Marino B, Vairo U, Corno A, et al. Atrioventricular canal in Down syndrome. Prevalence of associated cardiac malformations compared with patients without Down syndrome. Am J Dis Child 144:1120, 1990.

25. Newfeld EA, Sher M, Paul MH, et al. Pulmonary vascular disease in complete atrioventricular canal defect. Am J Cardiol 39:721, 1977.

26. Piccoli GP, Ho SY, Wilkinson JL, et al. Left-sided obstructive lesions in atrioventricular septal defect. J Thorac Cardiovasc Surg 83:453, 1982.

27. Rastelli G, Kirklin JW, Titus JL. Anatomic observations on complete form of persistent common atrioventricular canal with special reference to atrioventricular valves. Mayo Clin Proc 41:296, 1966.

28. Rastelli GC, Ongley PA, Kirklin JW, et al. Surgical repair of complete form of persistent common atrioventricular canal. J Thorac Cardiovasc Surg 5:299, 1968.

29. Rastelli GC, Ongley PA, McGoon DC. Surgical repair of complete atrioventricular canal with anterior common leaflet undivided and unattached to ventricular septum. Mayo Clin Proc 44:335, 1969.

30. Rastelli GC, Weidman WH, Kirklin JW. Surgical repair of the partial form of persistent common atrioventricular canal, with special reference to the problem of mitral valve incompetence. Circulation 31,32(suppl I):I–:31, 1965.

31. Ross DA, Nanton M, Gillis DA, et al. Atrioventricular canal defects: Results of repair in the current era. J Cardiac Surg 6:367, 1991.

32. Sellers RD, Lillehei CW, Edwards JE. Subaortic stenosis caused by anomalies of the atrioventricular valves. J Thorac Cardiovasc Surg 48:289, 1964.

33. Silverman N, Levitsky S, Fisher E, et al. Efficacy of pulmonary artery banding in infants with complete atrioventricular canal. Circulation 68(suppl II):148, 1983.

34. Soudon P, Stijfns M, Tremouroux-Wattiez M, et al. Precocity of pulmonary vascular obstruction in Down's syndrome. Eur J Cardiol 2:473, 1975.

35. Van Mierop LHS, Alley RD, Kansel HW, et al. The anatomy and embryology of endocardial cushion defects. J Thorac Cardiovasc Surg 43:71, 1962.

36. Van Praagh S, Antoniadis S, Otero-Coto E, et al. Common atrioventricular canal with and without conotruncal malformations: An anatomic study of 251 postmortem cases. In Takao A, Nora JJ (eds). Congenital Heart Disease: Causes and Processes. Mount Kisco, NY, Futura Publishing, 1984, pp 599–639.

37. Vargas FJ, Coto ED, Mayer JE Jr, et al. Complete atrioventricular canal and tetralogy of Fallot: Surgical considerations. Ann Thorac Surg 42:258, 1986.

38. Wakai CS, Edwards JE. Pathologic study of persistent common atrioventricular canal. Am Heart J 56:779, 1958.

39. Watkins E Jr, Gross RE. Experiences with surgical repair of atrial septal defects. J Thorac Cardiovasc Surg 30:469, 1955.

40. Williams WH, Guyton RA, Michalik RE, et al. Individualized surgical management of complete atrioventricular canal. J Thorac Cardiovasc Surg 86:838, 1983.

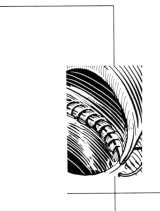

11 chapter

Ventricular Septal Defect

A ventricular septal defect (VSD) is a hole (or multiple holes) between the left and right ventricles. This chapter deals with VSD as an isolated lesion; VSDs associated with other congenital cardiac defects will be discussed separately. However, because closure of a VSD is the most commonly performed operation for congenital heart disease and the technical steps required are applicable to many different lesions, pertinent anatomic and technical aspects will be discussed in detail in this chapter.

ANATOMIC CLASSIFICATION

Because VSDs are almost exclusively closed from a right-sided approach, the landmarks of the right ventricular septal surface must be familiar to the surgeon. The following principal anatomic components of the right ventricular septum are shown in Figure 11–1:

1. The atrioventricular (AV) canal (Fig. 11–1A).
2. The muscular septum (or sinus septum) (Fig. 11–1B).
3. The septal band (proximal conal septum or trabecula septomarginalis) (Fig. 11–1C).
4. The conal septum (infundibular septum or parietal band) (Fig. 11–1D).

VSDs occur either within or between these four main ventricular septal components (Fig. 11–2).

Atrioventricular Canal Type Ventricular Septal Defect

In this variety (also called inlet septal defect), part or all of the septum of the AV canal is absent.

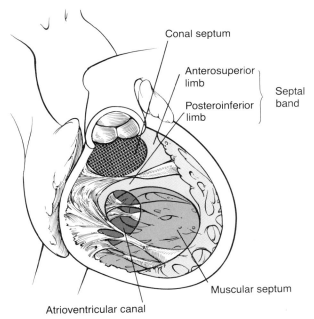

FIGURE 11–1. ☐

Schematic representation of the four principal components of the morphologic right ventricle: septum of the atrioventricular canal; muscular ventricular septum; septal band (trabecula septomarginalis) with anterosuperior and posteroinferior limbs; and conal septum.

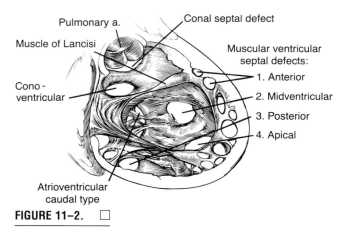

FIGURE 11–2. ☐

Classification of ventricular septal defects: ventricular septal defect, atrioventricular canal type; muscular ventricular septal defects—midventricular (1), apical (2), anterior (3), and posterior (4); conoventricular septal defect, which includes paramembranous and malalignment conoventricular septal defects; and conal septal defect.

The VSD lies beneath the tricuspid valve and is limited upstream by the tricuspid valve annulus, without intervening muscle (Fig. 11–2A).

Muscular Ventricular Septal Defects

A muscular defect is defined as one whose rim is totally made up of muscle (Fig. 11–2B). It can occur virtually anywhere in the trabecular portion of the septum. Midventricular defects often extend to or beyond the junction between the muscular septum and the septal band. From the right ventricular aspect these defects often seem multiple, as they are traversed by coarse trabeculae. When viewed through the left ventricle, they lie within the nontrabeculated or smooth portion of the ventricular septum and rarely exceed two or three in number. Muscular VSDs also may occur within the apical portion of the septum, lie anteriorly, be partially hidden behind the septal band, or be posterior and inferior to the tricuspid valve.

Conoventricular Septal Defects

Conoventricular septal defects are situated between the conal septum (Fig. 11–2C) and the ventricular septum, centered within the membranous septum. Conoventricular defects may be exclusively membranous, in which case both the conal and the ventricular septums are anatomically normal. However, these defects often extend beyond the confines of the membranous septum in anterior, inferior or superior positions; then they become paramembranous defects. The conal septum may be malaligned

anteriorly (as seen typically in conjunction with tetralogy of Fallot) or posteriorly (as is seen in conjunction with an interrupted aortic arch).

Most commonly, conoventricular defects abut the tricuspid valve annulus in the region where the septal and anterior tricuspid leaflets meet (anteroseptal commissure), immediately inferior to the infundibular septum and involving the area of the membranous ventricular septum. Usually the ventricular portion of the membranous septum is completely absent, in which case the VSD extends to the base of the noncoronary cusp of the aortic valve. The posteroinferior margin is then formed by the confluence of the septal and anterior leaflets of the tricuspid valve, the aortic valve, and the central fibrous body. Occasionally these defects may extend anteriorly into the area of the muscular septum, inferiorly into the area of the atrioventricular canal, or, as is the case in tetralogy of Fallot, superiorly because of associated hypoplasia of the infundibular septum. The medial papillary muscle (muscle of Lancisi) usually is located below the defect, and chordae from both the anterior and the septal leaflets of the tricuspid valve insert into it. In our experience, true aneurysms of the membranous septum are extremely rare. In most instances the radiologic image is created by a spinnaker-like anterior leaflet (or accessory leaflet) of the tricuspid valve that is fixed by chordae anchored to two or more quadrants of the VSD. In rare instances the anterior and septal leaflets of the tricuspid valve adhere to the edges of the conoventricular defect, forming a channel between the left ventricle and the right atrium. These so-called left ventricular-to-right atrial defects occur in less than 1% of conoventricular septal defects.

Conal Septal Defects

Conal septal defects (referred to also as *subpulmonary, supracristal,* or *outlet VSDs*) result from a defect within the conal septum (septal band or infundibular septum) (Fig. 11–2D). Characteristically, these defects are limited upstream by the pulmonary valve and are otherwise surrounded by muscle of the conal septum.

This classification of VSDs, proposed by Van Praagh et al.,[10] is useful for clear communication among surgeons, echocardiographers, angiographers, and radiologists. There are other useful classifications, but they will not be discussed here. There have been 427 infants with isolated VSD operated on since 1973 at Children's Hospital in Boston. The VSDs were single in 386 (90.4%) and multiple in 41 (9.6%). They were conoventricular in 337 cases (79%), muscular in 46 (11%), AV canal type in 26 (6%), and conal in 18 (4%). Thirty-nine patients (9.1%) had Down syndrome, 6 (1.4%) had duodenal atresia, 5 (1.2%) had cleft lip and another 5 patients had malformations of the central nervous system.

Atrioventricular Conduction Tissue

The atrioventricular node of Aschoff-Tawara occupies the apex of the triangle of Koch, which is limited by the ligament of Todaro posteriorly, the orifice of the coronary sinus inferiorly, and the tricuspid valve annulus superiorly (Fig. 11–3). The bundle of His originates from the AV node, penetrates the central fibrous body near the posteroinferior rim of the VSD, almost immediately traverses the septum, and then courses along the left ventricular aspect of the rim of the ventricular septum. The anterior and posterior left bundle branches spread along the left ventricular surface of the septum, while the right bundle branch travels back along the septum toward the right ventricular surface. At the anteroinferior border at the level of the muscle of Lancisi, the right bundle branch descends toward the right ventricular apex.

PATHOPHYSIOLOGY

The size of the VSD determines the initial pathophysiology of the disease. "Large" VSDs are the same size as or larger than the aortic valve orifice. They offer little or no resistance to flow and thus are often termed *nonrestrictive*. Consequently, right ventricular systolic pressure is equal to left ventricular pressure, and the pulmonary-to-systemic flow ratio (QP/QS) is inversely dependent on the ratio of pulmonary vascular resistance to systemic vascular resistance.

"Small" VSDs offer resistance to passage of flow across the defect, and therefore, right ventricular pressure is either normal or only minimally elevated and QP/QS rarely exceeds 1.5. These VSDs may be called *restrictive*.

"Moderate-sized" VSDs fall between these two groups; right ventricular systolic pressure is elevated, generally not exceeding half of left ventricular pressure, and QP/QS ranges between 2.5 and 3.0.

When there are multiple VSDs, the sum of the cross-sectional area of all defects determines the magnitude of QP/QS and the pressure difference across the septum.

During the first few weeks of life, it is rarely necessary to close an isolated VSD. However, as soon as the pulmonary vascular resistance decreases, the

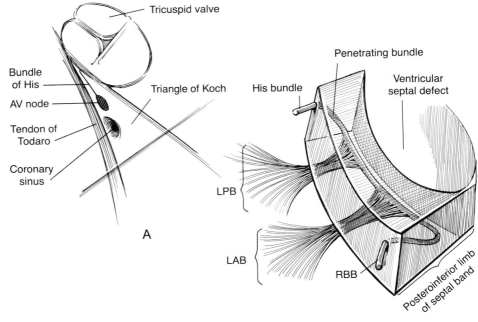

FIGURE 11–3. ☐

Schematic representation of the conduction system. *A,* The atrioventricular node lies embedded within the triangle of Koch, close to the orifice of the coronary sinus and between the annulus of the tricuspid valve and the tendon of Todaro. The bundle of His originates from the AV node, extends toward the commissure between the septal and anterior leaflets of the tricuspid valve, and *(B)* penetrates along the posteroinferior margin of the membranous septum and across the muscular ventricular septum, giving rise to the left posterior branch (LPB) and left anterior branch (LAB); the right bundle branch (RBB) then travels back along the ventricular septum toward the right ventricular septal surface. At the level of the muscle of Lancisi, the right bundle branch descends toward the right ventricular apex.

left-to-right shunt increases, and congestive heart failure may develop, requiring treatment. In some cases this includes closure of the VSD.

PREOPERATIVE EVALUATION AND MANAGEMENT

Previously, preoperative cardiac catheterization was necessary to (1) quantitate the left-to-right shunt, (2) measure pulmonary artery pressure, and (3) calculate pulmonary vascular resistance. A left ventricular cineangiogram can be useful to precisely define both the location and the number of VSDs. Two-dimensional echocardiography and color Doppler flow studies add substantially to the anatomic and functional diagnosis of VSDs. Reliable echocardiography has essentially supplanted preoperative cardiac catheterization in the infant with single or multiple VSDs, unless uncertainties remain about whether the VSD is restrictive and about pulmonary artery pressure and pulmonary vascular resistance.

INDICATIONS FOR SURGERY

Symptoms

Approximately 30% of infants with severe symptoms from VSDs require operation within the first year of life because of intractable congestive heart failure or, more commonly, failure to thrive. Because the majority of membranous and muscular VSDs tend to close spontaneously, surgical closure early in life is indicated only if the infant has failed aggressive medical management with digitalis and diuretics. In our experience spontaneous closure does not occur in infants with a large AV canal type VSD or a malalignment conoventricular defect, and therefore, closure at the time of first diagnosis is recommended for these patients, irrespective of age or weight.[2]

Older infants (<1 year) with VSDs and calculated pulmonary-to-systemic vascular resistance ratios greater than 0.7 are still considered surgical candidates because the likelihood that the elevated pulmonary vascular resistance reflects irreversible pulmonary vascular changes within the first year of life is extremely small. However, beyond infancy, a pulmonary-to-systemic vascular resistance ratio greater than 0.7 requires that a number of other criteria be met before the patient is considered for VSD closure.

An asymptomatic infant with a persistent VSD should undergo cardiac catheterization toward the end of the first year of life. The VSD should be closed at that time, if the pulmonary artery pressure exceeds half of the systemic pressure, to avoid development of irreversible pulmonary vascular disease. Early closure of VSDs should virtually eliminate the tragic development of irreversible pulmonary vascular obstructive disease.

Associated Lesions

Lesions in which the VSD is an intrinsic component of a more complex anomaly will not be discussed here. A large patent ductus arteriosus is present in about 25% of symptomatic neonates or infants with a VSD. A hemodynamically significant coarctation coexists in approximately 10% of cases. Other left-sided obstructive lesions are less common. For example, congenital mitral valve stenosis occurs in approximately 2% of patients with VSD, whereas congenital valvar or subvalvar aortic stenosis of hemodynamic importance is rarely seen within the first year of life.

The syndrome of aortic valve incompetence with a VSD is more common with conal septal defects than with conoventricular defects. It includes a congenital component (VSD) and an at least partially acquired lesion—namely, prolapse of the right, and occasionally noncoronary, aortic cusp. This syndrome is rare before 3 years of age and consequently will not be discussed further.

SURGICAL MANAGEMENT OF VENTRICULAR SEPTAL DEFECTS

Historical Note

In 1952, Muller and Dammann[6] described banding of the pulmonary artery for palliation of VSDs. This procedure is designed to prevent the development of pulmonary vascular obstructive disease and also to decrease left-to-right shunting and consequent left-sided volume overload. During the 1950s and 1960s, pulmonary artery banding was favored over primary closure of VSDs because of the lower mortality and morbidity. Now, because of improved cardiopulmonary bypass techniques (including deep hypothermia with or without circulatory arrest) and advances in intensive care of neonates and infants, primary closure of the VSD is favored in most specialized centers. Closure of a VSD was achieved for the first time in 1954 by Lillehei and associates[4] at the University of Minnesota, utilizing controlled cross circulation between the child and the parent. Between 1954 and 1955, 27 patients had VSDs closed by this method; 19 survived. Five of the first eight patients were infants; three of these five survived the operation. Kirklin and associates[3] at the Mayo Clinic first closed a VSD using a heart-lung machine in 1955. Transatrial closure was reported by Stirling and coworkers in 1958.[9] Routine closure of VSDs in infants, using profound hypothermia and total circulatory arrest with rewarming by a pump oxygenator, was first reported by Okamoto in 1969.[7] In 1969, Barratt-Boyes et al.[1] popularized primary repair in symptomatic infants with the use of deep hypothermia and circulatory arrest along with cooling and rewarming on cardiopulmonary bypass.

Operative Technique

Closure of Conoventricular Septal Defects

Preferably, all isolated conoventricular septal defects, AV canal type VSDs, and most muscular VSDs are repaired through the right atrium. In infants weighing less than 8 kg, we prefer to use deep hypothermia to 18°C (rectal temperature) and total circulatory arrest (see Chapter 2). Cardiopulmonary bypass and hypothermia at low flow with direct cannulation of the superior and inferior venae cavae is an alternative technique unless the infant weighs less than approximately 2.5 kg. Air can enter the systemic circulation through a patent ductus arteriosus (even if it is small enough not to be identified at cardiac catheterization) when the right side of the heart is opened; therefore, the ductus arteriosus is routinely ligated immediately after the patient is placed on cardiopulmonary bypass (see Chapter 12).

During the early phase of cooling, and with a decompressed heart, exposure of the ductus is facilitated. First the main pulmonary artery is retracted caudally, and the ductus, the pulmonary artery, and the undersurface of the aortic arch are cleared of pericardial and adventitial tissue. If it is large, the ductus is divided between ligatures; if it is small, the ductus is closed with a single ligature. The importance of visualizing the left pulmonary artery and the aortic arch cannot be overstated. Unfortunately there are instances in which patients have had inadvertent ligation of the distal left pulmonary artery and, even more disastrously, ligation of the distal aortic arch.

After circulatory arrest has been established and cardioplegic solution has been delivered (see Chapter 2), the right atrium is opened from the inferior vena cava toward the atrial appendage to avoid the area of the sinus node or its blood supply (Fig. 11–4A). After retracting the septal and anterior leaflets of the tricuspid valve, adequate exposure is achieved (Fig. 11–4B). The entire circumference of the defect must be readily visible. Commonly, the posteroinferior margin of the VSD lies hidden behind the commissure separating the septal and anterior leaflets of the tricuspid valve. The chordal attachments responsible for the poor exposure can be cut at the base of their insertion into the papillary muscle, allowing reflection of the leaflet posteriorly. They are reattached to the papillary muscle once the VSD is closed. The challenge is to close the VSD completely and, at the same time, avoid damage to the conduction system. Pledgetted, interrupted, nonabsorbable 5-0 or 6-0 suture material is used in neonates and infants. The first suture is placed into the mid-portion of the ventricular septal crest approximately 3 mm from the rim of the defect (Fig. 11–4C[1]). Each subsequent suture aids in exposing the margin of the defect.

When the septal leaflet of the tricuspid valve is reached, this leaflet is retracted anteriorly and caudally, and one or two sutures are placed underneath the leaflet, taking shallow bites of the septum (Fig. 11–4C[2,3]). At the point where the leaflet fuses with the crest of the VSD, sutures (Fig. 11–4C[4,5]) are placed within the fibrous tissue formed by this confluence. Because conduction tissue is composed of specialized muscle cells, fibrous tissue offers a safe area to place sutures. The use of Teflon pledgets permits more superficial placement of sutures to decrease the risk of encircling and damaging the bundle of His and the left bundle branches and to reduce the risk of suture line disruption (Fig. 11–4D). As a rule, there is little tissue separating the aortic valve from the posterosuperior margin of the defect. Therefore, to ensure secure closure of this potentially deficient area and also to avoid damage to the aortic valve cusps, three or four sutures are placed from the right atrial side through the tricuspid valve annulus, simultaneously retracting the anterior leaflet of the tricuspid valve while guiding the passage of the needle through the rim of the defect (Fig. 11–4C[6,7,8]). Infusion of small amounts of cardioplegic solution will fill the aortic root and allow accurate delineation of the insertion of the aortic valve cusps to prevent injury. Within the remaining anterosuperior rim of the defect, deeper bites can be taken without concern for injury to conduction tissue. All sutures are then passed through an appropriately tailored (slightly larger than the defect) Dacron patch and tied in place (Fig. 11–4E). If the curtain of chordae is so dense as to severely hinder complete and safe closure of the VSD, it is useful to incise the tricuspid valve along the base of the septal and anterior leaflets (Fig. 11–4F). By reflecting the incised leaflets anteriorly, satisfactory exposure of the posteroinferior rim is obtained.

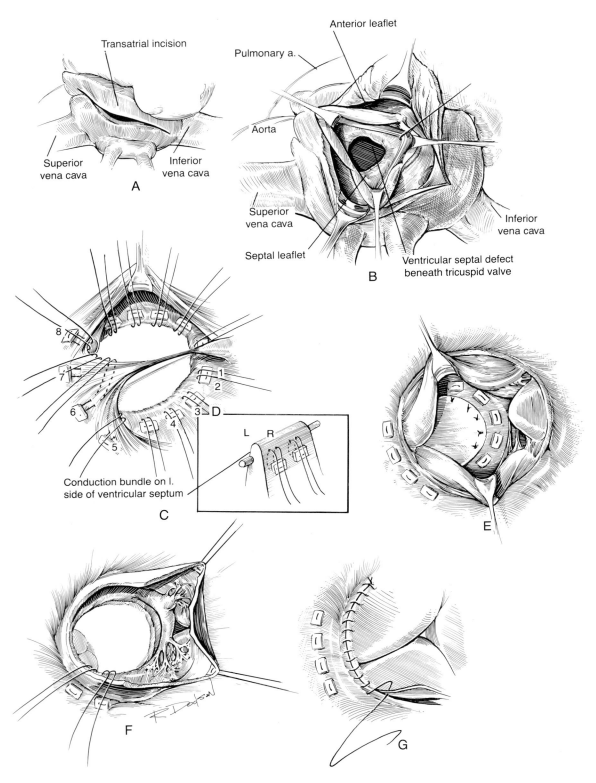

FIGURE 11–4. ☐

Trans–right atrial exposure of conoventricular VSD: *A*, Incision in the right atrium. *B*, Exposure of conoventricular VSD with retraction of the anterior and septal leaflets of the tricuspid valve. *C*, Sutures 1, 2, 3, and 4 are placed within the ventricular septal wall, approximately 3 mm from the rim of the defect. *D*, Suture 5 is placed where the leaflet fuses with the crest of the VSD, and sutures 6, 7, and 8 are passed from the right atrial side through the tricuspid annulus; the remainder of the sutures are placed within the anterosuperior rim of the VSD. *E*, Completed closure of the VSD with a Dacron patch and pledgetted sutures. *F*, If chordae and papillary muscles obliterate the view of the VSD, the septal and anterior leaflets of the tricuspid valve are incised along the base, permitting complete exposure of the VSD. *G*, Septal and anterior leaflets of the tricuspid valve resutured after closure of the VSD with a patch.

After closure of this VSD, the septal band and anterior leaflet of the tricuspid valve are resutured (Fig. 11–4*G*).

Closure of Atrioventricular Canal Type Ventricular Septal Defect

The AV canal type VSD lies beneath the septal leaflet of the tricuspid valve and extends to the tricuspid valve annulus (Fig. 11–5*A*). In general, it can be adequately exposed, without incising the septal leaflet of the tricuspid valve, by simply retracting the valve leaflet and the chordae (Fig. 11–5*B*). To close this defect effectively, a continuous suture technique is sometimes preferred, as it allows weaving in and out between the various chordae and papillary muscles (Fig. 11–5*C*). The first suture is placed within the base of the mid-portion of the septal leaflet of the tricuspid valve and is carried as a continuous horizontal mattress suture (within the

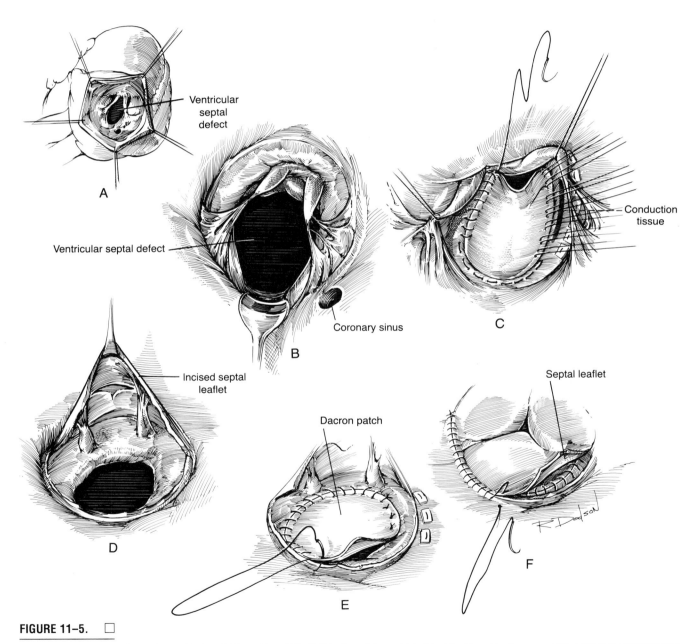

FIGURE 11–5.   ☐

Closure of AV canal type VSD. *A*, Transatrial view of AV canal type VSD. *B*, Retraction of the septal leaflet of the tricuspid valve exposes the defect to the tricuspid valve annulus. *C*, Closure of AV canal defect with the continuous suture technique. (Note the continuous horizontal mattress suture within the septal leaflet tissue and also the interrupted horizontal mattress sutures along the posteroinferior portion of the VSD, placed approximately 4 mm from the VSD to avoid damage of the conduction bundle.) *D*, If dense chordae obstruct the view of the defect, the septal leaflet of the tricuspid valve is incised along its base, providing exposure of the entire circumference of the AV canal type VSD. *E*, Patch closure of the AV canal type VSD. *F*, The incised leaflet of the tricuspid valve is reattached with continuous suture.

valve leaflet tissue), starting toward the superior rim of the defect. In this area, sutures can be placed without concern for the conduction tissue, as the bundle of His and its branches follow a posteroinferior course. To avoid damage to the His bundle and the right bundle branch while attaching the patch to the posteroinferior portion of the VSD, the four to five interrupted, pledgetted stitches are placed approximately 4 mm from the edge of the VSD. If an excessive number of chordae obstruct the view of the VSD and interfere with exposure and adequate closure, it is preferable to incise the leaflet along the base of the septal and anterior leaflets (Fig. 11–5D). After reflecting the incised valve anteriorly, complete exposure of the entire rim of the AV canal type VSD is obtained. The patch is then sewn in place according to the technique discussed earlier (Fig. 11–5E). The incised leaflets are reattached with a continuous 6-0 polypropylene suture (Fig. 11–5F).

Closure of Conal Septal Defects

When not associated with other anomalies, the conal septal defect or subpulmonary VSD can be approached through the right ventricle or through the pulmonary artery and valve. If this VSD is part of a more complex anomaly, such as truncus arteriosus, the conal septal VSD can be closed through a conventional ventriculotomy or, in case of transposition of the great arteries, through the aortic valve.

Transventricular Approach. Excellent exposure of the defect is obtained through a longitudinal infundibulotomy (Fig. 11–6A). Commonly, there is no intervening muscle between the superior edge of the defect and the pulmonary valve. Instead, a narrow, fibrous rim separates the pulmonary valve anteriorly from the aortic valve posteriorly. To avoid injury to one of the aortic leaflets, it is useful to fill the ascending aorta with blood or cardioplegic solution; this aids greatly in defining the cusps and placing the sutures. The initial sutures are placed within the fibrous rim separating the two semilunar valves (Fig. 11–6B). This is the only critical part of the operation, as the remainder of the rim of the VSD is infundibular septum and thus is distant from the conduction tissue. (The conduction tissue travels caudally between the infundibular and trabecular ventricular septum.) Occasionally the area between the aorta and the pulmonary cusps is too tenuous to support sutures. In this case, interrupted pledgetted mattress sutures are passed within the right and left pulmonary sinuses (Fig. 11–6C). The Dacron patch is anchored with a continuous suture to the remainder of the VSD (Fig. 11–6D).

Transarterial Closure. The pulmonary artery is incised transversely just above the valve commis-

sures, and the anterior pulmonary valve cusp is retracted, exposing the defect, which is characteristically located underneath the right and left pulmonary cusps. Interrupted mattress sutures reinforced with Teflon pledgets are placed from within the right and left pulmonary sinuses to close the upstream portion of the VSD. The remainder of the defect is closed using a continuous suture technique.

Closure of Muscular Ventricular Septal Defects

A muscular ventricular septal defect can exist (1) as a single defect, (2) with other muscular defects, or (3) in association with other types of VSDs such as a conoventricular or AV canal type. The location of muscular defects varies and includes the sinus portion of the ventricular septum. These so-called "mid-muscular defects" can be close to the AV valve but are always separated from the tricuspid annulus by muscle. Single and multiple mid-muscular defects can also be found at the junction between the muscular septum and the septal band. A cluster of muscular defects in the midventricular septum is, by preference, closed through the right atrium with a single patch (Fig. 11–7A). Because of the friability of the muscle and the many trabeculations within the right-sided surface of the ventricular septum, we prefer interrupted horizontal mattress sutures reinforced with Teflon pledgets, which allow a more secure anchoring of the stitches (Fig. 11–7B). When conoventricular and midmuscular ventricular septal defects coexist (Fig. 11–8A), the conduction bundle may traverse the bar of muscle separating both defects. Therefore, stitches within this muscle bar must be avoided, and a single patch is used instead (Fig. 11–8B).

Because the coarse multiple trabeculations in the region of the apex of the right ventricular septum make exposure difficult through the right side, closure of these apical defects was performed through a left ventricular apical incision, parallel to the left anterior and posterior descending coronary arteries, until 1988. When examined from the left ventricular surface, these seemingly multiple defects usually appear as a single or, maximally, as two or three distinct orifices easily recognizable within the smooth surface of the left ventricular septal surface. However, because left ventricular global dyskinesia, large apical aneurysms, or significant residual left-to-right shunts (>2:1) have been observed at late follow-up in 54% of patients who received left ventriculotomies, percutaneous transcatheter closure of apical ventricular septal defects has been carried out in the cardiac catheterization laboratory since 1988,[5] thus avoiding a left ventricular incision. In smaller infants, in whom percutaneous access is im-

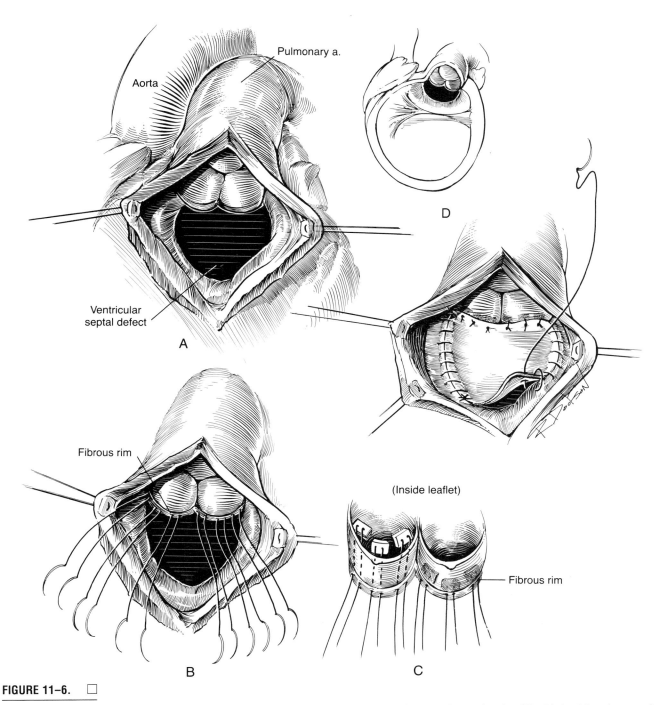

Aorta

Pulmonary a.

Ventricular
septal defect

A

D

Fibrous rim

B

(Inside leaflet)

Fibrous rim

C

FIGURE 11–6. ☐

Transventricular approach for closure of a conal septal defect. *A*, Commonly there is no intervening muscle between the superior edge of the defect and the pulmonary valve. *B*, Initial sutures placed within the fibrous rim separating the two semilunar valves. *C*, If the area between the aorta and the pulmonary cusps is tenuous, interrupted pledgetted mattress sutures are passed within the right and left pulmonary sinuses. *D*, The Dacron patch is anchored to the remainder of the VSD with a continuous suture.

possible, the umbrella device has been placed under direct vision in the operating room at the time of surgical closure of other more surgically accessible defects (see Chapter 7). This technique, using a modified double umbrella, has proven extremely effective in closing not only apical muscular defects,

but also multiple muscular defects partially hidden behind the septal band.

Anterior muscular defects, most commonly found as additional defects associated with tetralogy of Fallot, are best approached through a right ventriculotomy (Fig. 11–9A). Occasionally they are difficult

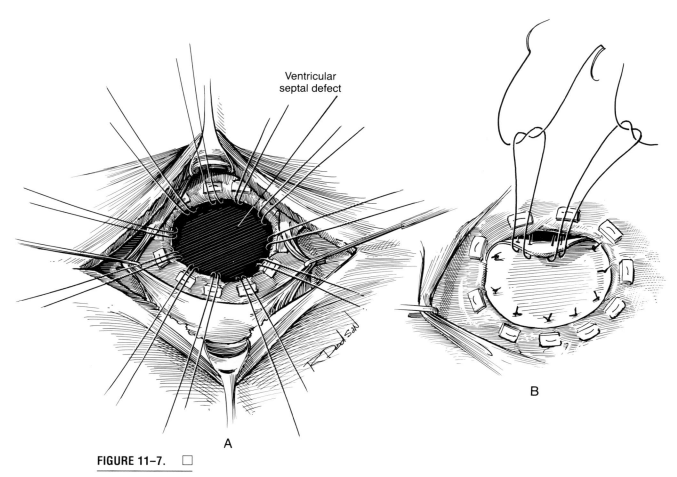

FIGURE 11–7. ☐

Transatrial closure of a midmuscular VSD. *A,* The defect is rimmed with pledgetted stitches. *B,* The VSD is closed with a patch.

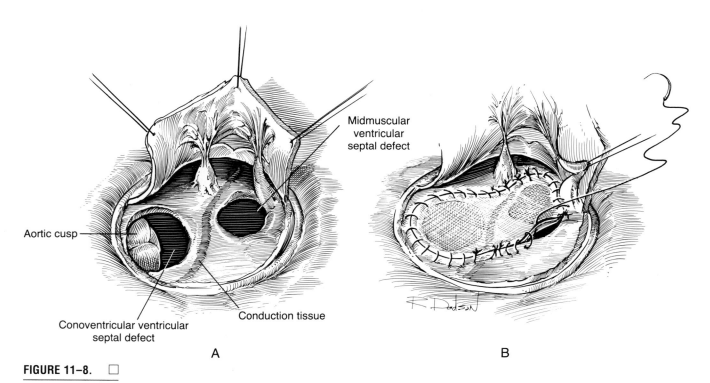

FIGURE 11–8. ☐

Transatrial closure of multiple VSDs (conoventricular and midmuscular). *A,* The septal and anterior leaflets of the tricuspid valve are incised parallel to the tricuspid valve annulus, allowing complete exposure of the conoventricular and midmuscular VSDs. *B,* A single patch is used to close both defects.

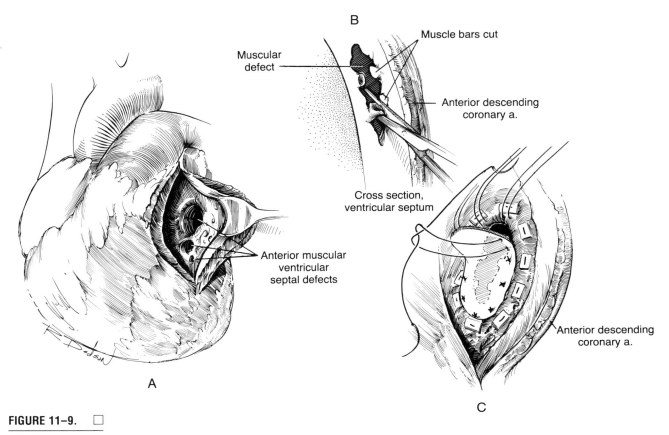

FIGURE 11–9. ☐

Transventricular exposure of anterior muscular VSDs. *A,* Approach through a right ventriculotomy. *B,* Division of muscle bundles binding the septal band to the free right ventricular wall to expose the entire VSD. (Note the anterior descending coronary artery coursing immediately anterior to the defect.) *C,* Interrupted horizontal mattress sutures reinforced with Teflon pledgets rim the anterior VSD and are placed through a Dacron patch used to close the defect.

to find, because they can be partially hidden behind the septal band and heavy trabeculae. It is important to divide the muscle bundles binding the septal band to the free right ventricular wall to expose the entire VSD (Fig. 11–9*B*). When placing interrupted horizontal mattress sutures reinforced with Teflon pledgets along the anterior margin of the defect, the surgeon must avoid deep sutures, which can distort or occlude the anterior descending coronary artery. Although occasionally it is tempting to close this defect primarily, a patch should always be used, as disruption of a primary suture line is fairly common when the heart starts to contract (Fig. 11–9*C*). At Children's Hospital in Boston, we do not favor closure of this defect by compression sutures brought through the anterior ventricular wall because distortion of the left anterior descending coronary artery is difficult to avoid with this technique.

Posterior and inferior muscular VSDs are best approached through the right atrium and tricuspid valve. These defects usually are partially hidden behind the posterior leaflet of the tricuspid valve. If a posterior muscular VSD coexists with an AV canal type VSD, the separating bar of muscle may carry

the conduction tissue. Therefore, a single patch should be used to close both defects. Otherwise, interrupted horizontal mattress sutures reinforced with Teflon pledgets are placed around the rim of the defect. A patch is routinely used to secure complete closure.

MANAGEMENT OF VENTRICULAR SEPTAL DEFECT WITH ASSOCIATED ANOMALIES

Ventricular Septal Defect and Coarctation of the Aorta

A large VSD and a coexisting severe coarctation usually cause severe symptoms early in infancy. In the past, management of these combined lesions included (1) initial repair of the coarctation alone, (2) coarctation repair and simultaneous banding of the pulmonary artery, or (3) VSD closure alone. At Children's Hospital in Boston, the protocol for many years was coarctation repair and simultaneous banding of the pulmonary artery. Subsequently this changed to coarctation repair of the aorta alone as the initial operation and, if symptoms persisted, early (same hospitalization) closure of the VSD. However, after gaining more experience with primary repair of interrupted aortic arch and also with the first-stage palliative procedure for aortic atresia, we have become more adept at dealing with the distal aortic arch, isthmus, and descending thoracic aorta through a midline incision. Consequently, we currently favor simultaneous repair of both the coarctation and a large VSD that is judged to be unlikely to close spontaneously. The technique of coarctation repair through a midline sternotomy is described in Chapter 21. For smaller VSDs, a clinical decision is made as to the significance of the VSD. If it appears that a pulmonary artery band would otherwise be necessary, simultaneous VSD closure is then undertaken. On the other hand, if the VSD appears restrictive and has a reasonable potential to close spontaneously, we consider coarctation repair only. The location of the VSD also plays a role in this decision. An AV canal type VSD or a large malaligned conoventricular VSD will (in our experience) not close spontaneously, whereas muscular VSDs are much more likely to do so.

EARLY RESULTS

Hospital Mortality

From January 1973 through December 1990, the hospital mortality rate for infants after repair of 427 VSDs not associated with other anomalies was 2.3% (10 of 427) (Table 11–1). There were no hospital or late deaths in 161 infants operated on from January 1984 through December 1990. Before that time, five of 337 infants (1.4%) died after repair of conoventricular VSDs, three of 46 (6.5%) after muscular (single or multiple) VSD closure, two of 18 (11.1%) after conal VSD, and none of 26 after repair of AV canal type VSD.[8] The hospital mortality rate for single VSDs was 1.8% (seven of 386) and for multiple VSDs, 7.3% (three of 41). The hospital mortality rate for neonates was initially higher (9%), but very

young age has been virtually eliminated as a risk factor since the late 1980s. Neither preoperative hemodynamics nor results of lung biopsy proved predictive of outcome in the infant group. Hospital mortality tended to be highest among infants with pre-existing respiratory problems or with hemodynamically significant residual lesions postoperatively.[11]

Pre-, Intra-, and Postoperative Causes of Mortality

Preoperative respiratory problems contributed significantly to the death of four patients. Three patients required preoperative intubation for pneumonia. The third infant with pneumonia also had a urinary tract infection. Despite preoperative antibiotic therapy, blood cultures revealed a generalized gram-negative sepsis. The fourth patient had episodes of severe bronchospasm preoperatively and required chronic ventilatory support postoperatively. Eventually, laryngeal polyps were demonstrated and successfully excised. Nonetheless, the patient died. None of the survivors required preoperative intubation, and none were known to have had preoperative pneumonia. In two infants preoperatively unrecognized additional lesions contributed to mortality. One had multiple ventricular septal defects that were unsuspected preoperatively and required a second operation for closure of a conal VSD. The other patient had a double-orifice mitral valve and a small left ventricle that had not been recognized preoperatively.

One 2-month-old infant suffered a laceration of a pulmonary vein at the time of left atrial line placement, this required a separate right thoracotomy to achieve hemostasis. The patient died 6 hours postoperatively. Another 2-month-old infant had an uncontrollable junctional tachycardia with a heart rate of up to 240 beats per minute; he died with low cardiac output 3 days after surgery. Two infants who appeared to be in relatively good health preoperatively died suddenly and unexpectedly on the second

TABLE 11–1. ☐ HOSPITAL AND LATE MORTALITY AFTER PRIMARY CLOSURE OF VSDs DURING INFANCY (JANUARY 1973 THROUGH DECEMBER 1990)

AGE AT OPERATION (months)	1973–1990			1984–1990		
	No. Patients	Hospital Mortality	Late Mortality	No. Patients	Hospital Mortality	Late Mortality
0–1	22	2 (9.0%)	0	7	0	0
2–3	83	2 (2.4%)	0	37	0	0
4–6	126	3 (2.3%)	1 (0.8%)	47	0	0
7–12	196	3 (1.5%)	2 (1%)	70	0	0
TOTAL	427	10 (2.3%)	3 (0.7%)	161	0	0

and third day after surgery. No cause of death was identified.

Late Deaths

Three patients (0.7%) died after discharge from the hospital. Two of the deaths were sudden and unexpected, suggesting an arrhythmic event. One of the two patients, 4 months old at the time of operation, died 6 weeks after the VSD closure. He had electrocardiographic evidence of an anterolateral myocardial infarction. The third late death occurred in a patient in whom a double-chambered right ventricle and complete heart block developed 5 years after successful closure of a conoventricular VSD. This patient died at another institution during surgery to relieve the right ventricular outflow obstruction and implant a pacemaker.

POSTOPERATIVE FINDINGS

Electrocardiography

The most typical preoperative findings were right axis deviation and biventricular hypertrophy. In 17% of the patients, there was a superior frontal plane axis, and one patient had congenital complete heart block preoperatively. Postoperatively, complete right bundle branch block developed in 62% of the patients. Nine percent of the infants had bifascicular block (complete right bundle branch block and left axis deviation) that was not present preoperatively. In two infants, complete heart block developed in the operating room, while in a third, complete heart block developed late postoperatively. All three infants had conoventricular VSDs; one had a conoventricular VSD combined with a midmuscular defect.

Complete right bundle branch block appears to be well tolerated in the short term by infants and children, although long-term implications of its presence await future clarification. Surgically induced bifascicular block has been suggested as a risk factor for sudden death after repair of tetralogy of Fallot and, more recently, after VSD closure as well. However, during a follow-up period of 275 patient-months, none of the patients with acquired bifascicular block in this series died or showed symptoms.

Lung Biopsy

Lung biopsy specimens were obtained from 49 patients. Pulmonary vascular abnormalities were identified in all tissue samples. Twenty-nine percent showed a reduction in the number of arterioles (morphometric grade C) with or without intimal proliferation (Heath-Edwards grade II). The calculated preoperative pulmonary vascular resistance in patients with grade B changes was not significantly different from that in patients with grade C changes. Four patients with grade C changes underwent cardiac catheterization 1 year after the operation, and none had elevated pulmonary vascular resistance.

These findings suggest that the morphometric technique for grading lung histology does not have strong predictive value for the assessment of hemodynamically significant pulmonary vascular changes in infants with VSD. Importantly, none of the infants was found to have Heath-Edwards changes beyond grade II.

Neurologic Complications

Transient abnormalities were recognized in 14 patients (5%). Twelve had generalized seizures postoperatively, one had a transient left hemiparesis, and one had irritability and hypertonia. No patient had a persistent neurologic deficit that was not present before surgery.

LATE HEMODYNAMIC MEASUREMENTS AND CATHETERIZATION FINDINGS

Pulmonary Artery Pressure and Pulmonary Resistance

Preoperatively, the mean pulmonary artery pressure was higher than 40 mm Hg in 96% of patients. Of the 148 patients who had 24-hour postoperative measurements, 51% continued to have elevated pulmonary artery pressures. Postoperative catheterization studies taken 1 year later showed that mean pulmonary artery pressure in this group of patients had decreased to a mean of 14 mm Hg (Fig. 11–10). There were only two infants who had values greater than 25 mm Hg; both had residual shunts with a PQ/PS greater than 2:1. Of the 148 patients in whom preoperative pulmonary resistance was calculated, only 30% had a value greater than 3.0 Wood units. At follow-up catheterization 1 year later, only three patients had residual, mildly elevated pulmonary vascular resistance; two of these were the patients with large residual VSDs (Fig. 11–11). The third patient had elevated pulmonary artery pressure and pulmonary vascular resistance that, became normal when he breathed 100% oxygen.

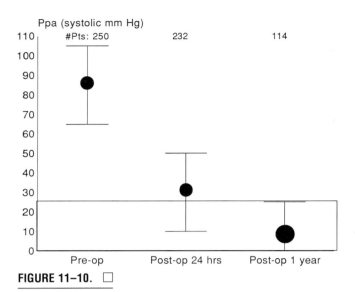

FIGURE 11–10. ☐

Early and late postoperative changes in pulmonary artery pressure after closure of VSDs in infants.

Intracardiac Shunt

Of the 148 infants who underwent cardiac catheterization 1 year after surgery, the VSD was found to be completely or virtually closed in 146 (98%). Two infants had residual shunts with a QP/QS greater than 2:1. Both patients underwent subsequent surgical repair.

Aortic regurgitation developed in four patients postoperatively. In two, the murmur of aortic regurgitation appeared immediately, while in the other two, murmurs became audible several months after surgery. However, angiographically, aortic regurgitation was severe in only one patient and mild in the other three.

Double-chambered right ventricle, which was identified after VSD closure, developed in four patients. In two, subaortic stenosis developed, with peak systolic ejection gradients of 62 and 30 mm Hg, respectively. One has undergone resection of a discrete subaortic membrane. Three patients were found to have coarctation of the aorta that had not been apparent preoperatively. One infant had a partial anomalous pulmonary venous connection to the right atrium that was not recognized before the postoperative cardiac catheterization.

At late follow-up, with the exception of patients who had either residual lesions or newly acquired intracardiac or extracardiac pathology (i.e. subaortic stenosis, coarctation, or double-chambered right ventricle), none had any cardiovascular symptoms.

Eleven patients remained below the third percentile for weight after 18 months of age. Seven of these had hemodynamically significant residual lesions:

severe aortic regurgitation (one), moderate subaortic stenosis (one), partial anomalous pulmonary venous connection (one), and a residual left-to-right shunt (three); the seventh patient had multiple congenital anomalies, including seizures and motor retardation, that had been recognized before operation. The remaining four children had no recognizable abnormalities.

IMPLICATIONS

Primary surgical closure of VSDs during the first year of life is a low-risk and effective option for most symptomatic infants. Infants with preoperative respiratory complications or hemodynamically significant residual lesions have higher mortality and morbidity rates. However, invasive and noninvasive diagnostic techniques have improved greatly over the years. Additional lesions that are undiagnosed preoperatively have become exceedingly rare. After successful VSD closure, the majority of infants demonstrate a prompt reduction in pulmonary artery pressure and relief of symptoms. Early VSD closure in infancy prevents the development of irreversible pulmonary vascular obstructive disease. The incidence of surgically induced complete heart block or complete right bundle branch block is not higher among infants than that reported after surgery in older patients. Successful VSD closure in the first year of life can be expected to result in near-normal growth and development and, hopefully, a normal life expectancy.

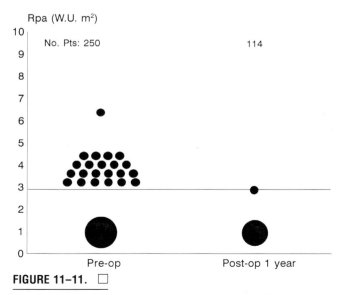

FIGURE 11–11. ☐

Changes in pulmonary vascular resistance 1 year after closure of VSDs in infants.

REFERENCES

1. Barratt-Boyes BG, Simpson M, Neutze JM. Intracardiac surgery in neonates and infants using deep hypothermia with surface cooling and limited cardiopulmonary bypass. Circulation 43(suppl I):25, 1971.
2. Castaneda AR, Lamberti J, Sade RM, et al. Open heart surgery during the first three months of life. J Thorac Cardiovasc Surg 68:719, 1974.
3. Kirklin JW, Harshbarger HG, Donald DE, et al. Surgical correction of ventricular septal defect: Anatomic and technical considerations. J Thorac Surg 33:45, 1957.
4. Lillehei CW, Cohen M, Warden HE, et al. The results of direct vision closure of ventricular septal defects in eight patients by means of controlled cross circulation. Surg Gynecol Obstet 101:446, 1955.
5. Lock JE, Block PC, McKay RG, et al. Transcatheter closure of ventricular septal defects. Circulation 78:361, 1988.
6. Muller WH Jr, Dammann JF Jr. The treatment of certain congenital malformations of the heart by the creation of pulmonic stenosis to reduce pulmonary hypertension and excessive pulmonary blood flow: A preliminary report. Surg Gynecol Obstet 95:213, 1952.
7. Okamoto Y. Clinical studies for open heart surgery in infants with profound hypothermia. Arch Jpn Chir 38:188, 1969.
8. Rein JG, Freed MD, Norwood WI, et al. Early and late results of closure of ventricular septal defect in infancy. Ann Thorac Surg 24:19, 1977.
9. Stirling GR, Stanley PH, Lillehei CW. The effects of cardiac bypass and ventriculotomy upon right ventricular function with report of successful closure of ventricular septal defect by use of atriotomy. Surg Forum 8:433, 1958.
10. Van Praagh R, Geva T, Kreutzer J. Ventricular septal defects: How shall we describe, name and classify them? J Am Coll Cardiol 14:1298, 1989.
11. Yeager SB, Freed MD, Keane JF, et al. Primary surgical closure of ventricular septal defect in the first year of life: Results in 128 infants. J Am Coll Cardiol 3:1269, 1984.

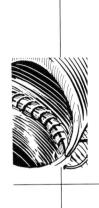

12

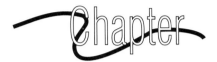

Patent Ductus Arteriosus

Patent ductus arteriosus is the persistence in post-natal life of the normal fetal vascular conduit that connects the central pulmonary and systemic arterial systems.

This lesion can be thought of as occurring in four distinct clinical forms: as an isolated cardiovascular lesion in otherwise healthy infants and children; as an isolated cardiovascular lesion in premature infants; as a relatively incidental finding associated with more significant structural cardiovascular defects; and as a critical compensatory structure in many forms of cyanotic or left-sided obstructive lesions.

This chapter will deal with patent ductus arteriosus in the first three forms; the last form is covered in the chapters that deal specifically with the primary cyanotic or obstructive lesions. When it occurs as an isolated lesion in an otherwise healthy patient, patent ductus arteriosus is among the simplest of all congenital cardiovascular anomalies to correct; however, it may increase considerably the complexity of a number of clinical situations (for example, the clinical management of the premature infant and the interpretation of physiologic data in patients with more complex heart disease).

ANATOMY

Developmental Considerations

Fetal cardiovascular development has an important impact on the configuration of the postnatal ductus arteriosus. The ductus is derived from the distal aspect of the embryologic left sixth arch. In a normal fetal cardiovascular system, ductal flow is considerable (about 60% of the combined ventricular output[21]) and is directed exclusively from the pulmonary artery to the aorta. Therefore, the ductus is equal in width to the descending aorta and appears as a smooth and direct extension of the main pulmonary artery into the descending aorta. As a result the proximal angle of the insertion of the ductus into the aorta is sharp, and the distal angle of insertion is obtuse.[3, 35] In essence the ductus runs almost parallel to the isthmus as it approaches the aorta. When intrauterine ductal flow is exclusively in the right-to-left direction (i.e., normal), it is not unusual for duct-like vascular cells to inhabit the wall of the isthmus and the aorta beyond the site of the ductal insertion. Postnatally, these cells may contribute to the formation of aortic coarctation. This normal configuration of the ductus arteriosus is usually preserved, but it may be further exaggerated when associated left-sided obstructive anomalies (e.g., aortic coarctation, interrupted arch, the hypoplastic left heart syndrome, and aortic or subaortic stenosis) are present.

If severe right-sided, obstructive cardiovascular lesions are present in utero, the configuration of the ductus arteriosus may be much more variable.[37] In fact the ductus arteriosus can be completely absent (as in tetralogy of Fallot with absence of the pulmonary valve and in some forms of simple tetralogy of

Fallot, tetralogy of Fallot with pulmonary atresia, and truncus arteriosus). In these cases the normal parallel circuitry of the fetal left and right ventricles is preserved by the large ventricular septal defect. Commonly, however, the ductus is present. In the fetus the blood flows exclusively from the aorta to the pulmonary artery; the volume is relatively small, as blood is supplied only to the high-resistance, pulmonary vascular bed (5% to 10% of the combined ventricular output). As a result the ductus is often smaller than the descending aorta, arises more proximally on the undersurface of the aortic arch, and forms an obtuse proximal angle and a sharp distal angle at its aortic insertion.[3, 35] In addition, when intrauterine ductal blood flow is exclusively left to right (i.e., abnormal), ductal vascular cells can be found in the pulmonary artery beyond the true site of ductal insertion. These cells may contribute to coarctation of the pulmonary artery in the postnatal period as the duct constricts.

Morphologic Features

The ductus arteriosus is a tube of specialized vascular tissue that connects the central pulmonary arterial system to the central systemic arterial system. The sites of the anatomic connection to the great vessels are usually quite consistent; however, some variability can exist. Typically the ductus arteriosus arises as a continuation of the main pulmonary artery or from the proximal portion of the left pulmonary artery. It then connects to the descending aorta just distal to the origin of the left subclavian artery, defining the distal end of the aortic isthmus. This is the exclusive configuration in the infant with an otherwise normal cardiovascular system. The pulmonary end of the ductus arteriosus is intrapericardial, and the aortic end is extrapericardial. The left recurrent laryngeal nerve is slung around the aortic end of the ductus just outside the pericardial reflection.

When other cardiovascular anomalies are present, variations in the length, orientation, origin, and insertion of the ductus arteriosus may occur. For a systemic-to–pulmonary artery connection to be considered a patent ductus arteriosus, it must contain the typical histologic structure of the vessel wall, it must arise centrally from the main, left, or right pulmonary artery, and it must insert into the systemic arterial system at the level of the transverse arch, proximal arch vessels, or aortic isthmus. In some forms of complex heart disease, it may be difficult to distinguish between a true ductus arteriosus and a large, central, systemic-to–pulmonary artery collateral vessel if histologic proof is not

available. The ductus arteriosus is almost always a left-sided structure; however, right-sided and bilateral ductus can also occur, usually in association with aortic arch anomalies.

The histologic structure of the ductus arteriosus is unique in the arterial system. The wall thickness of the ductus is similar to that of the aorta and pulmonary artery in the neonate, and there is a relatively intact internal elastic lamina. The media is deficient in elastic fibers and consists of layers of muscle cells arranged in a somewhat disorganized spiral pattern rather than in circumferential or longitudinal patterns. The intima of the ductus is thicker than that of the nearby aorta or pulmonary artery and holds an increased complement of mucoid substance.[14, 16, 17]

PATHOPHYSIOLOGY

Fetal and Transitional

Locally produced and circulating prostaglandin $E_2(PGE_2)$ and prostaglandin $I_2(PGI_2)$[5, 6, 8, 9] induce active relaxation of the ductal musculature, maintaining maximal patency during the fetal period. This allows the ductus to carry the major portion of the high volume of blood required by the low-resistance placenta. At birth, increased pulmonary blood flow metabolizes these prostaglandin products, and absence of the placenta removes an important source of them. Consequently there is a marked decrease in these substances, which actively relax the ductus arteriosus. In addition, circulating vasoconstrictive substances may be produced at the time of, and shortly after, birth.[28, 31]

However, the most important stimulus to ductal closure at birth is the increase in partial pressure of oxygen in the blood circulating through the ductus.[28, 31] The constriction of the smooth muscle within the ductus leads to functional closure as the thickened intima bulges into the lumen. In the great majority of term infants, this occurs within the first 24 hours after birth. Over the next several weeks, degeneration and fibrosis of the subintimal layers result in fibrosis and permanent closure.[14] In preterm infants the immature ductal tissue is much less reactive to oxygen, and postnatal ductal closure is less likely to occur.

The role of prostaglandins in both patency and closure of the ductus arteriosus forms the basis for the clinical use of exogenous prostaglandin $E_1(PGE_1)$ to prolong ductal patency postnatally in certain forms of cyanotic congenital heart disease and left-sided obstructive lesions and also for the use of indomethacin to effect ductal closure in premature infants with patent ductus arteriosus.

Postnatal

After birth, in an otherwise normal cardiovascular system, a patent ductus arteriosus results in an arterial level left-to-right shunt as pulmonary vascular resistance drops. Because the lumen of the patent ductus arteriosus varies and the structure also has length, the degree of resistance to flow varies. However, unrestrictive flow commonly occurs, with the size of the shunt then determined by the relative resistances in the pulmonary and systemic circulations. As a general rule, the shunt will increase over the first month or two after birth, as pulmonary vascular resistance naturally falls.

The hemodynamic consequences of an unrestrictive ductal shunt are left ventricular volume overload, elevated left atrial pressure, increased left pulmonary artery pressure, right ventricular pressure overload, and pulmonary edema. These changes result in increased sympathetic discharge, tachycardia, and tachypnea and lead to ventricular hypertrophy. The diastolic shunt results in lower aortic diastolic pressure and the potential for myocardial ischemia and underperfusion of other systemic organs, while the increased left atrial pressure and pulmonary blood flow may lead to pulmonary edema with a resultant increase in the work of breathing and a decrease in respiratory gas exchange. Unrestrictive flow through a patent ductus can lead to pulmonary vascular obstructive disease within the first year of life. These changes will be significantly attenuated if the size of the ductus arteriosus is only moderate and completely absent if the ductus is small.

Patent ductus arteriosus in the premature infant deserves special comment. With advancing fetal maturity, the vasoconstricting effect of oxygen on the ductus becomes more prominent, and the dilating effect of prostaglandins becomes less effective in preparation for the transition at birth to an "in-series" circuitry of the left and right ventricles; therefore, it is no surprise that patent ductus arteriosus is much more common in premature infants.[6, 28] In addition, two common therapeutic maneuvers in premature infants (mechanical ventilation and the use of furosemide) are both associated with increased production of circulating PGE_2 and its metabolites.[8, 18] It has been estimated that the ductus is patent in as many as 45% of infants with birth weights less than 1750 gm and 80% with birth weights less than 1200 gm.[20] Because many of these premature infants have accompanying severe

lung disease in the form of the respiratory distress syndrome secondary to ineffective surfactant production, elevated pulmonary vascular resistance may be present, and the degree of left-to-right shunting may be variable. The use of surfactant to treat the respiratory distress syndrome in premature infants has been shown to improve the lung disease, cause a decrease in pulmonary vascular resistance, and unmask the presence of a patent ductus arteriosus.[7] It is often difficult to separate the symptoms of a patent ductus arteriosus from those of primary lung disease in this patient population.

In addition to exacerbating underlying parenchymal disease of the lungs, the hemodynamic consequences of a patent ductus arteriosus (retrograde descending aortic flow to the pulmonary runoff) may also promote renal failure, induce intestinal ischemia (precipitating necrotizing enterocolitis), promote intracerebral problems, and affect function of the diaphragmatic muscles.[1, 24, 29, 39] Chronic lung disease (bronchopulmonary dysplasia) commonly develops in premature patients treated with aggressive ventilator support for a combination of primary lung disease and patent ductus arteriosus.

NATURAL HISTORY

The incidence of patent ductus arteriosus is approximately one in every 200 births[30]; however, the incidence increases markedly with increasing prematurity. The estimated death rate for infants with isolated, untreated patent ductus arteriosus is approximately 30%.[4] The leading cause of death is congestive heart failure, with respiratory infection as a secondary cause. Endocarditis is more likely to occur with a small patent ductus and is rarely fatal if aggressive antibiotic treatment is instituted. In contrast to premature infants, in whom spontaneous closure of a persistently patent ductus arteriosus frequently occurs as maturation continues postnatally, spontaneous closure of a persistently patent ductus arteriosus in term infants is not common.[6] This is because each of the appropriate closures in the term infant is not maturation-related but indicates an intrinsic abnormality of ductal responsiveness. Delayed spontaneous closure may occasionally occur in term infants in the first several months of life but is thought to be unusual after this time. In term infants, patent ductus arteriosus is more common in females than in males and is associated with maternal contraction of the rubella virus during the first trimester.[20]

In otherwise normal infants, if the patent ductus is small, hemodynamic manifestations are minimal, and the only finding may be a typical murmur on physical examination. With a moderate patent ductus, signs and symptoms of congestive heart failure are often seen, and these progress over the first three months of life. After this, compensatory mechanisms may improve the patient's clinical status and a condition of compensated congestive heart failure may develop. With a large patent ductus, an unrestrictive, arterial level, left-to-right shunt is produced, and severe congestive heart failure develops. This can result in death if no treatment is given.[4] However, some patients do manage to compensate enough to survive. Elevated pulmonary vascular resistance can develop by as early as 6 months of life, reducing the shunt and improving the clinical status. The pulmonary vascular resistance may progress to systemic levels within the first year of life, followed by the development of Eisenmenger's physiology.[20]

DIAGNOSIS

The diagnosis of a large patent ductus arteriosus is often suggested by a physical examination that reveals a combination of all of the nonspecific findings associated with any large left-to-right shunt and, in addition, a wide pulse pressure and a systolic murmur that may extend slightly into diastole.[20] The electrocardiogram is nonspecific, suggesting left ventricular strain and hypertrophy, left atrial enlargement, and possibly right ventricular hypertrophy. The chest radiograph is typical of any large right-to-left shunt, with the additional subtlety of an enlarged ascending aorta. Echocardiography can reliably document the patency of the ductus with color mapping, and evaluation of left-sided cardiac chamber sizes and the flow characteristics of blood in the aorta beyond the ductus can provide an estimate of the size of the shunt. Cardiac catheterization is rarely indicated for infants and is contraindicated for premature infants. In unusual cases in late infancy in which markedly elevated pulmonary vascular resistance is suggested (either by minimal shunting in the presence of a physically large patent ductus arteriosus or by differential cyanosis of the lower body if ductal flow becomes right to left), cardiac catheterization may be necessary to assess the status of the pulmonary vasculature.

With a moderate-size patent ductus, the physical findings of left-to-right shunting and congestive heart failure may be somewhat attenuated, and the classic loud, continuous murmur will be present. Electrocardiograms and chest radiographs are less distinctive, but the echocardiogram is usually definitive. A small patent ductus arteriosus may be detected only by the typical murmur. Electrocardio-

grams and chest radiograms are normal; echocardiography will document the patency of the ductus.

When cardiac catheterization is necessary to define the status of the pulmonary vasculature, caution must be exercised, as oximetry data may give unreliable information when attempts are made to calculate the magnitude of the shunt because of streaming and preferential ductal flow to one or the other pulmonary arteries.[36]

The differential diagnosis of patent ductus arteriosus in the neonate and infant includes truncus arteriosus, aortopulmonary window, origin of the left or right pulmonary artery from the aorta, peripheral pulmonary stenosis, venous hum, and a centrally positioned arteriovenous malformation. Echocardiography can distinguish patent ductus arteriosus from these lesions quite reliably.

INDICATIONS FOR MANAGEMENT

In term infants, because the likelihood of spontaneous closure of a large patent ductus arteriosus is extremely small after the first several weeks of life, intervention to accomplish physical closure is recommended once the diagnosis is established. If symptoms are present, the procedure should be performed immediately. If no symptoms are present, elective closure should be planned within 3 months.

In premature infants, early closure of patent ductus arteriosus has been shown to be beneficial[11, 27, 40]; therefore, aggressive intervention (initially pharmacologic with indomethacin, if no contraindications are present) is indicated as soon as the diagnosis is made. Because premature infants with patent ductus arteriosus often have multisystem problems, especially primary pulmonary disease, signs and symptoms that are present can often not be attributed to the patent ductus arteriosus with certainty. It has been recommended that echocardiographic screening of all high-risk premature infants (i.e., those with respiratory distress syndrome and very low birth weight) be performed to document the presence of a patent ductus arteriosus and that aggressive treatment with indomethacin be administered if patency is documented.[13, 40]

TREATMENT

Historical Perspective

In 1938, Gross performed the first successful surgical procedure for a congenital heart defect when he ligated a patent ductus arteriosus in a child.[19] After this Gross recommended division and oversewing of both ends of the ductus. In 1946, Blalock described the triple ligation technique currently used commonly in infants.[2] In 1963, DeCanq reported the repair of a patent ductus in a premature infant weighing 1400 gm.[12] Surgery provided the only definitive therapy for patent ductus arteriosus in premature infants until 1976, when Heymann introduced the clinical use of indomethacin (after extensive laboratory investigation) to close a patent ductus arteriosus pharmacologically.[22]

Management of Isolated Patent Ductus Arteriosus in Term Infants

In the term infant, indomethacin and other medical maneuvers are not effective forms of therapy; therefore, some form of mechanical closure is necessary (Fig. 12–1). Previously, the exclusive approach was surgical ligation, but current forms of therapy involve transluminal placement of various occlusive devices, such as umbrellas or clamshell devices[33, 34, 38] (see Chapter 7). The transluminal approach, however, is not applicable in young infants, as the peripheral vascular injuries probably outweigh the morbidity of traditional direct closure using a thoracotomy. Videoassisted thoracoscopic occlusion, using metal clips,[25] has also been described but has been performed in only a small number of patients. Its usefulness will be judged in comparison with the technique of thoracotomy and ligation.

The standard surgical approach to the patent ductus arteriosus is through a left thoracotomy. The patient is placed in the right lateral decubitus position. An incision is made in the skin just inferior to the lower tip of the left scapula and is extended both anteriorly and posteriorly with upward concavity. The latissimus dorsi and anterior serratus muscles are incised, and the thoracic cavity is entered through the fourth intercostal space. After placement of a rib retractor, the superior portion of the left lung is gently retracted anteriorly and inferiorly to expose the mediastinum. The vagus and phrenic nerves are identified, and the pleura overlying the aortic isthmus is incised longitudinally posteriorly and parallel to the vagus nerve, directly overlying the isthmus and descending aorta. In infants, exposure of the ductus arteriosus is not greatly improved by controlling the immobilized pleural edges with stay sutures; however, this is optional.

Using careful dissection, either with electrocautery or with dissecting instruments, the area is exposed until the aortic isthmus, descending aorta, distal aortic arch, left subclavian artery, ductus arteriosus, and recurrent laryngeal nerve coursing around the ductus are clearly identified. The ductus

is then exposed over most of its length and a right angle clamp used to bluntly clear a circumferential space around the structure. The patent ductus is then triply ligated. Monofilament permanent suture ligatures (size 4-0 or 5-0) are placed at both the aortic and pulmonary ends of the ductus, inserting the needle very superficially in the adventitia at several intervals circumferentially, just enough to hold the sutures in place. These sutures are then tied in sequence to ligate the ductus, taking care not to tie so tightly that the delicate and friable ductal tissue is disrupted. These ligatures then leave a central mass of ductal tissue. A heavy braided ligature (size 2-0) is then used to ligate the central portion of the ductus. This heavy ligature may be tied more tightly, as the lumen has already been obliterated, and the heavy material is less likely to cut the ductal tissue. This triple ligation technique serves several purposes: it minimizes ductal recanalization, which can occur with a simple ligature; it eliminates the use of vascular clamps on the ductus; and it avoids the need for division of the ductus, thereby minimizing bleeding complications. Occasionally a short, broad patent ductus arteriosus is encountered, although this is rare in infants. If the width of the structure approaches its length, division between specially designed Potts patent ductus clamps should be performed. This is followed by oversewing both the aortic and pulmonary arterial ends of the ductus.

Management of Isolated Patent Ductus Arteriosus in Premature Infants

The treatment for premature infants is more complex than for term infants (Fig. 12–2). Traditionally, these infants were treated with a course of supportive therapy that included blood transfusion to provide red cell mass and adult hemoglobin, nutritional support, volume restriction, diuretic therapy, inotropic support, afterload reduction, and pulmonary management, which often included ventilator support. If this failed to adequately support the infant until the natural maturing process closed the ductus, surgical ligation was performed. After the introduction of indomethacin in 1976, several multicenter trials were carried out to test various medical protocols. However, none of these protocols included a primary treatment arm using surgical ligation. In aggregate, the 1-year follow-up results of these trials failed to show any convincing advantage for either primary traditional medical management with indomethacin or surgical backup or primary use of indomethacin with traditional medical management.[15, 32] Short-term results suggested a

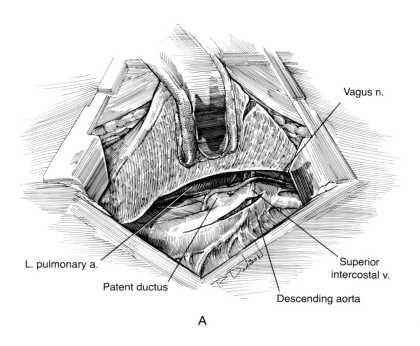

Vagus n.

L. pulmonary a.

Patent ductus

Superior
intercostal v.

Descending aorta

A

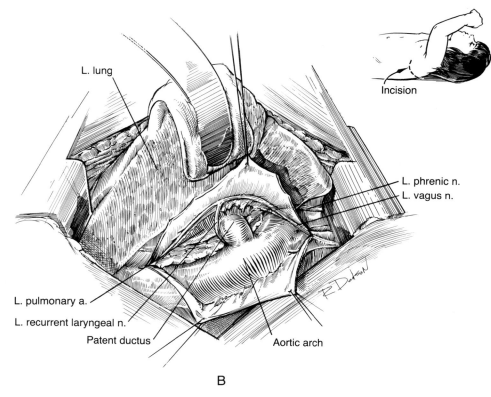

L. lung

Incision

L. phrenic n.
L. vagus n.

L. pulmonary a.

L. recurrent laryngeal n.

Patent ductus

Aortic arch

B

FIGURE 12–1.   ☐

A, Surgeon's perspective of infant patent ductus arteriosus (PDA) exposed via a left thoracotomy. *B,* The pleura over the aortic isthmus is incised and mobilized.

higher incidence of pneumothorax and retrolental fibroplasia in the group that had surgical backup.[15] More recent studies suggest that the aggressive use of echocardiographic screening to detect and treat "silent" patent ductus arteriosus early with indo-methacin may yield superior results.[40] It must be emphasized that randomized multicenter trials testing this approach have not yet been performed. With regard to indomethacin, there is still some uncertainty related to pharmacokinetic issues, such as

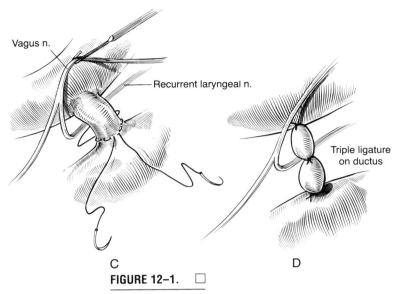

Vagus n.

Recurrent laryngeal n.

Triple ligature on ductus

C

D

FIGURE 12–1. □

Continued. C and *D*, Technique of triple ligation.

route of administration, appropriate levels, amount of dosage, and length and timing of treatment. To add to the uncertainty, a number of reports (nonrandomized) on the use of primary surgical ligation suggest outcomes that are at least as good as those with medical or indomethacin protocols.[10, 23, 41]

At the present time a well-accepted approach is to aggressively diagnose with echocardiography, to address all of the supportive issues, and also to treat the patient aggressively with either oral or intravenous indomethacin unless contraindicated. A dose of 0.2 mg/kg is given, followed by a second and third

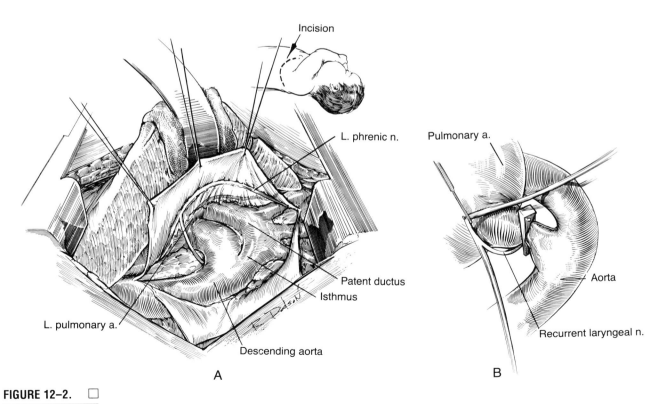

Incision

L. phrenic n.

Pulmonary a.

Patent ductus

Isthmus

Aorta

L. pulmonary a.

Descending aorta

Recurrent laryngeal n.

A

B

FIGURE 12–2. □

A, Surgeon's perspective of neonatal PDA exposed via a left thoracotomy with the pleura incised and mobilized. Note the differences in the relative sizes of the PDA and the aortic isthmus and differences in orientation compared with infant PDA. *B,* Surgical closure using a metal clip.

dose of similar or lesser quantity, depending on age. These doses are given 12 to 24 hours apart, depending on renal function. In some cases in which a beneficial response is obtained initially, the ductus may reopen. Judgment must then be used as to whether a second course of indomethacin should be given or surgical ligation should be performed. This decision will be influenced by the likelihood of side effects from the additional indomethacin and by the need for rapid closure of the ductus for hemodynamic reasons. Contraindications to the use of indomethacin include azotemia, evidence of gut ischemia, thrombocytopenia, intracerebral or other hemorrhage, and sepsis. Birth weight below 1000 gm is considered a contraindication by some[27]; however, at many centers, including Children's Hospital in Boston, infants who have very low birth weights are treated with indomethacin.[26]

If surgical ligation is to be performed, the approach is as described previously for term infants; however, in very small premature infants (less than 1500 gm) who require surgical ligation, the size and tissue integrity of the ductus are such that the triple ligature technique is dangerous. A single central ligature is effective if circumferential dissection can be easily accomplished. Alternatively, a medium-size metal clip is equally effective, especially in cases in which circumferential dissection is deemed difficult.

When compared with term infants, however, much greater attention to perioperative management is required for premature infants. In the great majority of cases, the patient will be mechanically ventilated at the time of consideration. The surgical procedure can be performed in the intensive care nursery or in the operating room. If the operation is to be performed in the operating room, careful attention to patient transport is required. The major problems to which these very small infants are vulnerable during transport are temperature instability and mechanical disruption of life-supporting lines. In the operating room the procedure may be performed on the transport isolette, or the patient may be transferred to the standard operating table. If the operation is to be performed with the patient in the isolette, the patient should be placed in the right lateral decubitus position, with all lines positioned appropriately for surgery in the intensive care nursery before transport to the operating room. If the operation is to be performed on the standard operating table, the surgeon and anesthesiologist should spend considerable time in the intensive care nursery before transfer, simplifying all lines and monitoring equipment to facilitate eventual transfer of the patient from the isolette to the operating room table. Transportation from the intensive care

nursery should be orchestrated to keep the time to an absolute minimum, and the patient should enter the operating room with the ambient room temperature preset as high as can be tolerated by the surgical team. The operation should then proceed expeditiously.

The basics of the operation proceed as described for the term infant; however, a number of precautions must be taken. Special care must be taken when retracting the left lung to expose the ductus. The lungs are often edematous, friable, and noncompliant; therefore, mechanical lung injury, gas exchange compromise, and cardiac tamponade can all be easily induced. To maintain acceptable hemodynamics and gas exchange, it may be necessary to work intermittently for 30- to 60-second periods, interrupted by equal periods of time during which full left lung expansion is achieved. The most important monitor for the surgeon during this period is the tone and rate of the pulse oximeter. Decreased systemic oxygenation and bradycardia are sensitive indicators that suggest that the infant is compromised, signaling that the dissection should be interrupted, retractors removed, and full attention focused on ventilation. It is not uncommon for these patients to require continuous hand ventilation by the anesthesiologist from the time the patient leaves the intensive care nursery until the patient is returned. In severely compromised infants, it may be expedient to simply dissect a small area of pleura on both the upper and lower margins of the patent ductus arteriosus and to carefully place a medium metal clip to ligate it. In more stable cases a heavy braided ligature, followed by a medium metal clip, can be used to increase the security of the closure, although some do not practice this "double ligature" technique. It should be emphasized that misidentification of the ductus is much more likely in premature infants because of the more limited surgical exposure and the emphasis on minimizing the length of the procedure. If an arterial catheter is present, a change in the pulse pressure should be observed when the correct structure is test-occluded with forceps. Also, a pulse oximeter or arterial catheter on the lower body can be used to ensure patency of the isthmus and the descending aorta. After ligation the pleura is usually left open and the ribs approximated with a single ligature after placing a small drainage catheter in the left pleural space to evacuate fluid and air. The soft tissues are closed in two layers with running sutures. Transportation back to the intensive care nursery is conducted with the same care as the initial transport. After a chest radiograph in the intensive care nursery, if full lung expansion is present and there is no air leak, the pleural catheter may be removed or left until the first postoperative day. Primary care of the patient is usually administered by the intensive care nursery team, as the patent ductus arteriosus often is only one of many problems relating to prematurity.

Management of Patent Ductus Arteriosus Associated with Intracardiac Lesions

In the clinical setting in which a patent ductus arteriosus accompanies a more complex intracardiac lesion that is to be corrected, the ductus is usually approached via a median sternotomy (Fig. 12–3). After the sternotomy is performed and the thymus gland is mobilized and partially resected, the pericardium is opened longitudinally. The main pulmonary artery is retracted inferiorly, and the cut edge of the left side of the pericardium is retracted superiorly and to the left. The pericardial reflection onto the ductus and left pulmonary artery is thereby put on tension. The pericardial reflection is carefully dissected superiorly off the ductus arteriosus, exposing its length. The acute angle between the origin of the ductus and the left pulmonary artery must be carefully exposed, and the vagus and recurrent laryngeal nerves, which are in close proximity to the tissue in this angle, are identified and spared. The right-angle clamp is used to create a circumferential plane around the pulmonary end of the ductus, and a ligature is placed at this point. During this procedure, potential compromise of the origin of the left pulmonary artery must be kept in mind. Care must also be taken that the ligature does not impinge on the aortic isthmus or distal aortic arch. The surgeon then proceeds with the intracardiac portion of the operation.

POSTOPERATIVE CARE

Postoperative care in the otherwise healthy infant is routine. The drainage tube in the chest is re-

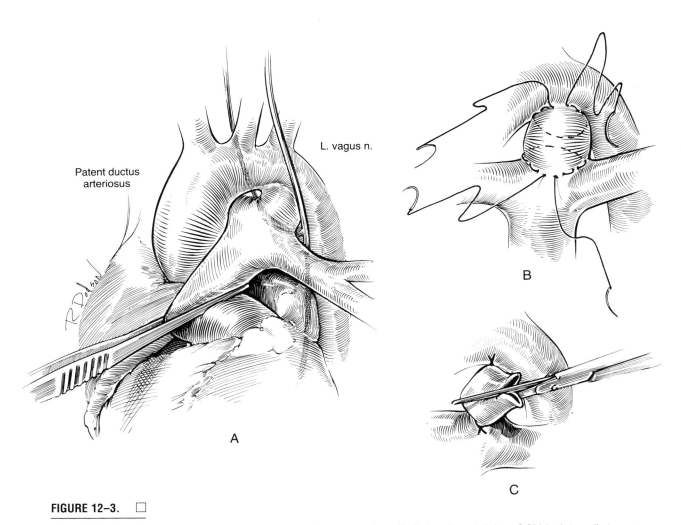

FIGURE 12–3. ☐

A, PDA seen from the surgeon's perspective after exposure via a median sternotomy. *B*, Double ligature closure technique. *C*, Division between ligatures.

moved on the first postoperative day. Potential complications after ligation of the ductus arteriosus in infants include residual patent ductus arteriosus, recurrent laryngeal or vagus nerve injury, trauma to the lungs (with or without pneumothorax), chylothorax, pneumonia, and infection of the wound. A particularly morbid complication is accidental ligation of the wrong structure, including such major structures as the aortic isthmus, left pulmonary artery, and left bronchus.

RESULTS

Our experience with surgical closure of patent ductus arteriosus is largely limited to three groups: (1) premature infants in whom indomethacin is ineffective or contraindicated; (2) term infants in whom indomethacin is not effective or indicated; and (3) larger infants and children in whom transcatheter device closure has not been successful or is contraindicated (i.e., because of very large diameter or patient or family preference).

Between 1985 and 1991, 103 cases of patent ductus arteriosus were surgically ligated in infants less than 1 year old at Children's Hospital in Boston. Table 12–1 shows the age distribution and incidence of premature infants. Approximately half of the infants were premature. In the majority of these, ligation was performed within the first month of life; however, a significant number were not referred for ligation until the second month. The age range for ligation in premature infants was 7 to 56 days (mean, 22 days); the mean age of ligation in premature infants who survived was 20 days and in those who died was 33 days ($P < .01$). Some of these patients received as many as five three-dose courses of indomethacin before referral for surgery. During this period a total of 365 premature infants were treated with indomethacin for a clinical diagnosis of patent ductus arteriosus.

There have been four deaths in term infants, all of whom had multisystem anomalies such as tracheoesophageal fistula or congenital diaphragmatic hernia. None of these deaths were attributable to

the patent ductus arteriosus ligation. In the premature infant group, three deaths occurred within 7 days of patent ductus ligation, all in patients with multisystem disease. None of these deaths were attributable to the surgical procedure.

Two other cases deserve special mention. These involved ligation after failed attempts at transcatheter occlusion of the patent ductus arteriosus. In both cases Rashkind or clamshell devices were used initially, and at the time of surgery the arms of the device had either migrated transluminally or had significantly distorted the wall of the ductus, making dissection particularly treacherous. Ligation was successful in both of these cases and did not induce embolization of the device or significant hemorrhage.

SUMMARY

Patent ductus arteriosus in the otherwise healthy, full-term infant can be surgically ligated with little morbidity and a mortality rate of essentially 0%. Newer techniques, including transcutaneous intraluminal occlusion and thoracoscopy-directed ligation, have not yet been fully proven; however, they appear to offer the possibility of further reduction in morbidity. As our experience indicates, these procedures can also present new technical challenges for the surgeon when complications occur.

Ligation of a patent ductus arteriosus in the premature infant can be effectively performed as well, with very little morbidity and mortality directly related to the surgical procedure. The degree of prematurity or multisystem compromise, however, does have an important influence on the ultimate outcome for these patients. These complications make the clinical situation for premature infants much more complex than that for term infants, particularly when decisions must be made regarding the alternative therapeutic options of medical therapy, pharmacologic closure with indomethacin, and surgical closure. It should be emphasized that the form of therapy most beneficial for premature infants has not been definitively established.

The premature infant with a patent ductus arteriosus presents a unique situation in that it is the only significant congenital cardiovascular lesion that, once identified, is not managed primarily by pediatric cardiologists and cardiac surgeons but by neonatologists. Ligation at a mean age of 22 days (and older in patients who died), in our experience, indicates either a delay in diagnosis or a delay in referral for consideration of surgical ligation; this observation is of some importance, as most studies show that early removal of the ductus results in the

TABLE 12–1. □ AGE DISTRIBUTION AND INCIDENCE OF PREMATURITY IN INFANTS UNDERGOING LIGATION OF PATENT DUCTUS ARTERIOSUS

AGE	TOTAL NO.	PREMATURE INFANTS		FULL-TERM INFANTS	
		No.	%	No.	%
<30 days	58	41	71	17	29
1–3 mo	26	8	31	18	69
4–12 mo	19	0	0	19	100
	103	49	48	54	52

best outcome. A prospective study examining early echocardiographic screening and early treatment, using various protocols (including primary surgical ligation), may address a number of as-yet-unsettled issues related to optimal management of the premature infant with patent ductus arteriosus.

REFERENCES

1. Alpan G, Mauray F, Clyman RI. The effects of the patent ductus arteriosus on diaphragmatic blood flow and function. Pediatr Res 28:437, 1990.
2. Blalock A. Operative closure of the patent ductus arteriosus. Surg Gynecol Obstet 82:113, 1946.
3. Calder AL, Kirker JA, Netuze JM, et al. Pathology of the ductus arteriosus treated with prostaglandins: Comparisons with untreated cases. Pediatr Cardiol 5:85, 1984.
4. Campbell M. Natural history of persistent ductus arteriosus. Br Heart J 30:4, 1968.
5. Clyman RI. Ontogeny of the ductus arteriosus response to prostaglandins and inhibitors of their synthesis. Semin Perinatol 4:115, 1980.
6. Clyman RI, Heymann MA. Pharmacology of the ductus arteriosus. Pediatr Clin North Am 28:77, 1981.
7. Clyman RI, Jobe A, Heymann M, et al. Increased shunt through the patent ductus arteriosus after surfactant replacement therapy. J Pediatr 100:101, 1982.
8. Clyman RI, Mauray F, Roman C, et al. Circulating prostaglandin E2 concentrations and patent ductus arteriosus in fetal and neonatal lambs. J Pediatr 97:455, 1980.
9. Coceani F, Olley PM. Role of prostaglandins, prostacyclin, and thromboxanes in the control of prenatal patency and postnatal closure of the ductus arteriosus. Semin Perinatol 4:109, 1980.
10. Coster DD, Gorton ME, Grooters RK, et al. Surgical closure of the patent ductus arteriosus in the neonatal intensive care unit. Ann Thorac Surg 48:386, 1989.
11. Cotton RB, Stahlman MT, Bender HW, et al. Randomized trial of early closure of symptomatic patent ductus arteriosus in small preterm infants. J Pediatr 93:647, 1978.
12. DeCanq HE Jr. Repair of patent ductus arteriosus in a 1417g infant. Am J Dis Child 106:402, 1963.
13. De Simone L, Cecchi F, Favilli S, et al. Usefulness of pulsed Doppler echocardiography in the diagnosis and medical therapy of patent ductus arteriosus in the newborn with respiratory distress. G Ital Cardiol 21:409, 1991.
14. Fay FS, Cooke PH. Guinea pig ductus arteriosus. II. Irreversible closure after birth. Am J Physiol 222:841, 1972.
15. Gersony WM, Peckham GJ, Ellison RC, et al. Effect of indomethacin in premature infants with patent ductus arteriosus: Results of a national collaborative study. J Pediatr 102:895, 1983.
16. Gittenberger-De Groot AC, Strengers JLM, Mentink M, et al. Histologic studies on normal and persistent ductus arteriosus in the dog. J Am Coll Cardiol 6:394, 1985.
17. Gittenberger-De Groot AC, Van Ertgrugen I, Moulaert AJ, et al. The ductus arteriosus in the preterm infant: histologic and clinical observations. J Pediatr 96:88, 1980.
18. Green TP, Thompson TR, Johnson D, et al. Furosemide use in premature infants and appearance of patent ductus arteriosus. Am J Dis Child 135:239, 1981.
19. Gross RE, Hubbard JP. Surgical ligation of a patent ductus arteriosus. Report of first successful case. JAMA 112:729, 1939.
20. Heymann MA. Patent ductus arteriosus. In Adams FA, Emmanouilides GC, Reimenschneider TA, (eds). Moss' Heart Disease in Infants, Children and Adolescents. 4th ed. Baltimore, Williams & Wilkins, 1989.
21. Heymann MA, Rudolph AM. Control of the ductus arteriosus. Physiol Rev 55:62, 1975.
22. Heymann MA, Rudolph AM, Silverman NH. Closure of the ductus arteriosus in premature infants by inhibition of prostaglandin synthesis. N Engl J Med 295:530, 1976.
23. Hubbard C, Rucker RW, Realyvasquez F, et al. Ligation of the patent ductus arteriosus in newborn respiratory failure. J Pediatr Surg 21:3, 1986.
24. Ichihashi K, Shiraishi H, Endou H, et al. Cerebral and abdominal arterial hemodynamics in preterm infants with patent ductus arteriosus. Act Paediatr Jpn 32:349, 1990.
25. LaBorde F, Noirhomme T, Karam J, et al. A new video thoracoscopy surgical technique for management of patent ductus arteriosus in infants and children. Abstract. Presented at the American Association of Thoracic Surgery Annual Meeting, Los Angeles, CA, 1992.
26. Leonhardt A, Isken V, Kuhl PG, et al. Prolonged indomethacin treatment in preterm infants with symptomatic patent ductus arteriosus: Efficacy, drug level monitoring, and patient selection. Eur J Pediatr 146:140, 1987.
27. McCarthy JS, Zies LG, Gelband H. Age dependent closure of the patent ductus arteriosus by indomethacin. Pediatrics 62:706, 1978.
28. McMurphy DM, Heymann MA, Rudolph AM, et al. Developmental change in constriction of the ductus arteriosus: Response to oxygen and vasoactive substances in the isolated ductus arteriosus of the fetal lamb. Pediatr Res 6:231, 1972.
29. Meyers RL, Alpan G, Lin E, et al. Patent ductus arteriosus, indomethacin, and intestinal distention: Effects on intestinal blood flow and oxygen consumption. Pediatr Res 29:569, 1991.
30. Mitchell SC, Korones SB, Berendes HW. Congenital heart disease in 56,109 births. Incidence and natural history. Circulation 43:323, 1971.
31. Oberhansli-Weiss I, Heymann MA, Rudolph AM, et al. The pattern and mechanisms of response to oxygen by the ductus arteriosus and umbilical artery. Pediatr Res 6:693, 1972.
32. Peckham GJ, Miettinen OS, Ellison RC, et al. Clinical course to 1 year of age in premature infants with patent ductus arteriosus: Results of a multicenter radomized trial of indomethacin. J Pediatr 105:285, 1984.
33. Portsmann W, Wirny L, Warnke H, et al. Catheter closure of patent ductus arteriosus: 62 cases treated without thoracotomy. Radiol Clin North Am 9:203, 1971.
34. Rashkind WJ, Cuaso CC. Transcatheter closure of patent ductus arteriosus. Pediatr Cardiol 1:3, 1979.
35. Rudolph AM, Heymann HA, Spitznas U. Hemodynamic considerations in the development of narrowing of the aorta. Am J Cardiol 30:514, 1972.
36. Rudolph AM, Mayer FE, Nadas AS, et al. Patent ductus arteriosus: A clinical and hemodynamic study of patients in the first year of life. Pediatrics 22:892, 1958.
37. Santos MA, Moll JN, Drumond C, et al. Development of the ductus arteriosus in right ventricle outflow tract obstruction. Circulation 62:818, 1980.
38. Sato K, Fujino M, Kozuka T, et al. Transfemoral plug closure of patent ductus arteriosus: Experience in 61 consecutive cases treated without thoracotomy. Circulation 51:337, 1975.
39. Wong SN, Lo RN, Hui PW. Abnormal renal and splanchnic arterial Doppler pattern in premature babies with symptomatic patent ductus arteriosus. J Ultrasound Med 9:125, 1990.
40. Zanardo V, Milanesi O, Trevisanuto D, et al. Early screening and treatment of "silent" patent ductus arteriosus in prematures with RDS. J Perinat Med 19:291, 1991.
41. Zerella JT, Spies RJ, Deaver DC III, et al. Indomethacin versus immediate ligation in the treatment of 82 newborns with patent ductus arteriosus. J Pediatr Surg 18:835, 1983.

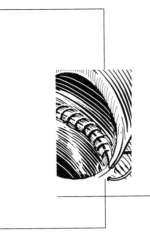

13

Tetralogy of Fallot

In 1672 Stensen[37] described for the first time the anatomic features of what is now termed *tetralogy of Fallot*. In 1888 Fallot[11] published his astute clinical observations correlating what he considered to be the four primary lesions: a ventricular septal defect, infundibular pulmonic stenosis, right ventricular hypertrophy, and dextroposition of the aorta with the clinical finding of progressive cyanosis. Presently, from a pathophysiologic standpoint, the dominant features of tetralogy of Fallot (TOF) are the ventricular septal defect (VSD) and the degree of right ventricular outflow tract obstruction (RVOTO). In its extreme form the anatomy, pathophysiology, and operative repair of TOF with pulmonary stenosis (TOF-PS) are sufficiently different from those of TOF with pulmonary atresia (TOF-PA) to warrant separate considerations.

ANATOMIC DESCRIPTION

Tetralogy of Fallot With Pulmonary Stenosis

Fallot's original concept of four primary defects has been challenged by Van Praagh and colleagues,[39] who introduced the notion that TOF is actually a monology resulting from underdevelopment or hypoplasia of the right ventricular infundibulum or conus. The hypoplastic infundibulum is shortened, narrow, and shallow. The infundibular septum (parietal band or crista), which normally

follows a posterior, inferior, and rightward course (Fig. 13–1*A*, *B*), remains in a superior, anterior, and leftward position in TOF, thus crowding the right ventricular outflow tract (Fig. 13–1*C*). By remaining anterior and superior, the infundibular septum also fails to occupy the space above the ventricular septum between the left anterosuperior and right posteroinferior limbs of the septal band or trabecula septomarginalis, resulting in the typical large VSD of TOF that is posterior and inferior to the infundibular septum (Fig. 13–1*D*). This primary infundibular hypoplasia is particularly evident in the young infant with TOF in whom the malpositioned infundibular septum and the septal band have not yet undergone secondary hypertrophic changes. Although there is a wide spectrum of RVOTO in TOF-PS, the characteristic lesion, particularly in symptomatic infants, includes hypoplasia of the right ventricular outflow tract accompanied by stenosis of the pulmonary valve and hypoplasia of both the pulmonary annulus and pulmonary trunk. Discontinuity of pulmonary arteries is rare in simple TOF-PS, as are arborization abnormalities of either the left or right pulmonary arteries. It must be emphasized that the right and left pulmonary arteries in TOF-PS are almost never prohibitively hypoplastic, even in the presence of severe narrowing of the right ventricular outflow tract. However, extension of the hypoplasia of the right ventricular infundibulum and pulmonary valve annulus to the pulmonary trunk, including its distal portion, is common. In this case

215

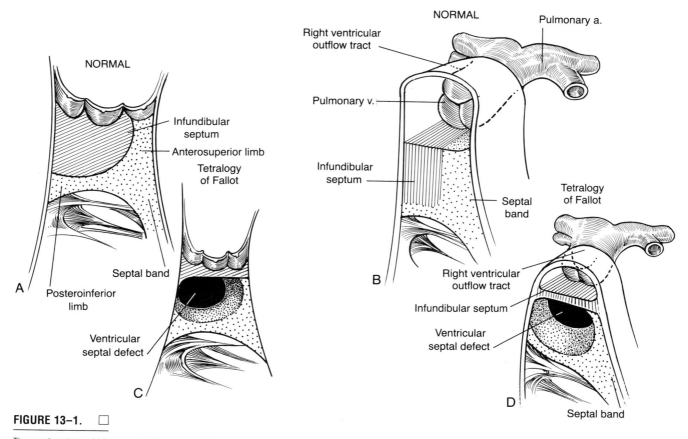

FIGURE 13–1. ☐

The conal septum, which normally follows a posterior and rightward course (A, B), has a superior, anterior, and leftward position in tetralogy of Fallot (TOF), thus crowding the right ventricular outflow tract (C, D). By remaining anterior and superior, the conal septum fails to occupy the space above the ventricular septum between the left anterosuperior and right posteroinferior limbs of the septal band, resulting in the typical malalignment ventricular septal defect seen in TOF.

the pulmonary valve itself is often dysmorphic, cartilaginous in consistency, and immobile, representing an additional and significant obstruction to pulmonary blood flow.

The malaligned conoventricular VSD is limited posterosuperiorly by the infundibuloventricular fold and the aortic valve annulus, superiorly by the hypoplastic infundibular septum, anteriorly by the anterosuperior limb, and inferiorly by the posteroinferior limb of the septal band and the membranous septum. Surgically, the most important variant concerns the posteroinferior rim of the VSD. In a relatively small percentage of patients, the posteroinferior limb is well developed, essentially forming a continuous muscular border. This well-defined muscle bar even covers the membranous septum. In this case the bundle of His penetrates and crosses the ventricular septum some distance from the posteroinferior edge of the VSD and is deeply embedded within muscle. The right bundle travels between the posteroinferior limb and the trabecular septum. In the other (more frequent) anatomic variant, the posteroinferior border of the VSD is capped by a fibrous

rim formed by the confluence of the membranous septum, attachments of the tricuspid and mitral valves, and the aortic valve annulus. The posteroinferior limb of the septal band is hypoplastic and therefore does not extend to the posteroinferior border. In this case the bundle of His penetrates and traverses the septum near the fibrous posteroinferior rim of the VSD. The right bundle branch travels subendocardially along the right-sided anteroinferior border of the defect. Consequently, both the bundle of His and the right bundle branch are more susceptible to surgical trauma.

In a small subset of patients, the infundibular septum is extremely hypoplastic or even absent; consequently, the VSD extends into the subpulmonary area. The aortic and pulmonary valves are separated by a thin band of fibrous tissue. In about 50% of these patients, the pulmonary annulus is also significantly reduced in size.

In approximately 3% of infants with TOF-PS, a second ventricular septal defect may be present. In our experience the most common additional defect is an anterior muscular VSD.

FIGURE 13–2. ☐

Depiction of the histologic characteristics of an aortopulmonary collateral artery (APCA) before it enters the lung parenchyma and within the lung parenchyma. Before entering the pulmonary parenchyma, the APCA retains the characteristics of a muscular artery with a well-developed muscular media and adventitia. Within the normal lung, the medial muscle is gradually replaced by a thin elastic lamina (*upper vessel*). In an unobstructed APCA, changes of pulmonary vascular obstructive disease (PVOD) are mostly due to increased pressure and blood flow (*middle vessel*). In an obstructed APCA, normal histologic anatomy is preserved with a thin elastic layer (*lower vessel*).

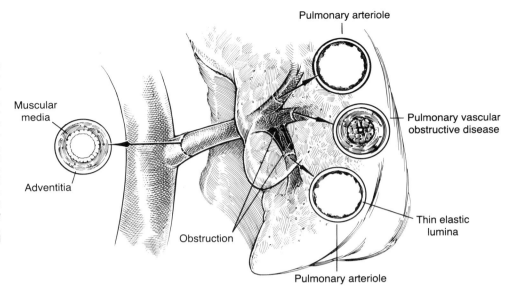

Various coronary artery anomalies, related to either origin or distribution, have been described in TOF.[12, 42] However, the most surgically relevant coronary anomalies include an anterior descending coronary artery arising from the right coronary and a single coronary artery with origin of the right coronary from a normally arising left coronary. The former occurs in approximately 3% of patients; here, the anterior descending coronary artery crosses the right ventricular outflow tract at varying distances from the pulmonary valve annulus and therefore can interfere with the placement of a transannular patch. Aortopulmonary collateral arteries (APCAs) are rare in TOF-PS. A persistent ductus-like vessel, originating from either the left or the right subclavian artery, or direct APCAs usually indicate rare hypoplasia of the pulmonary artery branches.

Tetralogy of Fallot With Pulmonary Atresia

The coexistence of pulmonary atresia poses additional therapeutic challenges, primarily because of the wide range of origin, size, and distribution of the pulmonary blood supply. The most favorable subset of TOF-PA consists of those patients with valvar pulmonary atresia and a duct-dependent pulmonary circulation. In this condition the pulmonary arteries are usually normal. At the other end of the spectrum are patients with TOF-PA, no patent ductus arteriosus, and diminutive or absent central pulmonary arteries; in these patients, pulmonary blood flow is supplied exclusively by APCAs.

Embryologic Considerations

Early during fetal development, the vascular plexus within the lung buds connects with systemic segmental arteries originating from the dorsal aorta. By the 40th day of gestation, the vascular plexus has differentiated into pulmonary segmental arteries, supplying the terminal bronchopulmonary units. For a short time, the pulmonary parenchyma receives a dual blood supply (from the right ventricle and the pulmonary arteries that originate from the sixth branchial arches and from the previously described systemic segmental arteries). However, by the 50th day of gestation, the systemic arterial supply normally involutes, and during subsequent normal fetal development, flow to the developing lungs is delivered exclusively by the pulmonary arteries. In the more complex forms of TOF-PA, this normal development is affected; some bronchopulmonary segments or lobes can be supplied by true pulmonary arteries and others by APCAs. It is important to note that before entering the lung parenchyma, these systemic collaterals retain the histologic characteristics of muscular arteries, whereas after penetrating the pulmonary parenchyma, the median muscular layer gradually changes into an elastic lamina, structurally resembling true pulmonary arteries (Fig. 13–2).[38] Unobstructed flow through APCAs can lead to pulmonary vascular obstructive disease (PVOD), while stenosis within APCAs protects against the development of PVOD.

Gross Anatomy

The intracardiac lesion in TOF-PA usually resembles that of conventional TOF except that there is complete obliteration of the distal portion of the right ventricular–pulmonary outflow tract. The complexity of this malformation is dependent on the anatomy of the pulmonary circulation, principally the origin, size, course, and final destination of the pulmonary blood supply. From a therapeutic standpoint, it is useful to divide TOF-PA patients into four anatomic subgroups based on the pulmonary artery anatomy. Figure 13–3 depicts the major anatomic subsets of this anomaly.

Groups I and II. Patients in groups I and II have TOF-PA with well-developed pulmonary arteries; the pulmonary blood flow is almost always supplied principally by a large patent ductus arteriosus. In these patients the pulmonary arteries tend to connect to all bronchopulmonary segments, and it is exceedingly uncommon to find diminutive pulmonary arteries. In group II patients the main pulmonary artery may be absent.

Group III. In these infants the patent ductus is either absent or very small. Consequently, the pulmonary arteries are hypoplastic or diminutive, connecting to a variable number of bronchopulmonary segments. Commonly, the APCAs are the more important source of pulmonary flow. Discontinuity between the diminutive left and right pulmonary arteries occurs in approximately 30% of these patients. Frequently when this happens, one of the diminutive pulmonary arteries originates from a left- or right-sided patent ductus arteriosus, depending on the orientation of the aortic arch.

Group IV. Patients in group IV have no true mediastinal arteries; all bronchopulmonary segments are exclusively supplied by APCAs, although there may be remnants of parenchymal pulmonary arteries.

As a general rule, in the presence of large APCAs, both central and peripheral pulmonary arteries

tend to be hypoplastic. Also, in approximately 60% of the APCAs, significant stenosis can be identified either at the origin from the aorta or at the junction where the systemic collateral connects with the pulmonary artery. The majority of the APCAs originate from the descending thoracic aorta, usually in the vicinity of the left main bronchus (left aortic arch) or close to the carina in the case of a right aortic arch. In some cases, the APCAs can originate from a common aortic trunk; occasionally a large left or right APCA, distant from its aortic origin, may give rise to an APCA that crosses over to the contralateral lung. Finally, APCAs can also originate from branches of the aorta such as the left and right subclavian and internal mammary arteries or, occasionally, even from intra-abdominal branches (indirect APCAs).

APCAs may (1) connect outside the lung with central pulmonary arteries (Fig. 13–4A), (2) connect within the lung with lobar or segmental pulmonary arteries (Fig. 13–4B), or (3) not connect with any pulmonary arteries, supplying the lung independently (Fig. 13–4C). Haworth, who has contributed much to the understanding of pulmonary blood supply in TOF-PA, demonstrated that, on average, central pulmonary arteries supply 50% while APCAs supply 45% of the bronchopulmonary segments.[14] In the remaining 5% pulmonary blood supply is dual, although toward the periphery, these arteries tend to diverge, each accompanying a different airway to supply a different portion of the bronchopulmonary segment.

The source of pulmonary blood flow, whether diminutive pulmonary arteries or APCAs, signifi-

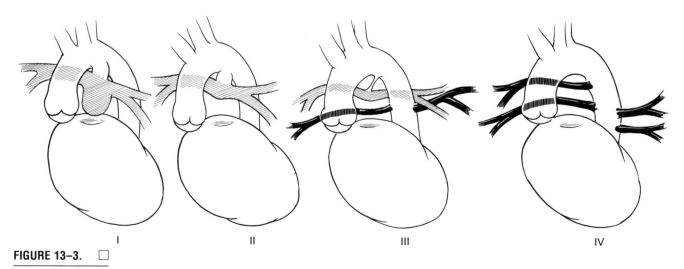

| I | II | III | IV |

FIGURE 13–3. ☐

Tetralogy of Fallot with pulmonary atresia (TOF-PA) is classified into four groups. In groups I and II, the pulmonary arteries are well developed, and blood flow is supplied by a large patent ductus arteriosus. The main pulmonary artery is absent in group II. In group III, the ductus is either absent or very small. Both left and right pulmonary arteries are diminutive, connecting to variable numbers of bronchopulmonary segments; the more important sources of pulmonary blood flow are APCAs. In group IV, there are no mediastinal pulmonary arteries, and all bronchopulmonary segments are supplied entirely by APCAs.

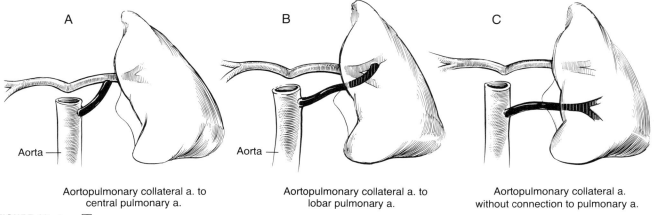

FIGURE 13–4. ☐

APCAs connect to either central pulmonary arteries within the mediastinum (*A*) or lobar or segmental pulmonary arteries within the lung (*B*) or do not connect with any pulmonary artery supplying the lung independently (*C*).

cantly affects the anatomy and function of the pulmonary microcirculation. In infants who have TOF-PA, preacinar vessels tend to be abnormally small; perhaps even more importantly, the intra-acinar arteries, which normally continue to develop during the first 3 years of life, are fewer in number and also have a thinner media and a smaller external diameter. Rabinovitch et al.[32] also documented a corresponding decrease in the number of pulmonary alveoli when pulmonary blood supply was decreased early in life. Therefore, in patients with TOF-PA, an increase in pulmonary vascular resistance calculated early in life is likely a result of the decreased number of intra-acinar arteries, while at a later age, an increase in pulmonary vascular resistance is more likely caused by pulmonary vascular obstructive changes secondary to increased pressure and flow through unobstructed APCAs. Stenosis within APCAs protects the pulmonary vascular bed; however, decreased pulmonary blood flow limits pulmonary vascular and parenchymal development and will prove equally limiting in the long term.

PATHOPHYSIOLOGY

Tetralogy of Fallot With Pulmonary Stenosis

The pathophysiology of patients with TOF-PS depends primarily on the degree of RVOTO and secondarily on the level of systemic vascular resistance. Because there is almost always a large VSD, the two ventricles are functionally a single pumping chamber, and the distribution of the ventricular output depends on the relative resistance to blood flow of the RVOTO and the systemic arterial bed.

The presence of TOF does not influence fetal cir-

culation adversely. Infants are usually well developed at birth, but after birth, depending on the degree of RVOTO, the flow of blood from the right ventricle to the lungs is restricted. As long as the ductus arteriosus is patent, pulmonary blood flow is usually adequate. However, it is important to remember that increasing levels of oxygen in the blood tend to constrict the ductus arteriosus, which in turn decreases pulmonary blood flow. As long as ductal tissue remains responsive, a decrease in arterial Po_2 may again increase the size of the ductus. This phenomenon may explain intermittent episodes of hypoxemia in the neonate. However, once the duct closes definitively, systemic arterial saturation falls, and the degree of cyanosis then depends mostly on the degree of RVOTO. If the obstruction is severe, arterial saturation falls precipitously, leading to severe hypoxemia and even acidemia. However, if RVOTO is mild or moderate, pulmonary blood flow is adequate to meet the oxygen requirements of the tissue and, in some rare instances, it may even become excessive. Because of the large VSD that results in a functional single ventricle, the systemic and pulmonary circuits are parallel, and therefore, changes in systemic vascular resistance also affect pulmonary blood flow. A decrease in systemic vascular resistance decreases pulmonary blood flow, while an increase has the opposite effect. Also, the high hemoglobin levels in neonates (18 gm/100 ml) decrease to approximately 12 gm/100 ml during the first few months of life. Persistent hypoxemia after birth stimulates bone marrow production of red blood cells. Because iron stores and dietary supply are limited in infants, these neonates tend to have microcytic and hypochromic anemia. Eventually the body adapts to hypoxemia by increasing the oxygen-carrying capacity of blood, developing polycythemia and increased hemoglobin concentration of the individual red cells. Cyanotic patients also tend to be hypervolemic, mostly because of an increase in red cell volume with a normal or decreased plasma volume. A hematocrit higher than 65% or 70% raises blood viscosity, impedes capillary flow, and decreases delivery of oxygen to tissues.

Cerebral abscesses in infants are extremely rare, but cerebrovascular accidents can occur. The most effective prevention of this dreaded complication is early operation. Early repair should also make the other late complications of TOF (e.g., brain abscesses, bacterial endocarditis, hemorrhagic disorders, gout, and pulmonary artery hypertension secondary to aortopulmonary shunts) of historical interest only.

Tetralogy of Fallot With Pulmonary Atresia

By force, there is an obligatory right-to-left shunt of all right ventricular blood into the aorta. Pulmonary blood flow is exclusively dependent on either a patent ductus arteriosus or APCAs. The degree of arterial unsaturation depends on the extracardiac sources of pulmonary blood supply. In TOF-PA with a ductus-dependent circulation, closure of the duct can lead to rapid death during the neonatal period. APCAs usually provide adequate pulmonary blood flow during the early months of life; in fact, in the case of unobstructed APCAs, the neonate or young infant may be in congestive heart failure.

PREOPERATIVE DIAGNOSIS

Tetralogy of Fallot With Pulmonary Stenosis

The central clinical feature of TOF is cyanosis, which is mostly continuous but can be intermittent, and the infant may develop hypoxic spells. During a hypoxic crisis, the typical short, harsh systolic ejection murmur along the left sternal border may be absent. The chest radiograph shows a normal-size heart with a prominent right ventricular contour, an absent or deficient pulmonary artery segment, and an upwardly displaced apex (coeur en sabot). Peripheral pulmonary markings are usually diminished. Frequently, the aortic arch is on the right side (25%). The electrocardiogram is nonspecific, although a persistent upright T wave in the right precordial leads indicates right ventricular hypertrophy. With recent advances in echocardiography, particularly with the addition of color Doppler techniques, the echocardiographic diagnosis makes an appropriate operative strategy possible in the ma-

jority of patients with TOF-PS. Echocardiography has proved remarkably accurate in demonstrating additional VSDs, defining the origin and the course of the proximal right and left coronary arteries, evaluating atrioventricular valve anatomy and function, and also outlining the anatomy of the central pulmonary artery, including the origin of the left pulmonary artery. Only if the echocardiographer feels unsure about any of these issues are cardiac catheterization and cineangiography undertaken at this time in neonates and infants. However, if the infant has a history of one or more previous palliative operations, and if there is concern about iatrogenic pulmonary artery distortion, the presence of APCAs, or pulmonary vascular obstructive disease, cardiac catheterization is still indicated.

Tetralogy of Fallot With Pulmonary Atresia

The diagnostic challenge for the surgeon in these cases is to identify preoperatively the presence, size, and continuity of native pulmonary arteries and then to detail the origin, the course, and the distribution of all APCAs. It is virtually always necessary to make selective injections into all direct and indirect APCAs to obtain a complete and detailed map of the entire pulmonary blood supply. Only then can the physician design an appropriate treatment strategy.

Pulmonary Artery Size

Accurate measurement of the size of a pulmonary artery preoperatively presents a number of problems. First, with diminished pulmonary blood flow, the maximal capacity or compliance of the undistended pulmonary arteries cannot be accurately assessed. Consequently, the potential postoperative size of a pulmonary artery carrying a normal volume of blood is difficult to predict. Nevertheless, several methods to quantitate pulmonary artery size and its effect on the postrepair outcome have been used. One popular formula was suggested by Piehler and associates.[29] Known as the *McGoon ratio*, it is based on the diameter of the right and left pulmonary arteries, normalizing these by relating them to the diameter of the descending thoracic aorta at the level of the diaphragm. Right and left pulmonary arteries are considered to be nonrestrictive when the combined diameter is about 2 or greater, while a combined diameter of less then 0.8 is supposed to indicate severely restrictive central pulmonary arteries. One drawback of the McGoon ratio is that the descending aorta at the diaphragm tends to be more narrow in patients with TOF than in normal individuals, making the McGoon ratio falsely more favorable. Nakata and colleagues[28] measured the diameter of the right and left pulmonary arteries immediately proximal to their first branching. Magnification errors are corrected either by using previously determined values from the catheterization laboratory or by relating vessel size to the known size of an appropriate catheter. Pulmonary artery size is reported as the sum of the cross-sectional areas of the right and left pulmonary arteries, indexed to body surface area. The normal cross-sectional index is 330 ± 30 mm^2/m^2. At Children's Hospital in Boston, the pulmonary arteries are considered diminutive when the pulmonary artery index (PAI) is less than 150 mm^2/m^2.

Kirklin, Blackstone, and colleagues[2, 18] stated that prediction of postoperative P$_{RV}$:$_{LV}$ is best obtained by using both the dimensions of components of the right ventricular outflow tract and the size of the pulmonary arteries, excluding peripheral pulmonary artery branches. If the pulmonary valve annulus is hypoplastic, it tends to remain so throughout life. Therefore, Blackstone and Kirklin expressed the annular size relative to the child's size as a Z value which represents the number of standard deviations that the patient's pulmonary valve annulus deviates from a mean normal value for age and size (measured diameter − the mean normal diameter ÷ the standard deviation of the mean normal diameter).

As already mentioned, however, all of these angiographic assessments contain the intrinsic limitation that the size of the pulmonary arteries after repair may be significantly larger, given the increased volume and the distending pressure after establishing right ventricular–to–pulmonary artery continuity. On the other hand, there clearly is a small subset of patients in whom the mediastinal pulmonary arteries are indeed so diminutive (1 to 2 mm in diameter) that they cannot carry right ventricular output, and therefore, closure of the VSD is contraindicated.

INDICATIONS FOR OPERATION

Tetralogy of Fallot With Pulmonary Stenosis

Nearly 70% of patients with TOF and pulmonary stenosis require an operation during the first year of life because of hypoxic spells or persistent hypoxemia (resting arterial oxygen saturation less than 70%). Approximately 30% of neonates with TOF-PS die within the first year of life if untreated. In the past, palliative aortopulmonary shunt operations were favored because of high mortality and morbidity from primary repair in the very young. As a result of the development of hypothermic circulatory arrest or low-flow hypothermic cardiopulmonary bypass, improved anesthetic management of neonates and infants, and advances in postoperative care (including the availability of specialized pediatric cardiac intensive care units), both mortality and morbidity after early one-stage repair of TOF have decreased dramatically, and such repair is currently favored in many centers. This approach avoids the additional risk of two operations and eliminates early and late complications of shunt operations such as a nonfunctioning shunt, partial or complete occlusion of a pulmonary artery, or development of PVOD. Because of our gratifying experience at Children's Hospital in Boston with repair of TOF-PS in symptomatic infants,[5–7] we have also steadily decreased the age of elective repair.

There is increasing evidence that early repair of congenital heart anomalies minimizes secondary damage to vital organs, particularly of the heart itself, the lungs, and the brain. In TOF-PS, it is hoped that by eliminating or reducing RVOTO early in life, the stimulus for pathologic right ventricular hypertrophy will be eliminated, thus preserving ventricular systolic and diastolic function and also electrical stability of the myocardium.[27, 40] Furthermore, by establishing early antegrade pulmonary blood flow, postnatal pulmonary angio- and alveologenesis should also be enhanced. Finally, by eliminating cyanosis as early as possible, the adverse effects of cyanosis on the central nervous system should also be reduced. In a review by Kirklin and associates[18] of 196 patients with TOF, including 100 consecutive patients from Children's Hospital in Boston, very young age proved to be a general risk factor for death after repair. However, with favorable anatomy allowing satisfactory relief of right ventricular hypertension, with or without the use of a transannular patch, young age remained only as a very small incremental risk factor. Also, we are convinced that young age is not an immutable risk factor, as there has already been a considerable decrease in surgical mortality in the very young after repair of TOF when compared with earlier time periods. Observations in the past that neonatal hearts have less ability to adapt to sudden increases in stroke volume or that neonates are more susceptible to the damaging effects of cardiopulmonary bypass are true; nevertheless, they remain within the range of biologic tolerance, as evidenced by the excellent results obtained with neonatal arterial switch operations for anatomic repair of transposition of the great arteries. It is likely that, excluding patients who have TOF-PA or other significant associated anomalies (such as the absent pulmonary valve syndrome), results of early repair of TOF in neonates will soon parallel those obtained in infants beyond the first month of life.

It is important to emphasize once more that TOF-PS is different from TOF-PA and pulmonary circulation dependent on APCAs. It must also be understood that very young patients with TOF-PS are still at a greater risk of dying within the first year of life than are older patients; the risk is significantly greater for those who have severe cyanosis or cyanotic spells. The current slightly increased mortality after repair in the first few months of life is still significantly less than the mortality associated with the natural history of this disease in this age group. Therefore, primary repair at the time of presentation is indicated in such patients. Aside from extracardiac causes (e.g., intracerebral bleeding, generalized sepsis, or acute necrotizing enterocolitis), the only contraindication to primary repair in the very young is anomalous origin of the anterior descending coronary artery from the right coronary artery. In this case, a systemic-to-pulmonary shunt (preferably a modified Blalock-Taussig shunt) is recommended, followed later by interposition of a conduit.

Tetralogy of Fallot With Pulmonary Atresia

Most patients who have TOF-PA and a ductus-dependent pulmonary circulation have sufficiently large pulmonary arteries (PAI > 150 mm^2/m^2) that they can be successfully repaired at a low operative risk with good late hemodynamic and electrophysiologic results. However, a therapeutic challenge is presented by the subset of patients with diminutive pulmonary arteries (PAI < 100 mm^2/m^2) and large APCAs that supply a variable number of bronchopulmonary segments.

The ultimate therapeutic goal in these patients is to establish a right ventricular–dependent pulmonary circulation, ideally including all 20 bronchopulmonary segments. Hemodynamically, the aim is to achieve a postoperative PRV/LV ratio of less than 0.6 with no residual left-to-right shunt at any level or any ventricular ectopic activity. Until relatively recently, this ideal result has been achieved only extremely rarely, mostly because of surgical technical limitations in dealing with these varied complex anatomic features (many of which can currently be dealt with by invasive catheterization techniques) and probably because of a delay in treating these lesions aggressively during early infancy.

In the past, these patients were managed somewhat haphazardly by a variety of medical or surgical approaches, including primary repair or staged operations such as preliminary systemic-to–pulmonary artery shunts or establishment of right ventricular–to–pulmonary artery continuity. These procedures were primarily aimed at providing relief of cyanosis and stimulating enlargement of the hypoplastic central pulmonary arteries, with the expectation that later the VSD would close and eliminate any remaining functionally important APCAs. As already mentioned, most of these attempts proved unsuccessful. By 1984, it had been shown that hypoplastic or stenotic pulmonary arteries could be enlarged by transcatheter balloon dilatation and also that APCAs could be successfully interrupted by transcatheter placement of coils.[25] Consequently, a new staged approach to the management of patients with TOF-PA and diminutive pulmonary arteries evolved at Children's Hospital in Boston. This approach consists of early surgical relief of RVOTO, leaving the VSD open, followed by interventional catheterization to dilate stenotic peripheral pulmonary arteries and occlude redundant APCAs[8] with coils. Whenever indicated, unifocalization procedures are added, connecting as many aortopulmonary collaterals to the true pulmonary arteries as possible. These preliminary procedures are then followed by surgical relief of any residual RVOTO and closure of the VSD. Interposition of a valved homograft between the right ventricle and the pulmonary artery during early infancy not only stimulates enlargement of the pulmonary arteries, but also provides an avenue for balloon dilatation of stenotic peripheral pulmonary arteries, which are common in this entity. It also facilitates angiographic delineation of the blood supply in peripheral pulmonary arterial segments.

SURGICAL MANAGEMENT OF TETRALOGY OF FALLOT

Historical Note

Surgical treatment of TOF was initiated by Blalock and Taussig[3] in 1945 with the establishment of the subclavian artery–to–pulmonary artery anastomosis. Klinner et al., in 1962,[20] were the first to interpose a prosthetic conduit between the subclavian artery and the pulmonary artery, a technique that was further refined by de Leval and colleagues.[22] Laks and Castaneda[21] added an occasionally helpful modification of the Blalock-Taussig shunt, using the subclavian artery ipsilateral to the aortic arch. In 1946, Potts et al.[30] introduced the descending aorta–to–left pulmonary artery anastomosis, in 1955 Davidson[9] reported the first central aortopulmonary shunt by direct suture, and in 1962 Waterston[41] performed the ascending aorta–to–

right pulmonary artery anastomosis, an important alternative to the Blalock-Taussig and Potts operations. In 1948, both Sellors[35] and Brock[4] expanded the scope of palliative operations by adding closed pulmonary valvotomy and infundibulotomy.

In an imaginative and daring effort, on April 31, 1954, Lillehei and collaborators,[23] using controlled cross circulation in a 10-month-old boy, carried out the first intracardiac repair of tetralogy of Fallot; this included closure of the VSD and relief of the RVOTO under direct vision. In Lillehei's original cross-circulation series of 11 TOF repairs, six patients were less than 2 years old. In fact, remarkably, the first, and youngest, patient (10 months old at the time of operation) is well and working as a physician. The first successful repair of TOF using a heart-lung machine was accomplished by Kirklin and associates in 1955.[17] Lillehei recognized the need for enlarging the right ventricular infundibulum with a patch and extended the patch across a stenotic pulmonary valve annulus as early as 1956.[13] The use of a nonvalved prosthetic conduit from the right ventricle to the pulmonary artery for the treatment of TOF-PA was first reported by Klinner.[19] Ross and Somerville[33] first reported the interposition of a valved aortic homograft for repair of TOF-PA in 1966. However, after the initial success with TOF repair in infancy, subsequent attempts at early repair carried a high mortality rate, and the two-stage repair became universally favored. In 1969, Barratt-Boyes and Neutze[1] successfully reinitiated primary repair of symptomatic infants with TOF-PS. In 1972, at Children's Hospital in Boston, we began our experience with early repair of symptomatic infants with TOF, including infants within the first three months of life.

In addition to the important contributions by surgeons in the use of nonvalved and valved conduits for repair of TOF-PA, and the innovative techniques of percutaneous balloon dilatation and occlusion of collateral arteries developed by cardiologists, much is owed to Edwards and McGoon,[10] Thiene et al.,[38] Haworth and Macartney,[14] and Rabinovitch et al.[31, 32] They significantly advanced our knowledge of the anatomy and histology of APCAs, their intraparenchymal connections with pulmonary artery branches, and the effect of a decreased (or increased) pulmonary flow on the pulmonary parenchyma.

Operative Technique

Tetralogy of Fallot With Pulmonary Stenosis

Through a median sternotomy, cardiopulmonary bypass is instituted using an ascending aortic cannula and a venous cannula placed through the right atrial appendage. The ductus arteriosus is ligated if patent. Pericardium is excised before the infant is placed on cardiopulmonary bypass and is pretreated with 0.6% glutaraldehyde for 10 minutes for subsequent use in the reconstruction of the right ventricular outflow tract. During cooling, the main pulmonary artery is dissected free from the ascending aorta as well as from the right and left pulmonary arteries. At 18°C rectal temperature, the ascending aorta is clamped, and cardioplegic solution is instilled. The circulation is then stopped, and the right atrial cannula is removed.

A vertical incision is made into the free wall of the infundibulum. If the pulmonary valve annulus is hypoplastic, the incision is extended to the bifurcation of the main pulmonary artery. If the pulmonary valve leaflets are thickened or dysplastic, they are excised. If there is narrowing at the orifice of the left or right pulmonary artery, the incision is extended into one of these vessels. Proximally, the incision is carried to the level of the infundibular septum. Deep hypothermia and cardioplegia render the heart quite flaccid, facilitating intracardiac exposure and therefore allowing for a shorter ventriculotomy. Because there is virtually no secondary hypertrophy of the infundibular structures and heavy muscular trabeculations are not present so early in life, resection of muscle mass from the outflow tract should be avoided. A small tangential incision is made where the infundibular septum fuses with the anterior (parietal) right ventricular wall (ventriculoinfundibular fold); this facilitates exposure of both the posteroinferior and posterosuperior margins of the VSD (Fig. 13–5A).

The large malalignment type of VSD is closed with a Dacron patch using either a continuous suture technique or, preferably, interrupted horizontal mattress sutures (6-0 Teflon-coated Dacron) reinforced with Teflon pledgets. It is convenient to place the first suture into the mid-portion of the infundibular septum and to progress clockwise (Fig. 13–5B); each subsequent suture aids in exposing the margin of the defect. When the level of the papillary muscle of the conus (Lancisi) is reached, the septal and anterior leaflets of the tricuspid valve are retracted caudally. Depending on the type of anatomy, sutures are placed within the posteroinferior muscular limb of the septal band, which is free of conduction tissue (Fig. 13–5B,C), or preferably, if the posteroinferior rim of the defect is fibrous, the stitches are anchored either within this tough tissue (Fig. 13–5 D, E) or within the muscular septum, distant from the edge of the VSD (Fig. 13–5E). Fibrous tissue is a safe anchor for sutures, as conduc-

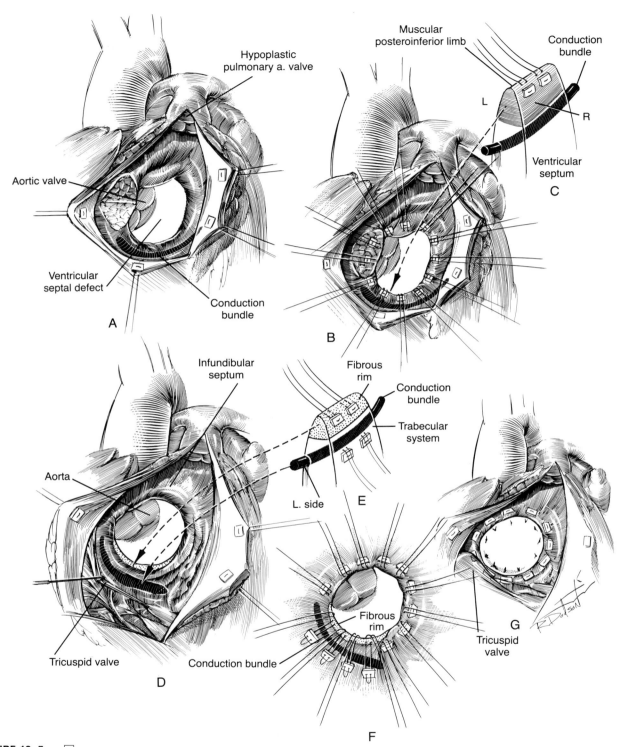

FIGURE 13–5. ☐

A, To improve exposure and access to the posteroinferior quadrant of the ventricular septal defect (VSD), the parietal extension of the infundibular septum is partially incised. *B,* The malalignment VSD is closed. *C,* In this schema, the posteroinferior limb of the trabecular septa marginalis is well developed, and the atrioventricular bundle is more deeply embedded within muscle and also more closely related to the left ventricular aspect of the septal crest. Sutures are placed safely within this muscle, avoiding encircling the crest of the ventricular septum. *D,* In this schema, the posteroinferior limb of the septal band is hypoplastic and is reduced to a fibrous rim formed by the confluence of the aortic valve annulus and endocardial cushion tissue of the tricuspid valve, establishing aortic valve–triscuspid valve continuity. *E,* Because of the hypoplasia of the posteroinferior limb, the bundle of His is less deeply embedded and thus lies closer to the right ventricular surface of the septal crest. In this anatomic variant, the sutures are either anchored within the fibrous rim to avoid the bundle of His or placed approximately 5 mm from the ventricular crest. *F,* All interrupted sutures reinforced with pledgets are in place. *G,* The VSD is completely closed with a Dacron patch anchored with interrupted horizontal mattress sutures reinforced with Teflon pledgets.

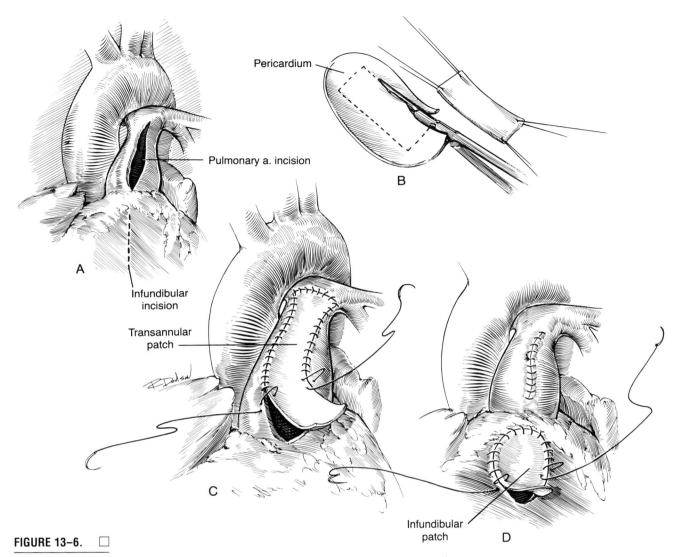

Pericardium

Pulmonary a. incision

Infundibular
incision

Transannular
patch

Infundibular
patch

A   B   C   D

FIGURE 13–6.   □

A, The pulmonary artery incision is extended across the pulmonary valve annulus, into the right ventricular infundibulum, and to the bifurcation of the main pulmonary artery. Dysplastic pulmonary valve leaflets are excised. A rectangular segment of glutaraldehyde-pretreated pericardium (*B*) is sutured with continuous 5-0 Prolene suture to the edges of the pulmonary artery and the right ventriculotomy (*C*). If the pulmonary valve is stenotic but not dysplastic and the valve annulus is of adequate size, a pulmonary valvotomy is carried out through the main pulmonary artery from above. A segment of pericardium is then sutured into the infundibular incision to avoid narrowing of the outflow tract by primary closure, while the pulmonary arteriotomy is closed primarily (*D*).

tion tissue, being specialized muscle, always courses within muscle. The use of Teflon pledgets permits a more superficial placement of sutures to decrease the risk of encircling and damaging the bundle of His, while at the same time avoiding suture line disruption. Sometimes it is difficult to visualize the posteroinferior and posterosuperior rim of the defect. Exposure of this area is facilitated by having the first assistant place a fine suction tip through the VSD and retracting it toward the left. Once all sutures are in place (Fig. 13–5*F*), an appropriately tailored Dacron patch is used to close the defect (Fig. 13–5*G*). In patients with a subpulmonary extension of the VSD (i.e., absence of the conal sep-

tum), sutures must be placed with much care within the fibrous band separating the pulmonary valve from the aortic valve. Next, the ventricular septum is searched for additional defects. The muscular portion anterior to the septal band is particularly suspect. If an anterior muscular VSD is present, it is preferable to use a patch instead of primary closure to avoid tearing this often very friable tissue.

If the pulmonary annulus is hypoplastic, a transannular patch is necessary (Fig. 13–6*A*). If the annulus is nonrestrictive, the patch can be limited to the right ventricular outflow tract without crossing the annulus (Fig. 13–6*B*).

It is important to fashion the pericardial right ventricular outflow patch to be wide rather than tapered, both proximally and distally (rectangular shape) (Fig. 13–6C), and to extend the patch into the left pulmonary artery whenever necessary to eliminate any obstruction at that level (Fig. 13–6C). Proximally, the length of the patch should be limited to about a third of the right ventricular length (measured from apex to pulmonary valve), and the width should approximate the normal size of the pulmonary valve annulus according to age. After anchoring the patch distally with one or two sutures, the atrial septum is examined. Small patent foramen ovales are left open to allow right-to-left decompression in case of temporary postoperative right-sided failure and also to facilitate transseptal left-sided catheterization studies later, after surgery. The right heart is then filled with saline, and the patient is placed back on cardiopulmonary bypass, again using a single cannula in the right atrium, the tip of which is positioned close to the junction of the superior vena cava and the right atrium. This technique allows for effective decompression of the right heart and limits the period of circulatory arrest to approximately 15 to 20 minutes. During rewarming, the patch on the right ventricular outflow tract is sutured with a continuous 5-0 Prolene suture to the edges of the pulmonary artery and the right ventriculotomy incision. Before the pericardial patch is fixed entirely, a pursestring suture is placed within the epicardium in the right ventricular free wall and a 19-gauge catheter is guided into the left pulmonary artery to make it possible to monitor the infant postoperatively and also to obtain a pullback tracing, usually within 24 to 48 hours after the operation.

Before removing the aortic crossclamp, a generous hole is made in the proximal ascending aorta to allow air to escape. The lungs are inflated vigorously to expel possible air trapped in the pulmonary veins. Cold saline can be infused into the left atrium to aid in removal of air from the left side of the circulation. The right coronary artery is temporarily occluded, and the aortic clamp is then removed.

The heart usually defibrillates spontaneously or is defibrillated at an esophageal temperature between 27°C and 30°C.

Hudspeth and associates, in 1963,[15] demonstrated that TOF could be repaired exclusively through the right atrium. The appeal of this approach is the theoretical advantage of minimizing or eliminating entirely the need for a right ventriculotomy, with consequent "preservation" of right ventricular function. The surgical technique includes closure of the VSD through the right atrium and tricuspid valve and also relief of RVOTO through the tricuspid and

pulmonary valves. However, if enlargement of the pulmonary valve annulus is required, an incision is necessary across the valve ring, extending the incision only minimally into the right ventricular outflow tract.

The operative mortality rate after transatrial repair of TOF in older children has been low, and the reported early postoperative hemodynamic measurements are certainly encouraging. Although we have had little experience with this technique at Children's Hospital in Boston, we believe it is unlikely that it is applicable to the broad spectrum of patients with TOF, particularly those with severe infundibular hypoplasia, who represent a large proportion of symptomatic neonates or young infants. Also, late follow-up studies are required to critically assess the function of the right ventricle and to determine whether late differences indeed persist between this transatrial method and the classic transventricular repair. It should also be noted that even though a ventriculotomy is avoided, this technique nevertheless requires extensive resection of muscle within the right ventricular outflow tract.

Postoperative Management. All neonates and infants remain connected to a volume-cycled respirator. The patient is weaned from the mechanical ventilator by decreasing intermittent mechanical ventilation, usually over a 24-hour period. Catheters in the right atrium, left atrium, and pulmonary artery facilitate volume replacement, detection of any residual intracardiac shunting, and measurement of right ventricular–pulmonary artery pressure gradients during the immediate postoperative period.

Most neonates and infants, particularly if they have received a transannular patch, are given a low dose of inotropic support, most commonly 5 μg/kg/min of dopamine, during and after weaning from the bypass. The drug is usually discontinued within 24 to 48 hours. Diuretics and digitalis are commonly continued for 4 to 6 months after the operation.

Tetralogy of Fallot With Pulmonary Atresia

As discussed previously, the origin and the course of all APCAs must be clearly outlined preoperatively. In the majority of instances, they emerge from the posterior mediastinum, anterior to the left or right bronchus, to enter their respective hila (Fig. 13–7A). Before continuing with cardiopulmonary bypass, these vessels must be dissected and looped to prevent runoff from the systemic-to-pulmonary circulation, which would result in systemic hypoperfusion and left ventricular distention. In most instances, to approach these collaterals it is useful to dissect the area between the ascending aorta and

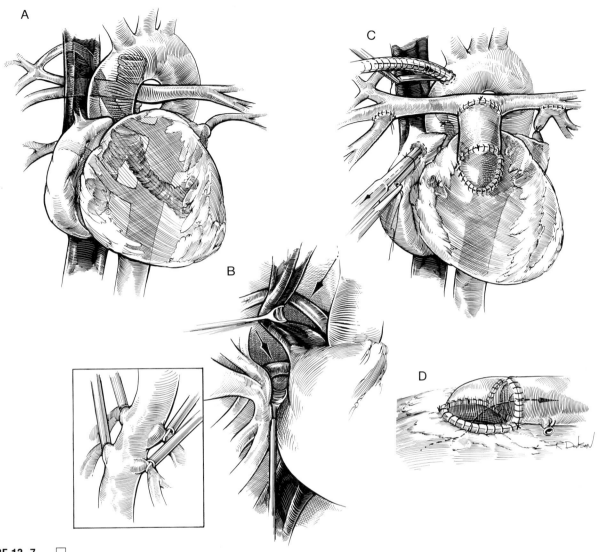

FIGURE 13–7. □

TOF-PA with diminutive pulmonary arteries. Most APCAs emerge from the posterior mediastinum anterior to the left or right bronchus (*A*). To expose these collaterals, it is useful to dissect the area between the ascending aorta and the right superior vena cava and also the area between the superior vena cava and the right pulmonary veins (*B*). In instances in which the APCA originates from the distal descending thoracic aorta or courses behind the left or right bronchus, a preliminary thoracotomy is often necessary to either temporarily or permanently interrupt these vessels (*insert*). Whenever an APCA is an end artery, it is detached from the aorta and anastomosed to the nearest branch of the pulmonary artery (*C*). Note the simple ligation of the right upper APCA, which connects with the right upper pulmonary artery and the unifocalization of the right lower APCA to the right lower lobe of the pulmonary artery; note also the side-to-side anastomosis of the left APCA to the left lower lobe of the pulmonary artery. The operation is completed by interposing a valved aortic allograft between the right ventricle and the diminutive pulmonary artery. The proximal anastomosis of the right ventricle to the homograft is augmented with a segment of glutaraldehyde-pretreated pericardium sutured to the remaining portion of the ventriculotomy and the homograft to avoid kinking (*D*).

the right superior vena cava through a midline sternotomy (Fig. 13–7*B*). Commonly, the more important APCAs can be found in this area, coursing anteriorly to the right bronchus. In the few instances in which the APCAs originate from the distal descending thoracic aorta or course behind the left or right bronchus, a preliminary thoracotomy is often necessary to either temporarily or permanently interrupt these vessels or to anastomose them to a pulmonary artery (unifocalization) (Fig. 13–7*C*).

Whenever an APCA is an end artery and supplies a significant area of lung parenchyma (for example, one entire lobe), the APCA is detached from the aorta and anastomosed to the nearest branch of the pulmonary artery (Fig. 13–7*D*). As a general rule, as many bronchopulmonary segments as possible are incorporated; generally it is necessary to establish flow to the equivalent of one whole lung (10 segments) before considering closure of the VSD. If the APCA is the principal blood supply to one lung and this collateral cannot be approached from the midline, a preliminary shunt operation may be necessary to ensure sufficient pulmonary blood flow during detachment of the APCA from the descending thoracic aorta. The vessel walls, particularly those of the pulmonary artery branches, are tenuous, and optimal surgical conditions are necessary to carry out an end-to-side anastomosis with 7-0 sutures. At Children's Hospital in Boston, it is the policy to confirm patency by obtaining an angiogram soon after unifocalization. Should additional unifocalization procedures be necessary on the opposite lung, this is accomplished, by preference, during the same hospitalization or soon thereafter.

If the APCAs can be approached through a midline sternotomy, the collaterals are first dissected and are occluded immediately as the patient is started on cardiopulmonary bypass. It is hoped this maneuver will diminish the threat of perioperative complications involving the central nervous system (e.g., acute or chronic choreoathetosis, which we have observed in a few patients with uncontrolled APCAs during cardiopulmonary bypass). Although the exact cause of this dreadful complication is not known, the possibility of a central nervous system "steal" phenomenon while the infant is on bypass, interfering with adequate blood supply to the globus pallidus and other related areas, seems a reasonable hypothesis. Because of this complication, every effort should be made to control as many APCAs as possible before commencing the bypass. Once the infant is on bypass and during cooling, the APCAs are either detached and anastomosed to the nearest pulmonary artery in an end-to-side fashion, as described previously, or ligated temporarily or permanently, depending on whether they are the sole blood supply or are part of a dual blood supply to an important segment of the lung. Also, because it is impossible to completely control all collateral flow on bypass, and to avoid ventricular distention, the left ventricle must be decompressed with a vent introduced through the junction of the right pulmonary vein and left atrium. At 20°C, tympanic temperature, flow is reduced to 50 ml/kg/min and P_{CO_2} is maintained at 45 mm Hg or more. A tangential vascular clamp especially designed for infants is placed on the confluence of the right and left diminutive pulmonary arteries. A longitudinal incision is made, and the distal end of a 7- to 10-mm aortic or pulmonary artery homograft is anastomosed to the pulmonary artery using a continuous 7-0 polydioxanone suture technique (Fig. 13–7D). At this reduced flow and with the atrial cannula directed toward the junction of the superior vena cava with the atrium, it is rarely necessary to induce circulatory arrest. A vertical ventriculotomy is then made to

allow for the anastomosis between the right ventricle and the proximal end of the homograft (Fig. 13–7E). Approximately 50% of the circumference of the homograft is anastomosed to the distal end of the right ventriculotomy, and the anastomosis is completed with a segment of glutaraldehyde-pretreated pericardium sutured to the remaining portion of the ventriculotomy and homograft (Fig. 13–7F). This pericardial baffle augments the anastomosis and prevents kinking or obstruction of the homograft. At this point, the patient is rewarmed; the VSD is left open. With the improvements in transcatheter closure of midmuscular or apical VSDs, we at Children's Hospital in Boston are currently suturing a perforated Dacron patch into the conoventricular VSD, facilitating later percutaneous catheter closure of the VSD with a clamshell device.

Although small pulmonary arteries can be enlarged by systemic-to–pulmonary artery shunts, on numerous occasions we have observed significant iatrogenic damage to these small branches of pulmonary arteries after a classic or modified Blalock-Taussig shunt, and even more often after a Waterston shunt. Frequently these hypoplastic pulmonary arteries kink, reducing or completely obstructing ipsilateral or contralateral pulmonary blood flow. By establishing early right ventricular–to–pulmonary artery continuity with a conduit, leaving the VSD open, the surgeon achieves antegrade and more even flow into both right and left pulmonary arteries. Results after the use of cryopreserved, valved homografts are impressive. These offer significant advantages over prosthetic grafts with regard to technical ease of anastomosis to these very small pulmonary arteries and their long-term patency rate.

Discontinuous Diminutive Right and Left Pulmonary Arteries or Absent Mediastinal Pulmonary Arteries. In a few patients, diminutive pulmonary artery branches are present but are discontinuous; indeed, even fewer patients have no mediastinal pulmonary arteries (Fig. 13–8A). However, in the majority of these patients there is a pulmonary artery within the hilum, albeit small, that is suitable for anastomosis. In that case, through a lateral thoracotomy, a 3.5- or 4-mm Gore-Tex graft is interposed between the right subclavian artery and the stump of the hilar pulmonary artery (Fig. 13–8B1). Usually, during the same hospitalization, this procedure is repeated on the opposite side (Fig. 13–8B2). The objective is to (1) stimulate growth of these pulmonary arteries, (2) eventually connect the left and right pulmonary arteries, and (3) connect the reconstituted pulmonary arteries to the right ventricle using a valved homograft. Therefore, after angiographically documented enlarge-

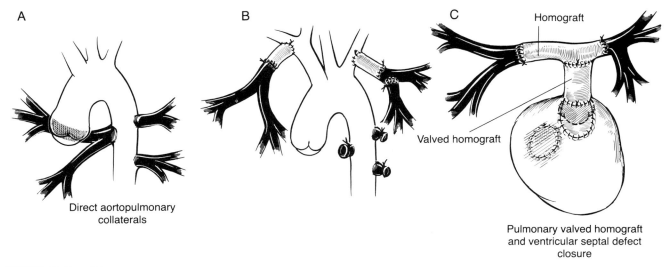

Direct aortopulmonary
collaterals

Homograft

Valved homograft

Pulmonary valved homograft
and ventricular septal defect
closure

FIGURE 13–8. ☐

TOF-PA and absent mediastinal pulmonary arteries. *A,* The pulmonary blood supply is exclusively from APCAs. Through a lateral thoracotomy, the APCAs are detached from the descending thoracic aorta, followed by interposition of a graft and anastomosis to branches of the ascending aorta (*B*). This procedure is repeated on the opposite side within the same hospitalization. Note the unifocalization of the left inferior APCA to the left superior APCA. Through a midline sternotomy incision, the previously positioned Gore-Tex conduits are detached and removed. The left and right distal pulmonary arteries are connected with a nonvalved aortic allograft. A valved aortic allograft is then interposed between the right ventricular outflow tract and the reconstructed left and right pulmonary arteries (*C*). The VSD was also closed during this second stage of the operation.

ment of both left and right intraparenchymal pulmonary branches (usually after 6 to 12 months), through a midline sternotomy and on cardiopulmonary bypass, a 12-mm conduit (preferably a nonvalved aortic homograft) is interposed between the right and left hilar pulmonary arteries, and a valved aortic homograft is made to connect the right ventricle with the nonvalved aortic homograft (Fig. 13–8*C*).

In patients with absent mediastinal pulmonary arteries, the aortopulmonary collaterals are detached from the descending aorta through a right thoracotomy and are connected to the right subclavian artery or to the ascending aorta (Fig. 13–8*B*) using a 4- or 5-mm Gore-Tex graft, depending on age and size. During the same hospitalization, through a left thoracotomy, the left APCAs are likewise detached from the descending thoracic aorta, adding unifocalization if necessary (as depicted in Figure 13–8*B*), and anastomosed to the left subclavian artery using a 4- or 5-mm Gore-Tex graft. To avoid development of PVOD, these children are brought back for cardiac catheterization in 6 months. This is followed by surgery, at which time the modified Blalock-Taussig shunts are detached from the ascending aorta and subclavian artery. The Gore-Tex shunts are removed, and, preferably, a valved homograft is placed between the right ventricular outflow tract and the left pulmonary artery directly, often as depicted in Figure 13–8*C*. An ad-

ditional extension of nonvalved aortic homograft is required to connect the valved homograft to the right pulmonary artery. The VSD is closed only if both peripheral pulmonary arteries have enlarged sufficiently and the combined left and right blood supply exceeds that in 10 bronchopulmonary segments. Otherwise, the VSD is left open and is closed at a third operation. It is often advisable to transect the ascending aorta to facilitate anastomosis of the graft to the right pulmonary artery and also to place the graft in a retroaortic position, which avoids retrosternal compression and allows for a shorter graft.

RESULTS

Tetralogy of Fallot With Pulmonary Stenosis

Fourteen of 330 infants (4.2%) died early after the operation (Table 13–1). The highest mortality rate occurred among the 32 neonates. For infants older than 1 month, the hospital mortality rate averaged 3%. Note that the results improved after 1985, including those for neonates.

Only five of the 14 hospital deaths were primarily related to repair of tetralogy of Fallot. Among the remaining nine deaths, one patient had preoperative necrotizing enterocolitis, another had myocardial infarction after postoperative cardiac catheterization, and yet another had idiopathic hypertrophic

TABLE 13–1. ☐ TETRALOGY OF FALLOT WITH PULMONARY STENOSIS

AGE (mos)	JANUARY 1973–DECEMBER 1990					JANUARY 1985–DECEMBER 1990			
	No. of Infants	Deaths				Number of Infants	Deaths		
		Hospital		Late			Hospital		Late
		No.	%	No.	%		No.	%	
0 to <1	32	4	12.5	1	3.1	16	1	6.2	0
1 to <3	68	2	2.9	0		24	0		0
3 to <6	104	5	4.8	1	0.9	33	1	3.0	0
6 to <12	126	3	2.3	1	0.7	47	1	2.1	0
Total	330	14	4.2	3	0.9	120	3	2.5	0

subaortic stenosis associated with tetralogy of Fallot. One patient died from hyperkalemia; one neonate developed fever and pericardial effusion and died during an attempt at a pericardial tap. Of the four remaining deaths, two were caused by sepsis and two by pulmonary complications. The use of a transannular patch did not affect the hospital mortality rate (5% with and 4% without transannular patches).

Five of the 14 deaths were directly related to technical matters concerning the operation. However, pulmonary artery size (PAI < 120) was the cause of death in only one neonate. In retrospect, this patient should have had the VSD patch perforated immediately after the operation.

There were three late deaths. One patient with trisomy 21 died 6 months after surgery from endocarditis. The second patient died 14 months after surgery from an adenovirus, necrotizing pneumonitis, and encephalitis. The third patient, with a large aortopulmonary collateral, developed PVOD and died 8 years postoperatively from progressive cyanosis and left heart failure. The actuarial survival rate, including hospital deaths, was 93% at 15 years.

Reoperations

Twenty-six infants (7.8%) required reoperation, 18 because of residual RVOTO ($\Delta P > 40$ mm Hg). The causes of the residual obstruction included infundibular patches that did not extend across hypoplastic pulmonary valve annuli (four patients) and retained dysplastic pulmonary valve tissue (two patients). Four patients had obstructing anomalous muscle bundles in the proximal right ventricular outflow tract. The remaining eight had residual stenosis at the distal end of the patch to the pulmonary artery anastomosis. Residual VSDs were closed in eight other patients, four of whom had additional VSDs located within the anterior muscular ventricular septum. Two other patients required ligation of aortopulmonary collaterals, and one needed mitral

valve replacement for severe mitral stenosis caused by a parachute mitral valve. The actuarial freedom rate from reoperation was 85% at 15 years.

Electrocardiographic Holter Monitoring and Electrophysiologic Studies

Of 183 patients with late electrocardiographic follow-up, 91% had right bundle branch block and 6% had an additional left anterior hemiblock. Arrhythmias included sinus bradycardia in one patient and infrequent uniform ventricular ectopic activity (Lown 1 VEA) in 6% of the patients. Holter data recorded from 41 patients approximately 15 months after operation revealed a 25% incidence of Lown 1 VEA; none had greater than Lown 2 VEA.

Electrophysiologic studies in the same 41 patients revealed a prolonged corrected sinus node recovery time in only one patient. The AH interval was prolonged in two patients and the HV interval in three. Delayed activation of the right ventricular apex, consistent with central right bundle branch block, was observed in 20 patients. None of the surviving patients received antiarrhythmic drugs, nor were any of the three late deaths related to an arrhythmic event.

Primary or Two-Stage Repair

The surgical strategy of primary repair of TOF-PS early in life has given excellent early and late results and compares favorably with two-stage approaches. Encouraged by our results with primary repair for symptomatic infants who have TOF-PS, we at Children's Hospital in Boston have begun to operate electively on asymptomatic young infants with this abnormality.

Although a two-institution review of 196 patients with TOF-PS revealed that age less than 3 months was a risk factor for death after repair, we have found that this risk has decreased in neonates since 1988. It is also true that death was more often associated with an intraoperative event in the very young; however, these initial difficulties have also decreased significantly since 1988. We are certain that with increasing experience and improved surgical techniques, the slightly higher risk of repairing TOF-PS in the neonate will soon be overcome.

Most reoperations were related to residual RVOTO. The majority of these were necessitated by technical problems (e.g., not carrying the outflow patch across a hypoplastic pulmonary annulus or leaving dysplastic pulmonary valve tissue behind). Of interest are the patients whose residual stenosis was at the distal end of the patch, despite the effort to fashion a rectangular patch and to carry the anastomosis beyond the left pulmonary artery take-off. In three of these patients the gradient was eliminated by carrying the anastomosis beyond the stenotic junction of the main and left pulmonary arteries. However, the other patient continues with significant right ventricular hypertension.

Use of a Transannular Patch

The question of when to use a transannular patch (TAP) can be resolved in several ways. Kirklin and associates[16] identified a close correlation between the preoperative Z value of the annulus and postoperative $P_{RV:LV}$ ratios. In the presence of nearly normal right and left pulmonary arteries, they recommended using a TAP whenever the Z value is -2 or less. Another practical option is to measure the size of the annulus with a Hegar dilator and compare it with normal pulmonary annulus diameters based on Rowlatt and associates' data.[34] Over the years, most of us at the Children's Hospital in Boston have depended on a subjective, visual evaluation (before and during the operation) of the need for a transannular patch. Interestingly, results of a comparison between our empiric approach and the quantitative approach of surgeons at the University of Alabama concerning the need for a TAP correlated surprisingly well. In general, there is also a correlation between the postoperative elevated $P_{RV:LV}$ ratios and hypoplasia of the annulus (i.e., the smaller the pulmonary valve annulus [by inspection or by Z value], the greater the probability of a higher postrepair $P_{RV:LV}$ ratio even when using a TAP). Clearly, if a TAP is not necessary, its use should be avoided. We have lately decreased the use of TAPs, partly because we are operating on a larger number of asymptomatic infants who have more favorable anatomy. However, TAPs are still needed in nearly 100% of symptomatic neonates or young infants operated on during the first 3 months of life in our institution.

Because of the known risks of residual RVOTO, some of us have opted toward a more liberal use of TAPs. In our experience, the use of a TAP does not increase the operative risk, and clear-cut evidence of a deleterious effect of isolated pulmonary valvular insufficiency on right ventricular function after TOF repair has not been reported. Most experiences indicate that both acute and chronic right ventricular volume overloads secondary to pulmonary valve insufficiency are well tolerated over a long period of time. Also, many postoperative catheterization studies done decades after TOF repair do not identify pulmonary valve insufficiency as a contributing factor to poor late hemodynamic results. In fact, the presence of a TAP does not seem, in itself, to increase the need for a pulmonary valve insertion unless there is residual stenosis or hypoplasia of one or both pulmonary arteries. Clearly, one of the important questions that remains to be answered (regardless of the method used to predict the need for a transannular patch) is whether, in borderline cases, the risk of chronic mild pulmonary valve insufficiency outweighs the risk of moderately elevated residual right ventricular hypertension ($P_{RV:LV}$ between 0.5 and 0.75).

Tetralogy of Fallot With Pulmonary Atresia

Between 1984 and 1990 at the Children's Hospital in Boston, we treated 27 patients who had TOF-PA and diminutive but continuous pulmonary arteries. These patients were managed according to the previously outlined protocol. Of these, 11 were younger than 9 months of age at initial treatment, and six were neonates. In all, aortic or pulmonary cryopreserved, valved homografts were interposed between the right ventricle and the junction of the right and left diminutive pulmonary arteries. Six patients died early or late after the operation (three shortly after the operation, two within 6 months, and one 1 year later because of rupture of a dilatation-induced aneurysm of the right pulmonary artery). In six of these 27 patients, a separate lateral right thoracotomy was required to control aortopulmonary collaterals before continuing with cardiopulmonary bypass. In nine patients unifocalization procedures were carried out (six unilateral and three bilateral). Of the surviving 21 patients, 10 have since undergone closure of the VSD. Seven of these patients have good hemodynamic results proved at cardiac catheterization. One has residual right ventricular hypertension (two thirds systemic), and two have not yet been studied postoperatively. The 10 repaired survivors are all alive at an average of 31 months after the operation. Seven of the 10 surviving repaired patients also had successful coil embolization of residual systemic collaterals and dilatation of pulmonary artery stenosis. Of the remaining 11 unrepaired patients, two are currently deemed unrepairable because of inadequate distal pulmonary arteries, three await additional unifocalization procedures, and the remaining six are candidates for repair. So far, important pulmonary artery growth has been achieved after interposition of the first-stage homograft in all patients, including one with an initial PAI of 10 mm²/m².

Our experience with the subset of patients who have TOF-PA and discontinuous and diminutive or absent mediastinal pulmonary arteries is much more limited. So far, of seven patients with absent mediastinal pulmonary arteries, four have survived the initial left and right modified Blalock-Taussig shunt operations and subsequent connection of left and right pulmonary hila, with additional interposition of a valved homograft between the right ventricle and the reconstructed pulmonary arteries. In two of the four survivors, the ventricular septal defects have been closed during a third operation.

IMPLICATIONS

Encouraged by early and late (as much as 20 years of follow-up) experience with primary repair of TOF in symptomatic infants, at Children's Hospital in Boston we currently electively repair tetralogy of Fallot in infancy. This is consistent with the notion that early repair minimizes secondary damage of vital organs and also allows for normal postnatal developmental changes. Elective repair in the neonate looms as a realistic therapeutic goal in the not-too-distant future.

Concerning TOF-PA and diminutive pulmonary arteries, we are not yet in a position to draw any final conclusions from our present experience with this complex subject because of the small number of patients subjected to this staged and combined approach and the diverse nature of this entity. However, we are encouraged by the results with early establishment of right ventricular–to–pulmonary artery continuity using a valved homograft, subsequent pulmonary artery dilatations, and embolization of the APCAs. This has led to successful second-stage repair in a number of patients. We expect that this staged approach, if started early in life (preferably in neonatal or early infancy period), should enhance normal development of pulmonary vascular and parenchymal structures and, consequently, should lead to a more successful late outcome in the majority of patients.

TETRALOGY OF FALLOT WITH ABSENT PULMONARY VALVE

This variant of tetralogy of Fallot includes massively enlarged pulmonary arteries, a typical malalignment type of VSD, usually aplasia or rudimentary development of the pulmonary valve, and also, commonly, a mildly hypoplastic pulmonary valve annulus.

An additional intriguing feature of this syndrome is absence of the ductus arteriosus. In reported cases of TOF with absent pulmonary valve and continuous pulmonary arteries, no ductus arteriosus remnants have been identified. The only cases in which a ductus arteriosus has been found are those in which the left pulmonary artery is discontinuous and is supplied solely by the ductus.

The development of pulmonary artery aneurysms in this syndrome has been ascribed to the absence of the ductus in combination with pulmonary regurgitation and high pulmonary vascular resistance in utero. Because the main pulmonary artery cannot be decompressed into the aorta because of the absent ductus, there are increased pulmonary artery pressure and volume overload. The pulmonary regurgitation causes additional widening of the main pulmonary arteries. The implication of this argument is that development of the aneurysm is dependent on the absence of the ductus.

However, this argument seems flawed. The presence of a nonrestrictive VSD in this syndrome mandates that right ventricular pressure cannot exceed left ventricular pressure. Similarly, main pulmonary artery pressure cannot rise above aortic pressure. Therefore, in the presence of a nonrestrictive VSD in utero, the main pulmonary artery and aortic pressures will be equal regardless of whether the ductus arteriosus is present. Therefore, we believe that absence of the ductus arteriosus has little to do with the development of the pulmonary artery aneurysm. Why, then, is a ductus arteriosus not found in this syndrome?

Possibly the ductus arteriosus is just as likely to be present in TOF when the pulmonary valve is absent as in typical TOF (i.e., 80% to 90% of the time). However, if a ductus arteriosus forms when the pulmonary valve is absent, the fetus cannot survive for reasons outlined later, while those fetuses fortunate enough to develop without a ductus arteriosus survive. The reason a patent ductus in this condition causes fetal death is that the ductus allows unrestricted regurgitant flow from the aorta retrograde through the main pulmonary artery and across the absent pulmonary valve. In addition, the large VSD provides more capacitance in diastole so that regurgitant flow can occur into both ventricles.

This combination of absent pulmonary valve with a ductus arteriosus is physiologically comparable to unrestrictive aortic regurgitation.

Some evidence exists to support this argument. First, as mentioned, a ductus arteriosus has been described in cases of tetralogy of Fallot with absent pulmonary valve, but only in those cases where it is the sole supplier to an otherwise discontinuous left pulmonary artery. This observation proves that a ductus can exist with this syndrome. It also suggests that the reason these infants have survived is because the ductus is discontinuous with the main pulmonary artery and the absent pulmonary valve. Therefore, there is no aortic regurgitation equivalent. Second, absence of the pulmonary valve has been reported with an intact ventricular septum and a ductus arteriosus. These fetuses can survive but are critically ill (i.e., hydropic) in late gestation and in the neonatal period. These cases confirm the contention that the combination of a ductus and pulmonary regurgitation is a life-threatening, hemodynamic lesion for the fetus and neonate. With an intact ventricular septum, however, the smaller capacitance of the right ventricle may restrict regurgitant flow enough so that some fetuses can survive, although barely, until birth. With the increased capacitance in diastole of the left ventricle (provided by the nonrestrictive VSD in TOF with absent pulmonary valve), the volume of regurgitation will increase significantly and thereby preclude fetal survival. This hypothesis is not mutually exclusive with an intrinsic pulmonary arterial wall abnormality.

In fact, the histologic abnormalities described in the pulmonary arteries (e.g., thickened and fragmented elastic laminae or medial hypertrophy of pulmonary arterioles) and also compression of bronchi by tufts of segmental arteries, which entwine and compress the intrapulmonary bronchi, could all conceivably be secondary to the altered intrauterine hemodynamics.[31] Momma and associates[26] demonstrated experimentally in rats that bronchial compression starts in the fetus and that ventricular dilatation is associated with diastolic volume overload resulting from massive pulmonary valve regurgitation. Whether the absent pulmonary valve syndrome is caused primarily by some teratogenic effect on neural crest cells or occurs secondary to the absence of the ductus arteriosus, causing pulmonary valve insufficiency, has not been clearly established.

Symptoms

The principal symptoms of airway obstruction and secondary pulmonary infections are mostly due to compression of the mainstem bronchi by the markedly enlarged central pulmonary arteries. However, as mentioned previously, branching anomalies of intraparenchymal pulmonary arteries can contribute to the pathophysiology of this syndrome.

Symptoms can range from life-threatening respiratory difficulties at birth to few, if any, cardiorespiratory symptoms. This latter group can safely undergo elective cardiac surgery later in childhood. This discussion will concentrate on the symptomatic neonate or young infant with this syndrome.

Operative Technique

Various surgical procedures have been proposed in the past. In 1973 Litwin and associates[24] recommended a two-stage approach in which the tracheobronchial tree first was decompressed by interposing a conduit between sections of the divided right pulmonary artery. At the second stage, performed later in childhood, the conduit was replaced by a larger one, and the TOF was repaired. At Children's Hospital in Boston, we have abandoned this technique because of the large initial risk and the complexity of the second-stage operation. Clearly, the aim of any procedure has to prominently include the elimination of bronchial compression by the aneurysmally dilated pulmonary arteries.[36] Therefore, we currently excise a generous portion of both the anterior and posterior walls of the main, left, and right pulmonary arteries. We have found this to be the only technique that allows effective and uniform reduction in size of the pulmonary arteries. The malalignment type of VSD is closed, as described previously for repair of tetralogy of Fallot. Finally, we also consider it important to provide these critically ill neonates or young infants with a functioning pulmonary valve; therefore, we have used an orthotropically positioned homograft valve within the right ventricular outflow tract.

Implications

Although our experience with this extensive approach is still limited, we are nevertheless persuaded that the results will improve. Until 1989 we had had no symptomatic neonates with TOF and an absent pulmonary valve survive attempts at various types of repair, but since adopting the operative strategy just described, two of three neonates survived the operation and are doing well.

REFERENCES

1. Barratt-Boyes BG, Neutze JM. Primary repair of tetralogy of Fallot in infancy using profound hypothermia with circula-

tory arrest and limited cardiopulmonary bypass: A comparison with conventional two-stage management. Ann Surg 178:406, 1973.

2. Blackstone EH, Kirklin JW, Bertranou EG, et al. Preoperative prediction from cineangiograms of postrepair right ventricular pressure in tetralogy of Fallot. J Thorac Cardiovasc Surg 78:543, 1979.

3. Blalock A, Taussig HB. The surgical treatment of malformations of the heart in which there is pulmonary stenosis or pulmonary atresia. JAMA 128:189, 1945.

4. Brock RC. Pulmonary valvulotomy for relief of congenital pulmonary stenosis. Report of 3 cases. Br Med J I:1121, 1948.

5. Castaneda AR. Classical repair of tetralogy of Fallot: Timing, technique, and results. Semin Thorac Cardiovasc Surg 2:70, 1990.

6. Castaneda AR, Freed MD, Williams RG, et al. Repair of tetralogy of Fallot in infancy. J Thorac Cardiovasc Surg 74:372, 1977.

7. Castaneda AR, Lamberti J, Sade RM, et al. Open heart surgery during the first three months of life. J Thorac Cardiovasc Surg 68:719, 1974.

8. Castaneda AR, Mayer JE Jr, Lock JE. Tetralogy of Fallot, pulmonary atresia and diminutive pulmonary arteries. Prog Pediatr Cardiol 1:50, 1992.

9. Davidson JS. Anastomosis between the ascending aorta and the main pulmonary artery in the tetralogy of Fallot. Thorax 10:348, 1955.

10. Edwards JE, McGoon DC. Absence of anatomic origin from heart of pulmonary arterial supply. Circulation 54:117, 1973.

11. Fallot A. Contribution al'Anatomie pathologique de la Maladie Bleue (Cyanose Cardiaque). Marseille, Barlatier-Feissat, 1888.

12. Fellows KE, Freed MK, Keane JR, et al. Results of routine preoperative coronary angiography in tetralogy of Fallot. Circulation 51:561, 1975.

13. Gott VL. C. Walton Lillehei and total correction of tetralogy of Fallot. Ann Thorac Surg 49:328, 1990.

14. Haworth SG, Macartney FJ. Growth and development of pulmonary circulation in pulmonary atresia with ventricular septal defect and major aortopulmonary collateral arteries. Br Heart J 44:14, 1980.

15. Hudspeth AS, Cordell AR, Johnston FR. Transatrial approach to total correction of tetralogy of Fallot. Circulation 27:796, 1963.

16. Kirklin JK, Kirklin JW, Pacifico AD. Transannular outflow tract patching for tetralogy: Indications and results. Semin Thorac Cardiovasc Surg 2:61, 1990.

17. Kirklin JW, DuShane JW, Patrick RT, et al. Intracardiac surgery with the aid of a mechanical pump-oxygenator system (Gibbon type): Report of eight cases. Proc Staff Meet Mayo Clin 30:201, 1955.

18. Kirklin JW, Blackstone EH, Jonas RA, et al. Morphologic and surgical determinants of outcome events after repair of tetralogy of Fallot and pulmonary stenosis: A two-institution study. J Thorac Cardiovasc Surg 103:706, 1992.

19. Klinner W. Indikationsstellung und operative technik fur die korrektur der Fallotschen tetralogie. Langenbecks Archiv fur Klinische Chirurgie 308:40, 1964.

20. Klinner VW, Pasini M, Schaudig A. Anastomose zwischen System- und Lungenarterie mit hilfe von Kunststoffprothesen bei Cyanotischen Herzvitien. Thoraxchirurgie 10:68, 1962.

21. Laks H, Castaneda AR. Subclavian arterioplasty for the ipsilateral Blalock-Taussig shunt. Ann Thorac Surg 19:319, 1975.

22. de Leval MR, McKay R, Jones J, et al. Modified Blalock-Taussig shunt. Use of subclavian artery orifice as flow regulator in prosthetic systemic-pulmonary artery shunts. J Thorac Cardiovasc Surg 81:112, 1981.

23. Lillehei CW, Cohen M, Warden HE, et al. Direct vision intracardiac surgical correction of the tetralogy of Fallot, pentalogy of Fallot and pulmonary atresia defects: Report of first ten cases. Ann Surg 142:418, 1955.

24. Litwin SB, Rosenthal A, Fellows K. Surgical management of young infants with tetralogy of Fallot, absence of pulmonary valve and respiratory distress. J Thorac Cardiovasc Surg 3:65:117, 1981.

25. Lock JE, Castaneda-Zuniga WR, Fuhrman BP, et al. Balloon dilation angioplasty of hypoplastic and stenotic pulmonary arteries. Circulation 67:962, 1983.

26. Momma K, Ando M, Takao A. Fetal cardiac morphology of tetralogy of Fallot with absent pulmonary valve in the rat. Circulation 82:1343, 1990.

27. Murphy JD, Freed MD, Keane JF, et al. Hemodynamic results after intracardiac repair of tetralogy of Fallot by deep hypothermia and cardiopulmonary bypass. Circulation 62(suppl 1):168, 1980.

28. Nakata S, Imai Y, Takanashi Y, et al. A new method for the quantitative standardization of cross-sectional areas of the pulmonary arteries in congenital heart diseases with decreased pulmonary blood flow. J Thorac Cardiovasc Surg 88:610, 1984.

29. Piehler JM, Danielson GK, McGoon DC, et al. Management of pulmonary atresia with ventricular septal defect and hypoplastic pulmonary arteries by right ventricular outflow obstruction. J Thorac Cardiovasc Surg 80:552, 1980.

30. Potts WJ, Smith S, Gibson S. Anastomosis of the aorta to a pulmonary artery. JAMA 132:627, 1946.

31. Rabinovitch M, Grady S, David I, et al. Compression of intrapulmonary bronchi by abnormally branching pulmonary arteries associated with absent pulmonary valves. Am J Cardiol 50:804, 1982.

32. Rabinovitch M, Herrera-deLeon V, Castaneda AR, et al. Growth and development of the pulmonary vascular bed in patients with tetralogy of Fallot with or without pulmonary atresia. Circulation 64:1234, 1981.

33. Ross D, Somerville J. Correction of pulmonary atresia with a homograft aortic valve. Lancet 2:1446, 1966.

34. Rowlatt JF, Rimoldi HJA, Lev M. The quantitative anatomy of the normal child's heart. Pediatr Clin North Am 10:499, 1963.

35. Sellors TH. Surgery of pulmonary stenosis (a case in which pulmonary valve was successfully divided). Lancet 1:98, 1948.

36. Stellin G, Jonas RA, Goh TH, et al. Surgical treatment of absent pulmonary valve syndrome in infants: Relief of bronchial obstruction. Ann Thorac Surg 36:468, 1982.

37. Stenson N. Hafniencia Acta Med Philosoph 1:200, 1671–1672.

38. Thiene G, Frescura C, Bini RM, et al. Histology of pulmonary arterial supply in pulmonary atresia with ventricular septal defect. Circulation 60(5):1066, 1979.

39. Van Praagh R, Van Praagh S, Nebesar RA, et al. Tetralogy of Fallot: Underdevelopment of the pulmonary infundibulum and its sequelae. Am J Cardiol 26:25, 1970.

40. Walsh EP, Rockenmacher S, Keane JF, et al. Late results in patients with tetralogy of Fallot repaired during infancy. Circulation 77:1062, 1988.

41. Waterston D. Leceni Fallotovy tetralogie u deti do jednoho roku veku. Rozhl Chir XLI:3, 1962.

42. White RI Jr, Frech RS, Castaneda AR, et al. The nature and significance of anomalous coronary arteries in tetralogy of Fallot. Am J Roentgenol 114:350, 1972.

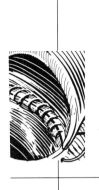

14

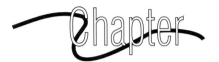

Pulmonary Atresia With Intact Ventricular Septum

The term *pulmonary atresia with an intact ventricular septum* (PA-IVS) is used to describe those patients who have "isolated" atresia of the outlet semilunar valve from the right ventricle without an associated ventricular septal defect and who have normal (concordant) relationships between the atria and ventricles and between the ventricles and the great vessels (S,D,N). Since the advent of surgical approaches to this and other cardiac defects, numerous reports on both the pathologic aspects of this disorder[6, 8, 9] and the clinical management of these patients have appeared.[3, 5, 7, 10] These clinical results have shown continuing improvement, but the results of surgical therapy remain imperfect. This chapter will focus on the important anatomic variations within the diagnosis of PA-IVS and will describe the ways in which current management is tailored to these anatomic variations.

ANATOMIC CONSIDERATIONS

Despite the implication from the terminology that PA-IVS is simply a defect of the pulmonary valve, this diagnosis encompasses a spectrum of disorders that have important anatomic variations involving not only the pulmonary valve, but also the tricuspid valve, the right ventricle, and the coronary circula-

tion. These anatomic variations have important implications for the surgical approaches to be employed.

The morphology of the pulmonary valve is somewhat variable, but most valves share the common feature of a diaphragm-like structure in the normal position of the pulmonary valve. This diaphragm appears to be formed by the fusion of the three commissures of the valve,[9, 16] and the fusion lines between the rudimentary leaflets are generally readily apparent when the valve is visualized. The consistency of the leaflets varies from thin and relatively pliable to markedly thickened and myxomatous. In a minority of cases, the pulmonary valve is much less well developed, and the valve is represented only by a dimple at the base of the main pulmonary artery. These cases are almost always associated with atresia or severe hypoplasia of the infundibulum. Becker suggested that when there is a patent infundibulum, the leaflet morphology consists of a valve containing a dome-shaped central area with peripheral raphes, whereas in infundibular atresia, the annulus is more hypoplastic, and the valve tissue is characterized by prominent commissural ridges that meet at the center of the pulmonary root.[2] The pulmonary annular size is also variable and ranges from nearly normal to quite hypoplastic.[2, 9] The main pulmonary artery is generally of normal or near-normal size, although there is a

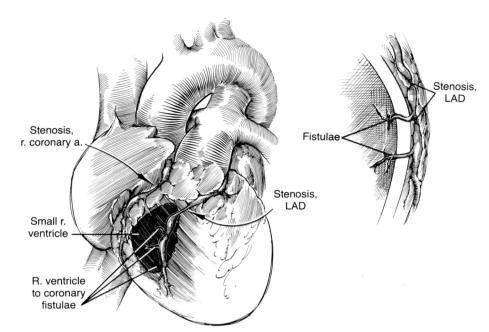

Stenosis, r. coronary a.

Small r. ventricle

R. ventricle to coronary fistulae

Fistulae

Stenosis, LAD

Stenosis, LAD

FIGURE 14–1. ☐

Depiction of coronary artery stenoses in right and anterior descending systems associated with a markedly hypoplastic right ventricle and tricuspid valve. The insert shows that stenoses (or atretic areas) may occur proximal or distal to coexisting right ventricle–to–coronary artery fistulae. LAD, Left anterior descending artery.

subset of patients with infundibular atresia and poorly formed, severely hypoplastic pulmonary valves that tend to have much smaller main pulmonary artery segments.[16]

The tricuspid valve generally has a reasonably normal leaflet structure, but in as many as 30% of these patients, the interchordal spaces are obliterated, which can result in functional tricuspid stenosis.[21] In a few cases the leaflet tissue is actually muscularized,[21] and rarely the tricuspid leaflets may be absent.[21] An important subgroup are those with PA-IVS and Ebstein's malformation of the tricuspid valve (see Chapter 16). The tricuspid annulus is frequently hypoplastic to varying degrees,[21] and the size of the tricuspid annulus generally correlates with the degree of hypoplasia of the right ventricular cavity.

The size and structure of the right ventricle are also variable, ranging from extremely diminutive to larger than normal. In an autopsy series at Children's Hospital in Boston, only 18% of the right ventricles were of normal size or larger; the remainder had varying degrees of hypoplasia.[21] Similar results were noted by Bull and coworkers.[5] The right ventricle almost always shows marked hypertrophy of the wall because of the outflow obstruction.[5, 9, 21] The normal right ventricle is generally thought to consist of three parts:[8, 15] the inlet, or sinus; the trabecular portion; and the infundibulum. On an angiogram or echocardiogram, the trabecular or infundibular portions of the right ventricle in PA-IVS may appear to be "absent,"[5] but on pathologic examination, the right ventricle generally contains an inlet, trabecular, and infundibular portions.[21]

The varying degrees of cavity obliteration by hypertrophied trabecular muscle bundles account for the variations in the cavitary volume of the trabecular and infundibular parts.[2] Bull and coworkers[5] found that in nearly half of the cases in their autopsy series, there was obliteration of either the trabecular or trabecular and infundibular portions of the right ventricular cavity. Van Praagh and coworkers found that 30 of 37 autopsied hearts with PA-IVS had moderate to extreme hypoplasia of the right ventricular cavity.[21] The inlet portion of the ventricle is virtually always present (unless there is tricuspid atresia—see Chapter 15), and its size is related to the size of the tricuspid annulus. The infundibular portion of the right ventricle is also generally present, but one subgroup of patients with the most severe hypoplasia of the right ventricle appears to have atresia not only of the pulmonary valve but also of the distal infundibulum. This atresia of the infundibular cavity also appears to be secondary to severe hypertrophy of the septoparietal musculature of the infundibulum.[14]

There is essentially always a large atrial septal defect with leftward herniation of the septum primum into the left atrium,[21] and frequently there are prominent remnants of the venous valve in the right atrium (20% of patients).[21]

Perhaps the most surgically significant anatomic abnormalities involve the coronary circulation. Approximately 10% of patients with PA-IVS have either major stenoses or atresia of one or more of the major coronary arteries (Fig. 14–1).[21] The portions of the coronary arteries that are distal to these narrowed or atretic areas generally receive their blood supply via fistulous communications between the right ventricle and the coronary artery bed. Calder and Sage[6] found that such fistulae were present in more than 60% of autopsy cases. However, as a comparison of the incidences of right ventricular-to-coronary artery fistulae and coronary stenoses would imply, the presence of right ventricular-to-coronary artery fistulae does not necessarily mean that obstruction will be found in the native coronary arteries. We have observed clinically that coronary anomalies are most frequently seen in patients with the smallest tricuspid valve annuli and right ventricular volumes (unpublished observations); these findings are in agreement with the findings in autopsy series.[6, 9] These ventriculocoronary fistulae appear to occur only when the right ventricular pressure is greater than systemic pressure. The embryologic origins of these fistulous communications are unclear, but they are presumed to result from persistence of the intertrabecular sinusoidal channels, which are the pathways by which blood is supplied to the myocardium during the early pre-coronary artery phase of the development of the heart. It is noteworthy that the formation of the pulmonary valve (during the division of the truncus arteriosus into separate aortic and pulmonary roots) occurs several stages (horizons) before the appearance of the coronary circulation.[13, 20] However, because the interventricular foramen is still patent at this stage, there is not likely to be right ventricular hypertension before the development of the coronary arteries. Therefore, it seems likely that the right ventricle–to–coronary artery fistulae and the coronary artery anomalies must form later in development. From a therapeutic standpoint, it is the stenoses and atresias of the native coronary arteries and the amount of myocardium supplied only via the right ventricle that have the greatest significance among the coronary anomalies, as will be described subsequently. In addition to stenotic coronary lesions, 17% of patients in one autopsy series[6] were found to have a single coronary artery, and in most of these cases the aberrantly arising coronary crossed the right ventricular outflow tract.

PATHOPHYSIOLOGY

The neonate with PA-IVS is typically cyanotic from birth, as there is an obligatory right-to-left shunt at the atrial level. The neonate is able to survive only as long as the ductus arteriosus remains patent, as this is the sole source of pulmonary blood flow. In almost all patients the ductus undergoes normal constriction and occlusion within the first few days of life. When this occurs, the child becomes severely hypoxemic and acidotic, and death will follow soon thereafter without some intervention. The right ventricular pressure is commonly suprasystemic, and there is also usually at least mild tricuspid valvar regurgitation. Only if the tricuspid regurgitation is severe will the right ventricular pressure be in the normal range, and in these cases the right ventricular volume is frequently normal or increased. Generally, however, right ventricular volume is less than normal, and right ventricular compliance is low secondary to the accompanying right ventricular hypertrophy. Therefore, in most patients, continued cyanosis can be anticipated even after relief of the right ventricular outflow tract obstruction (unless the atrial septal defect is closed), as the compliance of the massively hypertrophied right ventricle is less than left ventricular compliance.

The presence of either stenoses or atretic segments in the coronary circulation has no immediate consequences for the neonate as long as the coronary bed distal to the stenoses continues to be supplied by the high-pressure right ventricle. However, if the right ventricle is decompressed by relief of the right ventricular outflow tract obstruction, the coronary segments that are supplied only via the right ventricle will be underperfused, and ischemia (particularly of the left ventricle) will result.

DIAGNOSIS

The presence of a significant congenital heart defect is generally suspected in patients with PA-IVS because of cyanosis and the presence of a systolic or continuous murmur from the ductus arteriosus. The chest radiograph will generally show diminished pulmonary blood flow and a normal heart size unless there is massive tricuspid regurgitation. In this case, the overall heart size will be enlarged, with most of the enlargement along the right border. The electrocardiogram (ECG) generally shows a normal axis (between 0 and 120 degrees) and absence of the right ventricular dominance usually seen in the neonatal electrocardiogram. These findings are in contrast to those seen in other forms of right-sided obstruction, such as tricuspid atresia (ECG axis <0 degrees) or pulmonary stenosis or atresia with a ventricular septal defect (right ventricular dominance by voltages).

The definitive diagnosis is generally made by two-dimensional echocardiography, which demonstrates the atretic right ventricular outflow tract and the morphology of the right ventricle and tricuspid valve. Doppler examination can confirm the absence of forward flow through the pulmonary valve, identify and quantify tricuspid valvar regurgitation, delineate anatomic abnormalities of the tricuspid valve, and demonstrate the flow of blood from the aorta to the pulmonary artery via the ductus. Peak right ventricular pressure can be estimated from the velocity of the tricuspid regurgitant jet. In some patients who have severe pulmonary valvar stenosis and a patent ductus arteriosus with elevated distal pulmonary artery pressure, the Doppler evaluation may not detect any forward flow through the pulmonary valve, and therefore, the echocardiogram cannot absolutely distinguish between these two related entities. With improved echocardiographic equipment and software for image processing, flow in right ventricle–to–coronary artery fistulae can also frequently be identified.

At Children's Hospital in Boston, we currently believe that all patients with PA-IVS should undergo cardiac catheterization, primarily to identify abnormalities in the coronary circulation. Angiograms should include both a right ventriculogram and an aortic root injection to demonstrate areas of stenosis or atresia in the native coronary bed and also to demonstrate which areas of the myocardium receive their blood supply exclusively from the right ventricle (right ventricular–dependent coronary circulation). If this information is not obtained from aortic root angiography, either selective coronary injections or a "balloon occlusion" aortic root injection should be performed.[17] Catheterization will also provide information on the right ventricular pressure, the magnitude of tricuspid valvar regurgitation, and the pulmonary artery anatomy. If significant coronary stenoses or atretic segments are identified by catheterization or angiography, operative interventions that will decompress the right ventricle should be avoided.

MANAGEMENT IN THE NEONATAL PERIOD

Medical Management

The goals of medical management of the neonate with PA-IVS are to establish the correct diagnosis and an optimal hemodynamic and metabolic state so that the patient will be in good condition to undergo operative intervention. Once it is suspected that the patient is dependent on the ductus arteriosus as the source of pulmonary blood flow, an infusion of prostaglandin E_1 (PGE_1) should be started to maintain patency of the ductus. A dose of 0.05 µg/kg/min is generally sufficient to maintain ductal patency. Many of these children require endotracheal intubation and mechanical ventilatory support because of the tendency for PGE_1 to cause apnea. The

general approach to the resuscitation of the cyanotic neonate is detailed in Chapter 5. Arterial saturations of 75% to 85% should be relatively easily attained after the first hour or two of the infusion, and once this level of arterial oxygenation is attained, metabolic acidosis (if present) should clear relatively rapidly. Infusions of sodium bicarbonate ($NaHCO_3$) and inotropic agents (e.g., dopamine) may be necessary initially if the diagnosis has been made late, after severe hypoxemia and acidosis have occurred. Arterial saturations greater than 85% suggest an excessive pulmonary-to-systemic blood flow ratio and should be managed with the techniques outlined in Chapter 15 for the preoperative management of patients with single-ventricle physiology. Every effort should be made to establish a stable metabolic and hemodynamic state before operative intervention.

Surgical Management

Multiple management schemes have been suggested for the neonate with PA-IVS, but most series have contained relatively small numbers of patients who do not appear to represent the entire spectrum of this disorder. It has become clear to us that no single management scheme is appropriate for the entire spectrum of these patients, and we currently believe that different strategies must be used depending on the individual anatomic variations.

Rationale

Survival of the Patient. The primary objective of initial management is to achieve survival of the patient; this requires the establishment of a reliable (non–ductus-dependent) source of pulmonary blood flow. In the majority of patients, a systemic-to–pulmonary artery shunt is required to provide adequate pulmonary blood flow, even if the obstruction of the right ventricle-to-pulmonary artery pathway is relieved. The reason a shunt is commonly required, despite relief of the obstruction of the right ventricular outflow tract, is related to the initial inability of the hypertrophied, small-volume right ventricle and the hypoplastic tricuspid valve to carry a normal cardiac output to the lungs. As noted earlier, the compliance of the right ventricle can be expected to be significantly less than normal, and therefore, normal output cannot be attained without markedly elevated filling pressures. The need for a systemic-to-pulmonary artery shunt in patients with obstruction of the right ventricular outflow tract (pulmonary stenosis or atresia) has been retrospectively related to echocardiographically measured right ventricular volume and tricuspid annular diameter in a study by Trowitzsch and coworkers.[18] Those patients with the smallest right ventricular volumes and tricuspid annular diameters all required systemic-to–pulmonary artery shunts to have acceptable oxygenation. Other groups have advocated reconstruction of the right ventricular outflow tract without a shunt, and inadequate oxygenation is treated with continued infusion of prostaglandin E_1 until the right ventricle becomes capable of delivering sufficient pulmonary blood flow to ensure adequate oxygenation.[10] Because there currently are catheterization techniques for the occlusion of systemic-to-pulmonary artery shunts, the disadvantages of placing a shunt seem to be outweighed by the necessity to give prolonged infusions of PGE_1 to maintain ductal patency and by the inability to control the size of the ductus and, therefore, the size of the pulmonary-to-systemic flow ratio. There may be a very small subset of patients with PA-IVS who have nearly normal right ventricular volumes and tricuspid valve size and function and who might be candidates for right ventricular outflow tract reconstruction and closure of the atrial septal defect without a shunt; however, at Children's Hospital in Boston, we have not seen such a patient since 1987.

Another aspect of ensuring survival is to avoid decompression of the right ventricle when a significant amount of myocardium is dependent on the right ventricle as the source of its coronary blood supply. It is clear that a significant proportion of neonates with PA-IVS have significant stenoses or atretic segments in the coronary arteries (see "Anatomic Considerations"). Therefore, before the right ventricle is decompressed, it is important to be sure that significant myocardial ischemia will not result. At present, angiographic visualization of the coronary arteries is the only reliable means of defining the coronary anatomy. If there are significant areas of the myocardium that will be at risk for ischemia with right ventricular decompression, reconstruction of the right ventricular outflow tract should be avoided. As a general rule, we have found that involvement of more than one of the three major epicardial coronary systems implies an unacceptable amount of myocardium at risk, although the important (but not currently measurable) variable is really the amount of myocardium at risk. It is also useful to note that in our experience those patients with right ventricular–dependent coronary circulations have been found exclusively among those with the smallest right ventricular volumes and the smallest tricuspid annular diameters (Fig. 14–2). In this group of patients with right ventricular–dependent coronary circulations, initial surgical treat-

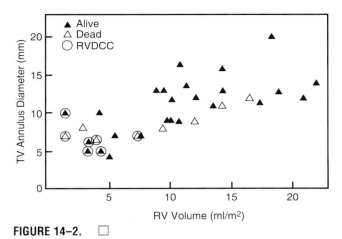

FIGURE 14–2.   □

Relationship of right ventricular (RV) volume and tricuspid valve (TV) annular diameter to survival and the presence of right ventricular–dependent coronary circulation (RVDCC).

ment should only create a systemic-to–pulmonary artery shunt with a view toward ultimately creating a Fontan type of circulation. Alternatively, consideration can be given to cardiac transplantation for these patients, but the long-term outcome of patients with PA-IVS undergoing either a Fontan repair or transplantation is unknown. One controversial group of patients consists of those with right ventricle–to–coronary artery fistulae without coronary artery stenoses. Freedom and Harrington believe that this anatomy may frequently lead to the secondary development of coronary stenoses because of the effects of high-pressure (high shear stress) ejection of right ventricular blood into the coronary artery.[11] They advocated either direct ligation of the right ventricle–to–coronary artery fistulae or, if the right ventricle is deemed to be hopelessly small, obliteration of the right ventricular cavity by "thromboexclusion."[19] We have not yet identified a patient in whom this mechanism of coronary artery disease has occurred, and we have not used thromboexclusion thus far in treating patients with PA-IVS.

Decompression of the Right Ventricle. The second important goal of neonatal surgical intervention is to decompress the right ventricle (when consistent with survival) to provide an optimal opportunity for the right ventricle and tricuspid valve to grow. As shown by Bull and coworkers,[5] the diameter of the tricuspid valve does not increase as the patient grows unless the right ventricle is decompressed. Right ventricular decompression is most consistently accomplished by placement of a transannular patch with resection of the dysplastic valve tissue. If the pulmonary annulus is truly normal in size and the leaflet tissue is thin and pliable, an

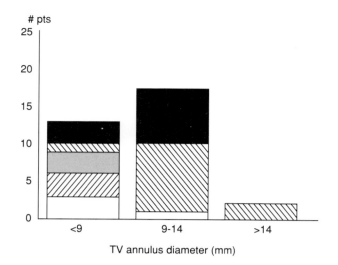

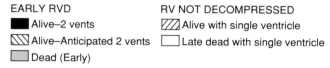

FIGURE 14–3. ☐

Neonatal tricuspid valve (TV) annular diameter for 33 patients with pulmonary atresia and intact ventricular septum. RV, Right ventricle; RVD, right ventricular depression; vents, ventricles.

incision in the pulmonary valve along the rudimentary commissures or excision of the valve tissue may provide a sufficient valve orifice. However, frequently there is significant subvalvar muscular obstruction in the infundibular region that will continue to restrict emptying of the right ventricle,[1] and only a very small percentage of patients can be managed by valvotomy alone. There may also be some advantage to inducing pulmonary valvar regurgitation, as the regurgitant blood volume may encourage growth of the right ventricle. At Children's Hospital in Boston, we believe it is important to decompress the right ventricle whenever possible, because at least some of these patients with very small right ventricles can grow sufficiently to allow a two-ventricle circulation later in life (Figs. 14–3 and 14–4). The atrial septal defect should almost always be left open at the time of initial relief of the right ventricular outflow tract obstruction. With currently available techniques, it is possible to close at least some atrial septal defects with a device in the catheterization laboratory, and the systemic-to–pulmonary artery shunt can be coil embolized as well (see Chapter 7). Therefore, it has been possible in several cases to have the neonatal operation be the only operation (although not the only intervention) that is necessary.

In addition to patients with right ventricular–de-

pendent coronary circulations, there is a second group of patients in whom relief from obstruction of the right ventricular outflow tract by transannular patching is probably unwise. These are patients with massive tricuspid valvar regurgitation and a large, thin-walled right ventricle. In this group, the creation of pulmonary valvar regurgitation in addition to the existing tricuspid valvar regurgitation will likely lead to severe right-sided heart failure and inadequate pulmonary blood flow. At the extreme end of this spectrum are patients with Ebstein's anomaly of the tricuspid valve and pulmonary valvar atresia; these clearly constitute an extremely high-risk group (see Chapter 16). Currently, patients with the combination of severe tricuspid regurgitation and PA-IVS are managed with placement of a systemic-to–pulmonary artery shunt, and the right ventricular outflow tract is reconstructed only when tricuspid valve annuloplasty can be carried out to reduce the regurgitation.

Size of the Right Ventricle and Tricuspid Annulus. A third consideration in the design of neonatal treatment is the question of whether a group of patients can be identified in the neonatal period who have right ventricles, tricuspid annuli, or both that are too small to ever provide all of the necessary pulmonary blood flow. In our own experience, several patients with small tricuspid annular diameters (<9 mm) (Fig. 14–3) or small right ventricular volumes (<8 ml/m²) (Fig. 14–4) either have

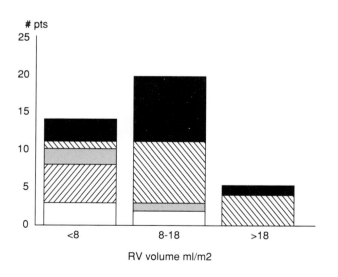

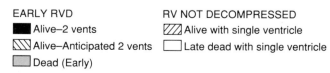

FIGURE 14–4. ☐

Neonatal right ventricular (RV) volume for 37 patients with pulmonary atresia and intact ventricular septum. RVD, right ventricular decompression; vents, ventricles.

progressed to have a two ventricle circulation or appear likely to be good candidates for a two-ventricle circulation in the future. Data from the Congenital Heart Surgeons Society (CHSS) multicenter study have shown that thus far no patient with a tricuspid annular diameter of more than four standard deviations below normal has progressed to a two-ventricle circulation, and that the mortality rate for a shunt alone is less than that if reconstruction of the right ventricular outflow tract is also carried out. Interpretation of both our own data and the CHSS data is limited by relatively short follow-up time, which makes it difficult to truly conclude that a two-ventricle repair is not possible for a given patient. Data from deLeval and coworkers[7] show that almost all patients (16 of 19) with tricuspid valve diameters larger than three standard deviations below normal (Z value greater than −3) survived two-ventricle repairs beyond the neonatal period. Therefore, it appears appropriate to attempt to decompress the right ventricle and provide optimal conditions for growth of the tricuspid valve and right ventricle, regardless of the neonatal size of these structures, unless the coronary anatomy or massive tricuspid regurgitation preclude this approach. It should be recalled that patients with the smallest right ventricles and tricuspid annular diameters are the most likely to have a right ventricular–dependent coronary circulation, which contraindicates right ventricular decompression.

To summarize the initial surgical management of the neonate with PA-IVS, the following scheme has been adopted at Children's Hospital in Boston:

1. All patients should undergo right ventricular decompression using a transannular patch (or, very rarely, a valvotomy) unless there is either a right ventricular–dependent coronary circulation or massive tricuspid regurgitation.
2. Most patients should have an additional systemic-to–pulmonary artery shunt to augment pulmonary blood flow (unless the right ventricle is of nearly normal size with a well-functioning tricuspid valve).
3. Patients with right ventricular–dependent coronary circulations (more than one coronary artery system involved or a significant portion of the left ventricular mass supplied only via the right ventricle) should have only a systemic-to–pulmonary artery shunt. These patients are candidates for either a subsequent Fontan repair or perhaps cardiac transplantation.
4. In essentially all cases, the atrial septal defect should be left open to prevent systemic venous hypertension.

Technical Aspects

Shunt Alone. Systemic-to–pulmonary artery shunts have generally been constructed with polytetrafluoroethylene (PTFE) (Impra or Gore-Tex), with the origin from the right subclavian or innominate artery and the distal anastomosis to the right pulmonary artery. When only a shunt is to be placed, the approach may be carried out through either a right thoracotomy or a median sternotomy (Fig. 14–5). More recently we have used a median sternotomy approach to reduce later problems with aortopulmonary collateral formation across chest wall adhesions in patients who are potential candidates for a Fontan type of definitive operation. The midline approach also allows the prompt institution of cardiopulmonary bypass if the hemodynamic condition deteriorates, although this is a relatively unusual situation in the well-prepared neonate with PA-IVS. After the sternotomy, the thymus is subtotally resected, leaving either the left lobe or the cervical extensions. The pericardium is opened only over the great vessels. The innominate and right subclavian arteries are dissected free. Control of the subclavian artery is obtained with a side-biting clamp placed across the entire vessel. An end-to-side anastomosis is then constructed between a 3.5- to 4-mm PTFE tube graft and the incision in the subclavian artery with running monofilament suture; a similar technique is used to construct the shunt-to–right pulmonary artery anastomosis. The ductus arteriosus is not disturbed until after the shunt has been inserted so as not to jeopardize the source of pulmonary blood flow during the occlusion of the right pulmonary artery. After shunt placement and release of the occluding clamps, the ductus arteriosus is temporarily occluded with a tourniquet, and if the arterial saturation is adequate (>80%), the ductus may be ligated.

Reconstruction of the Right Ventricular Outflow Tract. After a midline sternotomy and subtotal resection of the thymus, a rectangular peri-

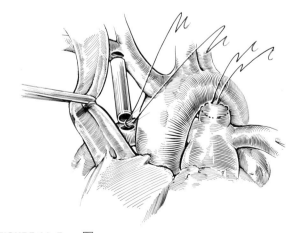

FIGURE 14–5. □

Technique of a right-sided modified Blalock-Taussig shunt via a midline sternotomy incision.

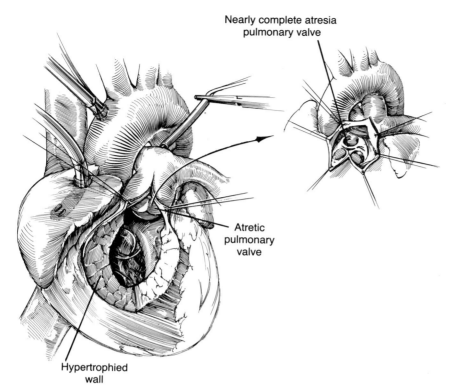

Nearly complete atresia
pulmonary valve

Atretic
pulmonary
valve

Hypertrophied
wall

FIGURE 14–6. □

The heart is shown after a transannular infundibular incision has been made, using a single arterial and a single venous cannula for cardiopulmonary bypass. The ductus arteriosus is controlled as bypass is initiated. The inset shows the atretic pulmonary valve with commissural fusion.

cardial patch (1.5 to 2 cm in width) is removed, treated in 0.6% glutaraldehyde for 10 to 15 minutes, and then thoroughly rinsed in saline solution. The glutaraldehyde treatment cross-links the collagen fibers to increase the strength of the pericardium and improves its handling characteristics by increasing its stiffness. After all preparations for the initiation of bypass have been completed, including placement of pursestring sutures in the aorta and right atrial appendage, the ductus arteriosus is gently dissected and surrounded with a ligature, which is left loose. Cannulation for bypass is accomplished with an arterial cannula in the ascending aorta and a single venous cannula (No. 20 French) in the right atrial appendage.

After bypass is established, the ductus is either ligated or controlled with a tourniquet. Temperatures are reduced to 30°C to 34°C; if this is accomplished gradually, using a normothermic and normocalcemic pump priming solution, the heart will usually remain beating. The pulmonary artery is incised, and the incision is extended across the pulmonary annulus into the infundibulum (except in the extremely rare case in which a valvotomy alone is to be performed) (Fig. 14–6). As noted earlier, valvotomy alone has been very rarely employed in our experience. The pericardial patch to enlarge the outflow tract is then sewn into the incisions in the pulmonary artery and right ventricle with continu-

ous monofilament suture material (Fig. 14–7). The modified Blalock-Taussig shunt is constructed as described earlier, and rewarming is started during the construction of the distal shunt-to–pulmonary artery anastomosis. Alternatively, the shunt can be placed before the initiation of bypass if arterial saturations remain satisfactory. When the shunts are placed during the time that the patient is heparinized, 7-0 Gore-Tex suture can be used for the anastomoses to reduce bleeding from suture holes. The Gore-Tex suture material is actually larger than the needle onto which it is "swaged," and thus there tends to be less needle hole bleeding from the graft material. The shunt is kept occluded until a few minutes before the discontinuation of bypass to prevent a "steal" of systemic blood flow from the pump into the pulmonary circuit. Alternatively, the shunt may be opened several minutes before ceasing bypass, but there must be transfusion from the bypass circuit to the patient to provide adequate filling of the left ventricle to force the heart to eject so that systemic perfusion is preserved. A fall in perfusion pressure as the shunt is opened is a good indicator of satisfactory patency of the shunt. A monitoring line for administering drugs and monitoring pressure is placed through the free wall of the right atrium, and bypass is discontinued, usually with low-dose inotropic support (dopamine, 5 μg/kg/min).

Continuous monitoring of arterial saturation by a

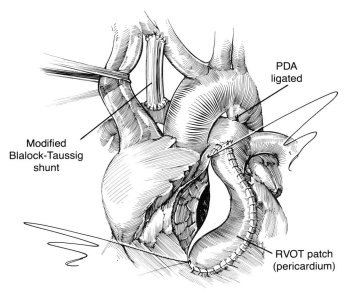

Modified
Blalock-Taussig
shunt

PDA
ligated

RVOT patch
(pericardium)

FIGURE 14–7. □

A transannular patch is placed to enlarge the right ventricular outflow tract (RVOT), and a right-sided modified Blalock-Taussig shunt is placed from the right subclavian–innominate artery to the right pulmonary artery. (Bypass cannulas in the aorta and right atrium are not shown.) PDA, Patent ductus arteriosus.

pulse oximeter is useful to gauge the adequacy of pulmonary blood flow; this is supplemented with arterial blood gas determinations. Arterial Po_2 of 35 to 40 mm Hg and an arterial oxygen saturation of >75% are acceptable values. Once the hemodynamic and ventilatory state is stable, the bypass cannulas are removed, and the heparin is reversed with protamine. If the ductus arteriosus has previously been controlled only with a tourniquet, it can be ligated at this stage. Frequently, it is useful to place a second right atrial monitoring catheter in the atrial appendage cannulation site for use in postoperative monitoring and as a route for intravenous nutrition.

If the right ventricle and tricuspid valve have been judged to be suitable to carry the entire cardiac output, based on preoperative assessment (a rare occurrence), the operative procedure is altered to include closure of the atrial septal defect using the techniques described in Chapter 8.

MANAGEMENT BEYOND THE NEONATAL PERIOD

Rationale

With regard to most forms of congenital heart disease, it has been our policy at Children's Hospital in Boston to achieve a complete repair as early in life as feasible and to avoid, whenever possible, the use of multiple palliative procedures. For patients with PA-IVS these same principles apply, and an attempt is made to achieve complete separation of systemic venous return from pulmonary venous return within the first year or two of life. The primary goal continues to be a two-ventricle circulation with closure of atrial level communications and systemic-to–pulmonary artery shunts. This approach minimizes the effects of a chronic volume load on the left ventricle and of persistent cyanosis on the developing heart and central nervous system. In general, the anatomic considerations previously discussed for the newborn still apply later in the first year of life, particularly with regard to the coronary vascular bed and the size of the right ventricle and tricuspid valve. The presence of right ventricle–to–coronary artery fistulae and obstructive lesions in more than one of the major coronary arteries should still preclude an attempt at decompression of the right ventricle. Study of the coronary anatomy by repeating catheterization is advisable whenever right ventricle–to–coronary artery fistulae are known to exist either by previous catheterization or by echocardiogram. If a significant amount of left ventricular myocardium will be placed at risk by decompression of the right ventricle, a single-ventricle repair (Fontan type) should be the ultimate goal of future therapy.

Once the issue of the coronary anatomy is settled, the predominant consideration dictating further therapy is the size of the right ventricle and the tricuspid valve. As noted previously, the right ventricle and tricuspid valve may be considerably smaller than normal and still allow a two-ventricle circulation to be created. Although exact criteria have not been defined, the guidelines for tricuspid valve diameter suggested by deLeval and coworkers[5, 8] have seemed to provide a reasonable estimate of adequate-size, right-sided structures. In addition, for those patients with previous reconstruction of the right ventricular outflow tract, the adequacy of the right-sided structures can be evaluated in the catheterization laboratory with balloon occlusion of the atrial septal defect and systemic-to–pulmonary artery shunt (if present). If the right atrial pressures remain less than 18 to 20 mm Hg without a significant decrease in cardiac output when the atrial septal defect and shunt are occluded, it is likely that operative or catheterization laboratory occlusion of both structures will be well tolerated. If the catheterization data suggest that closure of the septal defect and shunt will not be tolerated but the right ventricular outflow tract is patent, a choice must be made between a single-ventricle Fontan approach and a "1½-ventricle" repair for patients without significant coronary artery lesions. The 1½-ventricle option employs a combination of the right ventricle and a direct venous-to–pulmonary artery (modified Glenn) connection to provide pulmonary blood flow. If the right-sided structures are judged to be too small, a Fontan approach is used. Current data suggest that when favorable pulmonary vascular resistance and pulmonary artery anatomy are present, a Fontan approach can be safely carried out despite young age. In the presence of unfavorable anatomy or physiology, a bidirectional cavopulmonary shunt can be employed as an interval step before a subsequent Fontan operation. For patients with right ventricular–dependent coronary circulations or with a truly diminutive right ventricle and tricuspid valve, a Fontan type of approach is undertaken.

Technique

If the atrial septal defect is not amenable to closure in the catheterization laboratory, it is closed using the techniques described in Chapter 7. In patients in whom there is a significant question about the adequacy of the right heart structures, a small residual defect can be left in the atrial septal defect closure; this can then be closed later in the catheterization laboratory. If catheterization closure of these defects is not available, an alternative strategy (which was used before the availability of catheterization closures) is to only partially close the atrial septal defect. The remaining defect is encircled by a pursestring type suture, and the ends of the pursestring suture are brought out through the right atrial wall near the interatrial groove. The suture can be tied to occlude the defect after the patient is weaned from bypass, while right atrial and systemic arterial pressure are monitored. If the right atrial pressure exceeds 20 mm Hg or if significant systemic hypotension occurs, then the suture can be loosened to leave a small atrial septal defect to serve as an "escape valve" for the systemic venous return. This idea was reported by Billingsley et al.[3] and is conceptually similar to the "fenestrated" Fontan procedure used in our own institution.[4]

If catheterization laboratory occlusion of the shunt is not available or has been technically unsuccessful, takedown of the systemic-to–pulmonary artery shunt is a relatively straightforward surgical procedure for a right-sided Blalock-Taussig shunt. It involves careful identification and dissection of the shunt between the aorta and the superior vena cava and division of the shunt between surgical clips or ligatures. Division of the shunt is preferred, as it seems, intuitively, less likely to result in late "tenting up" and distortion of the pulmonary artery. Left-sided shunts are more difficult to take down and should be placed only in the rare case of a right aortic arch.

For a 1½-ventricle circulation, a direct connection is made between the superior vena cava and the right pulmonary artery to supplement the pulmonary blood flow provided by the right ventricle. One technique for the venous-to–pulmonary artery connection is to divide the right pulmonary artery and connect it to the side of the superior vena cava, leaving the superior vena cava–right atrial junction open. In this way, right atrial blood may either traverse the tricuspid valve to reach the left pulmonary artery via the right ventricle or pass directly into the right pulmonary artery. An alternative approach, which also obviates the need for all of the systemic venous return to pass through the tricuspid valve and right ventricle, is to divide the superior vena cava and connect the cranial end to the undivided right pulmonary artery. This procedure leaves the pulmonary arteries in continuity so that the right ventricular output can be distributed to both lungs, but it requires that all blood from the inferior vena cava pass through the tricuspid valve and right ventricle. It is unclear thus far whether either of these procedures has an advantage over the other, but each can be used as a "backup" option if the patient does not seem to be tolerating partial or complete closure of the atrial septal defect in the operating room.

Techniques for the creation of cavopulmonary connections and for the modified Fontan operation are described in Chapter 15. These techniques include constructing a lateral caval-caval pathway within the right atrium to segregate systemic venous return and making the systemic venous-to–pulmonary artery connection using the superior vena cava and the right pulmonary artery. This approach has the additional advantage that the inflow to the right ventricle will be mostly pulmonary venous (oxygenated) blood that crosses the native atrial septal defect, and therefore, all of the coronary artery blood supply (whether through the right ventricle or the native coronary arteries) will be nearly fully oxygenated.

POSTOPERATIVE CARE

The general principles of postoperative care are similar to those outlined in Chapter 5. The only special considerations after neonatal operations relate to the patient with reconstruction of the right ventricular outflow tract and a systemic-to–pulmonary artery shunt in whom the hemodynamic effects of the shunt are potentially more difficult to assess than they are in the patient with single-ventricle and shunt physiology. Signs of "overshunting" include a wide systemic arterial pulse pressure and manifestations of low systemic output, including oliguria, cool extremities, and metabolic acidosis. A high arterial saturation alone (>90%) may be an indication that the right ventricle and tricuspid valve are adequate to carry most of the systemic venous return (avoiding right-to-left atrial level shunting) and not necessarily that the shunt is physiologically too large. Cardiac catheterization with test occlusion of the shunt may be the only way to resolve problematic cases.

In older patients undergoing operations to close the atrial septal defect and take down the systemic-to–pulmonary artery shunt, close observation for signs of right-sided heart failure is important. Right atrial pressure should be monitored and the patient carefully observed for the development of low cardiac output secondary to right-sided heart failure. The patient should also be carefully monitored for the development of pleural effusions and ascites. Significant right heart failure and low cardiac output are indications for either "fenestrating" the atrial septal defect closure or converting to a 1½-ventricle physiology.

RESULTS

Results of the entire experience with all patients who had PA-IVA managed by a number of different protocols from 1973 to 1987 at Children's Hospital in Boston have been summarized by Fyler.[12] The 1-year survival rate was 45% for the period from 1973 to 1977 and 82% for the 1983 to 1987 time frame. More recently, the CHSS multi-institutional results in 171 patients managed with multiple different protocols have shown a 1-month survival rate of 77% and a 4-year survival rate of 58%. Overall, the best results appear to have been achieved with neonatal placement of a transannular patch with a systemic-to–pulmonary artery shunt or with a neonatal pulmonary valvotomy with a shunt, although this analysis excluded patients with Ebstein's anomaly and those with right ventricular–dependent coronary circulation. The need for a shunt was inversely related to the size of the tricuspid annulus, as might be expected from our earlier experience.[18]

The Children's Hospital experience with PA-IVS was also reviewed in an attempt to answer two additional questions regarding these patients:

1. What is the impact of right ventricle–to–coronary ar-

tery fistulae and coronary obstructive lesions on survival if the right ventricular outflow tract is reconstructed?
2. What is the impact of the neonatal anatomy of the tricuspid valve and right ventricle on subsequent survival and suitability for a two-ventricle circulation?

To address the first question regarding the impact of right ventricle–to–coronary artery fistulae and coronary stenoses, angiograms from 82 patients with PA-IVS who were seen between January 1979 and January 1990 were reviewed. Right ventricle-to–coronary artery fistulae were found in 26 patients, and in 23 the quality of the angiograms was adequate to allow visualization of the coronary arteries. In 16 of these 23, the right ventricle was decompressed by reconstruction of the right ventricular outflow tract. Seven patients had fistulae but no coronary obstruction, and all survived decompression of the right ventricle. Six additional patients had obstructive lesions in one major coronary vessel, but four survived operations to decompress the right ventricle. In one of these six patients, there was probably progression of coronary stenosis despite the decompression of the right ventricle. In three patients, more than one coronary artery had obstruction, and all three died of myocardial dysfunction after decompression of the right ventricle. In the six patients with right ventricle-to–coronary artery fistulae in whom the right ventricle remained hypertensive because either a valvotomy did not relieve obstruction or a choice was made not to decompress the right ventricle, there was progression of the coronary lesions in only one patient. In patients who had right ventricle–to–coronary artery fistulae and in whom the right ventricle was decompressed, the fistulae remained patent but were visualized only by aortic injection and not by right ventriculography. In conclusion, the presence of right ventricle–to–coronary artery fistulae does not preclude reconstruction of the right ventricular outflow tract unless there are associated significant coronary artery stenoses that place a significant amount of myocardium at risk for ischemia if the right ventricle is decompressed. As a general rule, involvement of more than one of the major coronary arteries precludes reconstruction of the right ventricular outflow tract.

The second question tried to address whether there is a subset of patients with right ventricles and tricuspid valves that are so small in the neonatal period that reconstruction of the right ventricular outflow tract reconstruction will not lead to adequate growth of the right-sided structures. The neonatal echocardiograms of 37 patients seen at Children's Hospital in Boston in the neonatal period were reviewed to measure tricuspid valve diameter

(33 patients) and right ventricular volume (37 patients). The results of these studies are shown in Figures 14–2, 14–3, and 14–4. In the group of 14 patients with the smallest right ventricular volumes (<8 ml/m²) (see Fig. 14–4), three have had complete two-ventricle repairs, and five are alive with single-ventricle physiology. Similarly, in the 13 patients with the smallest diameters of the tricuspid valve annulus (see Fig. 14–3), three have two-ventricle circulations, and three have single-ventricle physiology. Again, it is noteworthy that the major coronary anomalies occurred in the patients with the smallest right ventricles and tricuspid annuli (see Fig. 14–2).

Although the numbers of patients in this subset are relatively small and experience with the 1½-ventricle repair and the modified Fontan operation is relatively limited, all but one of these patients have survived these definitive operations. These include one patient who underwent the 1½-ventricle repair and two patients who underwent the Fontan repair. Two other patients, not included in the 37 patients shown in Figures 14–2, 14–3, and 14–4, are also doing well after the 1½-ventricle repair.

COMPLICATIONS

Low cardiac output can be a complication of neonatal operations involving reconstruction of the right ventricular outflow tract and the placement of a systemic-to–pulmonary artery shunt in two ways. First, there can be excessive shunt flow, which results in low systemic cardiac output. As described in the section on postoperative care, signs of low output, including oliguria and metabolic acidosis, will be present along with a wide pulse pressure. In some patients with significant tricuspid regurgitation, the mechanism for low output will be the regurgitation of pulmonary artery blood backward through both the right ventricular outflow tract and the tricuspid valve, resulting in a volume load on the left ventricle without an excessive amount of blood traversing the pulmonary capillary bed. In this case the arterial saturation may not seem excessively high, but blood flow is still excessive through the shunt. In these cases, closure of the right ventricular outflow tract may be necessary if the tricuspid regurgitation cannot be reduced. The more common cause of low cardiac output is inadequate coronary blood flow owing to a right ventricular–dependent coronary circulation. Accurate preoperative delineation of the coronary artery anatomy should avoid this complication, but the accuracy of angiography in the neonate has not been perfect in our experience, and this complication may

still occur. Electrocardiographic evidence of ischemia may be present, along with elevated left atrial pressures. Generally, this problem becomes apparent in the operating room, and re-establishment of pulmonary atresia by ligating the right ventricular outflow tract to increase right ventricular pressure may be the only means of re-establishing coronary blood flow.

SUMMARY

Results with PA-IVS have shown continuing improvement since the 1970s, and these improvements have seemed to reflect an improved understanding of the anatomic and physiologic considerations in these patients, along with the introduction of PGE₁ for preoperative resuscitation and restoration of adequate oxygenation. Continuing improvements are likely to result from further refinements in the understanding of these patients and from continuing improvements in intraoperative and postoperative management, particularly of the neonate with a shunted single-ventricle physiology.

REFERENCES

1. Arom KV, Edwards JE. Relationship between right ventricular muscle bundles and pulmonary valve. Circulation 54(suppl 3):III-79, 1976.
2. Becker AE. Surgical pathology of pulmonary atresia with intact ventricular septum. In Crupi G, Parenzan L, Anderson RH (eds). Perspectives in Pediatric Cardiology: Pediatric Cardiac Surgery. 2nd ed. Mount Kisco, NY, Futura, 1990, p 93.
3. Billingsley AM, Laks H, Boyce SW, et al. Definitive repair in patients with pulmonary atresia and intact ventricular septum. J Thorac Cardiovasc Surg 97:746, 1989.
4. Bridges ND, Lock JE, Castaneda AR. Baffle fenestration with subsequent transcatheter closure: Modification of the Fontan operation for patients at increased risk. Circulation 82:1681, 1990.
5. Bull C, deLeval MR, Mercanti C, et al. Pulmonary atresia and intact ventricular septum: A revised classification. Circulation 66:266, 1982.
6. Calder AL, Sage MD: Coronary arterial abnormalities in pulmonary atresia with intact ventricular septum. Am J Cardiol 59:436, 1987.
7. deLeval M, Bull C, Hopkins R, et al. Decision making in the definitive repair of the heart with a small right ventricle. Circulation 72(suppl II):II-52, 1985.
8. deLeval M, Bull C, Stark J, et al. Pulmonary atresia and intact ventricular septum: Surgical management based on a revised classification. Circulation 66:272, 1982.
9. Edwards JE. Congenital malformations of the heart and great vessels: C. Malformation of the valves. In Gould SE (ed). Pathology of the Heart and Blood Vessels. 3rd ed. Springfield, IL, Charles C Thomas, 1968, p 312.
10. Foker JE, Braunlin EA, St Cyr JA, et al. Management of pulmonary atresia with intact ventricular septum. J Thorac Cardiovasc Surg 92:706, 1986.
11. Freedom RM, Harrington DP. Contributions of intramyocardial sinusoids in pulmonary atresia and intact ventricular

septum to a right sided circular shunt. Br Heart J 36:1061, 1974.

12. Fyler DC. Pulmonary atresia with intact ventricular septum. In Fyler DC (ed). Nadas' Pediatric Cardiology. Philadelphia, Hanley & Belfus, 1992, p 635.

13. Goor DA, Lillehei CW. The embryology of the heart. In Congenital Malformations of the Heart. New York, Grune & Stratton, 1975, p 38.

14. Goor DA, Lillehei CW. Obstruction of the pulmonary arterial pathways. In Congenital Malformations of the Heart. New York, Grune & Stratton, 1975, p 312.

15. Goor DA, Lillehei CW. The anatomy of the heart. In Congenital Malformations of the Heart. New York, Grune & Stratton, 1975, p 1.

16. Kutsche LM, VanMierop LHS. Pulmonary atresia with and without ventricular septal defect: A different etiology and pathogenesis for the atresia in the 2 types? Am J Cardiol 51:932, 1983.

17. Mandell V, Lock JE, Mayer JE, et al. The "laid-back" aortogram: An improved angiographic view for demonstration of coronary arteries in transposition of the great arteries. Am J Cardiol 65:1379, 1990.

18. Trowitzsch E, Colan SD, Sanders SP. Two-dimensional echocardiographic evaluation of right ventricular size and function in newborns with severe right ventricular outflow tract obstruction. J Am Coll Cardiol 6:388, 1985.

19. Trusler GA, Williams WG, Freedom RM, et al. Experience with pulmonary atresia and intact ventricular septum from 1968 through 1987. In Crupi G, Parenzan L, Anderson RH (eds). Perspectives in Pediatric Cardiology. Vol 2: Pediatric Cardiac Surgery. 2nd ed. Mount Kisco, NY, Futura, 1989, p 108.

20. Van Mierop LHS. Morphological development of the heart. In Berne RM (ed). Handbook of Physiology: The Cardiovascular System. Vol 1: The Heart. 2nd ed. Baltimore, Williams & Wilkins, 1979, p 1.

21. Van Praagh R, Ando M, Van Praagh S, et al. Pulmonary atresia: Anatomic considerations. In Kidd BS, Rowe RD (eds). The child with congenital heart disease after surgery. Mount Kisco, NY, Futura, 1976, p 103.

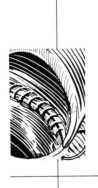

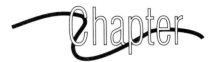

15
Chapter

Single-Ventricle Tricuspid Atresia

A wide variety of congenital defects share the common characteristic that there is functionally only a single ventricular chamber. These defects include tricuspid atresia and single right and left ventricles, but other defects such as double-outlet right ventricle with an inlet (uncommitted) ventricular septal defect and many of the forms of heterotaxia (asplenia/polysplenia) are included as well. The special case of the hypoplastic left heart syndrome is discussed in a separate chapter. All of these other defects will be considered as forms of single ventricle, as they currently are not suitable for a two-ventricle repair either in the neonatal period or later in life. In addition, they share other similarities such as the frequent coexistence of obstruction of one outlet valve or of the aortic arch. Because these anatomically dissimilar defects share such a large number of functional characteristics, they are grouped together into this single chapter.

ANATOMY

Terminology

The Van Praagh segmental approach to the description of these defects is used throughout this discussion.[30] When the terms *left* and *right* are used in reference to a ventricle, they refer to the morphology of the ventricle and not to position.[32] Left ventricles have relatively smooth (nontrabeculated) internal walls and do not have chordal attachments of the atrioventricular valves to the septal surface.[32] In contrast, right ventricles are more heavily trabeculated and generally have some chordal attachments of the atrioventricular valve to the septal surface.[32]

The determination of the ventricular looping pattern (D or L) is made after morphologic identification of the right and left ventricles, and then the relationship between the two ventricular chambers (even if one is rudimentary) is determined. The concept of chirality (or handedness) of the ventricle is useful in determining the ventricular looping pattern as described by Van Praagh.[33] Briefly, if the palm of the right hand is placed on the septal surface of the morphologic right ventricle, then, in a D ventricular looping pattern, the thumb will point toward the inlet (tricuspid) valve, and the index finger will point toward the outlet valve. The left hand placed on the septal surface of the left ventricle in D looping will fulfill the same criteria. Conversely, the morphologic right ventricle in an L-loop pattern is "left-handed," so that when the left palm is placed on the septal surface of the morphologic right ventricle (which is left-sided), the thumb points to the inlet valve and the index finger points to the outlet valve.[33] The actual position of the ventricles within the thorax is irrelevant to these considerations of ventricular loop.

The determination of the pattern of ventricular looping can generally be made based on echocardiographic and angiographic data. The anatomy of the great arteries can vary independently of the ventricular anatomy, and in each of the defects the aorta may be anterior or posterior to the pulmonary artery, or the great vessels may be side by side. Similarly, the atrial anatomy may be variable with either solitus atria (right-sided right atrium, left-sided left atrium) or inverted atrial situs. In some cases of heterotaxia syndrome (asplenia and polysplenia), the atrial situs will be ambiguous. The anatomic arrangements at these three levels (atrial, ventricular loop, and great vessel) are then combined to form various anatomic combinations that can be described in a shorthand system using alphabetic symbols[30]; this system will be used in the remainder of this discussion.

Tricuspid Atresia

In tricuspid atresia, there is no opening from the right atrium into either ventricle, and in the majority of patients there is no identifiable valve tissue or valve remnant.[8] Rather, the floor of the right atrium is completely muscular, and this floor is separated from the ventricular mass by the fibrofatty tissue of the atrioventricular sulcus.[8] Scalia and coworkers have argued that in hearts with atresia of the right atrioventricular valve, the ventricular looping pattern (D or L) does not alter the internal appearance of the right atrium, and therefore, they included those hearts with an L ventricular loop and right atrioventricular valve atresia in their report.[23] For the purposes of the current discussion, however, only patients with a D ventricular loop and atrial situs solitus (or L loop with inverted atrial situs) will be classified as having "classic" tricuspid atresia; the remainder will be considered under the discussion of single ventricle. Generally, in association with the atretic right atrioventricular valve, there are total absence of the inlet and varying degrees of deficiency of the trabecular portions of the right ventricle. The only part of the right ventricle that is consistently present is the infundibulum, although there are variations in the extent of its development.[8] A communication is generally (but not always) present between the left ventricle and this infundibular chamber (bulboventricular foramen), but an interventricular communication may also occur more toward the apex of the ventricle.[8] In the majority of hearts, the interventricular communication is a site of obstruction to blood flow, but obstruction may also occur at the level of the outlet valve or in the subvalvar infundibulum.[5] The great vessels may be normally related (aorta arising from the left ventricle and the pulmonary artery from the

infundibular chamber) or transposed (aorta arising from the infundibular chamber and the pulmonary artery from the left ventricle). The great vessel relationship forms the basis for the most commonly used classification system for tricuspid atresia: type I, normally related great arteries; type II, transposed great arteries.[25] Both great arteries may also originate from the morphologic left ventricle.[23] Types I and II are further subclassified by the degree of obstruction to pulmonary blood flow[8]: a, atresia of the pulmonary valve; b, stenosis of the pulmonary valve; c, unrestricted pulmonary blood flow. The most common patterns seem to be types Ib, Ia, IIc, and IIb. In the absence of a patent bulboventricular foramen in type I, the pulmonary valve is generally, but not always, atretic. A significant number of hearts with normally related great vessels also have infundibular or valvar pulmonary stenosis.[8] There is essentially always an atrial septal communication, and this generally occurs in the same region as a secundum atrial septal defect. However, there may also be an essentially common atrium and, less frequently, an atrial defect of the sinus venosus type. There is generally a patent ductus arteriosus at birth, but the ductus usually closes within a few days as in infants with normal circulation. Obstruction at the aortic arch and isthmus is not uncommon with type II tricuspid atresia[23, 25] and occurs most frequently in association with a small interventricular (subaortic) communication. In this situation, the ascending aorta and aortic annulus also tend to be smaller than normal.

Single Left Ventricle

The two most common forms of single left ventricle occur with normal (D) ventricular looping and with inverted (L) ventricular looping. In the former, the left ventricle is generally left-sided (and left-handed) with a right-sided infundibular chamber, and in the latter the left ventricle is right-sided (and right-handed), generally with a left-sided infundibular chamber. The rudimentary "ventricle" or infundibular chamber is connected to the left ventricle by a ventricular septal communication (bulboventricular foramen), which appears to be a persistence of the embryonic communication between the primitive ventricle and the bulbus cordis.[29] Both atrioventricular valves empty into the single left ventricle (double inlet), but either atrioventricular valve may be stenotic or atretic. The tricuspid valve may also straddle the ventricular septum with some attachments into the rudimentary right "ventricle."[31] Clearly, there is an anatomic spectrum ranging from two ventricles with a straddling tricuspid valve to a single left ventricle with a hypoplastic right "ventricle," depending on the degree of development of the right ventricle and the degree of overriding and straddling of the tricuspid valve. The great vessels may arise in either normally related or transposed fashion, and either or both great vessels may arise either from the single left ventricle or, more commonly, from the rudimentary right "ventricle." In our experience, the most common anatomic subset among patients with a single left ventricle is {S,L,L}, (i.e., atrial situs solitus, L ventricular loop, and L-transposition of the great arteries) (Table 15–1). Other common anatomic subsets are {S,D,D} and {S,D,N} (Holmes's heart). As observed in patients with tricuspid atresia, there is almost always obstruction to either systemic or pulmonary blood flow. Pulmonary valvar or subvalvar stenosis or atresia occurs in more than half of the patients, while obstruction to systemic blood flow occurs in many of the remaining ones. It is relatively uncommon for there not to be obstruction of one of the two outlets from the single ventricle. In those patients with obstruction to aortic outflow, there is a high incidence of coarctation of the aorta, hypoplasia of the aortic arch, or both.[17] Similarly, the presence of aortic arch hypoplasia or coarctation is highly associated with the presence of an intracardiac lesion that restricts systemic outflow,[17] a finding that has important implications for neonatal treatment of the patient with a single ventricle, in whom pressure gradients are not generally found if the ductus arteriosus is patent.

Single Right Ventricle

A single ventricle of right ventricular morphology is much less common than a single left ventricle if patients with the heterotaxia syndromes are not included. There may be a rudimentary left ventricle connected to the right ventricle by a ventricular septal defect, but it is rare for either great vessel to connect to this ventricle. The most common anatomic subtype of isolated single right ventricle is double-outlet right ventricle {S,D,D} (i.e., single right ventricle with D-transposition of the great arteries, with both arterial trunks arising from the right ventricle).[31] Stenosis of the outflow to the pulmonary circulation is much more common than restriction of systemic outflow.[31] There may be atresia or stenosis of one atrioventricular valve, most commonly the mitral valve.

Heterotaxia Variants

Heterotaxia patients are characterized by failure of many "right-left" differentiations, leading to ambiguities of visceral and atrial situs and characteristic anomalies of systemic or pulmonary venous return associated with splenic anomalies.[34] Not all such patients have a functional single ventricle, but in the majority there is a a single ventricle, typically of right ventricular morphology. An endocardial cushion defect is present in virtually all of these hearts.[34] Thus, the atrioventricular valve has an atrioventricular canal type of morphology (i.e., common atrioventricular valve), and generally there is an essentially common atrium.[34] Frequently there are anomalies of the systemic venous return, with a high incidence of bilateral superior venae cavae. In patients with the polysplenia type of heterotaxia, the infrahepatic portion of the inferior vena cava is frequently absent, and the venous return from the lower part of the body enters the superior vena cava via the azygos vein. In hearts from patients with asplenia, the right and left hepatic veins may enter the ipsilateral sides of the common atrium, remaining separate from the inferior vena caval entrance. Abnormalities of pulmonary venous return are also common in both asplenia and polysplenia; direct connection to the superior or inferior vena cava (sometimes with obstruction) is more frequent in asplenia, and anomalous pulmonary venous drainage into the same side of the atrium as the systemic venous drainage apparently is more frequent in polysplenia. However, Van Praagh suggests that in hearts of patients with polysplenia, the pulmonary

TABLE 15–1. ☐ OUTCOME AFTER NEONATAL MANAGEMENT OF SINGLE VENTRICLE

DIAGNOSIS	NO.	EARLY DEATHS	ALL LATE DEATHS	AWAITING SURGERY	BDCPS OR GLENN	FONTAN	LOST TO FOLLOW-UP
Single ventricle	63	11	9	8	12	20	3
Heterotaxia	47	7	14	6	9	8	3
Double-outlet right ventricle	22	5	7	2	4	3	1
Tricuspid atresia I	16	4	0	2	0	8	2
Tricuspid atresia II	14	0	1	0	2	10	1
Total	162	27 (16.7%)	31 (19.1%)	18 (11.1%)	27 (16.7%)	49 (30.2%)	10 (6.2%)

BDCPS, Bidirectional cavopulmonary shunt.

venous drainage is normal, and the appearance of an abnormal pulmonary venous connection is due to malattachment of the septum primum in an abnormally leftward position (leaving all of the pulmonary venous connections in what appears to be the right atrium).[34] Frequently there is outflow obstruction to pulmonary arterial blood flow at either the valvar or subvalvar level. Pulmonary atresia is more common with asplenia, whereas pulmonary stenosis is more common with polysplenia.[34] Pulmonary artery anomalies are not rare, particularly when there is pulmonary atresia with the ductus arteriosus as the only source of pulmonary blood flow. After the ductus closes, a "coarctation" commonly develops in the pulmonary artery just at the insertion of the ductus. The branching pattern of the pulmonary arteries generally assumes one of two forms, depending on whether an asplenia or polysplenia type of pattern is present. In asplenia, both right and left pulmonary arteries tend to look like a normal right pulmonary artery, with the bronchus for the upper lobe being above the first segmental artery for the right upper lobe (eparterial bronchus). In contrast, in the polysplenia form of heterotaxia, the bronchi are below the pulmonary artery at the hilum (hyparterial bronchi), as is the case for a normal left pulmonary artery.[34] In asplenia, both lungs tend to be trilobed, whereas in polysplenia both lungs tend to be bilobed. These features have contributed to the general rule (which has many exceptions) that asplenic patients tend to have bilateral "right-sidedness," while polysplenic patients tend to have bilateral "left-sidedness." Obstruction in the aortic arch is relatively uncommon, although when it is present, it usually is associated with subaortic obstruction.

Double-Outlet Right Ventricle

Certain anatomic forms of double-outlet right ventricle (DORV) require surgical approaches that are more closely related to those used for management of a single ventricle than to those used for the common forms of DORV. In some forms of DORV, the right ventricle is quite hypoplastic, and from a functional standpoint, the defect results in essentially a single ventricle. In this subgroup, there is frequently a straddling tricuspid valve and sometimes a superior-inferior ventricular relationship.[13] In other forms of DORV the left ventricle is hypoplastic, and frequently there is hypoplasia or atresia of the mitral valve.[13, 35] However, in still other patients there are two relatively well-formed ventricles, but the ventricular septal defect is in the inlet (atrioventricular canal) septum, and construction of

a baffle to divert the left ventricular output to the aorta may be extremely difficult without disruption of the tricuspid chordal attachments and anterior enlargement of the ventricular septal defect[24]; therefore, a single-ventricle approach may be elected. When a single-ventricle approach is considered, the critical surgical features are the function of the atrioventricular valves and obstruction to outflow from both ventricles into the aorta. There is a high incidence of obstruction to either the aorta or the pulmonary artery in patients with DORV.[13, 35] In our experience, straddling tricuspid valves and common atrioventricular valves may be regurgitant in patients with DORV.

HISTORY

The anatomic entities of tricuspid atresia and single ventricle were described in the late nineteenth century and were well recognized by clinicians such as Helen Taussig.[26, 27] Van Praagh made a significant conceptual contribution when he defined single-ventricle physiology as those hearts in which both atrioventricular valves empty into one ventricle.[31] Surgical therapy for patients with various forms of functional single ventricle began with palliative procedures such as pulmonary artery banding and the Blalock-Taussig shunt. Later, the concept of providing pulmonary blood flow with a direct connection between a systemic vein and the pulmonary arteries was reported by Glenn,[14] based on a body of experimental work that has since been reviewed by Sade and Castaneda.[22] In 1971, Fontan and Baudet described an operation on a patient with tricuspid atresia that became the definitive operation for this group of patients.[10] This operation, with numerous subsequent modifications, has remained the most widely employed operation for patients with this defect. Despite the encouraging report of a staged approach to septation of single-ventricle hearts reported by Ebert,[7] we have found that septation of the single ventricle has been possible only rarely in patients with favorable anatomic varieties of single ventricle, and therefore, it will not be considered further in this chapter.

PATHOPHYSIOLOGY

The pathophysiology of the patient with a single ventricle is determined primarily by obstruction of outflow to either the systemic or the pulmonary circulation and by the presence or absence of obstruction to pulmonary venous return. Assuming that there is no obstruction to pulmonary venous return, the relative resistance to blood flow into the systemic and the pulmonary circuits determines how the output from the single ventricle is distributed between the pulmonary and systemic circulations. This relative distribution, in turn, determines the clinical picture at the time of presentation. Thus, if there is severe obstruction to pulmonary blood flow, cyanosis will be present as a result of inadequate pulmonary blood flow, whereas obstruction to the systemic circulation frequently results in inadequate systemic perfusion and "shock." In the presence of subaortic obstruction there is a high incidence of aortic arch hypoplasia and coarctation as well, both of which contribute to inadequate systemic perfusion. The effects of outflow obstruction can be greatly influenced by the ductus arteriosus, which, when patent, will offset obstruction in either the systemic or pulmonary circuit. It is rare for there to be obstruction to outflow to both the pulmonary and systemic circulations; the patient with obstruction to the pulmonary circuit generally has adequate systemic output, whereas the patient with systemic outflow obstruction generally has excessive pulmonary blood flow. In a small subset of patients there is relatively little obstruction to either systemic or pulmonary blood flow. In these neonates, there may be a reasonably favorable balance between pulmonary and systemic blood flow initially, but as the normal postnatal reduction of pulmonary vascular resistance occurs, pulmonary blood flow progressively increases, leading to a progressive volume load on the single ventricle and reduction of systemic blood flow. Congestive heart failure with pulmonary edema will result unless compensatory mechanisms in the lung vasculature lead to elevated pulmonary vascular resistance. However, the compensatory increase in pulmonary resistance that occurs secondary to medial hypertrophy (and, later, intimal hyperplasia and fibrosis) in the pulmonary vasculature may significantly reduce the likelihood that the patient will ultimately be a candidate for a Fontan type of repair. In the presence of pulmonary venous obstruction, the patient is likely to be cyanotic, even if there is no anatomic obstruction to pulmonary blood flow, because of the elevated pulmonary resistance that results from the venous obstruction.

For the patient with a single ventricle to have sufficient oxygenation to survive without development of pulmonary vascular obstructive disease, there must be a significant degree of obstruction to pulmonary blood flow with relatively unimpeded systemic outflow from the single ventricle. Neonatal palliative operations are undertaken to achieve this hemodynamic state so that a subsequent Fontan operation can be carried out. However, the persist-ence of the palliated single-ventricle state, even if the pulmonary and systemic blood flows are well balanced, has potential deleterious effects on both the heart and the remainder of the body. These long-term effects on the heart include a chronic volume overload on the ventricle, as well as persistence of cyanosis. Both of these states can lead to impaired ventricular function over the long term. In addition, there are systemic risks of chronic venous admixture to the systemic circulation, including embolic stroke and the development of brain abscess. Notably, a risk factor for late death after Fontan operations is older age (and, implicitly, a longer time with palliated single-ventricle physiology) at the time of the Fontan operation.[11]

DIAGNOSIS

Diagnosis in the Neonate

The diagnosis of single ventricle in the newborn period is generally suspected because of the presence of either cyanosis or inadequate systemic perfusion, depending on whether there is obstruction to pulmonary or systemic outflow from the single ventricle. In some circumstances in which there is enough pulmonary stenosis to prevent excessive pulmonary blood flow without severe cyanosis, the presence of a murmur may be the only clue to the presence of a significant intracardiac defect. Also, as long as the ductus arteriosus is patent, obstruction to either systemic or pulmonary blood flow may be masked. In general, however, the ductus will close within the first few days of life, and the presence of a significant defect will become apparent. The appearance of the chest radiograph will depend on whether there is reduced pulmonary blood flow (dark, hypoperfused lung fields) or excessive pulmonary blood flow. The patient with obstruction to pulmonary venous return generally has an engorged pulmonary vasculature, although if there is coexisting obstruction to pulmonary blood flow, the chest radiograph may not have an appearance typical of that for obstructed pulmonary veins. Currently the anatomic diagnosis of the patient with single ventricle is readily made in the neonate and infant with the use of two-dimensional echocardiography, which will identify almost all of the morphologic problems in these patients. The identification of pressure gradients across areas of obstruction cannot be used to assess the severity of either aortic or pulmonary stenosis if the ductus arteriosus is patent, and imaging of these areas of narrowing is a much better means of assessing their potential significance. The presence of significant hypoplasia or coarctation in the aortic arch should prompt a thorough search for obstruction to systemic outflow within the heart. Angiography in the newborn period is generally not necessary to plan initial management. However, it may be difficult to completely evaluate the anatomy of the pulmonary arterial tree by echocardiography, and if there are any doubts about pulmonary artery anatomy, angiography should be performed. In the newborn period, there generally is relatively little need for the physiologic information that can be obtained from catheterization. Although it is particularly important to determine whether there is any restriction to pulmonary venous return, particularly across a restrictive interatrial communication, this assessment can almost always be made by Doppler echocardiography in conjunction with echocardiographic imaging.

Diagnosis Beyond the Neonatal Period

A critical aspect of the management of patients with single-ventricle anatomy is continuing, close follow-up with both echocardiographic and catheterization evaluation after the neonatal period, particularly when any palliative surgical interventions have been undertaken. This aggressive stance is necessary to identify and correct those problems that will adversely affect the patient's ability to have a Fontan procedure done in the future. Therefore, invasive studies should generally be undertaken by no later than 6 months of age, particularly if there have been palliative operations in the perinatal period.

In the assessment of patients for systemic venous–to–pulmonary artery operations (Fontan or bidirectional cavopulmonary shunt operations), the anatomy and physiology of the pulmonary vasculature must be investigated, but other physiologic aspects—including ventricular function, obstruction of pulmonary venous return, the presence of aortopulmonary collateral vessels, and atrioventricular valve function—must also be assessed. This information is generally best obtained at cardiac catheterization, although supplemental information (particularly regarding ventricular and atrioventricular valve functions) is also obtained by echocardiography. Pulmonary artery pressure and pulmonary arteriolar resistance (indexed to body surface area) have been strongly correlated with outcome after Fontan operations, as has distortion of the pulmonary arteries.[19] These data must be obtained as completely as possible at the diagnostic catheterization. It is important to keep in mind, however, that the physiologic data obtained at catheterization are only a "snapshot" of the patient's usual physiologic

state, and therefore are not to be relied on absolutely in making management decisions. Because many variables may influence pulmonary resistance, including pH and PCO_2, the significance of a particular calculation of pulmonary vascular resistance must be interpreted with these and other variables in mind. Thus, if the patient has required heavy sedation during catheterization and hypoventilates as a result, the calculated pulmonary vascular resistance may be artificially high. It should also be recalled that calculation of blood flows by the Fick method requires either the assumption of an oxygen consumption or the direct measurement of oxygen consumption. This measurement of oxygen consumption can be difficult to make accurately because of the technical problems involved in collecting all of the expired gases, particularly in small children, and therefore, the components of the calculation of pulmonary vascular resistance must be examined before this calculation is accepted with confidence. It should also be noted that when the source of pulmonary blood flow is nonpulsatile (e.g., after a bidirectional cavopulmonary shunt), calculations of pulmonary vascular resistance probably do not have the same meaning as when the source is pulsatile (e.g., through a banded native pulmonary artery or a systemic-to-pulmonary shunt). This difference results from the fact that the resistance calculation in a pulsatile system (which is based on the *mean* pulmonary artery pressure) does not account for the pulsatile nature of the waveform. Calculation of impedance from instantaneous measurements of flow and pressure would be more appropriate in a pulsatile system, but current technology does not allow the measurement of instantaneous flow. Therefore, assessments of the pulmonary vascular bed are currently made with calculations of resistance, but the comparability of the calculated resistances in pulsatile and nonpulsatile systems is questionable.

Unless relieved, pulmonary venous obstruction almost always precludes a successful Fontan operation, and if it is unilateral, it may be difficult to diagnose even with angiography and direct catheterization of the pulmonary veins. Radionuclide lung scans may be helpful in this situation and will show reduced flow on the side of the pulmonary venous obstruction. It is also important to identify collateral connections between the systemic and pulmonary circulations; these commonly exist in patients with reduced pulmonary blood flow. These collaterals may provide a significant amount of pulmonary blood flow. After Fontan or bidirectional cavopulmonary shunt operations, these collaterals may "compete" with systemic venous blood for access to the pulmonary circulation and thereby raise the systemic venous pressure. Therefore, we believe it is important to identify and control these collateral vessels (generally by coil occlusion in the catheterization laboratory) before procedures that provide pulmonary blood flow by systemic venous–to–pulmonary artery connections.

MANAGEMENT

Management in the Neonatal Period

Medical Management

Once the anatomic diagnosis is made in the newborn, surgical therapy will generally be necessary unless there is a good balance between pulmonary and systemic blood flow as a result of moderate restriction to pulmonary blood flow without obstruction to the systemic circulation. It is relatively unusual for this to be the case, however. Initial medical management is directed at resuscitation of the patient, increasing pulmonary blood flow if it is inadequate because of pulmonary stenosis or atresia, and increasing systemic blood flow if there is significant obstruction either within the heart or at the level of the aortic arch. Generally, administration of prostaglandin E_1 to re-establish or preserve ductal patency will accomplish these goals and will stabilize the patient before any operative intervention. Complete resuscitation of the patient with the restoration of normal acid–base status and renal and hepatic function is generally possible with the use of prostaglandin E_1. However, if there is obstruction to pulmonary venous return, medical management—other than temporary mechanical ventilation—has no place in the management of these patients, and urgent surgical intervention is necessary. The management of the patient with single-ventricle physiology before surgery involves attempts to balance pulmonary and systemic resistances and blood flows so that adequate oxygenation ($PO_2 > 30$ mm Hg) is maintained, along with adequate systemic blood flow to prevent damage to the abdominal viscera, the coronary circulation, and the brain. The details of the management of these patients are given in the section on intensive care management (see Chapter 5, section on Management of the Infant and Neonate with Congenital Heart Disease).

Surgical Management

Indications for Surgery. If pulmonary venous obstruction is not present, surgical management is dictated by whether there is inadequate or excessive pulmonary blood flow, with or without obstruction to systemic blood flow. All of these situations generally require surgical intervention in the first few days to weeks of life.

Surgery for Inadequate Pulmonary Blood Flow. A shunting procedure between a systemic artery and the pulmonary artery is used to provide adequate pulmonary blood flow, and at Children's Hospital in Boston, we have generally preferred a modified Blalock-Taussig shunt, using a 3.5-mm polytetrafluoroethylene (PTFE) graft. This operation can be undertaken either through a thoracotomy or a sternotomy, but more recently we have favored the sternotomy approach. This preference for the sternotomy is based on the finding that patients with previous thoracotomies seem to form aortopulmonary collateral connections across chest wall adhesions, which may complicate subsequent Fontan operations. Also, the sternotomy approach easily allows the institution of cardiopulmonary bypass if necessary to support oxygenation during the insertion of the shunt. The technique for placement of the shunt via a median sternotomy has been described in Chapter 14.

The technique for placement of a modified Blalock-Taussig shunt via a thoracotomy is relatively straightforward. As a general rule, it is preferable to place the shunt on the same side as the superior vena cava, as shunts in this position will be easier to control and to take down at any subsequent operation. However, if a neonatal patient is dependent on the ductus arteriosus for pulmonary blood flow, the position of the ductus must also be taken into account in choosing the site for the shunt. Because the ductus cannot be occluded until the shunt has been completed, it is difficult to place the distal end of the shunt in a location proximal enough to facilitate its subsequent takedown if it is on the same side as the ductus arteriosus. Therefore, it is preferable to place the shunt on the side opposite the ductus in situations in which pulmonary blood flow is ductal dependent. The technique of the typical shunting procedure is shown in Figure 15–1. It is important to preserve the recurrent laryngeal nerve, which arises as a branch from the vagus nerve and courses around the right subclavian artery when there is a left aortic arch and a usual branching pattern of the arch vessels. The subclavian artery is controlled with a vascular clamp, and a longitudinal arteriotomy is made. A standard end-to-end anastomosis is carried out between a PTFE graft and the subclavian artery. Then the clamp is removed from the artery, and the graft is occluded and cut to appropriate length. The distal end of the graft is then anastomosed to a longitudinal arteri-

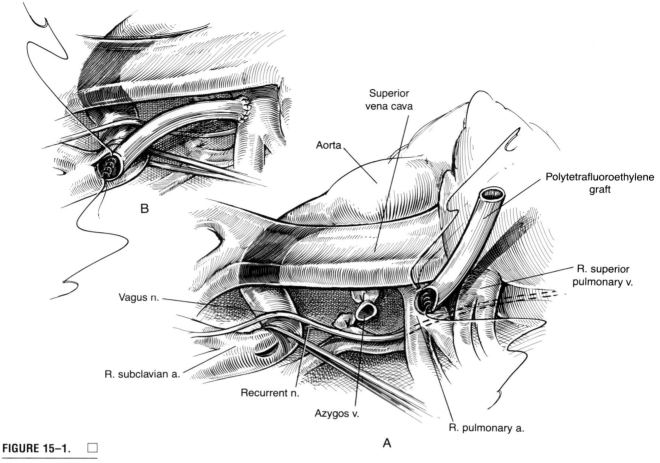

FIGURE 15–1. ☐

Placement of a modified Blalock-Taussig shunt via a right thoracotomy incision. *A,* The right subclavian, innominate, and carotid arteries are dissected out, being careful to avoid injury to the vagus and recurrent laryngeal nerves. The azygos vein is divided between suture ligatures to improve access to the proximal right pulmonary artery. The right pulmonary artery is mobilized, accurately identifying the first major bifurcation. The pulmonary artery anastomosis is placed well proximal to this bifurcation. *B,* The proximal anastomosis is made to the incision in the right subclavian artery.

otomy in the superior surface of the pulmonary artery with running suture. It has been our preference to use fine monofilament suture (6-0 or 7-0 Prolene) for these anastomoses in a nonheparinized patient because of the ease of passing the suture through the tissues and the graft. Care must be taken in occluding branches of the pulmonary artery to avoid injury that may lead to subsequent stenosis at the occlusion sites. It has been our preference to use Silastic "vessel loops" to obtain control of pulmonary artery branches, but atraumatic vascular clamps may be used as well. A relatively small dose of heparin ($\frac{1}{2}$ mg/kg) is given by some during shunt placement. At the completion of the shunt there should be an increase in the arterial saturation, but a thrill may not be immediately palpable if the ductus arteriosus is still patent and the pulmonary artery pressure is elevated. Closure of the ductus almost always occurs within hours after prostaglandin E_1 is discontinued.

Surgery for Excessive Pulmonary Blood Flow Without Obstruction to Systemic Arterial Flow. In this situation, the intent of the operation is to reduce the volume load on the systemic ventricle to treat congestive heart failure and to reduce the pulmonary artery pressure and flow to prevent the development of elevated pulmonary vascular resistance and pulmonary vascular obstructive disease. In general, limitation of pulmonary blood flow is accomplished by banding the pulmonary artery. In more recent years, we have generally carried out pulmonary artery banding via a median sternotomy approach. By using this incision, the pulmonary artery band may be placed in essentially all great vessel configurations (D- or L-transposition or normally related great vessels). The technique is shown in Figure 15–2.

One important technical element of this operation is to place the band proximal enough to avoid distortion of the pulmonary artery branches. Because the

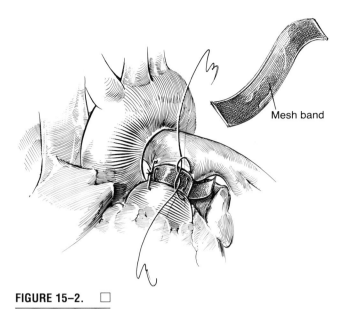

Mesh band

FIGURE 15–2. □

The pulmonary artery band is placed well proximal to the pulmonary artery bifurcation and is secured to the adventitia of the pulmonary artery to avoid distal "migration" of the band, which will distort the pulmonary artery bifurcation.

main pulmonary artery is generally short in the neonate, band placement is critical. It is useful to dissect only a short distance between the aorta and pulmonary artery to pass the banding material around the pulmonary artery and to help keep the band from migrating distally and impinging on the pulmonary artery bifurcation. Distal migration of the band can also be retarded with sutures that attach the band to the adventitia of the pulmonary artery proximally.

The banding material we have used is Silastic reinforced with a Dacron mesh. The Dacron mesh reduces the likelihood that the sutures that fix the diameter of the band will cut through the banding material. The choice of the appropriate diameter of the band can be difficult, but it has been found useful to mark the band according to the formula suggested by Trusler and Mustard for banding in patients with ventricular septal defects.[28] The general rule is that the circumference of the band in millimeters should be equal to the child's weight in kilograms plus 20. This circumference has proved to be useful as a starting point for banding, and additional adjustments to the band are made based on measurements of the pulmonary artery pressure distal to the band and on the changes in systemic arterial saturation and blood pressure as the band is tightened. As a general rule, the distal pulmonary artery pressure should be reduced to one third of systemic pressure with an arterial saturation no lower than 75%. It must be recalled that these measurements are being made in an anesthetized,

mechanically ventilated patient with an open chest, and the physiology is clearly quite different from that in an awake and spontaneously breathing child. These guidelines have generally proved to be useful, and the incidence of rebanding has generally been low. However, the difficulty in achieving an appropriate tightness of the band can be readily explained when it is recalled that Poiseuille's law predicts that blood flow is related to the fourth power of the radius of the vessel. Therefore, a minor alteration in diameter will have a large impact on flow and pressure gradient across the band site. It is also worthwhile to emphasize that banding the pulmonary artery to reduce pulmonary blood flow should be undertaken only when there is confidence that there is no obstruction to systemic outflow. Some observers have reported that pulmonary artery banding "causes" the development of subaortic obstruction in the patient with a single ventricle,[12] although, as outlined in the next section, it appears more likely that patients with a single ventricle and unrestricted pulmonary blood flow (i.e., those who require pulmonary artery banding early in life) also generally have the anatomic substrate that is conducive to the development of subaortic obstruction as the child grows.[17] Therefore, it seems inappropriate to condemn the pulmonary artery banding operation per se, although it is clear that close follow-up to identify the development of subaortic stenosis is mandatory in patients who undergo pulmonary artery banding operations.

Surgery for Excessive Pulmonary Blood Flow With Obstruction to Aortic Outflow. Patients in this group clearly are closely related to those patients with excessive pulmonary blood flow without systemic outflow obstruction. Patients with single ventricles without obstruction to pulmonary blood flow represent a spectrum of disorders, with no clear-cut points of demarcation between those with and those without obstruction to systemic outflow. Management of those patients with obvious intracardiac or valvar obstruction to systemic blood flow should be directed at relief of the obstruction and provision for limited pulmonary blood flow. The most common source of intracardiac obstruction to systemic blood flow is restriction at the bulboventricular foramen when the aorta arises from an infundibular chamber, although obstruction can also be found at the level of the subaortic conus or aortic valve annulus. When there is obstruction to systemic outflow within the heart, there frequently is obstruction in the aortic arch, and vice versa.[17] The approaches to these patients include bypass of the intracardiac obstruction to aortic outflow by connecting the proximal end of the divided main pulmonary artery to the aorta with a systemic-to–pulmonary artery shunt or by resecting of the subaortic stenosis (usually by enlargement of the bulboventricular foramen) and banding the pulmonary artery (see later discussion).

Patients without clear-cut physiologic evidence of an intracardiac systemic outflow obstruction but with a subaortic pathway that is smaller than the aortic annulus have been a more controversial group, as alluded to previously. At Children's Hospital in Boston, our treatment philosophy has been influenced by the data accumulated by Matitiau and colleagues,[17] in which the natural history of the subaortic bulboventricular foramen was determined by serial echocardiographic measurements of the dimensions of the bulboventricular foramen (indexed to the body surface area). As the body surface area increased with growth of the patient, the indexed cross-sectional area of the bulboventricular foramen progressively became smaller. Most importantly, those patients in whom the initial neonatal bulboventricular foramen area index was less than 2 cm²/m² all developed subaortic obstruction, regardless of the initial treatment, and subsequently required operative intervention to relieve the obstruction to systemic outflow. It was also clear that those patients with coarctation in the neonatal period had the smallest bulboventricular foramen areas. These data were obtained in patients with a single left ventricle and with the aorta arising from the infundibular chamber and thus do not represent the entire spectrum of patients with a single ventricle. Despite this limitation, it seems to be a useful principle that the patient with a single ventricle who has a coarctation or evidence of hypoplasia of the aortic arch is likely to have had some intracardiac restriction to systemic blood flow in utero and therefore is at risk for developing subaortic obstruction after the neonatal period, regardless of the initial management. Therefore, in these patients we have generally attempted to either directly relieve subaortic obstruction or bypass the subaortic area during the neonatal period.

The precise choice of an operation to treat existing or potential subaortic obstruction depends in part on the anatomic cause of the obstruction as well as on other anatomic factors, including the relationship of the great arteries and the aortic arch anatomy. We have generally employed operations to bypass the subaortic area by means of a pulmonary artery–to-aorta connection, relief of the aortic arch obstruction, and a modified Blalock-Taussig shunt. In patients with normally related great arteries, the operation is conducted in essentially the same manner as that described for the patient with the hypoplastic left heart syndrome (see Chapter 23). For those patients with L-transposition of the great ar-

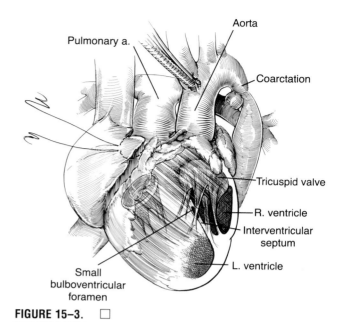

FIGURE 15–3.   □

L-transposition of the great arteries (LTGA), single left ventricle (right-sided) {S,L,L}, and coarctation of the aorta are shown. The communication (bulboventricular foramen [BFF]) that restricts blood flow to the subaortic infundibular chamber is shown.

teries and a left aortic arch (Fig. 15–3), the operation is conceptually the same, but some technical modifications are used. The operation is generally carried out using deep hypothermia and circulatory arrest with cannulation in the ascending aorta and the right atrium. If the arch obstruction is severe, two arterial cannulas are placed—one in the ascending aorta and the second in the main pulmonary artery—to provide perfusion to the descending aorta via the ductus arteriosus. If a single aortic cannula is used, the ductus arteriosus must be controlled with a ligature as soon as bypass is instituted to avoid runoff into the pulmonary circulation with systemic hypoperfusion. If descending aortic perfusion is provided via the pulmonary artery and ductus, the pulmonary artery branches must be occluded as bypass is initiated to prevent runoff into the pulmonary vascular bed. The cranial vessels should be controlled with tourniquets to minimize the chances for air embolism, and then the aorta is clamped, the circulation arrested, and the cardioplegic solution given. Next, the main pulmonary artery is divided just proximal to the bifurcation, and the distal orifice is closed primarily or with a pericardial patch (Fig. 15–4). This patch is placed to avoid stenosis of the pulmonary artery branches, although this is not always necessary. If a single aortic cannula has been used for perfusion, division and patching of the main pulmonary artery can be accomplished before arresting the heart and circulation. The aorta is incised along its rightward and

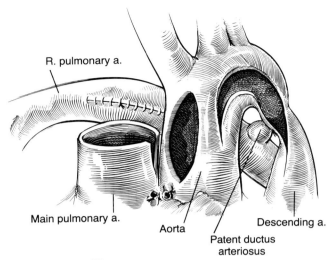

FIGURE 15–4. □

Incisions for the initial palliative operation for LTGA and aortic arch obstruction; note that the incisions on either side of the ascending aorta overlap. The incisions are extended proximally in the pulmonary artery and the aorta to allow a portion of the pulmonary artery–to-aorta connection to be "side to side."

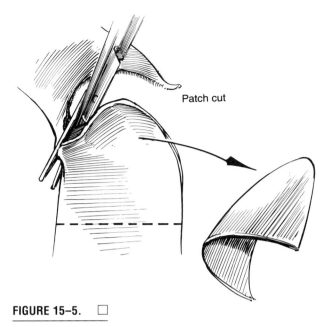

FIGURE 15–5. □

The patch to augment the pulmonary artery–to-aorta connection is cut so that it will form a "hemi-cone," which has a base equal to the circumference of the main pulmonary artery and a height equal to the distance between the top of the pulmonary artery and the distal end of the aortic incision.

posterior aspect, beginning inferiorly below the level of the pulmonary artery transection and extending superiorly nearly to the level of the origin of the innominate artery. Care must be taken inferiorly to avoid injury to the right coronary artery. Then the proximal pulmonary artery is incised longitudinally adjacent to the incision in the aorta, and these two incisions are joined with a side-to-side anastomosis using continuous absorbable monofilament suture. The remainder of the circumference of the pulmonary artery is connected to the remainder of the incision in the aorta by the use of an augmentation patch (Fig. 15–5), which is generally cut from autologous pericardium that has been treated with glutaraldehyde. A patch cut in the shape of a triangle with a base that is in the shape of an arc (rather than a straight line) will assume the shape of a half cone when sewn to the pulmonary artery and aortic incisions, as shown in Figure 15–5. The sides of the triangle should be roughly the length of the remaining aortic incision, and the length of the arc at the base of the triangle should be roughly equal to the circumference of the proximal pulmonary artery (Fig. 15–6). When the aortic arch is also to be augmented (which is very common for reasons outlined earlier), this is accomplished by placing a separate pericardial patch into an incision on the left lateral aspect of the ascending aorta; this is then carried around the aortic arch and into the descending aorta below the point of insertion of the ductus arteriosus (Fig. 15–7). It is important to make sure that these two patches on opposite sides of the ascending aorta overlap to avoid obstruction in the

segment of aorta (which may be moderately hypoplastic) between the patches. Alternatively, an approach similar to that employed in a stage I reconstruction for the hypoplastic left heart syndrome has also been used, with homograft tissue utilized to augment the aortic arch and the pulmonary

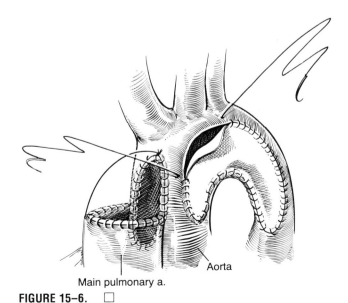

FIGURE 15–6. □

The pulmonary artery–to-aorta connection has been completed, and a separate patch is used to augment the aortic arch. The arch patch extends well down into the descending aorta.

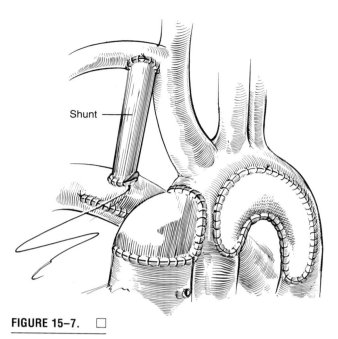

FIGURE 15–7. ☐

The operation is completed by placement of a right-sided modified Blalock-Taussig shunt.

artery–to-aorta anastomosis. The atrial septum should be inspected to be certain that there is a wide communication between the two atria, especially if there is atresia or stenosis of the left atrioventricular valve. Finally, the modified Blalock-Taussig shunt is constructed by the techniques previously described (Fig. 15–8). The shunt may be inserted after bypass has been resumed and the heart de-aired in an attempt to minimize the circulatory arrest time.

An alternative technique for the relief of subaortic obstruction caused by obstruction at the level of the bulboventricular foramen is to enlarge this interventricular communication and then to limit pulmonary blood flow by banding the main pulmonary artery. The advantage to this technique is that the patient is left with "banded physiology" rather than "systemic-to–pulmonary shunt" physiology. The difference between these two physiologic states is that in the banded patient, pulmonary blood flow occurs only during systole, and the aortic diastolic blood pressure is likely to be higher, which may lead to higher coronary blood flow. In contrast, the shunt-dependent patient has runoff from the systemic to the pulmonary circulation during essentially all phases of the cardiac cycle, and the diastolic blood pressure is likely to be lower, with the potential for lower coronary blood flow.

The technique for enlargement of the bulboventricular foramen has been described by Cheung and coworkers.[5] After the institution of bypass and in-

duction of moderate-to-deep levels of hypothermia, the aorta is clamped, and cardioplegic solution is given. It is sometimes possible to approach the bulboventricular foramen via an aortotomy and the aortic valve, but in the neonate it is frequently necessary to make an incision in the infundibular "outlet" chamber. An important consideration is the avoidance of heart block as the bulboventricular foramen is being enlarged. The location of the conduction system in relation to the bulboventricular foramen in both D- and L-loop ventricular patterns has been illustrated by Cheung and coworkers.[5] In general, the bulboventricular foramen should be enlarged inferiorly and toward the left (i.e., toward the obtuse margin of the heart). The infundibular incision should be closed with a patch, which will also serve to enlarge the subaortic outflow tract. Pulmonary artery banding can then be carried out during the rewarming period, and the band tightness can be adjusted after bypass is discontinued and hemodynamics have stabilized.

Postoperative Management

Management of the palliated patient with a single ventricle is outlined in Chapter 5 and is primarily concerned with achieving a favorable balance between systemic and pulmonary blood flow. If the postoperative course is unfavorable, with excessive cyanosis or inadequate systemic perfusion, a resid-

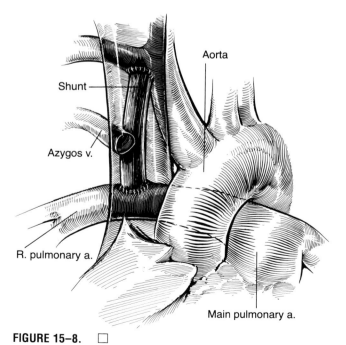

FIGURE 15–8. ☐

Anatomy of the single ventricle patient with a previous right Blalock-Taussig shunt.

ual anatomic defect must be aggressively sought by echocardiography, catheterization, or both.

Management Beyond the Neonatal Period

Medical Management

After the neonatal period, medical management of the patient with single-ventricle physiology is primarily concerned with control of congestive heart failure and attempting to ensure that the patient will be a candidate for a Fontan type of repair. Management of congestive heart failure generally relies on the use of digoxin and diuretics as the first line of treatment, and patients are routinely placed on these medications at the time of discharge from the hospital after neonatal interventions. If ventricular function is depressed, angiotensin-converting enzyme inhibitors (e.g., captopril or enalapril) are frequently helpful.

Identification of residual or newly developing anatomic problems that will adversely affect a subsequent Fontan operation is a critical aspect of management during this interval. The most commonly encountered problems are recurrent obstruction in the aortic arch, progression or new development of subaortic stenosis, distortion of the pulmonary arteries, deterioration of ventricular or atrioventricular valve function, and development of elevated pulmonary vascular resistance. Continuing difficulties in the management of congestive heart failure should particularly alert the clinician to the potential development of arch or subaortic obstruction. Echocardiography may identify some of these problems, but routine cardiac catheterization should be carried out in essentially all circumstances by the age of 6 months. In addition to measurement of pressures and flows and calculation of pulmonary resistance (outlined in the section on diagnosis), the presence of significant collateral vessels from the systemic to the pulmonary circulation should be aggressively sought at catheterization. We attempt to occlude all significant connections in the catheterization laboratory, using coils and other devices, as it has seemed that the presence of these collaterals would provide retrograde flow in the pulmonary arteries that would then retard the forward flow into the pulmonary arteries after a systemic venous–to–pulmonary artery anastomosis. Conclusive data to prove that these interventions are beneficial are not available.

Surgical Management

The major goals of surgical management of the patient with a single ventricle beyond the neonatal period are to minimize the pressure and volume loads on the single ventricle. The issue of relief of pressure load (afterload) on the ventricle by subaortic or aortic arch obstruction has been discussed in previous sections, and similar techniques of bypass of subaortic obstruction or enlargement of the bulboventricular foramen are used if these problems are recognized beyond the neonatal period. The relief of the volume load on the ventricle is accomplished by removal of systemic-to–pulmonary artery shunts or division of the main pulmonary artery and the creation of direct connections between the systemic venous circulation and the pulmonary arteries. The bidirectional cavopulmonary shunt and the Fontan operation itself accomplish this goal of relieving the volume load on the ventricle. It is important to recognize that the Fontan operation creates a physiologic situation in which all of the energy input into the cardiovascular system is provided by the single ventricle, and the systemic and pulmonary resistances to blood flow are in series rather than in parallel, as they were in the pre-Fontan state. It remains unknown (because truly long-term follow-up information on ventricular function after Fontan operations is not available) whether this rearrangement of the resistances from an in-parallel, volume-loaded circulation to an in-series circulation with reduced ventricular volume load is beneficial to the preservation of ventricular function.

The roles of the bidirectional cavopulmonary shunt and the Fontan operation continue to evolve, and the decision in specific patients has been based on a number of factors that have seemed to be risk factors for Fontan operations when our previous experience has been reviewed.[18, 19] In these analyses, pulmonary artery distortion, elevated pulmonary arteriolar resistance (>2 Wood units indexed to body surface area), elevated pulmonary artery pressure (>15 mm Hg), and the presence of either left atrioventricular valve atresia or a common atrioventricular valve have been associated with increased risk for a Fontan operation. Also, young age (<3 years) appeared to be a risk factor in the most recent analysis of the results, although it did not appear to be a risk factor in the original review of our experience up to 1985. In both reviews it has been clear that young age alone did not preclude a Fontan operation when there were no other associated risk factors. Therefore, when there appear to be significant risk factors for a Fontan operation during infancy, it is currently our practice to carry out an intermediate bidirectional cavopulmonary shunt, followed during the second year of life by a Fontan operation if there is improvement in the risk status of the patient. Only rarely is there a need for a

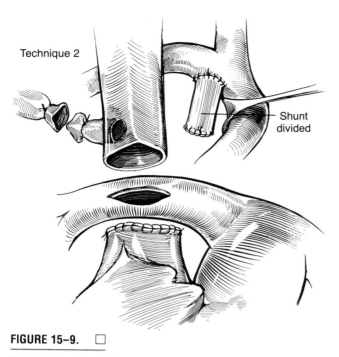

FIGURE 15–9. ☐

The right Blalock-Taussig shunt, superior vena cava, and azygos vein have been divided. The site of the previous shunt anastomosis to the right pulmonary artery had been enlarged to serve as the point for anastomosis of the cranial end of the superior vena cava.

the heart beating. However, later conversion to a full Fontan circulation may be more difficult, because the cardiac end of the superior vena cava must be dissected out to make a cavopulmonary connection, and there may be an increased risk of injury to the sinus node. An alternative approach is to make connections between both ends of the divided superior vena cava and the pulmonary artery and to place a patch within the right atrium at the entrance site of the superior vena cava during a brief period of cardioplegic arrest of the heart (Fig. 15–11). If the atrial septal defect is potentially restrictive, it is enlarged within the confines of the limbus. After closure of the atriotomy and de-airing of the heart, the crossclamp can be removed and the cavopulmonary anastomoses constructed with the heart reperfused. If this approach is used, the subsequent Fontan operation will involve only removal of the patch at the junction of the superior vena cava and the right atrium and placement of the intra-atrial baffle to divert the inferior vena caval blood up to the superior vena caval orifice. This approach may also be useful in situations in which there is localized stenosis in the right pulmonary artery (frequently at the site of a shunt); in this case the pulmonary artery, rather than the superior vena cava,

second systemic-to–pulmonary artery shunt if the patient "outgrows" a shunt placed in the neonatal period, as a second shunt may have a significant negative impact on candidacy for a later Fontan operation.[20]

Bidirectional Cavopulmonary Shunt. This procedure is routinely carried out through a midline sternotomy, with the establishment of bypass using cannulas placed in the ascending aorta, in the superior vena cava (or innominate vein), and in the right atrium near the entrance of the inferior vena cava. Before bypass it is useful to place marking sutures on the anterior surface of the superior vena cava and the pulmonary artery, because after the vessels are divided, it may be difficult to re-establish their normal orientation, and twisting or kinking of anastomoses may occur. As bypass is established, all existing systemic-to–pulmonary artery shunts are controlled, and the azygos vein is ligated and divided. The simplest method of establishing a bidirectional cavopulmonary connection is to divide the superior vena cava and anastomose its cranial end into a longitudinal incision in the superior margin of the right pulmonary artery. The cardiac end of the superior vena cava is then oversewn (Figs. 15–9 and 15–10). This approach has the advantage of being relatively simple to carry out and can be accomplished with mild degrees of hypothermia with

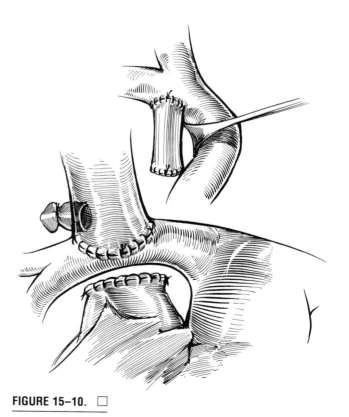

FIGURE 15–10. ☐

The superior vena cava–to–right pulmonary artery anastomosis is completed with running absorbable suture.

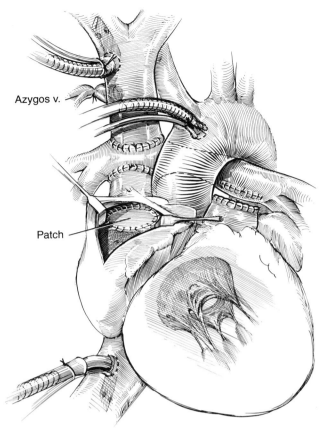

Azygos v.

Patch

FIGURE 15–11. ☐

Depiction of a bidirectional cavopulmonary artery shunt with patch occlusion of the superior vena cava–right atrial junction (hemi-Fontan procedure) using a single arterial cannula and direct cannulation of the superior and inferior venae cavae. The main pulmonary artery is shown divided and oversewn, but in some cases it may be allowed to remain patent.

is divided, and the cavopulmonary connections are made from the divided ends of the pulmonary artery to the sides of the superior vena cava (Fig. 15–12). Division of the pulmonary artery rather than the superior vena cava has also been useful when the pulmonary artery is smaller than the superior vena cava, as there seems to be less risk of distortion of a small pulmonary artery with this type of connection. At the conclusion of bypass, it is important to monitor both the superior vena cava pressure and the arterial oxygen saturation to determine whether the patient will tolerate the newly created physiology. In unusual circumstances the arterial saturation may be intolerably low, and then an explanation must be sought. If the superior vena cava pressure is significantly elevated or there is marked arterial desaturation, a technical problem with the anastomosis must be considered; this can be identified by direct measurement of pressures on either side of the anastomosis. Residual communications between the superior vena caval system and the

atrium should also be ruled out by echocardiography, particularly if the superior vena cava patch technique has been used. Finally, it can be useful to attempt to increase systemic cardiac output in order to increase the saturation of the inferior vena caval blood that is reaching the common atrium and mixing with the pulmonary venous return, as this will result in increased arterial saturation. If it is certain that there are no technical problems and no residual communication between the superior vena cava and the atrium, and that the arterial saturation is unresponsive to ventilatory and cardiac output manipulations, an additional source of pulmonary blood flow may be necessary. A small systemic-to–pulmonary artery shunt can be added to increase pulmonary blood flow. However, this maneuver will increase the volume load on the single ventricle and therefore will defeat one of the objectives of the bidirectional cavopulmonary shunt.

Modified Fontan Operation. This procedure is carried out via a midline sternotomy with venous cannulation directly into the superior vena caval system (superior vena cava or innominate vein) and at the junction of the inferior vena cava and the right atrium. All systemic artery–to–pulmonary artery shunts are controlled with the institution of bypass; cooling is generally carried out to 25°C but is carried to lower temperatures if it seems likely that circulatory arrest or markedly reduced pump flows will be necessary for exposure. Systemic venous–to–pulmonary artery connections are made in exactly the same manner as described in the section on bidirectional cavopulmonary shunts (Fig. 15–13). The portion of the atrial septum within the confines of the limbus of the fossa ovalis is excised, particularly if there is any concern about stenosis of the left atrioventricular valve. The systemic venous atrial blood is separated from the pulmonary venous return using the "lateral tunnel" technique, which has two advantages over previous methods of separating systemic from pulmonary venous return within the right atrium. deLeval and coworkers have presented data that suggest that there is a hydrodynamic advantage because energy losses resulting from turbulence are minimized.[4] Equally important, however, is the fact that this technique minimizes the size of the systemic venous pathway within the atrium and places the pathway relatively far away from the pulmonary venous pathway.[15] Both of these features reduce the chance that the systemic venous pathway will bulge into the pulmonary venous pathway and create pulmonary venous obstruction. This technique has proved to be particularly important in patients with left atrioventricular valve atresia or stenosis, in whom the pulmonary venous blood must cross from the left

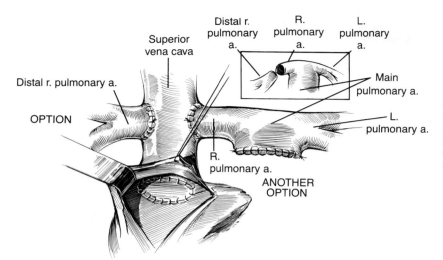

FIGURE 15–12. ☐

The hemi-Fontan procedure with division of the right pulmonary artery and anastomoses of the divided ends into the sides of the superior vena cava. This approach can be useful when there is stenosis of the right pulmonary artery at the site of a previous systemic-to–pulmonary artery shunt.

atrium to the right atrium to reach a right-sided systemic atrioventricular valve (e.g., in patients with the hypoplastic left heart syndrome).[18]

Placement of the baffle to direct the inferior vena caval blood flow to the superior vena caval orifice is

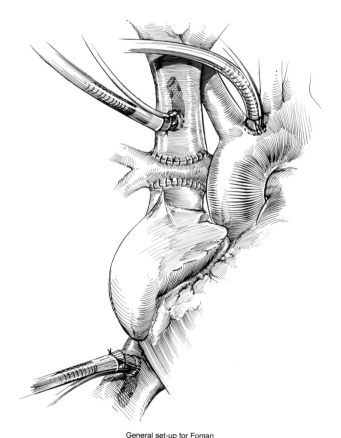

General set-up for Fontan

FIGURE 15–13. ☐

Cannulation for cardiopulmonary bypass for a Fontan operation with a single arterial cannula and direct cannulation of the superior and inferior venae cavae. (The cavopulmonary artery anastomoses are shown in completed form.)

detailed in Figure 15–14. The baffle is cut from a tubular piece of PTFE graft material, and both ends are beveled to allow for the fact that the intercaval distance is slightly shorter on the lateral wall of the atrium than between the medial aspects of the cavoatrial junctions. The baffle is sewn into position with running monofilament suture, beginning at the inferior vena caval entrance into the right atrium and proceeding superiorly, staying lateral and anterior to the entrance sites of the right pulmonary veins. If the posterior rim of the original atrial septum is present, this tissue is allowed to remain on the pulmonary venous side of the new baffle. This positioning of the baffle is important to prevent pulmonary venous obstruction. At the superior margin, the suture line is carried into the nontrabeculated tissue at the entrance site of the superior vena cava (beneath the crista terminalis) to minimize the possibility of any residual right-to-left communication in this area. This suture line is carried across to the lateral wall of the right atrium and stopped. Then the suture line is constructed around the entrance of the inferior vena cava into the atrium, leaving the coronary sinus on the pulmonary venous atrial side of the baffle. This positioning avoids potential injury to the atrioventricular node and is also important in ensuring unobstructed access of the pulmonary venous return to the right atrioventricular valve.

Once the lateral aspect of the inferior vena cava–atrial wall is reached with the suture line, the baffle may be tailored additionally to ensure an appropriate fit. If the baffle is to be fenestrated, a cruciate incision is made in the medial aspect of the baffle, and the fenestration is created with a 4-mm aortic punch. This size punch is rarely too large (i.e., resulting in excessive cyanosis) but is large enough to allow efficient systemic venous decompression and

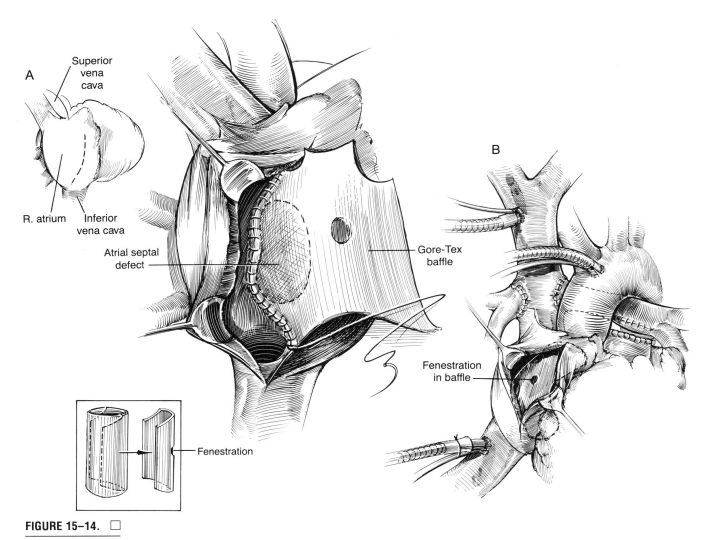

FIGURE 15–14. ☐

A, Placement of baffle to convey inferior vena caval blood along the lateral wall of the right atrium to the superior vena caval orifice. A 4-mm fenestration is made on the medial aspect of the polytetrafluoroethylene baffle. *B*, The cavopulmonary anastomoses are shown using the variation of division of the right pulmonary artery and end-to-side anastomoses between the divided ends of the right pulmonary artery and the sides of the superior vena cava.

to accommodate the catheterization laboratory devices used to close the fenestration in the postoperative period. Finally, the remainder of the baffle is sutured to the lateral wall of the atrium, air is removed from the heart, and the atriotomy is closed. The aortic crossclamp is then released, and rewarming is carried out while the cavopulmonary connections are being constructed. In situations in which reduced pump flow is needed because of excessive retrograde flow in the pulmonary arteries, removal of the aortic crossclamp is delayed until the need for hypothermia and reduced perfusion flow is absent. Also, in situations in which an additional anastomosis between the left superior vena cava and the left pulmonary artery is necessary, this anastomosis is more easily constructed with the heart arrested and decompressed.

Variations on these techniques of separation of

systemic and pulmonary venous return and creation of cavopulmonary connections have been used when there are variations in systemic and pulmonary connections, such as frequently occur in the heterotaxia syndromes. The most important consideration in choosing the route for the baffle to bring the inferior vena cava or hepatic venous drainage to the pulmonary arteries is the avoidance of pulmonary venous obstruction. In cases in which the pulmonary venous return joins the atrium in close proximity to the superior vena caval orifice, the baffle can be routed across the posterior wall of the atrium and the cranial end of the baffle connected to the orifice of the opposite atrial appendage, which in turn is joined to the adjacent pulmonary artery. Alternatively, the baffle can be brought to any point in the roof of the atrium, and an incision in the atrium can be connected to the pulmonary artery. Also, if placement of a baffle within the atrium is difficult, then an intra-atrial tube graft can be sewn around the inferior vena cava and hepatic vein orifices, and the superior end of the graft can be sewn to the atrio-pulmonary connection or to the superior vena cava orifice. One final anatomic option is the creation of an extra-atrial pathway from the inferior vena cava to the pulmonary artery with a tubular conduit, although both of these conduit techniques should be reserved for the older patient who does not require that growth potential in the inferior vena cava–to–pulmonary artery pathway.

During rewarming, monitoring catheters are placed into the left atrium and the systemic venous system (superior vena cava or right atrium), and bypass is discontinued while right- and left-sided filling pressures and systemic arterial oxygen saturation are monitored. We have found that atrium–pulmonary artery gradients are rarely present when cavopulmonary anastomoses are used, but some of us continue to place a pulmonary artery catheter so that the presence of an atriopulmonary gradient can be identified in the operating room or the intensive care unit.

Inotropic support in the form of dopamine (5 to 10 μg/kg/min) is frequently used. If the atrial septation baffle is fenestrated, arterial saturations of 80% to 90% are to be expected. If fenestration is not used, arterial saturations should be close to 100%. If saturations are significantly lower, a residual leak from the systemic venous to the pulmonary venous circulation is likely; this may be due to a defect in the baffle-to–atrial wall suture line. However, this leak may also be due to previously undocumented connections between the systemic and pulmonary venous chambers, particularly through coronary venous connections. If the patient is hemodynamically stable with arterial saturations greater than 75%, it may be best to conclude the operation and attempt to localize the site of the leak in the catheterization laboratory, where it may be able to be closed by interventional techniques. As long as the degree of arterial desaturation is not too severe, the physiologic state does not seem remarkably different from that seen with a fenestration in the atrial baffle.

The concept of the "fenestrated Fontan" was first reported in 1989 from Children's Hospital in Boston,[3] although leaving a residual right-to-left atrial shunt in situations where elevated right atrial pressure could be expected has been used when repairing tetralogy of Fallot in infants in this institution since the mid-1970s (by leaving the foramen ovale open). Application of this principle to patients who had pulmonary atresia with an intact ventricular septum was reported by Billingsley and coworkers in 1989,[1] although Edwards and Bargeron described

a similar concept for decompression of the superior vena cava after a classic Glenn operation in 1968.[9] The difference in the current concept from that previously described is the inclusion of elective catheterization laboratory closure (using a device) of the right-to-left communication under conditions in which the hemodynamic effects of closure can be tested before permanent occlusion (Fig. 15–15). Conceptually, the fenestration is useful to decompress the systemic venous pressure when there are transient and reversible physiologic increases in pulmonary vascular resistance or remedial (generally in the catheterization laboratory) distal anatomic obstructions to blood flow in the pulmonary artery tree.

To briefly summarize, in infancy a controlled source of pulmonary blood flow is established with either a shunt or a pulmonary artery band, and obstruction to systemic outflow from the ventricle to the aorta is relieved. Subsequently, patients undergo procedures that directly connect the systemic venous return to the pulmonary arteries. In young infants with increased risk factors for Fontan operations, the bidirectional cavopulmonary artery shunt is used. If the hemodynamics and anatomy of the pulmonary vascular bed are favorable, a fenestrated Fontan procedure is carried out at a later date.

Postoperative Management

In general terms, the postoperative management of the patient after a Fontan operation is similar to that after other open intracardiac repairs. However, there are some unique aspects of the care that are worthy of discussion. The first concept is that of attempting to reduce the total resistance to blood flow that the single ventricle must face (i.e., the afterload). As noted previously, after a Fontan operation the single ventricle faces resistances (i.e., the systemic and pulmonary resistances) in series. In addition, the blood passing through the mesenteric circulation must also pass through the resistance of the portal circulation. An additional theoretic factor that may contribute to elevation of the systemic vascular resistance after Fontan operations is the observation in isolated organ physiologic studies that elevation of the venous pressure results in a reflex rise in the tone of the arterioles. Because there is a generalized increase in the venous pressure after Fontan operations, it has seemed that such a mechanism may also be important in the post–Fontan surgery patient. Therefore, it has seemed logical that medications such as nitroprusside and amrinone that reduce the systemic resistance would be beneficial in the patient with Fontan physiology.

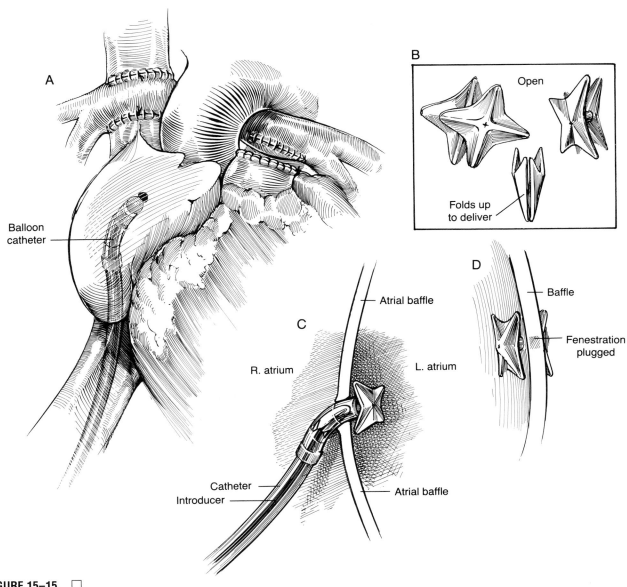

FIGURE 15–15. □

Catheter laboratory umbrella closure of fenestration.
A, A balloon catheter is placed into the fenestration to test the effects of fenestration closure on cardiac index and systemic venous saturation and pressure.
B, The umbrella is shown in "open" configuration (after delivery) and in "closed" configuration (within the delivery system before release).
C, The umbrella is shown connected to the delivery system with the left atrial "arms" deployed and the right atrial "arms" remaining within the delivery system.
D, The umbrella has been delivered with right and left atrial "arms" in appropriate positions on the right and left atrial sides of the Fontan baffle.

Also, interventions that minimize pulmonary vascular resistance can be expected to be useful, as pulmonary blood flow must occur with the systemic venous pressure as the driving force. Experimental studies suggest that pulmonary vascular resistance is minimized when the lung is operating near functional residual capacity. It remains debatable whether resistance is minimized by having the patient ventilate spontaneously or by using a mechanical ventilator, but it has been our preference to employ spontaneous ventilation soon after Fontan operations whenever the hemodynamic situation seems relatively stable.

It is also important to recognize that occasionally there are patients who cannot tolerate the physiology of a Fontan circulation, and these patients will expire unless their physiologic state is rapidly reversed. Therefore, the surgeon and cardiologist should be psychologically prepared to take down the Fontan procedure to a bidirectional cavopulmonary circulation if the patient seems to be failing after the operation. Manifestations of failure of the Fontan state include elevated systemic venous pressures (greater than 16 to 18 mm Hg), persistent low cardiac output with low mixed venous saturations, low urine output, poor peripheral perfusion, and continuing high inotropic requirements. Persistently elevated left (pulmonary venous) atrial pressures higher than 12 mm Hg are also an ominous sign. In these cases aggressive investigation by echocardiography and cardiac catheterization should be undertaken promptly, and any significant residual defects should be corrected, if possible. If this is not possible, strong consideration should be given to converting the circulation to a bidirectional cavopulmonary shunt. In our experience with the takedown of Fontan operations, this conversion can result in a dramatically improved hemodynamic state, with markedly improved perfusion and urine output occurring almost immediately. Takedown to a bidirectional cavopulmonary shunt has produced markedly better results than takedown to a systemic arterial–to–pulmonary artery shunt.

One final aspect of postoperative management after a Fontan operation concerns the development of pleural or pericardial effusion. In our first review of experience with the Fontan operation,[19] effusions that required chest tube drainage for more than 1 week developed in nearly 30% of the patients. The precise etiology of these effusions is incompletely understood, but it seems intuitively obvious that they are related to the elevated systemic venous pressures that exist after Fontan operations. Current evidence suggests that much of the fluid that is drained from the pleural space has its origin in the abdomen, most likely in the liver. In our own experience, the incidence of significant pulmonary effusions has been remarkably less in patients in whom only the superior vena caval pressure is elevated (bidirectional cavopulmonary anastomosis)[1] than in patients who have undergone a complete Fontan type of operation. In addition, both Lecompte and Norwood have had experience with Fontan operations in which one or more hepatic veins have been intentionally left draining to the pulmonary venous atrium; in their experience the incidence of pleural effusions has been remarkably reduced, with only mild reductions in arterial saturation (personal communications, June, 1992). It should also be recalled that the hepatic capillary bed is known to be the "leakiest" of the systemic capillary beds, and leaky capillary beds will theoretically result in the formation of the greatest amounts of interstitial fluid when venous pressure is elevated. Despite the advantage of reducing effusions by this diversion of some of the hepatic venous drainage, follow-up information from Lecompte has been unfavorable, as patients have become increasingly cyanotic with

time, presumably because of the formation of intrahepatic collateral vessels that divert increasing amounts of hepatic venous blood into the pulmonary venous atrium (personal communication, June 1992). Previous analysis has suggested that younger age at the time of the Fontan operation is also associated with a higher risk of persistent pleural effusions (unpublished data). In this context it should be recalled that there is evidence from at least two separate mammalian species that systemic capillaries are more permeable to fluid and protein in younger animals than in older members of the same species,[16, 21] and if this is also true in humans, a similar mechanism may be responsible for increased problems with effusions in younger Fontan patients. It has been rare in our experience, however, that a Fontan operation has required takedown because of persistent pleural effusion. While drainage is occurring it is important to replace the fluid and protein losses on a daily basis and to ensure adequate intake of nutrition to allow new protein synthesis to occur. The use of low-fat intake or parenteral nutrition has not made a consistent impact on reducing the formation of pleural fluid; ultimately patience seems to be rewarded in the vast majority of cases. If effusions persist for more than 2 to 3 weeks, we generally undertake catheterization to exclude any residual anatomic problems. Fenestration of the atrial baffle has reduced the percentage of patients with persistent effusions to approximately 10% and has also reduced the average hospital stay, presumably as a result of the somewhat lower right atrial pressures found in patients who have undergone the fenestrated Fontan approach.[4] One final occasional complication is a right-to-left shunt within the wall of the right atrium. These shunts seem to occur through Thebesian venous channels that enlarge with time. Several of these channels have been closed in the catheterization laboratory with devices, but a few have required reoperation with oversewing of the orifices.

RESULTS

One hundred sixty-two patients with functional single ventricle (as defined earlier) were seen at Children's Hospital in Boston between 1985 and 1991 at less than 1 year of age. A review of these patients forms the basis for the results presented in this section. The diagnoses and overall results are shown in Table 15–1. The initial hospital mortality rate was 16.7% (27 patients), and seven of these deaths occurred in association with early revisions of the initial operations. Thirty-one additional patients expired subsequently, 24 after the initial pal-

TABLE 15–2. ☐ LATE DEATHS (>30 DAYS) AFTER TREATMENT FOR SINGLE VENTRICLE

Before subsequent surgery	24
After revision of initial palliation	3/12
After bidirectional cavopulmonary shunt	1/28
During Fontan procedure	2/51
After Fontan procedure	1/49
	31

liation but before any other intervention and one late after a Fontan operation; the remaining six deaths were associated with later operations (Table 15–2). The results have been worse in patients with heterotaxia syndromes and in those with DORV. Among the heterotaxia patients, more than 50% (eight of 15) of those with anomalous pulmonary venous connections died in either the neonatal or follow-up periods. Patients with DORV are a heterogeneous group and were managed in a variety of ways. The only subgroup that seemed to be at markedly increased risk consisted of those with subaortic obstruction; three of four patients in this group are known to have died, and the fourth has been lost to follow-up.

Results of the neonatal management of patients with excessive pulmonary blood flow are shown in Table 15–3. There has been debate about the optimal form of management of patients with excessive pulmonary blood flow, particularly with regard to pulmonary artery banding versus anastomosis of the pulmonary artery to the aorta with a systemic-to–pulmonary artery shunt. The early mortality rate with pulmonary artery banding (with or without arch repair) is lower (three of 41, or 7.3%) when compared with the initial mortality rate of 17.2% (five of 29) for a pulmonary artery–to-aorta anastomosis with a systemic-to–pulmonary artery shunt (with or without arch repair). There was a signifi-

cant later mortality rate, with the total mortality rate reaching 26.3% of the survivors of neonatal operations with pulmonary artery banding compared with 37.9% (11 of 29) in the pulmonary artery–to-aorta anastomosis group. However, examination of Table 15–3 suggests that when the patients are divided into groups with or without associated aortic arch obstruction, the overall mortality rates are not remarkably different for the two different management strategies, although the numbers of patients in the isolated pulmonary artery–to-aorta anastomosis group and the pulmonary artery band–plus–arch reconstruction groups are relatively small. It is also noteworthy that the need for reoperation to revise the initial palliation is considerably higher in the groups having pulmonary artery banding than in the groups undergoing a pulmonary artery–to-aorta anastomosis. As shown in Table 15–2, the majority of these later deaths occur before any further surgical interventions.

Table 15–4 shows the results in patients with insufficient pulmonary blood flow in the neonatal period who were managed with a systemic-to–pulmonary artery shunt. The total mortality rate (early and late) in this group has been 34.9%, with a significant mortality rate after the initial palliative procedure.

Table 15–5 shows the mortality rates in the patients from this group managed from the neonatal period who later underwent either bidirectional cavopulmonary artery shunt or Fontan operations, according to the type of neonatal palliation. These data suggest that once patients become candidates for Fontan operations, the operative results are quite satisfactory, with survival rates comparable to those for all patients undergoing these operations.[18]

The lower age limit for a bidirectional cavopulmonary shunt is unknown, but experience with 14 patients under the age of 6.5 months who were op-

TABLE 15–3. ☐ OUTCOME AFTER NEONATAL MANAGEMENT OF EXCESSIVE PULMONARY BLOOD FLOW

	NO.	EARLY DEATHS	REOPERATION FOR SUBAORTIC STENOSIS OR ARCH	REOPERATION TO REVISE PBF	TOTAL DEATHS	AWAITING SURGERY	BDCPS OR GLENN	FONTAN	LOST TO FOLLOW-UP
Without arch obstruction									
PAB alone	35	2	6	6 (1)	9 (25.7%)	4	6	13	3
PA–Ao anastomosis	4	1	0	0	1 (25.0%)	0	0	1	1
SUBTOTALS	39	3 (7.7%)	6	6 (1)	10 (25.6%)	4	6	14	4
With arch obstruction									
PAB and arch repair	6	1	3 (3)	0	4 (66.7%)	1	0	1	0
PA–Ao and arch repair and MBTS	25	4	3 (2)	1 (1)	10 (40.0%)	0	6	8	1
Switch and arch repair	1	0	1 (1)	0	1 (100.0%)	0	0	0	0
SUBTOTALS	32	5 (15.6%)	7 (6)	1 (1)	15 (46.8%)	1	6	9	1
TOTAL	71								

Ao, Aorta; BDCPS, bidirectional cavopulmonary shunt; MBTS, modified Blalock-Taussig shunt; PA, pulmonary artery; PAB, pulmonary artery band; PBF, pulmonary blood flow.
Figures in parentheses are deaths.

TABLE 15–4. ☐ RESULTS OF SHUNTING PROCEDURES

DIAGNOSIS	NO.	EARLY DEATHS	ALL LATE DEATHS	AWAITING SURGERY	BDCPS OR GLENN	FONTAN
Single ventricle	20	3	4	3	3	7
Heterotaxia	22	4	7	0	5	5
Double-outlet right ventricle	4	0	1	1	1	1
Tricuspid atresia I	14	3	0	3	1	7
Tricuspid atresia II	3	0	0	0	0	2
TOTAL	63	10	12	7	10	22

BDCPS, Bidirectional cavopulmonary shunt.

erated on between 1989 and 1992 shows that 13 of the 14 survived this operation and had arterial saturations of 75% to 92% at the time of discharge. Three of these patients have subsequently had successful Fontan operations.

The lower age limit for Fontan operations is also unknown. Between January 1988 and July 1991, seven patients underwent Fontan operations at less than 1 year of age, and six of the seven survived. The relative roles of the bidirectional cavopulmonary artery shunt and the Fontan operation in these young patients remain incompletely defined.

COMPLICATIONS

Complications After Neonatal Management

As detailed in Table 15–1, both the short-term and intermediate-term results after neonatal palliative operations for single ventricle remain imperfect. Causes of perioperative mortality in patients who are dependent on systemic-to–pulmonary artery shunts generally seem to be related to difficulties in balancing the distribution of the output from the single ventricle between the systemic and pulmonary circulations. The significant intermediate-term mortality rate in patients with systemic-to–pulmonary artery shunts (most deaths occurred outside the hospital) suggests that thrombosis of the shunt is responsible, although this hypothesis remains unproved. The possibility that other extracar-

diac events upset the balance of systemic and pulmonary resistance and blood flows is an equally likely explanation for these out-of-hospital deaths in patients with palliated single ventricle. As noted in Table 15–3, pulmonary artery banding alone has required revisions of the band; in some cases, division of the pulmonary artery and substitution of a systemic-to–pulmonary artery shunt as a more controlled source of pulmonary blood flow have been required in 17% of patients who had a pulmonary artery banding procedure. In patients with associated aortic arch obstruction, 21.9% (seven of 32) required reoperation because of obstruction either in the aortic arch or at the level of the interventricular communication (in those with pulmonary artery banding operations).

Complications of Procedures Beyond the Neonatal Period

Complications after the bidirectional cavopulmonary shunt and Fontan operations have been relatively unusual except as noted previously. Inadequate pulmonary blood flow and excessive cyanosis have been rarely encountered after the bidirectional cavopulmonary shunt; when they occurred, the addition of a systemic-to–pulmonary artery shunt to supply the left pulmonary artery and interruption of the continuity between the right and left pulmonary arteries was employed in two cases. Alternatively, a systemic-to–pulmonary artery shunt with-

TABLE 15–5. ☐ OUTCOME OF BIDIRECTIONAL CAVOPULMONARY SHUNT (BDCPS) AND FONTAN OPERATIONS AFTER NEONATAL PALLIATION

	BDCPS OR GLENN			FONTAN			
	No.	Survived	Died	No.	Survived	Failed	Died
Shunt	13	12	1	28	24 (85.7%)	1	3
PA band	4	4	0	15	15 (86.7%)	2	0
PA–Ao anastomosis	7	7	0	8	8 (100%)	0	0
Other	4	4	0	4	4 (100%)	0	0
			0				
TOTAL	28	27	1	55	49 (89%)	3	3

Ao, Aorta; PA, pulmonry artery.

out separation of the pulmonary arteries can be used as long as the pressure in the superior vena cava does not exceed 20 mm Hg.

Complications of the Fontan operation have been discussed previously and include low cardiac output and persistent pleural effusions. One important late complication of the Fontan operation is the development of atrial arrhythmias. Although the exact incidence of this problem is currently unknown, these arrhythmias have occasionally proved to be difficult to treat medically (see Chapter 5, section on Management of Cardiac Arrhythmias). The use of the lateral atrial tunnel technique (cavocaval baffle) for the Fontan operation may reduce the incidence of atrial arrhythmias, as this technique exposes a smaller amount of the atrium to the elevated systemic venous pressures. However, currently there are no data from our institution to support this conclusion.

SUMMARY

Management of the patient with a functional single ventricle remains a surgical challenge, beginning at the time of birth. The continuing mortality and morbidity after neonatal palliative operations suggest that earlier reinterventions to establish a pulmonary circulation that is in series, rather than in parallel, with the systemic circulation may have the potential for reducing some of this mortality. However, because there is no long-term follow-up information on the Fontan operation, the lifetime outlook for the patient with a functional single ventricle currently remains unknown. Continued assessment of the "unnatural" history of the surgically treated patient with a single ventricle will be essential to refine the treatment of this difficult group of patients.

Fontan, after analyzing his considerable experience with his operation, sounded a cautionary note because of a late rise in the hazard function for survival.[11] Whether more appropriate patient selection or some of the previously outlined modifications of the original Fontan operation will have a more favorable impact on the long-term results remains to be seen. Clearly, there is a continuing need for improvements and, most importantly, for new ideas.

REFERENCES

1. Billingsley AM, Laks H, Boyce SW, et al. Definitive repair in patients with pulmonary atresia and intact ventricular septum. J Thorac Cardiovasc Surg 97:746, 1989.
2. Bridges ND, Jonas RA, Mayer JE Jr, et al. Bidirectional cavopulmonary anastomosis as interim palliation for high-risk Fontan candidates. Circulation 82 (suppl IV):IV-170, 1990.
3. Bridges ND, Lock JE, Castaneda AR. Baffle fenestration with subsequent transcatheter closure: Modification of the Fontan operation for patients at increased risk. Circulation 82:1681, 1990.
4. Bridges ND, Mayer JE, Lock JE, et al. Effect of fenestration on outcome of Fontan repair. Circulation 84(suppl II): II-120, 1991.
5. Cheung HC, Lincoln C, Anderson RH, et al. Options for surgical repair in hearts with univentricular atrioventricular connection and subaortic stenosis. J Thorac Cardiovasc Surg 100:672, 1990.
6. deLeval MR, Kilner P, Gewillig M, et al. Total cavopulmonary connection: A logical alternative to atriopulmonary connection for complex Fontan operations. J Thorac Cardiovasc Surg 96:682, 1988.
7. Ebert PA. Staged partitioning of single ventricle. J Thorac Cardiovasc Surg 88:908, 1984.
8. Edwards JE. Congenital malformations of the heart and great vessels: C. Malformations of the valves. In Gould SE (ed). Pathology of the Heart and Blood Vessels. 3rd ed. Springfield, IL, Charles C Thomas, 1968, p 312.
9. Edwards WS, Bargeron LM. The superiority of the Glenn operation for tricuspid atresia in infancy and childhood. J Thorac Cardiovasc Surg 55:60, 1968.
10. Fontan F, Baudet E. Surgical repair of tricuspid atresia. Thorax 26:240, 1971.
11. Fontan F, Kirklin JW, Fernandez G, et al. Outcome after a "perfect" Fontan operation. Circulation 81:1520, 1990.
12. Freedom RM, Benson LN, Smallhorn JF, et al. Subaortic stenosis, the univentricular heart, and banding of the pulmonary artery: An analysis of the courses of 43 patients with univentricular heart palliated by pulmonary artery banding. Circulation 73:758, 1986.
13. Fyler DC. Double-outlet right ventricle. In Fyler DC (ed): Nadas' Pediatric Cardiology. Philadelphia, Hanley & Belfus, 1992, p 643.
14. Glenn WWL. Circulatory bypass of the right side of the heart. II. Shunt between the superior vena cava and distal right pulmonary artery; report of a clinical application. N Engl J Med 259:117, 1958.
15. Jonas RA, Castaneda AR. Modified Fontan procedure: Atrial baffle and systemic venous to pulmonary artery anastomotic techniques. J Cardiac Surg 3:91, 1988.
16. Harake B, Power GC. Thoracic duct lymph flow: A comparative study in newborn and adult sheep. J Dev Physiol 8:87, 1986.
17. Matitiau A, Geva T, Colan SD, et al. Bulboventricular foramen size in infants with double-inlet left ventricle or tricuspid atresia with transposed great arteries: Influence on initial palliative operation and rate of growth. J Am Coll Cardiol 19:142, 1992.
18. Mayer JE Jr, Bridges ND, Lock JE, et al. Factors associated with improved survival after modified Fontan operations. J Am Coll Cardiol 17:33A, 1991.
19. Mayer JE Jr, Helgason H, Jonas RA, et al. Extending the limits for modified Fontan procedures. J Thorac Cardiovasc Surg 92:1021, 1986.
20. Mietus-Snyder M, Lang P, Mayer JE Jr, et al. Childhood systemic-pulmonary shunts: Subsequent suitability of Fontan operation. Circulation 76(suppl III):III-39, 1987.
21. Rosenthal SM, LaJohn LA. Effect of age on transvascular fluid movement. Am J Physiol 228:134, 1975.
22. Sade RM, Castaneda AR. The dispensable right ventricle. Surgery 77:624, 1975.
23. Scalia D, Russo P, Anderson RH, et al. The surgical anatomy of hearts with no direct communication between the right atrium and the ventricular mass—so-called tricuspid atresia. J Thorac Cardiovasc Surg 87:743, 1984.
24. Sridaromont S, Feldt RH, Ritter DG, et al. Double-outlet right ventricle associated with persistent common atrioventricular canal. Circulation 52:933, 1975.
25. Tandon R, Edwards JE. Tricuspid atresia. Am Heart J 87:511, 1974.

26. Taussig HB. A single ventricle and a rudimentary outlet chamber. In Congenital Malformations of the Heart. New York, Commonwealth Fund, 1947, p 278.
27. Taussig HB. Defective development of the right ventricle and tricuspid atresia. In Congenital Malformations of the Heart. New York, Commonwealth Fund, 1947, p 79.
28. Trusler GA, Mustard WT. A method of banding the pulmonary artery for large isolated ventricular septal defect with and without transposition of the great arteries. Ann Thorac Surg 13:351, 1972.
29. Van Mierop LHS. Morphological development of the heart. In Berne RM (ed). Handbook of Physiology: The Cardiovascular System. Vol 1: The Heart. 2nd ed. Baltimore, Williams & Wilkins, 1979, p 1.
30. Van Praagh R. Segmental approach to diagnosis. In Fyler DC (ed). Nadas' Pediatric Cardiology. Philadelphia, Hanley & Belfus, 1992, p 27.
31. Van Praagh R, Ongley PA, Swan HJC. Anatomic types of single or common ventricle in man. Am J Cardiol 13:367, 1964.
32. Van Praagh R, Van Praagh S. Morphologic anatomy. In Fyler DC (ed). Nadas' Pediatric Cardiology. Philadelphia, Hanley & Belfus, 1992, p 17.
33. Van Praagh R, Weinberg PM, Matsuoka R, et al. Malpositions of the heart. In Adams FH, Emmanouilides GC (eds). Moss' Heart Disease in Infants, Children, and Adolescents. 3rd ed. Baltimore, Williams & Wilkins, 1983, p 422.
34. Van Praagh S, Santini F, Sanders SP. Cardiac malpositions with special emphasis on visceral heterotaxy (asplenia and polysplenia syndromes). In Fyler DC (ed). Nadas' Pediatric Cardiology. Philadelphia, Hanley & Belfus, 1992, p 589.
35. Zamora R, Moller JH, Edwards JE. Double-outlet right ventricle: Anatomic types and associated anomalies. Chest 68:672, 1975.

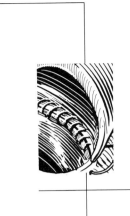

16

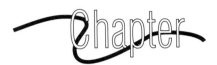

Ebstein's Anomaly

Because Ebstein's anomaly is an exceedingly rare condition, few surgeons have the opportunity to deal with its complete anatomic spectrum. If a child with Ebstein's anomaly is seen by a cardiologist during the first year of life, he or she is usually seen within hours of birth and is both cyanotic and acidotic. Until recently our experience, and the experience of others, with symptomatic neonates who have Ebstein's anomaly had been that both medical and surgical palliation were uniformly unsuccessful.

PATHOLOGIC ANATOMY

Carpentier et al.[2] described five anatomic characteristics that are relevant to the surgical management of this difficult condition (Fig. 16–1):

1. There is displacement of the septal and posterior leaflets of the tricuspid valve toward the apex of the right ventricle.
2. Although the anterior leaflet is attached at the appropriate level of the tricuspid annulus, it is larger than normal and may have multiple chordal attachments to the ventricular wall.
3. The segment of the right ventricle from the level of the true tricuspid annulus to the level of attachment of the septal and posterior leaflets is unusually thin and dysplastic and is described as "atrialized." The tricuspid annulus and the right atrium are extremely dilated.
4. The cavity of the right ventricle beyond the atrialized portion is reduced in size, usually lacks an inlet chamber, and has a small trabecular component.
5. The infundibulum is often obstructed by the redundant

tissue of the anterior leaflet as well as by the chordal attachments of the anterior leaflet to the infundibulum.

Carpentier et al. described four grades of Ebstein's anomaly. In type A, the volume of the true right ventricle is adequate; in type B, there is a large atrialized component of the right ventricle, but the anterior leaflet moves freely; in type C, the anterior leaflet is severely restricted in its movement and may cause significant obstruction of the right ventricular outflow tract; and finally, in type D, there is almost complete atrialization of the ventricle with the exception of a small infundibular component. The only communication between the atrialized ventricle and the infundibulum is through the anteroseptal commissure of the tricuspid valve (Fig. 16–2).

ASSOCIATED ANOMALIES

The most common associated anomaly is an atrial septal defect, which occurs in between 42% and 60% of cases.[16] In neonates at the severe end of the spectrum, survival is dependent on the presence of a patent ductus arteriosus. As already described, a variable degree of obstruction of the right ventricular outflow tract should be considered part of the basic anomaly.

A Wolff-Parkinson-White type of accessory pathway, with associated pre-excitation, is present in ap-

EXTERNAL APPEARANCE

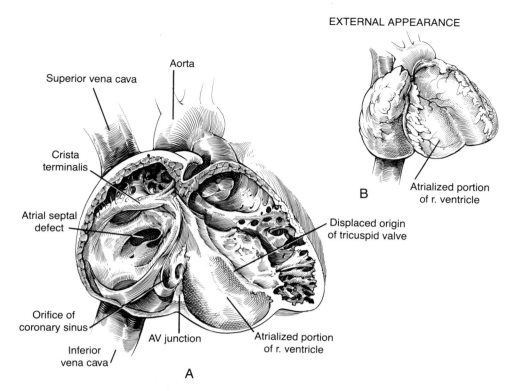

FIGURE 16–1. ☐

Ebstein's anomaly: Anatomic features. *A,* Displacement of the posterior and septal leaflets into the right ventricle results in a large atrialized chamber and tricuspid valve incompetence. *B,* External appearance.

proximately 10% of patients.[16] Other rare associations include ventricular septal defect, transposition of the great arteries, tetralogy of Fallot, and malformation of the mitral valve.[2, 8] An Ebstein-like malformation of the left-sided tricuspid valve is commonly associated with S, L, L (corrected) transposition, ventricular septal defect, and pulmonary stenosis; this is dealt with in Chapter 27.

Associated noncardiac anomalies include low-set ears, micrognathia, cleft lip and palate, absent left kidney, megacolon, undescended testes, and bilateral inguinal hernias.[8]

PATHOPHYSIOLOGY

As might be anticipated from the wide spectrum of anatomic severity, there are a similar wide spectrum of pathophysiology and associated symptoms. One fetal echocardiographic study revealed that this anomaly carries an extremely high rate of death in utero.[6] Neonates who are symptomatic from the time of birth have massive cardiac enlargement with corresponding hypoplasia of both lungs. There is no forward flow from the ineffective right ventricle, so there is physiologic pulmonary atresia, and the child is dependent on ductal patency for survival. All systemic venous return must pass from right to left, across the atrial septum and through the foramen ovale. Because left ventricular output

is also profoundly compromised in the sickest neonates, these children are both severely cyanosed and metabolically acidotic. It is speculated that the capacitance of the enormous right atrium and the to-and-fro flow into the ineffective right ventricle prevent effective filling of the left ventricle. Considering this, it is hardly surprising that simple palliative procedures such as systemic-to-pulmonary artery shunts carry an unacceptable mortality.

Neonates with less severe atrialization of the right ventricle and less pulmonary stenosis may have adequate pulmonary blood flow that will further improve as pulmonary resistance falls.[14] At the mildest end of the anatomic spectrum there may be only a very mild degree of cyanosis, which may not be noted until adult life and may result in few, if any, symptoms. In Watson's review of 505 cases only 35 children were seen in the first year of life.[16] Of these 35, more than half were neonates and were severely symptomatic.

PREOPERATIVE EVALUATION

Diagnosis

Anatomy

The plain chest radiograph of the neonate who is seen in extremis within hours of birth with cyanosis

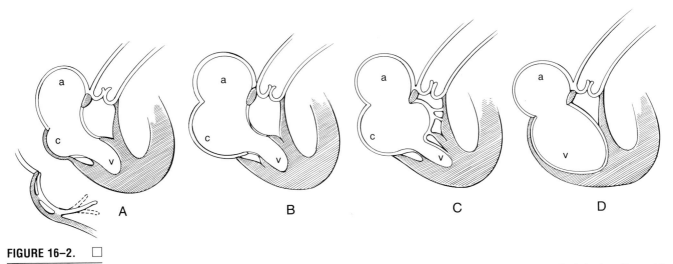

FIGURE 16–2. ☐

Four anatomic types of Ebstein's anomaly. *A,* Small, contractile, atrialized chamber (c) with mobile anterior leaflet. *B,* Large, noncontractile, atrialized chamber with a mobile anterior leaflet. *C,* Restricted motion of the anterior leaflet. *D,* "Tricuspid sac." Leaflet tissue forms a continuous sac adherent to the dilated right ventricle. (a, Atrium; v, ventricle). (Redrawn from Carpentier A, Chauvaud S, Mace L, et al. A new reconstructive operation for Ebstein's anomaly of the tricuspid valve. J Thorac Cardiovasc Surg 96:92, 1988.)

and acidosis is pathognomonic of Ebstein's anomaly. The cardiac silhouette almost completely fills the chest. Echocardiography should confirm the clinical diagnosis. Specific anatomic points of interest include the size of the right atrium and tricuspid annulus, the degree of atrialization of the right ventricle, the fixation of the anterior leaflet of the tricuspid valve, and the severity of pulmonary stenosis. Frequently, there is physiologic pulmonary atresia because of the inability of the right ventricle to generate sufficient pressure to open the pulmonary valve. The anatomy of the pulmonary artery should be examined, although it is unusual for there to be important distortion or hypoplasia of the central pulmonary arteries. It should not be necessary to undertake catheterization for anatomic definition of Ebstein's anomaly.

Hemodynamic Assessment

Before the availability of echocardiography, many reports documented the hazards of cardiac catheterization for children with Ebstein's anomaly.[8, 14, 16] Supraventricular and ventricular arrhythmias were common and often fatal. In the presence of a patent ductus arteriosus, no useful information regarding the function of the right ventricle or the degree of pulmonary stenosis can be derived. Nevertheless, our poor understanding of this anomaly and its continuing high mortality risk suggest the need to collect as much information as possible so that the pathophysiology may be better understood in the future, opening the way to a more rational approach to management.

In a 1971 report from Boston Children's Hospital, Kumar and colleagues[8] described the hemodynamic findings at catheterization in 36 patients, six of whom were less than 1 month old and nine of whom were between 1 and 24 months old. The five lowest saturations (<70%) occurred in infants. Arterial desaturation was correlated with inability to pass the catheter into the pulmonary artery. Right atrial mean pressure ranged from 2 to 11 mm Hg. The a wave ranged from 2 to 18 mm Hg and the v wave from 2 to 14 mm Hg. There was no consistent relation between right atrial pressure and right atrial size. In nine of 11 patients in whom a pullback gradient was obtained between the left and right atrium, the gradient was greater than 2 mm Hg. The highest right ventricular pressure in a patient with uncomplicated Ebstein's anomaly was 35 mm Hg. Right ventricular pressure was near systemic pressure in six patients with associated anomalies.

MEDICAL AND INTERVENTIONAL MANAGEMENT

The neonate who is in extremis within hours of birth requires extremely aggressive resuscitation if there is to be any chance of a successful surgical outcome. Pulmonary blood flow should be maintained by infusion of prostaglandin E_1 (PGE_1). The child should be anesthetized, intubated, and paralyzed. Pulmonary vascular resistance should be minimized by appropriate ventilation. Metabolic acidosis should be treated with bicarbonate infusion, and inotropic support should be given. The diagnosis of Ebstein's anomaly should be strongly suspected on the basis of the plain chest radiograph alone and then should be confirmed urgently by echocardiography. If it appears that the child is not responding to these supportive measures, it would seem reasonable to proceed immediately to the operating room, although because of the great rarity of this condition, there are no data to support such an approach.

Medical management of the older infant with a mild degree of cyanosis should be aimed at symptomatic relief only.

There are no useful interventional techniques in the management of critical Ebstein's anomaly in neonates. Balloon atrial septostomy serves to further increase the right-to-left shunt, which would be inappropriate in a child who is excessively hypoxic. The mechanism of right ventricular outflow tract obstruction suggests that balloon dilatation is unlikely to relieve this problem.

SURGICAL MANAGEMENT

History

Ebstein's anomaly was first described by Wilhelm Ebstein in 1866.[4] The diagnosis was not made during life until 1949, by which time a total of only 26 cases had been described at autopsy.[15] In 1963 surgical management by tricuspid valve replacement was first described by Barnard and Schrire.[1] In the following year Hardy and associates[5] reported successful tricuspid valve reconstruction using techniques previously described by Hunter and Lillehei.[7] The only large experience with the surgical management of Ebstein's anomaly has been described by Danielson and colleagues.[3] Carpentier et al.[2] have contributed new insights into the management of this difficult anomaly.

Indications for Surgery

In older children and adults, surgery has been reserved for those with important symptomatic limitation (New York Heart Association [NYHA] class 3 or 4), progressive cyanosis, and arrhythmias. There are few useful reports to guide the decision regarding the need for and timing of surgery in the infant and neonate. As stated previously, the neonate who fails to respond to aggressive resuscitation with PGE₁, intubation and ventilation, bicarbonate infusion, and inotropic support almost certainly will die without surgical intervention. However, the child who can be stabilized with this management has the possibility of improving over days and weeks as pulmonary resistance falls. Under such circumstances it might be reasonable to withdraw treatment with PGE₁ on a trial basis and observe the effect of ductal closure, particularly if the child appears to have an anatomically milder form of the anomaly (Carpentier grade A or B).[14] In our limited experience with this condition, however, it is only the children with the anatomically unfavorable form who are seen in extremis during the neonatal period.

The gloomy natural history of Ebstein's anomaly during infancy was documented in the 1971 report from Boston Children's Hospital.[8] Among patients with isolated Ebstein's anomaly, there was a 70% rate of survival to 2 years and a 50% rate of survival to 13 years of age. When associated anomalies were present, only 15% of infants survived to 2 years of age. Nevertheless, in general, patients who survive beyond early childhood can expect relatively few limitations. In his review of 505 cases of Ebstein's anomaly, Watson found that 73% of patients between 1 and 15 years of age had minimal disability, as did 69% of those between 16 and 25 years and 59% of those more than 25 years old.[16] Thus, for this anomaly, early diagnosis alone should not be an automatic indication to proceed to surgery, as there is a reasonable probability that the asymptomatic patient will have relatively normal biventricular function for many years.

Technical Considerations

Until recently there were no reports dealing specifically with the surgical management of neonates who have severe cyanosis and acidosis shortly after birth. Our experience has been that palliative procedures, such as closure of an atrial septal defect and Blalock shunt procedures, have been almost uniformly unsuccessful, particularly in the preprostaglandin era. In 1985, a 37-week-old fetus was delivered by cesarean section because of persistent fetal tachycardia following an in utero echocardiographic diagnosis of severe Ebstein's anomaly. The child remained persistently acidotic after birth despite administration of PGE₁, dopamine, and a bicarbonate infusion. The diagnosis of severe Ebstein's anomaly, including anatomic pulmonary atresia, was confirmed by two-dimensional echocardiography and was further verified by cardiac catheterization. It was concluded that the massive atrialization of the right ventricle was preventing effective flow into the left ventricle. Therefore, the child was taken urgently to the operating room, where the following procedure was performed.

The infant was placed on cardiopulmonary bypass

using an ascending aortic cannula and a single venous cannula in the right atrium. The ductus was ligated immediately after beginning bypass. The child was cooled to a rectal temperature of less than 18°C, at which time the ascending aorta was cross-clamped and crystalloid cardioplegic solution infused. Bypass was stopped and the venous cannula was removed. The right atrium was opened with an oblique incision, revealing the massively dilated tricuspid annulus. The foramen ovale was enlarged by excising the septum primum. A polytetrafluoroethylene (PTFE) baffle was sutured into the right atrium to direct blood from the superior vena cava, inferior vena cava, and coronary sinus exclusively to the left ventricle.

A 3-mm central shunt was constructed from the ascending aorta to the main pulmonary artery. Much of the redundant right atrial free wall was excised. Although the child initially did well after weaning from bypass, it became clear that the right ventricle was filling with blood, presumably from the Thebesian veins. This could be controlled by occasional aspiration of blood through an indwelling right ventricular catheter. However, over the first 6 hours in the intensive care unit, the child displayed worsening hemodynamic instability and eventually suffered a fatal cardiac arrest.

Postmortem examination confirmed that there was virtual valvar pulmonary atresia with only a pinhole opening in the valve. In retrospect it may have been sufficient to perform a limited pulmonary valvotomy to allow decompression of the right ventricle by enabling blood from the Thebesian veins to flow to the lungs. A similar concept has since been described and successfully executed by Pitlick and colleagues.[12] In 1988 and 1989, five neonates with a mean Po_2 of 30 mm Hg and a pH of 7.20 ± 0.05 were all found to be PGE_1 dependent. None of the neonates had *anatomic* pulmonary atresia, although all had *physiologic* pulmonary atresia. The mean age at the time of repair was 5 days. The procedure involved pericardial patch closure of the tricuspid valve, placing the coronary sinus on the ventricular side of the patch. The foramen ovale was enlarged, the right atrial free wall was plicated, and a 4-mm central shunt was placed between the ascending aorta and the main pulmonary artery. Interestingly, inotropic support with dopamine and epinephrine was required for right ventricular distention. Minimizing pulmonary vascular resistance with PGE_1 and hyperventilation was also useful in decreasing the tendency for right ventricular distention. There were no perioperative or late deaths over a mean follow-up period of 14 months. All infants were asymptomatic at the time of follow-up, with growth at the 50th percentile for height and the twentieth

percentile for weight. Two children underwent successful Fontan procedures approximately 2 years after their initial palliative procedure, while one child had a Glenn shunt placed.

Of particular interest in the report by Pitlick is the difficulty related to right ventricular distention despite excluding the right atrium from the right ventricle. In previous reports,[3, 5, 7] many authors dealing with an older and more elective population have emphasized the importance of obliterating the paradoxic motion of the atrialized portion of the right ventricle in addition to correcting tricuspid valve regurgitation. In 1958 Hunter and Lillehei[7] described the concept of tricuspid valve reconstruction for Ebstein's anomaly. This was further detailed by Hardy and colleagues,[5] who obliterated the atrialized portion of the right ventricle by transposing the displaced septal leaflet to the normal plane of the tricuspid valve and plicating the tricuspid annulus.

More recently, Danielson and colleagues have had considerable experience with a similar approach to tricuspid valve reconstruction.[3] By plicating the atrialized portion of the right ventricle from the apex toward the base (Fig. 16–3), the displaced leaflets come to lie at a more appropriate level relative to the rest of the tricuspid annulus. The atrial septal defect is closed, and the redundant right atrial wall is plicated. In addition, accessory conduction pathways, causing ventricular pre-excitation, are mapped and divided.[11] Using this approach Danielson reported an operative mortality rate of only 4.9% among 122 patients with Ebstein's anomaly. Sixteen (13%) of the patients underwent division of accessory conduction pathways for Wolff-Parkinson-White syndrome. Seventy-five percent underwent repair by plication and annuloplasty, while the remainder required plication and valve replacement with a bioprosthesis or Fontan reconstruction. There were no cases of complete heart block. It should be noted that there were no neonates in this series; patient age ranged from 11 months to 64 years.

Valve replacement for Ebstein's anomaly carried a high risk of complete heart block in many early series.[9] In their classic paper, Barnard and Schrire[1] described placement of a prosthetic valve on the atrial side of the coronary sinus, leaving the coronary sinus to drain into the ventricle. This technique appears to successfully minimize the risk of complete heart block. In a 1982 report, Westaby and associates described tricuspid valve replacement in 16 patients with Ebstein's anomaly.[17] Only two patients had plication of the atrialized ventricle. There was an early mortality rate of 25%. Complete heart block developed in one patient.

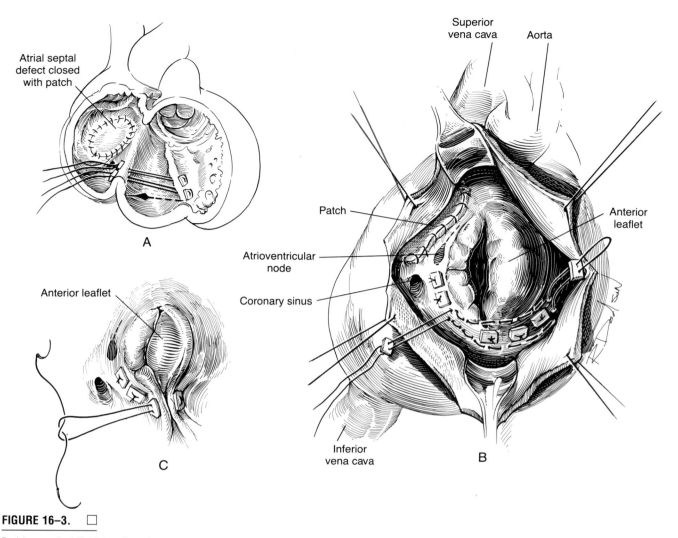

FIGURE 16–3. ☐

Danielson repair of Ebstein's malformation. *A*, Anterior cutaway drawing. The atrial septal defect is closed securely with a patch. Pledgeted sutures are placed so as to position the posterior leaflet at the annulus and imbricate the "atrialized" right ventricular chamber. *B* and *C*, Drawing of the right atrium showing the annuloplasty suture passed through two pledgets. Tying of this suture reduces dilatation of the tricuspid valve so that the large anterior leaflet can meet the two smaller cusps and constitute a functional, essentially monocusp valve.

In 1988 McKay and colleagues[10] described successful replacement of the tricuspid valve with an unstented pulmonary homograft in a 3½-year-old child with Ebstein's anomaly. The technique was essentially the same as that described by Yacoub and Kittle in 1969 for replacement of the mitral valve.[18] The allograft pulmonary valve is mounted within a Dacron tube graft with a generous skirt of pericardium, creating a "top hat" appearance. The coronary sinus is unroofed into the left atrium. The distal end of the homograft and the Dacron tube is anastomosed to the tricuspid annulus except in the region of the conduction bundle, where it is sutured directly to a remnant of septal leaflet tissue. The pericardial collar is sutured into the right atrium, creating a smooth pathway to the valve orifice.

Modifications of annuloplasty and plication pro-

cedures have been described by Carpentier et al.[2] and Quaegebeur and coworkers.[13] Carpentier based these modifications on extensive anatomic studies of Ebstein's anomaly. The major difference relative to the more classic procedure is that plication is performed in a circumferential fashion (Fig. 16–4), thereby preserving the apex-to-base dimension of the right ventricle. The anterior and posterior leaflets are detached and repositioned at the level of the tricuspid annulus. Finally, an annuloplasty ring is inserted to decrease the diameter of the dilated tricuspid annulus, thereby improving leaflet apposition and, therefore, competence of the valve. Carpentier suggested that the ring may be avoided in children. Carpentier[2] reported the results using this approach in 14 patients ranging in age from 9 to 51 years. There were no infants or neonates in the se-

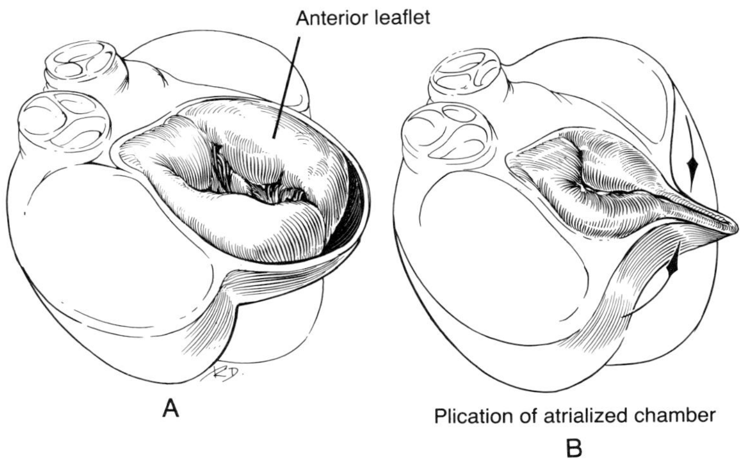

Anterior leaflet

A

Plication of atrialized chamber

B

FIGURE 16–4. □

Carpentier repair of Ebstein's malformation. *A,* Anterior and posterior leaflets of tricuspid valve are detached at annulus. *B,* Atrialized chamber is obliterated in a circumferential direction. The anterior and posterior leaflets are reattached to the new, smaller annulus.

ries. There were two operative deaths (14%), and complete heart block developed in one patient.

In 1991, Quaegebeur and coworkers[13] reported on a series of 10 patients in whom they used a technique similar to that used by Carpentier, except that an annuloplasty ring was not used. Transection and reimplantation of the papillary muscles also were not done. Mobilization of the anterior and posterior leaflets was achieved in all cases by freeing the attachments of these leaflets to the ventricular walls. There were no deaths, and all patients remained in sinus rhythm. Once again there were no infants or neonates in this series, and the mean age was 22 years (range, 4 to 44 years).

The dismal outlook for neonates who are seen in extremis soon after birth raises the issue of cardiac transplantation. However, we believe that few infants will be well served by this approach. For the neonate who cannot be stabilized by medical management, there is unlikely to be sufficient time in which to locate a suitable donor. Children who can be stabilized presumably have adequate left ventricular function. If, in addition, they have adequate right ventricular function, they are candidates for a biventricular repair. If the right ventricle does not function adequately, they require a Fontan operation.

POSTOPERATIVE MANAGEMENT

Points already emphasized that may be important in the management of the critically ill neonate include minimizing pulmonary vascular resistance with appropriate ventilation and sedation and support of the poorly functioning right ventricle with inotropic agents.

Surgical Results

Between 1982 and 1992, 18 children with Ebstein's anomaly have undergone surgery at Children's Hospital in Boston. Seven of the 18 children were less than 1 year old at the time of surgery. Of the four neonates, three died early. One child survived shunt placement alone, although his postoperative course was complicated by multiple supraventricular arrhythmias and prolonged hospitalization. Of the three children between 1 month and 1 year of age, there was one late death after placement of a right Blalock shunt. Of the 11 children who were older than 1 year of age at the time of surgery, there were no early deaths, although one child who underwent heart transplantation at 2 years of age died late after that procedure.

Complications

In the neonatal period, the most common postoperative problem (whether after a simple palliative procedure such as a Blalock shunt or after a more extensive procedure such as attempted exclusion of the right ventricle) has been low cardiac output. This may reflect the capacitance effect of the huge right atrium and the atrialized component of the right ventricle or, perhaps, some ventricular interaction between the left and right ventricle, resulting in poor systemic output. Experience with the hypoplastic left heart syndrome has shown that neonates poorly tolerate an extensive procedure employing hypothermia, cardiopulmonary bypass, and circulatory arrest when they are left with an exclusively shunt-dependent, pulmonary blood supply and a single-ventricle circulation.

Supraventricular arrhythmias have also been problematic in infants and neonates with Ebstein's anomaly. If a proven accessory conduction pathway is present, it may be necessary to ablate the pathway if the arrhythmias per se become life threatening. Complete heart block should be rare using the techniques described to avoid suturing between the coronary sinus and the tricuspid annulus.

There are so few survivors of neonatal and infant surgery for Ebstein's anomaly that there is little useful information regarding late complications. However, based on the natural history of this condition, which is remarkably benign for the majority of older children and adults, the outlook should be excellent for patients who have survived closure of an atrial septal defect with a plication and annuloplasty procedure.

SUMMARY

Ebstein's anomaly presents one of the widest anatomic, physiologic, and symptomatic spectra of all congenital heart anomalies. The dismal outlook for the fetus diagnosed to be in distress because of a severe malformation of this type during in utero development suggests that this is an area in which fetal surgery may play an important role in the future, especially in terms of right atrial plication to reduce heart size and allow adequate pulmonary parenchymal development before birth. The enlarging database of fetal echocardiography may allow a better understanding of the natural intrauterine history of this lesion, enabling early intrauterine identification of the infants at highest risk. Intrauterine listing for transplantation late in gestation may allow for controlled delivery by cesarean section as a donor heart becomes available in this small subset of critically affected infants. Whether surgical techniques described to date can be successfully applied to the neonate who cannot be stabilized with prostaglandin E_1 remains to be demonstrated. Surgery for the neonate who is ductal dependent but stable has been reported.[12] Refinement of valvuloplasty and plication techniques has opened the way to a satisfactory long-term outlook for the majority of adults and older children, who generally are only mildly symptomatic.

REFERENCES

1. Barnard CN, Schrire V. Surgical correction of Ebstein's malformation with prosthetic tricuspid valve. Surgery 54:302, 1963.
2. Carpentier A, Chauvaud S, Mace L, et al. A new reconstructive operation for Ebstein's anomaly of the tricuspid valve. J Thorac Cardiovasc Surg 96:92, 1988.
3. Danielson GK, Driscoll DJ, Mair DD, et al. Operative treatment of Ebstein's anomaly. J Thorac Cardiovasc Surg 104:1195–1202, 1992.
4. Ebstein W. Uber einen sehr seltenen Fall von Insufficienz der Valvula tricuspidalis, bedingt durch eine angeborene hochgradige Missbildung deselben. Arch Anat Physiol 33:238, 1866.
5. Hardy KL, May IA, Webster CA, et al. Ebstein's anomaly: A functional concept and successful definitive repair. J Thorac Cardiovasc Surg 48:927, 1964.
6. Hornberger LK, Sahn DJ, Kleinman CS, et al. Tricuspid valve disease with significant tricuspid insufficiency in the fetus: Diagnosis and outcome. J Am Coll Cardiol 17:167, 1991.
7. Hunter SW, Lillehei CW. Ebstein's malformation of the tricuspid valve with suggestions of a new form of surgical therapy. Dis Chest 33:297, 1958.
8. Kumar AE, Fyler DC, Miettinen OS, et al. Ebstein's anomaly. Am J Cardiol 28:84, 1971.
9. Lillehei CW, Kalke BR, Carlson RG. Evolution of corrective surgery for Ebstein's anomaly. Circulation 35(suppl I):111, 1967.
10. McKay R, Sono J, Arnold RM. Tricuspid valve replacement using an unstented pulmonary homograft. Ann Thorac Surg 46:58, 1988.
11. Oh JK, Holmes DR, Hayes DL, et al. Cardiac arrhythmias in patients with surgical repair of Ebstein's anomaly. J Am Coll Cardiol 6:1351, 1985.
12. Pitlick PT, Griffin ML, Bernstein D, et al. Followup on a new surgical procedure for Ebstein's anomaly in the critically ill neonate. Circulation 83(suppl III):716, 1990.
13. Quaegebeur JM, Sreeram N, Fraser AG, et al. Surgery for Ebstein's anomaly: The clinical and echocardiographic evaluation of a new technique. J Am Coll Cardiol 17:722, 1991.
14. Radford DJ, Graff RF, Neilson GH. Diagnosis and natural history of Ebstein's anomaly. Br Heart J 54:517, 1985.
15. Tourniaire A, Deyrieux F, Tartulier M. Maladie d'Ebstein: Essai de diagnostic clinique. Arch Mal Coeur 42:1211, 1959.
16. Watson H. Natural history of Ebstein's anomaly of tricuspid valve in childhood and adolescence. Br Heart J 36:417, 1974.
17. Westaby S, Karp RB, Kirklin JW, et al. Surgical treatment in Ebstein's malformation. Ann Thorac Surg 34:388, 1982.
18. Yacoub MH, Kittle CF. A new technique for replacement of the mitral valve by a semilunar valve homograft. J Thorac Cardiovasc Surg 58:859, 1969.

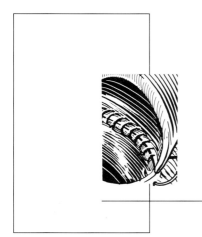

17

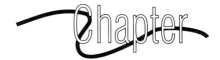

Truncus Arteriosus

Truncus arteriosus is a rare congenital heart defect in which a single great vessel arises from the heart, giving off the coronary arteries, true pulmonary arteries, and the ascending aorta. In virtually every case there is a ventricular septal defect and a single large semilunar valve. It should be noted, however, that in extremely rare cases there may be no ventricular septal defect, or there may even be remnants of two semilunar valves.[20] In the great majority of cases the pulmonary arteries arise from the truncal vessel above the coronary arteries but below the brachiocephalic vessels. Within these limits, however, the specific morphology of the pulmonary artery origins can vary, a fact that has stimulated various classifications of truncus arteriosus.

The two major classification systems are those of Collett and Edwards,[7] described in 1949 (Table 17–1), and Van Praagh and Van Praagh,[21] described in 1965 (Table 17–2). Each of these systems has contributed valuable information and provided insight into the nature of this lesion.

In this chapter a classification system will not be used; instead, morphologic details will be described to supply the necessary information. In the great majority of cases, one of two forms exists. Either the common trunk divides into the ascending aorta and a short main pulmonary artery segment, which then divides into the pulmonary artery branches, or, more commonly, the common trunk divides into the ascending aorta and the pulmonary artery branches, which arise adjacent to each other with-

out a well-defined main pulmonary artery segment (Collett and Edwards types I and II). These two morphologic subsets often merge, as the tissue contours may make it difficult to precisely identify a true main pulmonary artery segment. When the morphology varies from this general configuration, appropriate details will be given. At the present time, cases in which the lungs are supplied by large arteries arising from the descending aorta are not considered to be truncus arteriosus (Collett and Edwards type IV); at least one central pulmonary artery branch must arise directly from the trunk for the lesion to be considered truncus arteriosus (Van Praagh type A3).

TABLE 17–1. ☐ COLLETT AND EDWARDS CLASSIFICATION OF TRUNCUS ARTERIOSUS[7]

Type I	The common trunk gives rise to a main pulmonary artery, which then bifurcates into branch pulmonary arteries.
Type II	The branch pulmonary arteries arise directly and contiguously from the common trunk without a main pulmonary artery segment.
Type III	The branch pulmonary arteries arise from widely separated orifices on the common trunk.
Type IV	Pulmonary artery origin from a "common trunk" is absent, with pulmonary blood supply derived from the descending aorta. Currently this is not considered truncus arteriosus, but a form of tetralogy of Fallot with pulmonary atresia and nonconfluent central pulmonary arteries.

TABLE 17–2. ☐ VAN PRAAGH CLASSIFICATION OF TRUNCUS ARTERIOSUS[21]

Type A: VSD present
Type B: VSD absent

1. Partially formed aorticopulmonary septum (main pulmonary artery segment present)
2. Absent aorticopulmonary septum (no main pulmonary artery segment)
3. Absence of one branch of the pulmonary artery from the trunk
4. Underdeveloped aortic arch (hypoplastic or interrupted) with a large patent ductus arteriosus

VSD, Ventricular septal defect.
Subtypes 1–4 can occur with type A or B.

ANATOMY

Developmental Considerations

Embryologic deficiency of the aorticopulmonary septum combined with virtual absence of the subpulmonary infundibulum and partial or complete absence of pulmonary valve tissue results in truncus arteriosus. A number of lines of evidence implicate deficiencies in cardiovascular tissue derived from the neural crest as important in this process. The Van Praaghs' scholarly analysis of truncus arteriosus provides a more detailed description of the embryology of this lesion.[21] The degree of deficiency of the aorticopulmonary septum determines the variability of the origin of the pulmonary arteries. Development of the primitive arterial arches 4 and 6 varies inversely in this lesion. As a result the ductus is usually absent or extremely small when the aortic arch develops normally in truncus arteriosus, whereas a large ductus arteriosus is present when there is serious hypoplasia or interruption of the arch.

Morphologic Features

Truncus arteriosus is found almost exclusively with situs solitus and d-looped segmental anatomy. The atria are usually normal, and a patent foramen ovale or small secundum atrial septal defect occurs frequently enough to be considered almost a normal part of the lesion. The atrioventricular canal and inlets and bodies of both ventricles are usually normal, as is the left ventricular outflow tract.

In the great majority of cases the right ventricular infundibulum is deficient in the same manner as, but to a greater degree than, in tetralogy of Fallot, resulting in the typical ventricular septal defect. This defect is usually large and lies between the two limbs of the trabecula septomarginalis. These limbs form the anterior and inferior margins of the defect. In normal hearts the infundibular septum joins the muscular interventricular septum at this level, closing any potential interventricular communication. The absence of the infundibular septum in truncus arteriosus, then, results in this septal defect. The posterior margin of the septal defect is formed by the ventriculoinfundibular fold, the muscle mass that separates the truncal valve from the tricuspid valve. The ventriculoinfundibular fold merges with the posterior limb of the trabecula septomarginalis. In about two thirds of the cases of truncus arteriosus, this muscle is so well developed that the inferoposterior and posterior rims of the septal defect are completely made up of muscle. Therefore, the defect is relatively remote from the annulus of the tricuspid valve and from the proximal conduction system. In the other third the ventriculoinfundibular fold and its muscular connection to the posterior limb of the trabecula septomarginalis are deficient. If the deficiency is complete, the septal defect extends to the tricuspid annulus, and the proximal conduction tissue is vulnerable. The superior margin of the septal defect is invariably made up by the truncal valve itself, a result of the virtually absent infundibulum and infundibular septum. This essentially makes the septal defect "subarterial." Therefore, except for its superior margin, the septal defect is similar to that seen in tetralogy of Fallot.

The annulus of the truncal valve usually straddles the defect in a "balanced" fashion; however, it is not unusual for it to be positioned significantly further over the right ventricle, increasing the potential for restriction of the left ventricular outflow tract after repair.[5] The annulus is larger than a normal semilunar valve and is located in the normal aortic position with truncal-mitral fibrous continuity. In the great majority of cases the valve has two, three, or four leaflets; however, more than four leaflets occur rarely.[5] When four or more leaflets occur, the extra leaflet tissue represents incorporation of abnormal pulmonary leaflet tissue into the aortic valve. This is made possible by the absence of the aorticopulmonary septum at the level of the semilunar valve. Regardless of their number, the leaflets are often dysmorphic.

The coronary arteries may be normal; however, coronary anomalies are not unusual, occurring in about 50% of cases.[8] Many of these are relatively minor, although two variations are of practical importance. The left coronary ostium may arise high in the sinus of Valsalva or even from the truncal tissue at the margin of the pulmonary artery tissue. This coronary can be injured during repair when the pulmonary arteries are removed from the trunk or when the resulting truncal defect is closed. The right coronary artery can give rise to an important accessory (or sometimes to the sole) anterior descending coronary artery. This artery often passes across the right ventricle where the right ventriculotomy is most commonly performed during repair.

In the vast majority of cases the large truncal root gives rise to the ascending aorta and the origin of the pulmonary arteries. It is misleading to describe the pulmonary arteries as "arising from" the trunk; instead, the trunk bifurcates. At the bifurcation, the two pulmonary artery branches soon bifurcate as well, thus making it a somewhat subjective exercise to attempt to identify a true main pulmonary artery segment. Schematic diagrams comparing the Van Praagh types A1 and A2 or the Collett and Edwards types I and II are often somewhat idealized, making the distinction appear more clear than it really is.

The aortic-pulmonary bifurcation usually occurs with the pulmonary arteries forming to the left and posterior. The pulmonary artery branches are usually of normal caliber; however, stenosis of the orifices and diffuse hypoplasia can occur occasionally. Rarely one of the pulmonary arteries is absent and the affected lung is supplied by aortopulmonary collaterals or by a ductus arteriosus (Van Praagh classification type A3).

Generally the ascending aorta and arch are normal; however, frequent variations occur.[5] Most of these, such as the right aortic arch (occurring in 30% of patients) and the aberrant subclavian artery (5% to 10%) are of no practical consequence. Usually the ductus arteriosus is either totally absent or extremely small. One arch abnormality of considerable importance consists of a large ductus arteriosus associated with severe hypoplasia or interruption of the distal aortic arch. This occurs in about 10% to 15% of cases. In these cases origin of the pulmonary arteries from the trunk is usually more abnormal. The trunk appears to arise from the heart and continue on as a dominant main pulmonary artery segment that continues as the large ductus arteriosus to the descending aorta. The left and right pulmonary artery branches can arise from various sites on this large main pulmonary artery, resulting in a main pulmonary artery segment that can be very long or very short. The hypoplastic ascending aorta arises from the anterior right aspect of the trunk, appearing almost as a proximal branch off the dominant main pulmonary artery. Although these relationships appear unusual because of the discrepancy in size of the ascending aorta and main pulmonary artery, the morphology of the truncal and pulmonary artery bifurcations is really quite similar to that in simple truncus (Collett and Edwards types I and II; Van Praagh types A1 and A2).

In our series of 122 cases of truncus arteriosus accumulated since the 1970s, a number of other associated anomalies, determined by echocardiogra-

phy, catheterization or direct surgical inspection, have been identified. These are shown in Table 17–3.

PATHOPHYSIOLOGY AND NATURAL HISTORY

There are two important pathophysiologic consequences resulting from the morphology of truncus arteriosus. One is complete mixing of saturated and unsaturated blood at the levels of the ventricular septal defect and the single semilunar valve. This results in moderate cyanosis. The presence of marked cyanosis (<80% oxygen saturation in arterial blood) in an otherwise morphologically straightforward truncus should alert the physician to the possibility of pulmonary vascular obstructive disease. The other consequence is the presence of a nonrestrictive left-to-right shunt at the level of the great vessels. The position of the shunt above the semilunar valve results in a shunt that is pressure driven both in systole and diastole. This may be responsible in part for the early occurrence of pulmonary vascular obstructive disease in this lesion. The influence of cyanosis on the rate of development of pulmonary vascular obstructive disease is not well understood.

Other secondary pathophysiologic findings may accompany these two primary ones. Truncal valve stenosis or regurgitation, the presence of interrupted aortic arch, and stenosis of the pulmonary artery branches have the most important impact on the natural history. An interrupted aortic arch or significant stenosis or regurgitation of the truncal

TABLE 17–3. □ LESIONS ASSOCIATED WITH TRUNCUS ARTERIOSUS (*N* = 122)

LESION	NO. OF CASES	% OF TOTAL
Patent foramen ovale/secundum atrial septal defect	57	47
Mild tricuspid regurgitation/stenosis	56	46
Right aortic arch	27	22
Interrupted aortic arch and patent ductus arteriosus	13	11
Moderate/severe tricuspid regurgitation/stenosis	13	11
Peripheral pulmonary stenosis	7	6
Partial anomalous pulmonary venous connection	7	6
Anomalous coronary	7	6
Aberrant subclavian artery	5	4
Left superior vena cava	5	4
Multiple ventricular septal defects	4	3
Double-chambered right ventricle	3	2
Patent ductus arteriosus	3	2
Double-outlet mitral valve	2	2
Absent left pulmonary artery	2	2
Hypoplastic left pulmonary artery	2	2
Bicuspid tricuspid valve	2	2

One each: cervical arch, hypoplastic right ventricle, cleft mitral valve, hypoplastic left lung, total anomalous pulmonary venous connection, sinus venosus atrial septal defect, primum atrial septal defect valve leads to severe heart failure and cardiovascular instability early in life. Patients with these associated lesions rarely survive the neonatal period when untreated. Stenosis of the pulmonary artery branches, however, limits the left-to-right shunt, causing the early natural history to become more favorable.

Truncus arteriosus makes up only 2.8% of the cardiac anomalies in the cardiac registry at Children's Hospital in Boston.[6] The natural history of truncus arteriosus is one of relatively normal intrauterine physiology and overall fetal development. The alterations in fetal cardiovascular physiology are minor. Because of mixing at the ventricular and truncal levels, the coronary and cerebral vascular beds in fetuses with truncus arteriosus may not receive blood that is as highly oxygenated as that in the normal fetus. However, after birth the benign nature of truncus arteriosus changes dramatically. The drop in pulmonary vascular resistance induces a large, arterial-level, left-to-right shunt. Congestive heart failure or its sequelae resulting from this shunt are responsible for the extremely high mortality rate in these infants. A number of natural history studies suggest that 50% of patients die by 1 month of age, with the 1-year survival rate ranging from 10% to 25%. The vast majority of surviving patients are doomed to have severe pulmonary vascular obstructive disease, often by 6 months of age.

DIAGNOSIS AND INDICATIONS FOR SURGERY

The patient with truncus arteriosus has signs and symptoms of congestive heart failure and mild-to-moderate cyanosis. A wide pulse pressure may be present. The chest radiograph shows cardiomegaly and pulmonary overcirculation but is nonspecific; however, absence of the pulmonary knob may suggest truncus arteriosus. Electrocardiographic findings are also nonspecific.[6]

Echocardiography is usually diagnostic. The origin and configuration of the pulmonary arteries, the ventricular septal defect, the aortic arch and ductus arteriosus, the status of the truncal valve, and the position of the coronary arteries all can be defined reliably.

Cardiac catheterization may be performed to confirm anatomic details and provide physiologic data indicating the status of the pulmonary vasculature. However, at the present time, if echocardiography reveals straightforward anatomy and the patient is seen in the neonatal period, our practice at Children's Hospital in Boston is to undertake surgery without cardiac catheterization. Infants who are older than 3 months when first evaluated undergo

cardiac catheterization to define the status of the pulmonary vasculature. In neonates, catheterization is performed if echocardiography suggests abnormalities of the truncal valve, coronary anatomy, or associated lesions that need further characterization.

In the neonate, the differential diagnosis of truncus arteriosus includes aortopulmonary window and tetralogy of Fallot with pulmonary atresia; echocardiography can usually differentiate between these lesions.[6] The presence of truncus arteriosus is an absolute indication for surgery. Repair should be undertaken in the neonatal period or as soon as the diagnosis is established. Eisenmenger's physiology is the only absolute contraindication to correction.

SURGICAL MANAGEMENT

Historical Perspective

Truncus arteriosus was first managed with pulmonary artery banding as described by Armer and coworkers in 1961[1] and Smith and associates in 1964.[19] Experience with this technique resulted in only a modest improvement in the 1-year survival rate when compared with that of untreated patients. The first documented repair of truncus arteriosus was performed in 1962, as reported by Behrendt and colleagues in 1974.[3] This involved a valveless conduit from the right ventricle to the pulmonary artery and closure of the ventricular septal defect. In 1967, McGoon first used a valved allograft conduit to repair truncus arteriosus, basing the operation on the experimental work of Rastelli.[13] In the 1960s and 1970s, results of repair early in infancy were poor, with the mortality rate well over 50%. During this time valved allografts fell out of favor, a development that increased the technical risks of the repair, especially in small infants. However, results of repair in older infants, who were managed medically for the first 6 months of life before referral for surgical correction, were equally poor because of the morbidity that the prolonged arterial level shunt induced in the pulmonary vasculature. In 1984 Ebert and associates reported on a series of 100 infants repaired mainly before the age of 6 months; the mortality rate was 11%, emphasizing that repair early in infancy was critical in avoiding the development of pulmonary vascular obstructive disease.[9] This study also demonstrated that excellent results were achievable in infants when Dacron conduits containing porcine valves are used for the right ventricle–to–pulmonary artery reconstruction.

Over the past several years a number of groups,

including our own, have tended toward elective neonatal repair, with encouraging results,[4] while other groups have not had similar success.[15, 18] The renewed interest in valved allografts that occurred in the 1980s has allowed primary repair even in the youngest and smallest infants. At Children's Hospital in Boston we have successfully performed complete repair in one infant weighing less than 1.5 kg using a 7-mm aortic allograft.

Surgical Technique

Repair of Simple Truncus Arteriosus

After standard exposure of the heart through a median sternotomy incision, cardiopulmonary bypass is conducted in routine fashion, using either deep hypothermic circulatory arrest or low-flow continuous bypass (Fig. 17–1). The ascending aorta is cannulated well above the bifurcation of the truncus, and the venous system is cannulated through the right atrial appendage. A patch of autologous pericardium is harvested and fixed in glutaraldehyde. At the initiation of cardiopulmonary bypass, the pulmonary artery branches are snared and occluded. During the initial cooling phase of bypass, the coronary arteries are identified, and the bifurcation of the truncal root is carefully examined. After aortic crossclamping and administration of cardioplegic solution through the truncal root, the pulmonary artery snares are removed.

Under circulatory arrest, or alternatively at a reduced bypass flow rate of 50 ml/kg/min, the pulmonary arteries are carefully removed from the truncal root "in continuity," such that adequate tissue surrounding the orifices of the pulmonary artery branches is present for the distal conduit anastomosis. If there is a main pulmonary artery segment before the bifurcation of the pulmonary artery branches, this is easily performed. If there is little or no main pulmonary artery tissue, with both pulmonary artery branches forming just as they leave the trunk, it is necessary to remove some of the truncal tissue surrounding these branches to achieve this. (Alternatively, the truncal root may be transected just proximal and distal to the pulmonary artery origins to facilitate excision of the pulmonary artery, as well as to provide adequate tissue for the subsequent distal allograft–to–pulmonary artery anastomosis.)

The defect in the truncal root is then closed. This can usually be accomplished by primary closure. Most often the closure is oriented transversely to avoid narrowing the truncal root. An obliquely, or even longitudinally, oriented closure may be best,

however, depending on the shape and size of the defect created. In cases in which truncal tissue is taken with the orifices of the pulmonary artery branches, it may be necessary to close the truncal defect with a patch of glutaraldehyde-treated pericardium. In the case of truncal transection, a primary end-to-end anastomosis of the truncal root to the ascending aorta is performed. Closure is performed with a running polypropylene suture. Careful attention to the truncal valve and the coronary ostia is critical to this phase of the operation.

A longitudinal incision is then made in the right ventricle, beginning just below the truncal valve annulus. This exposes the ventricular septal defect. The incision is taken proximally onto the right ventricular free wall just far enough to adequately expose the septal defect and create a right ventricular opening of appropriate size for the conduit. If an anterior descending coronary artery or other large coronary branch crosses this area, the incision must be modified to preserve this vessel. The ventricular septal defect is inspected through the right ventriculotomy and all of its borders clearly defined. In the usual case, the posterior and inferior rims of the defect are muscular, and sutures in the base of the septal leaflet of the tricuspid valve can be avoided. When the ventricular septal defect extends to the tricuspid valve annulus, the posterior and inferior aspects of the patch are placed as described in Chapter 13 for tetralogy of Fallot. Because the infundibular septum is absent, the superior aspect of the defect is closed by applying the patch to the cut edge of the right ventriculotomy just below the truncal valve. The suture technique for closure of ventricular septal defects is described in Chapter 11.

The atrial septum is then inspected, looking either retrograde through the tricuspid valve or through a small right atriotomy. If a patent foramen ovale is present, it is left alone. If a large secundum atrial septal defect is present, it is partially closed by overlapping the septum primum to the left side of the limbus, thus creating a small defect (2 to 3 mm) in the form of a patent foramen ovale. After closure of the right atriotomy, the patient can be placed back on cardiopulmonary bypass and core rewarming begun.

A valved allograft is then used to construct a right ventricular outflow tract. The distal end-to-end anastomosis between the allograft and pulmonary artery "stoma" is performed first, using running 6–0 polypropylene suture. The proximal end of the allograft is then sutured to the edge of the right ventriculotomy, often incorporating ventricular muscle and the superior rim of the patch on the ventricular septal defect. About 30% to 40% of the circumference of the graft is sutured in this way. A

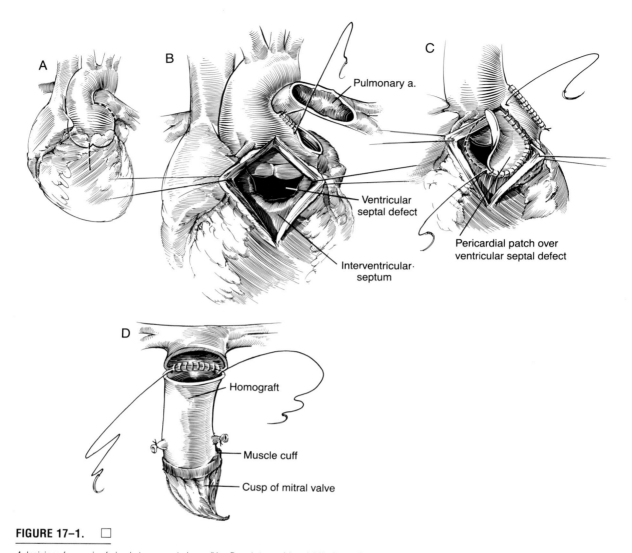

FIGURE 17–1. ☐

A, Incisions for repair of simple truncus arteriosus (Van Praagh types A1 and A2). *B* and *C*, Ventricular septal defect (VSD) closure. Note that the suture line makes a transition from the edge of the VSD to the cut edge of the infundibular free wall incision. *D* and *E*, Reconstruction of the right ventricular outflow tract using an allograft.

pericardial hood is then used to complete the reconstruction of the right ventricular outflow tract; the hood is attached to the remaining circumference of the allograft and to the remainder of the ventriculotomy incision.

An important point in the reconstruction is to leave the potential for interatrial shunting. This allows continued normal left-sided cardiac output during the phase of right ventricular dysfunction in the early postoperative period. Infants may have a significant right-to-left shunt at the atrial level, with systemic arterial Po_2 levels often below 40 mm Hg and occasionally as low as 30 mm Hg on the first postoperative day. This gradually improves during the first 24 to 48 hours after surgery. We believe that this maneuver is extremely important. The low systemic arterial Po_2 level is well tolerated, and the usual pathophysiologic consequences of right ventricular failure (i.e., ascites, pleural effusions, and low cardiac output) are avoided, or at least minimized.

Another important point in the neonatal truncus repair is to provide a right ventricle–to–pulmonary artery conduit with a competent valve. There are reports of successful neonatal truncus repair using nonvalved conduits;[16] however, in our opinion this approach, although successful in some cases, is likely to complicate early postoperative recovery. The obligatory pulmonary regurgitation in the setting of elevated neonatal pulmonary vascular resistance will compromise the outcome. There are reports of repair of truncus arteriosus using autologous tissue for part of the right ventricular outflow tract reconstruction. This is also likely to

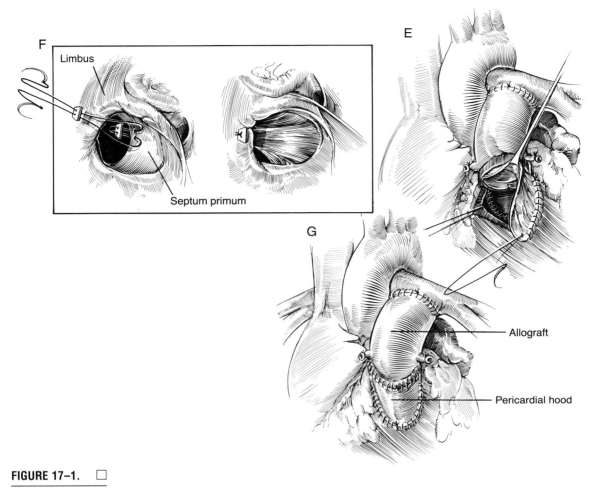

FIGURE 17–1. □

Continued. F, Partial closure of a patent foramen ovale or ostium secundum atrial septal defect (ASD). *G,* Completed repair of simple truncus arteriosus.

result in varying degrees of pulmonary regurgitation.[2] The theoretical advantage of such a technique is that reoperation for revision of the right ventricle–to–pulmonary artery conduit may be avoided. This approach may be tolerated in selected slightly older infants (2 to 6 months old) when pulmonary vascular resistance has reached a nadir. However, in the newborn the fetal pulmonary vascular musculature has not completely involuted; therefore, baseline pulmonary vascular resistance may be higher, and free pulmonary regurgitation will be less well tolerated.

Associated lesions may need to be addressed at the time of the initial repair. If stenosis of the pulmonary artery branches is present, the stenotic section is opened longitudinally before creating the anastomosis between the distal end of the allograft and the pulmonary artery. The distal end of the allograft is tailored with an extension that will augment the pulmonary artery orifice.

Repair of Truncus Arteriosus With Truncal Valve Replacement

If truncal stenosis is present, the judgment regarding whether or not to address this problem surgically may be quite difficult. Because of the massive flow across the truncal valve preoperatively, gradients usually overestimate the true degree of stenosis. Severe truncal stenosis postoperatively, after removal of the volume load, is unusual, and therefore, inspection at the time of surgery becomes critical. The size of the orifice and the mobility of the leaflets are given careful consideration. Mild or moderate stenosis is acceptable, but severe stenosis may require commissurotomy. This should not be undertaken lightly, as this procedure has the potential to result in significant truncal regurgitation. In borderline cases, an attempt can be made to wean the patient from cardiopulmonary bypass. Subsequent commissurotomy or valve replacement should be performed only if the hemodynamics are not acceptable. In our experience, truncal stenosis has not been a risk factor for death.[12]

Truncal regurgitation presents a more important problem. It is much more common than truncal stenosis and, when significant, complicates the hemodynamics of cardiopulmonary bypass. In contrast to stenosis, the degree of truncal regurgitation can be underestimated preoperatively because the pulmonary runoff produces a marked reduction in diastolic aortic pressure. Mild or moderate truncal regurgitation is acceptable; only severe regurgitation is surgically addressed. In our experience, severe truncal regurgitation is a risk factor for death.[12]

At the time of surgery the valve is carefully inspected through the defect in the truncal root that was created after removing the pulmonary arteries (Fig. 17–2). Occasionally the truncal regurgitation can be improved by the method used for reconstruction of this truncal root defect. Closure of the defect in a longitudinal manner can narrow the circumference of the trunk at the level of the tops of the commissures, allowing improved coarctation of the leaflets (essentially performing an annuloplasty). Valvuloplasty, using pledgetted sutures to resuspend commissures, may also be beneficial in selected cases. Conversely, insufficient care in the closure of the truncal root defect can exacerbate truncal valve regurgitation.

In more complex cases of insufficiency, truncal valve replacement is necessary. In neonates, this is best performed using a valved aortic allograft conduit.[10] The technique proceeds by transecting the ascending aorta just above the level of the origin of the pulmonary artery from the trunk. The truncal valve leaflets are excised, and the coronary artery ostia are mobilized in a manner similar to that used in the arterial switch operation. The standard right ventriculotomy incision for truncus is made; however, the incision is advanced through the truncal valve annulus. The aortic allograft tube is then attached proximally at the truncal annular level, using the anterior mitral leaflet of the graft to close the ventricular septal defect. The coronary ostial pods are attached to the side of the allograft, again as in the arterial switch operation. Finally, the distal aspect of the allograft tube is attached end to end to the ascending aorta. The right ventricular outflow tract is then reconstructed in standard fashion.

A particularly vexing problem with truncal regurgitation occurs during the conduction of cardiopulmonary bypass. Once the myocardium ceases to contract effectively during initial cooling, truncal regurgitation on bypass must be managed by venting the heart. The same situation may occur during rewarming from deep hypothermia. Although suc-

cessful venting of the heart may be achieved when severe truncal regurgitation is present, most of the pump flow is "short circuited" through the valve to the vent, resulting in inadequate systemic perfusion. In this case it may be necessary to manually compress the ventricle during the cooling phase to maintain adequate systemic perfusion. Alternatively, it may be necessary to clamp the truncal root at the start of bypass and provide cardioplegic solution directly to the coronary arteries. This latter technique can be technically difficult in very small infants and also may result in a prolonged period of myocardial ischemia, initially with relatively warm temperatures. Another option is early crossclamping with retrograde coronary sinus cardioplegia, which requires bicaval cannulation for venous return.

Repair of Truncus Arteriosus With Interrupted Aortic Arch

In the case of interrupted aortic arch associated with truncus arteriosus, cannulation and repair of the interrupted arch proceed differently than for isolated interrupted aortic arch (Fig. 17–3). The large main pulmonary artery component of the trunk or the distal ascending aorta may be used for arterial cannulation. Double arterial cannulation is unnecessary, as perfusion via the ductus and ascending aorta is achieved with one cannula. The pulmonary artery branches are snared as bypass is begun. When deep hypothermic circulatory temperatures are reached, the vessels to the head are occluded, circulatory arrest is achieved, the ductus arteriosus is ligated and divided, and the large main pulmonary artery component of the truncal root is transected just above the truncal valve. This provides a large main pulmonary artery with a single lumen for acceptance of the distal allograft anastomosis during the right ventricular outflow tract reconstruction performed later in the operation. Ductal tissue is then trimmed from the descending aorta, and continuity between the normal-size descending aorta and the small ascending aorta is established. This can be achieved in several ways. If adequate mobilization can be accomplished, and the gap that composes the interrupted segment is not great, direct anastomosis of the descending aorta to the distal end of the ascending aorta is performed. Alternatively, the left subclavian artery may be sacrificed as peripherally as possible and the central remnant turned proximally to the ascending aorta to bridge the interruption, as in the Blalock-Park procedure. Once ascending-to-descending aortic continuity is achieved, the entire hypoplastic aorta from the level of the truncal valve to the ductal

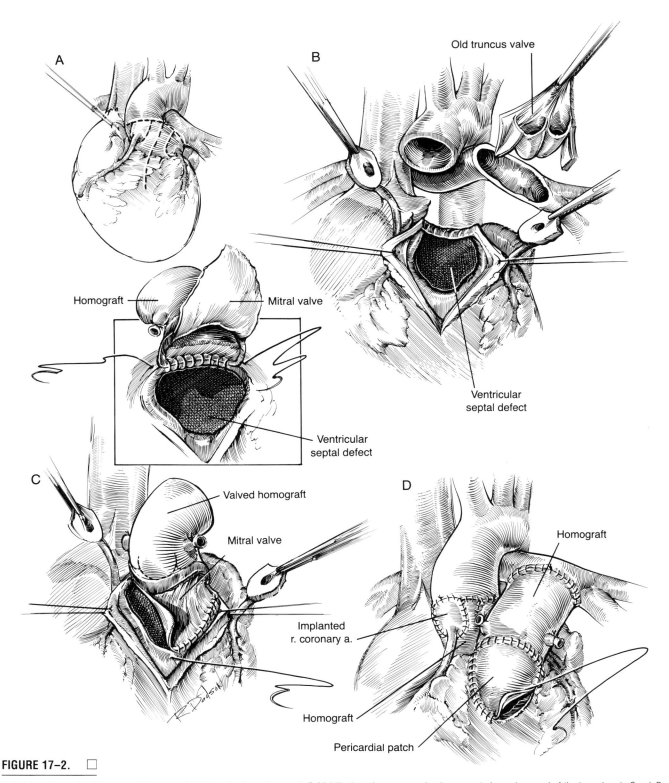

FIGURE 17–2. ☐

A, Incisions for repair of truncus arteriosus requiring truncal valve replacement. *B,* Mobilization of coronary and pulmonary arteries and removal of the truncal root. *C* and *D,* Allograft replacement of the aortic root with coronary implantation, VSD closure, and standard reconstruction of the right ventricular outflow tract using a valved allograft.

insertion is "filleted" open. With the large proximal truncal stoma left by transection of the main pulmonary artery, this leaves a large semilunar valve, small ascending aorta, and transverse "arch" analo-

gous to that in the hypoplastic left heart syndrome (see Chapter 23). An allograft or pericardial gusset is then used to augment the aorta from the level of the truncal valve to the descending thoracic aorta,

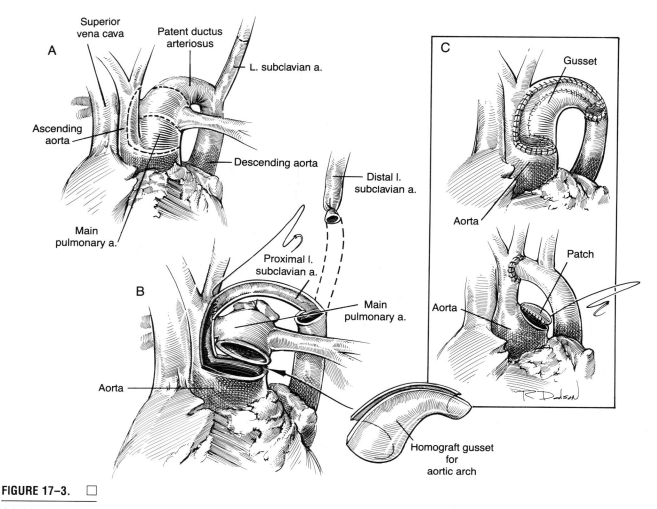

FIGURE 17–3. ☐

A, Incisions for repair of truncus arteriosus with an associated interrupted aortic arch. *B,* Reconstruction of an interrupted aortic arch with allograft gusset; repair of the VSD and the right ventricular outflow tract are as in Figure 17–1. *C,* Alternative repair of an interrupted aortic arch using an end-to-side primary aortic anastomosis.

exactly as is done in repair of hypoplastic left heart syndrome. Closure of the ventricular septal defect and reconstruction of the right ventricular outflow tract then proceed as in simple truncus arteriosus. This technique provides abundant tissue for a straightforward end-to-end anastomosis between the distal end of the conduit and the pulmonary artery without having to manipulate the orifices of the pulmonary artery branches. Other techniques for the repair of interrupted aortic arch in truncus arteriosus have been reported[11, 14, 17]; however, the approach described is less likely to result in obstruction of both the aorta and pulmonary arteries, tension on the suture line, or distortion of coronary artery orifices. In our experience, interrupted aortic arch associated with truncus arteriosus is a risk factor for death.[12]

In cases in which the left pulmonary artery is discontinuous with the trunk, arising instead from a ductus arteriosus, the reconstruction proceeds by ligating the ductus arteriosus and connecting the end of the left pulmonary artery to the side of the right ventricular outflow tract allograft, after first connecting the allograft end to end to the mobilized right pulmonary artery cuff.

Postoperative Care

The postoperative management of truncus arteriosus is similar to that for most reconstructed cardiac defects in neonates. Particular emphasis is placed on using measures to keep pulmonary vascular resistance minimized. Sustained pulmonary hypertension and acute pulmonary hypertensive crises have been difficult problems after truncus repair in the past. Maintenance of hypocarbia, respiratory alkalosis, continuous sedation, and paralysis, along with avoidance of unnecessary stimulation

TABLE 17–4. □ RESULTS OF TRUNCUS ARTERIOSUS REPAIR BETWEEN 1972 AND 1992

YEARS	NO. OF CASES	NO. OF DEATHS	MORTALITY RATE
1972–1976	11	7	64%
1977–1981	21	13	62%
1982–1986	33	13	39%
1987–1991	57	10	18%

TABLE 17–5. □ TRUNCUS ARTERIOSUS MORTALITY IN PATIENTS LESS THAN 3 MONTHS OLD

YEARS	NO. OF CASES	NO. OF DEATHS	MORTALITY RATE
1972–1976	7 (64%)	6	86%
1977–1981	11 (52%)	10	91%
1982–1986	20 (61%)	12	60%
1987–1991	41 (72%)	8	19%

Percentages in parentheses refer to all cases managed surgically during that time period, regardless of the patient's age.

such as routine tracheal suctioning, help to minimize these complications.

Early neonatal repair may markedly reduce the problems associated with a labile pulmonary vascular bed. At Children's Hospital in Boston, we have found that pulmonary vascular resistance is much more stable in patients who have undergone truncus repair in the neonatal period rather than later in infancy. Postoperative pulmonary hypertensive problems have been markedly reduced in our intensive care unit in patients with truncus arteriosus who underwent repair in the neonatal period, with an incidence of only 16%. This contrasts with an incidence of more than 50% in patients who are repaired after 30 days of life.[12] Absence of pulmonary vascular hypertensive problems has been associated with a much shorter period of ventilator dependence. We have inferred from these observations that it is beneficial to relieve the unrestricted, arterial-level left-to-right shunt in the first days of life.

RESULTS

Between 1972 and 1991, 122 patients with truncus arteriosus underwent surgical treatment at Children's Hospital in Boston. There were 45 early deaths (defined as occurring in the hospital or less than 30 days after surgery). Table 17–4 shows the total cases and mortality by 5-year intervals within this 20-year period. The improvement in mortality over time reflects a number of factors, but surgical technique figures most prominently.

Between 1972 and 1976, only five of 11 patients underwent primary repair. Even in this early period, however, seven of the 11 were addressed surgically before they were 3 months of age. Six of these seven patients died, four after primary repair and two after pulmonary artery banding was performed. From 1977 through 1981, fewer pulmonary artery band procedures were performed, with 19 of 21 patients undergoing primary repair. Eleven infants underwent surgery before they were 3 months of age, all for complete repair. There were 10 deaths in these 11 cases. In the decade from 1972 to 1981, therefore, two of 18 patients operated on before 3

months of age survived, one with a pulmonary artery band and one with primary repair.

From 1982 through 1986, 27 of the 33 patients underwent primary repair. Twenty were operated on before 3 months of age, with 18 of the 20 undergoing primary repair. The two patients receiving pulmonary artery bands died, while 10 of the 18 who underwent primary repair died. From 1987 through 1991, 57 of the 60 patients underwent primary repair; in the other three, palliative pulmonary arterial banding had been carried out at other institutions before referral. Forty-four of these patients were repaired before the age of 3 months. There were eight deaths in these 44 patients. Table 17–5 reviews the mortality by time periods for patients repaired at less than 3 months of age during these 20 years.

As can be seen from Table 17–5, surgical philosophy did not change dramatically over the 20-year period, with the majority of patients undergoing primary repair during early infancy in all time periods. However, the mortality did drop dramatically over time. Further analysis of the deaths reveals that the great majority occurred in the immediate perioperative period (i.e., on the day of surgery or the first postoperative day). These two observations suggest that technical factors were important in the improved outcome in later years. Improvements in myocardial protection and reintroduction of allograft valved conduits also occurred during this period. Further analysis of the period from 1987 through 1991 indicated a definite trend toward neonatal primary repair, with the outcome supporting this approach. Table 17–6 shows the number of pa-

TABLE 17–6. □ RESULTS OF TRUNCUS ARTERIOSUS REPAIR IN PATIENTS LESS THAN 3 MONTHS OLD

YEAR	NO. OF CASES	MEAN AGE (DAYS) OF REPAIR	NO. OF DEATHS (%)
1987	5	49	0
1988	5	47	2 (40%)
1989	12	40	2 (17%)
1990	11	29	3 (27%)
1991*	8	14	1 (12%)

*Data available for only 8 months of 1991.

tients operated on before the age of 3 months for the years 1987 to 1991. The age at surgery has dropped dramatically even within this 5-year period. From 1987 through 1989, there were no patients who underwent "elective" operation before 1 month of age. Only patients with significant truncal regurgitation or associated interrupted aortic arch underwent neonatal repair during these 3 years. By contrast, in 1990, five of 11 patients underwent "elective" neonatal repair, and in 1991, no patient was operated on after the neonatal period. As mentioned earlier, since 1991 we have noted a marked reduction in postoperative pulmonary hypertension and pulmonary vascular lability in these "elective" neonatal cases.

In our experience there are four important preoperative risk factors for death after repair in patients with truncus arteriosus: truncal valve regurgitation, associated interrupted aortic arch, coronary artery anomalies, and repair undertaken after 100 days of life.[12] Of the 10 deaths in the years 1987 through 1991, all occurred in patients with one or more of these associations. Three of the six patients with associated interrupted aortic arch died, while four of eight patients with significant truncal stenosis or regurgitation died. Patients with these two associated anomalies were much more likely to have coronary anomalies as well. The remaining three deaths occurred in patients who had isolated coronary anomalies or underwent repair late. One patient with an isolated coronary anomaly but otherwise excellent hemodynamics died suddenly on the first postoperative day, and one had severe myocardial dysfunction suggestive of an intraoperative myocardial infarction.

Long-term follow-up was available in all patients seen after 1986. There were four late deaths. Two of these were in patients with discontinuous right pulmonary arteries. One patient had scimitar syndrome and a severely hypoplastic right lung that was removed at the time of repair. The other patient had absence of the right pulmonary artery with multiple small, aortopulmonary collateral vessels to the right lung. Both patients underwent right ventricular outflow reconstruction to the left lung only, and both survived the perioperative period. The first patient died 4 months postoperatively from sudden hemorrhage into the left lung, and the other died suddenly at home 6 months postoperatively. These results suggest that single-lung truncus repair is not well tolerated over time. During long-term follow-up of all patients dating back to 1972, the following procedures associated with repair of truncus arteriosus have been documented without mortality: 21 right ventricular outflow tract revisions; three pulmonary artery surgical angioplasties; one

repair of an aneurysm of the right ventricular outflow tract; 11 balloon or stent pulmonary artery dilatations; two resections for double-chambered right ventricle; four closures of residual ventricular septal defects; seven truncal valve replacements; one Konno aortoventriculoplasty procedure; one resection of subaortic and supra-aortic obstruction; and placement of one pacemaker for complete heart block.

SUMMARY

Repair of truncus arteriosus is best undertaken within the first few days of life. The availability of small valved allografts for the right ventricle–to–pulmonary artery reconstruction, the realization that a patent foramen ovale is beneficial postoperatively, and increasing experience with complex neonatal surgery have contributed to the smoother postoperative course and improved outcome. Early repair appears to greatly reduce the incidence of pulmonary vascular hypertension and pulmonary hypertensive crises in the postoperative period. The excellent results with conduit revisions support the concept that early repair will allow long-term survival and also argue against attempts to repair truncus arteriosus using valveless, autologous tissue for the right ventricle–to–pulmonary artery reconstruction. This latter approach may have some merit in selected infants who are beyond the neonatal period and have markedly reduced pulmonary vascular resistance and severe heart failure. In the neonatal period, however, significant pulmonary regurgitation may not be routinely tolerated because of the immature pulmonary vasculature. Therefore, repair resulting in significant pulmonary regurgitation is likely to increase mortality. We believe that purposefully delaying surgery beyond the neonatal period, to a time when the pulmonary vascular resistance is low, in order to possibly have appropriate conditions for performing a partially autologous or valveless reconstruction of the right ventricular outflow tract, is incorrect. This may result in fewer reoperations for surviving patients, but the delay will create significant numbers of patients who develop a hyperactive pulmonary vasculature before surgery. This will increase perioperative mortality no matter what reconstructive approach is taken.

We recommend repair in the neonatal period as soon as the diagnosis is made, as this reduces pulmonary vascular problems. The repair should include closure of the ventricular septal defect, use of a valved allograft conduit for the right ventricle–to–pulmonary artery construction, and retained patency of the foramen ovale. Using this approach, we have repaired 33 consecutive neonates with truncus arteriosus (without associated complex lesions) without mortality. Patients with either severe truncal valve regurgitation or interrupted aortic arch remain at increased risk, as do patients who undergo surgery after 100 days of life. Newer methods of arch reconstruction and the use of allograft root replacement may improve the outcome of patients with complex morphologic variants.

REFERENCES

1. Armer RM, De Oliveira PF, Lurie PR. True truncus arteriosus. Review of 17 cases and report of surgery in 7 patients. Circulation 24:878, 1961.
2. Barbero-Marcial M, Riso A, Atik E, et al. A technique for correction of truncus arteriosus types I and II without extracardiac conduits. J Thorac Cardiovasc Surg 99:364, 1990.
3. Behrendt DM, Kirsch MM, Stern A, et al. The surgical therapy for pulmonary artery-right ventricular discontinuity. Ann Thorac Surg 18:122, 1974.
4. Bove EL, Beekman RH, Snider AR, et al. Repair of truncus arteriosus in the neonate and young infant. Ann Thorac Surg 47:499, 1989.
5. Butto F, Lucas RV Jr, Edwards JE. Persistent truncus arteriosus: Pathologic anatomy in 54 cases. Pediatr Cardiol 7:95, 1986.
6. Calder L, Van Praagh R, Van Praagh S, et al. Truncus arteriosus communis: Clinical, angiocardiographic, and pathologic findings in 100 patients. Am Heart J 92:23, 1976.
7. Collett RW, Edwards JE. Persistent truncus arteriosus. A classification according to anatomic subtypes. Surg Clin North Am 29:1245, 1949.
8. de la Cruz MV, Cayre R, Angelini P, et al. Coronary arteries in truncus arteriosus. Am J Cardiol 66:1482, 1990.
9. Ebert PA, Turley K, Stanger P, et al. Surgical treatment of truncus arteriosus in the first six months of life. Ann Surg 200:451, 1984.
10. Elkins RC, Steinberg JB, Razook JD, et al. Correction of truncus arteriosus with truncal valvar stenosis or insufficiency using two homografts. Ann Thorac Surg 50:728, 1990.
11. Fujiwara K, Yokota Y, Okamoto F, et al. Successful surgical repair of truncus arteriosus with interrupted aortic arch in infancy by an anterior approach. Ann Thorac Surg 45:441, 1988.
12. Hanley FL, Heinemann MK, Jonas RA, et al. Neonatal repair of truncus arteriosus. J Thorac Cardiovasc Surg 105:1047–1056, 1993.
13. McGoon DC, Rastelli GC, Ongley PA. An operation for the correction of truncus arteriosus. JAMA 205:69, 1968.
14. McKay R, Miyamoto S, Peart I, et al. Truncus arteriosus with interrupted aortic arch: Successful correction in a neonate. Ann Thorac Surg 48:587, 1989.
15. Pearl JM, Laks H, Drinkwater DC Jr, et al. Repair of truncus arteriosus in infancy. Ann Thorac Surg 52:780, 1991.
16. Peetz DJ, Spicer RL, Crowley DC, et al. Correction of truncus arteriosus in the neonate using a nonvalved conduit. J Thorac Cardiovasc Surg 83:743, 1982.
17. Raudkivi PJ, Sutherland GR, Edwards JC, et al. Truncus arteriosus with type B interrupted aortic arch: Correction in the neonate. Pediatr Cardiol 11:117, 1990.
18. Sharma AK, Brawn WJ, Mee RB. Truncus arteriosus. Surgical approach. J Thorac Cardiovasc Surg 90:45, 1985.
19. Smith GW, Thompson WM, Damman JF, et al. Use of pulmonary artery banding procedure in treating type II truncus arteriosus. Circulation 29(suppl 1):108, 1964.
20. Swift LH, Shimowura S, Ryan SF, et al. New type of truncus arteriosus communis with two semi-lunar valves, aortic valvular atresia, and no ventricular septal defect. Circulation 40(suppl III):199, 1969.
21. Van Praagh R, Van Praagh S. The anatomy of common aortico-pulmonary trunk (truncus arteriosus communis) and its embryonic implications. A study of 57 necropsy cases. Am J Cardiol 16:406, 1965.

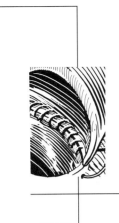

18

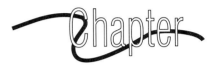

Aortopulmonary Window

Aortopulmonary window is a rare lesion consisting of a two-dimensional communication between the proximal ascending aorta and the main pulmonary artery in the presence of two normally formed semilunar valves. This lesion can be found in isolation but is commonly associated with other complex cardiovascular anomalies. This chapter will focus on the morphology, clinical presentation, and management of the isolated aortopulmonary window in neonates and infants. Associated lesions will also be discussed, especially if they affect neonatal management. Because an individual institution rarely sees more than one aortopulmonary window per year and because of the frequent association with other lesions, experience is limited. However, an understanding of the morphology and physiology provides a firm base for making management recommendations.

ANATOMY

Developmental Considerations

Abnormal development of the embryologic aorticopulmonary septum is thought to be caused by incomplete formation of the right and left conotruncal ridges, resulting in the aortopulmonary window. Some believe that this lesion represents one point along a spectrum of lesions resulting from various degrees of embryologic maldevelopment of the cono-

truncal septum.[7, 21] More complete conotruncal defects result in truncus arteriosus and less severe defects in isolated, anomalous origin of the right pulmonary artery from the aorta.[18] Others believe this lesion to be unrelated to truncus arteriosus, largely based on indirect evidence (i.e., that truncus and aortopulmonary window have a very different spectrum of associated lesions).[12]

Morphologic Features

The exact morphology of the defect may vary, but its position is limited to areas in which the left posterolateral and posterior aspect of the ascending aorta is contiguous with the right anterolateral aspect of the main pulmonary artery and the anterior aspect of the right pulmonary artery. From the perspective of the inside of the ascending aorta, therefore, the defect has been classically described as occurring in one of two positions: on the left posterolateral aortic wall just above the aortic valve or slightly more cephalad on the posterior aortic wall.[18] In the former case the defect opens into the facing right anterolateral wall of the main pulmonary artery, while in the latter it opens into the junction of the main and right pulmonary arteries or into the right pulmonary artery itself.

The size of the defect may vary also, but it is generally large enough to be nonrestrictive to flow. When the defect is large, the two morphologic variations mentioned previously may merge into one. This very large lesion may give the impression that the right pulmonary artery arises separately from the right posterior aspect of the aorta in association with a large confluence of the ascending aorta and the main pulmonary artery above the two semilunar valves.[2] Usually the defect is approximately circular or oval; however, when the right pulmonary artery is involved, more complex two-dimensional shapes may exist.

The coronary arteries usually arise normally, but on occasion the right, left, or all coronary arteries may arise anomalously from the confluence or from the pulmonary artery itself.[3, 5, 12, 13]

Reported series suggest that associated anomalies occur in approximately 50% of cases of aortopulmonary window.[12] Our experience suggests an even higher incidence, with only 6 of 18 cases not associated with some other major cardiovascular defect. Table 18–1 shows the associated lesions found in the 18 patients managed surgically at Children's Hospital in Boston over the last two decades. One syndrome that has been identified in the literature[2, 14] and that we have seen[8] involves a large, confluent, aortopulmonary window, with separate origin of the right pulmonary artery from the right posterolateral ascending aorta, combined with an interrupted aortic arch and patent ductus arteriosus. Interrupted aortic arch, almost exclusively type A, is a common associated lesion in most large series.[4, 12]

PATHOPHYSIOLOGY AND NATURAL HISTORY

The isolated aortopulmonary window results in an arterial-level, systemic-to-pulmonary artery shunt, similar to the pathophysiology of a large patent ductus arteriosus (see Chapter 12). However, when compared with patent ductus arteriosus, it is more likely that the patient with aortopulmonary window will have a large shunt, severe associated congestive heart failure, and failure to thrive. This is probably because the typical large size and two-dimensional configuration of the aortopulmonary window are less likely to restrict the shunt. Occasionally, smaller aortopulmonary windows provide some restriction to the flow, and as a result the magnitude of the left-to-right shunt and the signs and symptoms of congestive heart failure are correspondingly less severe.

Aortopulmonary window is a rare defect, both in our experience (18 cases over a 20-year period) and in that reported by others.[12, 16, 20] It is a highly lethal lesion. Untreated patients either die in infancy of intractable heart failure or survive beyond infancy only because of persistently elevated pulmonary vascular resistance. Pulmonary vascular obstructive disease develops rapidly in surviving patients (usually within the first year of life, although exceptions exist),[8] and ultimately it severely limits life expectancy. Typically, patients with isolated aortopulmonary window have worsening congestive heart failure shortly after the neonatal period, as pulmonary vascular resistance falls. If pulmonary vascular resistance does not fall, the congestive heart failure will be absent or less apparent.

Associated lesions may alter the natural history significantly. If interrupted aortic arch is present, patients typically are seen in profound cardiovascular collapse shortly after birth. This was the case in the single patient in our series with this associated lesion. Such patients require aggressive preoperative resuscitation with prostaglandin E$_1$, inotropic support, and mechanical ventilation.

DIAGNOSIS AND INDICATIONS FOR SURGERY

The physical findings, chest radiograph, and electrocardiogram of the infant with aortopulmonary window and associated congestive heart failure are similar to those of any patient with congestive heart failure secondary to a large, arterial-level, systemic-to-pulmonary artery shunt. The patient who has either a restrictive aortopulmonary window or elevated pulmonary vascular resistance may have attenuated signs or symptoms of the left-to-right shunt and of congestive heart failure. Subtle variations in the physical examination may suggest aortopulmonary window rather than the other major lesion in the differential diagnosis: large patent ductus arteriosus.[10] In infants, other lesions in the differential diagnosis include truncus arteriosus, anomalous origin of the pulmonary artery from the aorta, and possibly ventricular septal defect.

TABLE 18–1. ☐ LESIONS ASSOCIATED WITH AORTOPULMONARY WINDOW (18 CASES)

LESION	NUMBER
Secundum atrial septal defect	5
Patent ductus arteriosus*	4
Ventricular septal defect	4
Interrupted aortic arch	3
Double-outlet right ventricle	3
Tetralogy of Fallot	2
Tetralogy of Fallot with pulmonary atresia	2
Hypoplastic left ventricle	2
Right aortic arch	2
Peripheral pulmonary stenosis	2
Partial anomalous pulmonary venous return	1
Coarctation of the aorta	1
Anomalous right subclavian artery	1

*Patent ductus arteriosus occurred only with interrupted aortic arch or coarctation of the aorta.

Echocardiography can reliably distinguish aortopulmonary window from these other lesions.[1, 15, 17] The morphologic details of the defect (such as the size and position of the defect, the origin of the coronary arteries, the size and origin of the pulmonary artery branches, and associated lesions) can usually be defined. Echocardiography is considered the definitive preoperative study for the patient seen early in infancy with congestive heart failure, although some recommend routine cardiac catheterization.[22] If uncertainty remains regarding anatomic details or associated cardiovascular lesions after echocardiography, or if the patient is seen later in infancy or has had an examination that suggests elevated pulmonary vascular resistance, cardiac catheterization is indicated. The course of the catheter, oximetry data, and angiography can be diagnostic. The major role of catheterization is to define the physiologic status of the pulmonary vasculature.

Surgical correction is indicated at the time of diagnosis. Judgment may be necessary in the unusual case of an extremely small defect or when diagnosis has been delayed, resulting in pulmonary vascular obstructive disease. Eisenmenger-like physiology is the only absolute contraindication to closure of the defect.

SURGICAL MANAGEMENT

Historical Perspective

Gross first applied surgical methods to repair this lesion in 1952 when he performed closed surgical ligation.[9] Other closed techniques followed shortly, including closed division with oversewing of the resulting aortic and pulmonary artery defects.[19] The introduction of cardiopulmonary bypass allowed safer and more reliable open techniques to be used. These methods include external division and oversewing and various internal exposures (e.g., transaortic, transpulmonary artery) to either primarily close or patch the defect. In 1978, Johansson et al. reported making an incision directly into the front (anterior) part of the aortopulmonary window itself, which provides excellent internal exposure to both the aorta and the pulmonary artery adjacent to the defect.[11]

Surgical Technique

Simple Aortopulmonary Window

Cardiac exposure is gained through a median sternotomy, subtotal resection of the thymus, and a pericardotomy (Fig. 18–1). The aortopulmonary window is inspected externally to confirm the diagnosis. Two semilunar valves should be identified and the positions of the coronary artery origins noted. Extensive external dissection of the great vessels adds little information concerning the morphologic details of the defect and should be avoided. In preparation for cardiopulmonary bypass, the aorta is cannulated as cephalad as possible, and a single right atrial venous cannula is used. At the institution of cardiopulmonary bypass, the pulmonary artery branches are occluded. The procedure is performed using continuous cardiopulmonary bypass at moderately hypothermic temperatures; however, deep hypothermic circulatory arrest may occasionally be used, as it provides the surgeon with the flexibility of removing the aortic crossclamp to improve exposure by reducing distortion of the great vessels. If interrupted aortic arch is present, cannulation for cardiopulmonary bypass is similar to that described for truncus arteriosus with interrupted aortic arch (see Chapter 17), and deep hypothermic circulatory arrest is used for the entire reconstruction.

The isolated defect is best approached directly through an incision in the aortopulmonary window itself. An incision is made along the circumference of the anterior half of the defect and is performed carefully after fully assessing the origins of the coronary arteries and the pulmonary artery branches. Dacron or glutaraldehyde-treated pericardium can be used to patch the defect. For the most straightforward morphologic variant, this involves an oval patch tailored to the size of the defect itself. Using running polypropylene suture, the patch is sewn to the intact posterior half of the circumference of the window until the two ends of the original incision are reached. The anterior edge of the patch is then "sandwiched" between the cut edges of the original incision in the anterior aspect of the window by continuing the running sutures.

After completion of the reconstruction, the remainder of the operation—including reinstitution of cardiopulmonary bypass, core rewarming, and separation from cardiopulmonary bypass—is routine.

Aortopulmonary Window With Interrupted Aortic Arch

If an interrupted aortic arch is present, it should be addressed first, as described in Chapter 22. As mentioned previously, the aortopulmonary window itself is likely to be more complex in this situation (i.e., a very large window consisting of a central confluence of the aorta and main pulmonary artery, with an apparently separate origin of the right pulmonary artery from the right posterolateral area of

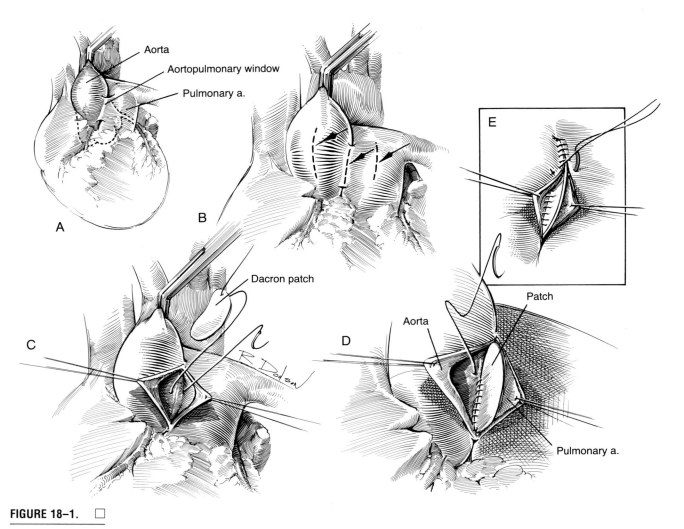

FIGURE 18–1. □

A, Surface morphology of a heart with an aortopulmonary window. *B,* Possible incisions for exposure of the aortopulmonary window. *C,* Exposure of defect via an incision in the anterior rim of the aortopulmonary window itself. *D* and *E,* Patch closure of the aortopulmonary window.

the aorta). The patch and its suture line must be configured to baffle the right pulmonary artery so that it is in continuity with the main pulmonary artery after the reconstruction. This must be carried out with care to avoid obstruction of the right pulmonary artery or obstruction of the ascending aorta.

Associated Coronary Artery Anomalies

The position of the coronary arteries is an important consideration. If anomalous origin of the right or left coronary ostium is present, the reconstruction may need to be modified. The basic approach is to leave the coronary ostia alone, if at all possible, and to modify the position of the patch so that the coronaries arise from the aortic side of the patch after reconstruction is completed. If the anterior (right) coronary ostium is anomalous, the initial in-

cision in the anterior aspect of the window may need to be slightly modified so that this coronary ostium remains on the aortic side of the patch. If the posterior (left) coronary ostium is anomalous, then the placement of the patch suture line on the intact posterior aspect of the aortopulmonary window may need to be modified to ensure that this ostium remains on the aortic side of the patch. Although we have not yet encountered a situation involving an anomalous coronary ostium not amenable to this approach, such a situation would most likely necessitate transfer of a coronary ostial button to the aorta.

Other associated cardiovascular lesions, if present, should be corrected. At the Children's Hospital in Boston, two cases of aortopulmonary window associated with tetralogy of Fallot were repaired before 1977.[6]

Postoperative Care

Several aspects of postoperative management should be emphasized. A catheter should be left in place to measure the pulmonary artery pressure in the early postoperative period. Episodes of pulmonary hypertension should be expected, given the preoperative pathophysiology of this lesion. Standard maneuvers for minimizing pulmonary vascular resistance, as described in Chapter 17, should be performed. The pulmonary artery catheter also allows oximetric detection of a residual systemic-to-pulmonary artery shunt if there is a leak in the patch. In cases involving complex windows with separate origin of the right pulmonary artery from the aorta, placing the distal tip of the pulmonary artery catheter into the right pulmonary artery allows determination of any right pulmonary artery pullback gradient in the postoperative period as a check for stenosis at this level.

RESULTS

Between 1972 and 1991, 18 cases of aortopulmonary window were seen at Children's Hospital in Boston. In six of these cases, the lesion was isolated or associated with only minor additional cardiovascular lesions. These included patent foramen ovale, secundum atrial septal defect, right aortic arch, peripheral pulmonary stenosis, aberrant left subclavian artery, and left superior vena cava. The major associated lesions are listed in Table 18–1. In the entire group there was only one early death. Late follow-up was available for nine patients, with one death occurring in a patient who was noted to have left pulmonary artery occlusion. Three other patients have since undergone either surgical or balloon angioplasty for obstructed pulmonary artery branches.

The age at operation ranged from 7 days to 6.5 months in the 15 cases with unrestrictive aortopulmonary windows. In three patients—one with tetralogy of Fallot, one with tetralogy of Fallot and pulmonary atresia, and one with hypoplastic left ventricle—the aortopulmonary windows were restrictive and provided the primary source of pulmonary blood flow. These patients underwent definitive surgery of both the aortopulmonary window and the associated lesion at between 1 and 2 years of age; repair was accomplished in two, and a Fontan modification in one. Another patient with a hypoplastic left ventricle underwent repair of the unrestrictive aortopulmonary window in infancy and subsequently received a classic Glenn shunt.

SUMMARY

Because of the rarity of this lesion, the time span over which these cases have been seen, and the number of associated major lesions, no consistent surgical approach was used in these 18 patients. At the present time, however, we recommend repair at the time of diagnosis, with the defect approached through an incision in the aortopulmonary window itself. Either Dacron or glutaraldehyde-treated pericardium can be used for the patch. Preferably, surgical correction should be performed in the neonatal period or early in infancy. Associated lesions, which are common, may modify the age at which the patient is seen and the severity of symptoms. These associated anomalies should be addressed at the time of the initial procedure. The patient with associated interrupted aortic arch is usually profoundly ill in the neonatal period and may need several days of preoperative resuscitation, including inotropic support and the administration of prostaglandins (see Chapter 22).

Our results at Children's Hospital in Boston suggest that long-term follow-up should be performed to carefully monitor for the development of pulmonary artery distortion. Excellent long-term results should be possible with treatment of this lesion as long as diagnosis and surgical correction are not delayed beyond early infancy.

REFERENCES

1. Balaji S, Burch M, Sullivan ID. Accuracy of cross-sectional echocardiography in diagnosis of aortopulmonary window. Am J Cardiol 67:650, 1991.
2. Berry TE, Bharati S, Muster AJ, et al. Distal aortopulmonary septal defect, aortic origin of the right pulmonary artery, intact ventricular septum, patent ductus arteriosus and hypoplasia of the aortic isthmus: a newly recognized syndrome. Am J Cardiol 49:108, 1982.
3. Bourlon F, Kreitmann P, Jourdan J, et al. Anomalous origin of left coronary artery with aortopulmonary window; a case report with surgical correction and delayed control. Thorac Cardiovasc Surg 29:91, 1981.
4. Braunlin E, Peoples WM, Freedom RM, et al. Interruption of the aortic arch with aorticopulmonary septal defect. An anatomic review. Pediatr Cardiol 3:329, 1982.
5. Brouwer MH, Beaufort-Krol GC, Talsma MD. Aortopulmonary window associated with an anomalous origin of the right coronary artery. Int J Cardiol 28:384, 1990.
6. Castaneda AR, Kirklin JW. Tetralogy of Fallot with aorticopulmonary window: Report of two surgical cases. J Thorac Cardiovasc Surg 74:467, 1977.
7. Collett RW, Edwards JE. Persistent truncus arteriosus: Classification according to anatomic types. Surg Clin North Am 29:1245, 1949.
8. Ding WX, Su ZK, Cao DF, et al. One stage repair of absence of the aortopulmonary septum and interrupted aortic arch. Ann Thorac Surg 49:664, 1990.
9. Gross RE. Surgical closure of an aortic septal defect. Circulation 5:858, 1952.
10. Heymann MA. Patent ductus arteriosus. In Adams FH, Em-

manouilides GC, Riemenschneider TA (eds). Moss' Heart Disease in Infants, Children, and Adolescents. 4th ed. Baltimore, Williams & Wilkins, 1989.

11. Johansson L, Michaelsson M, Westerholm CJ, et al. Aortopulmonary window: A new operative approach. Ann Thorac Surg 25:564, 1978.

12. Kutsche LM, Van Mierop LH. Anatomy and pathogenesis of aorticopulmonary septal defect. Am J Cardiol 59:443, 1987.

13. Lloyd TR, Marvin WJ Jr, Lee J. Total anomalous origin of the coronary arteries from the pulmonary artery in an infant with aorticopulmonary septal defect. Letter. Pediatr Cardiol 8:153, 1987.

14. Mendoza DA, Ueda T, Nishioka K, et al. Aortopulmonary window, aortic origin of the right pulmonary artery, and interrupted arch: Detection by two-dimensional and color Doppler echocardiography in an infant. Pediatr Cardiol 7:49, 1986.

15. Pieroni DR, Gingell RL, Roland JM, et al. Two-dimensional echocardiographic recognition and surgical management of aortopulmonary septal defect in the premature infant. Thorac Cardiovasc Surg 30:180, 1982.

16. Ravikumar E, Whight CM, Hawker RE, et al. The surgical management of aortopulmonary window using the anterior sandwich patch closure technique. J Cardiovasc Surg 29:629, 1988.

17. Rice MJ, Seward JB, Hagler DJ, et al. Visualization of aortopulmonary window by two-dimensional echocardiography. Mayo Clin Proc 57:482, 1982.

18. Richardson JV, Doty DB, Rossi NP, et al. The spectrum of anomalies of aortopulmonary septation. J Thorac Cardiovasc Surg 78:21, 1979.

19. Scott HW Jr, Sabiston DC Jr. Surgical treatment for congenital aortopulmonary fistula. Experimental and clinical aspects. J Thorac Surg 25:26, 1953.

20. Tiraboschi R, Salomone G, Crupi G, et al. Aortopulmonary window in the first year of life: Report on 11 surgical cases. Ann Thorac Surg 46:438, 1988.

21. Van Praagh R, Van Praagh S. The anatomy of common aorticopulmonary trunk (truncus arteriosus communis) and its embryologic implications. A study of 57 necropsy cases. Am J Cardiol 16:406, 1965.

22. van Son JA, Kaan GL, van Oort A, et al. Aortopulmonary window. The need for early surgical correction. Tijdschr Kindergeneeskd 59:32, 1991.

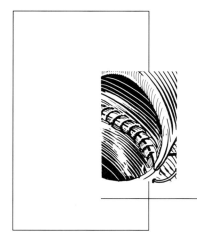

19
Chapter
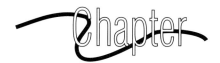

Coronary Artery Anomalies

ANOMALOUS LEFT CORONARY ARTERY FROM THE PULMONARY ARTERY

Anomalous left coronary artery from the pulmonary artery (ALCAPA) is a rare lesion, with an estimated incidence of between 1 in 30,000 and 1 in 300,000.[28] It is a unique congenital heart anomaly in several ways. For example, although infants are not usually brought to the cardiologist at the time of ductal closure, the anomaly is often lethal in early infancy, with some reports suggesting a mortality rate as high as 90% in the first year of life.[30] Diagnosis, even with the current quality of two-dimensional echocardiography and color Doppler, may be difficult.[21] False dropout, suggesting normal aortic origin of the left coronary artery as well as misinterpretation of the transverse sinus as the left main coronary artery,[18] has led to a failure of early diagnosis in many cases. Variable development of collateral vessels further complicates the diagnosis and management of this condition. Fortunately, surgical advances in the management of neonatal coronary arteries make this an eminently correctable lesion as long as surgery is performed sufficiently early in life.

PATHOLOGIC ANATOMY
Embryology

Normal development of the coronary arteries requires a connection between buds that arise from the aortic sinuses of Valsalva and the arterial plexus, which forms epicardially. The epicardial arterial plexus communicates with the intramyocardial plexus, which is derived from venous structures. Buds also grow out from the pulmonary trunk as part of normal development, but these usually regress. In the case of ALCAPA, there is a failure of normal communication to the left coronary bud in the aorta, with an abnormal connection to a pulmonary bud.[1]

Anatomy

The anomalous ostium of the left main coronary artery can be situated almost anywhere in the main pulmonary artery or in its proximal branches. The most common location is the leftward and posterior sinus of the pulmonary root,[25] followed by the rightward and posterior sinus, the posterior wall of the main pulmonary artery trunk, and the origin of the right pulmonary artery posteriorly. An anteriorly placed origin of the anomalous coronary from the main pulmonary artery is exceedingly rare.

There is variable development of collateral vessels, particularly between the right coronary artery and the left anterior descending coronary through the circle of Vieussens. In older patients, these vessels can become considerably dilated. There have been several reports of a conal coronary artery arising anteriorly from the aorta, separate from the right coronary artery and giving rise to collateral vessels to the left coronary artery system.[28] Often there is fibrosis and scarring of the left ventricle (related to the age of the patient), dominance of the left coronary artery, and some degree of collateral formation.[25] Endocardial fibroelastosis is prominent in some patients,[9] and the left ventricle is very dilated, often massively, unlike that in patients with obstructive left heart problems who have endocardial fibroelastosis. Left ventricular dilatation and papillary muscle dysfunction are responsible for the mitral regurgitation that is frequently present. Structural abnormalities of the mitral valve are unusual.

Associated Anomalies

The association of ALCAPA with other anomalies is particularly rare, although such an association may be functionally important. For example, surgical ligation of a persistently patent ductus arteriosus[21] or closure of a ventricular septal defect[9] (both of which present better oxygenated blood to the ALCAPA) without preoperative recognition of the associated ALCAPA is likely to lead to a fatal outcome. ALCAPA has also been reported in association with tetralogy of Fallot[17, 31] and pulmonary valve stenosis.[9]

PATHOPHYSIOLOGY

In 1964, Edwards[11] proposed the pathophysiologic mechanism that accounts for the common clinical presentation of young infants at approximately 6 weeks of age, a presentation that includes evidence of angina associated with feeding or an established infarct, massive left ventricular dilatation, and mitral regurgitation. During in utero development, pulmonary artery pressure and aortic pressure are similar because of ductal patency, and there is satisfactory perfusion of the anomalous left coronary artery, albeit at a slightly reduced oxygen saturation. After ductal closure after birth, pulmonary artery pressure and, consequently, left coronary artery perfusion progressively decline as pulmonary vascular resistance decreases. Normally during the first weeks of life, hyperplasia and hypertrophy of myocytes, as well as coronary angiogenesis, are present to maintain appropriate wall stress as the left ventricle grows. With inadequate coronary perfu-

sion, these things cannot happen, so the left ventricle becomes progressively dilated and thin walled.[22] Left ventricular dilatation, as well as papillary muscle dysfunction or infarction, results in functional mitral regurgitation. These events are modified by the relative dominance of the right and left coronary arteries, as well as the rapidity with which collateral vessels form between the two coronary trees.

If the infant survives this early crisis, there may be continuing collateral development that eventually results in an important left-to-right shunt[32] secondary to retrograde flow through the anomalous coronary into the main pulmonary artery. Under such circumstances, diagnosis becomes more simple as color flow mapping or angiography demonstrates flow into the pulmonary artery, and an oxygen step-up can be measured. Such patients may be asymptomatic, but in adult life they may suffer from arrhythmias, angina, or sudden death. There is one case report[12] of a child who had severe symptoms at the age of 4 years and who was well, with a normal-sized heart, by the age of 10 years without surgical intervention.

PREOPERATIVE EVALUATION

The young infant who is brought to the cardiologist with dilated left ventricular cardiomyopathy must undergo exhaustive exclusion of ALCAPA. Often there is classic electrocardiographic evidence of left ventricular ischemia and infarction. Mitral regurgitation, as shown by two-dimensional echocardiography, can be massive, as is the left ventricular end-diastolic volume. In a group of six infants described by Rein and coworkers,[22] the mean left ventricular end-diastolic volume was four times normal. Various indices of left ventricular function are profoundly depressed. Visualization of the anomalous ostium may be particularly difficult and may be complicated by false dropout when the pulmonary artery lies close to the aorta—suggesting aortic origin—as well as by misinterpretation of the transverse pericardial sinus as a left main coronary artery passing posterior to the main pulmonary artery. Occasionally, evidence by color Doppler of flow from the anomalous coronary into the pulmonary artery will aid the echocardiographic diagnosis, although this sign is often absent in the infant without much collateral development. If there is any doubt, cardiac catheterization should be undertaken, including an aortic root injection as employed for the definition of coronary artery anatomy in neonates with transposition. Undoubtedly, cardiac catheterization carries a greater risk than usual in these very compromised infants, so if the diagnosis can be made conclusively by two-dimensional echocardiography alone, it is preferable to avoid catheterization.

MEDICAL THERAPY

The high surgical mortality among symptomatic infants led Driscoll et al.,[10] in 1981, to adopt a conservative approach to surgery, particularly because they noted an 87% survival rate in 15 patients treated medically. There have also been occasional reports of spontaneous improvement.[12] However, we believe that in the current era there is no place for medical therapy for this anomaly. Diagnosis should be made as early in life as possible and followed by surgery as soon as it is practical. Even in asymptomatic older children and adults, the risk of a gradual deterioration of left ventricular function, as well as the risk of sudden death, justifies creation of a dual coronary system at the time of diagnosis. Similar recommendations have been made by many authors over the last decade.

SURGICAL MANAGEMENT

History

Many surgical techniques have been described for both palliation and correction of ALCAPA after the first description of this anomaly by Bland and coworkers in 1933.[4] The aim of early palliative operations was to increase pulmonary artery pressure and thereby increase coronary perfusion pressure. Banding of the main pulmonary artery, as well as creation of an aortopulmonary window, was attempted. Another palliative approach was to decrease the "myocardial steal." This was achieved by ligation of the anomalous left coronary artery, although there was a tendency for the ligated coronary to recanalize.[19] Physiologically corrective techniques have included creation of a dual coronary system with bypass grafting, using the left subclavian artery, left common carotid artery, internal mammary artery, and saphenous vein. In 1979, Takeuchi and colleagues[27] described creation of an aortopulmonary window and an intrapulmonary artery baffle to direct aortic blood to the anomalous ostium. Most recently, increasing experience with the manipulation of neonatal coronary arteries has led a number of centers, including Children's Hospital in Boston, to use an anatomically and physiologically corrective procedure: direct reimplantation of the left coronary artery into the aorta.

Indications

The diagnosis alone should be the indication for surgery in all patients, with the aim to preserve as many myocytes as possible. It is possible that a small subset of patients with profoundly depressed ventricular function and massive mitral regurgitation may be better served by heart transplantation than by corrective surgery. With early diagnosis and application of the techniques described later, this should very rarely be necessary.

Technical Considerations

ALCAPA is one of the few congenital heart anomalies in which myocardial function is likely to be profoundly compromised preoperatively, before the additional insult of intraoperative myocardial ischemia. In addition, the unusual anatomic and physiologic circumstances require that some extremely important changes be made in conducting the bypass as well as in the techniques of myocardial protection. However, to the child's advantage, the postoperative circulation will be essentially a normal, in-series, biventricular circulation, albeit with a variable degree of mitral regurgitation. It may well be appropriate in the case of the most severely compromised children to plan an elective period of postoperative left ventricular assistance using whatever system the surgical team is most familiar with.

Approach is by a median sternotomy, with high cannulation of the ascending aorta and a single venous cannula. Immediately after commencing bypass, the tourniquets that have been placed around the right and left pulmonary arteries should be tightened. Surprisingly, this highly important step has not been previously described, although it serves several important functions. First, there is always some collateral flow between the two coronary systems. If runoff is allowed into the decompressed pulmonary arteries, there will be compromised perfusion of both the right and left coronary systems. In addition, blood passing into the left coronary system and pulmonary artery will pass through the pulmonary veins into the left atrium and left ventricle. The compromised left ventricle will be unable to cope with this left heart return, resulting in serious left heart distention. Distention of the left heart must be assiduously avoided during the procedure. Often it is convenient to amputate the tip of the left atrial appendage. Alternatively, a small vent may be inserted through the right superior pulmonary vein.

During cooling, the main pulmonary artery and its branches should be mobilized after carefully visualizing the external course of the anomalous coronary. At a rectal and tympanic membrane temperature of less than 18°C, bypass flow is reduced to 50 ml/kg/min, and the ascending aorta is clamped. Cardioplegic solution is infused into the root of the aorta. Although some have recommended simultaneous infusion of cardioplegic solution into the pulmonary artery root, we have observed satisfactory blanching of the left ventricle using aortic cardioplegia only. In fact, the pulmonary artery root is soon seen to fill with clear cardioplegic solution and equilibrate with aortic root pressure, the latter also having been observed during the cooling phase on bypass. This anomaly may also represent an appropriate situation for retrograde infusion of cardioplegic solution into the coronary sinus. If adequate visualization is not achieved at any time during the procedure because of collateral return, deep hypothermic circulatory arrest may be established.

Coronary Reimplantation

A transverse incision is made in the main pulmonary artery at the level of the anomalous coronary ostium, as determined both preoperatively and by visualization of the course of the left main coronary artery during the operation. After identification of the ostium, the main pulmonary artery is transected at the level of the ostium, and the anomalous coronary is excised, including a generous button of the wall of the main pulmonary artery, just as for the arterial switch procedure. Not uncommonly, the ostium will lie close to the top of the posterior commissure of the pulmonary valve, and therefore, it may be necessary to detach the very top of this commissure to achieve a suitable button. This does not appear to result in serious pulmonary regurgitation postoperatively.

Just as for the arterial switch operation, the left main coronary artery is mobilized sufficiently to allow a tension-free anastomosis to the posterior and leftward wall of the ascending aorta. Early in our experience the aortic site was prepared by a simple stab incision in the aorta, followed by use of a 2.5- or 4-mm punch. However, it would seem that the relative levels of the aorta and pulmonary valves may be altered in this anomaly, with the pulmonary valve being lower than anticipated relative to the aortic valve. Thus, blind creation of the aortic defect places the aortic valve at risk. Accordingly, our current practice is to make a separate vertical anterior and rightward aortotomy. The aortic defect is made with direct visualization of the aortic valve.

The coronary button is sutured into the aortotomy using continuous 7-0 polydioxanone or polypropylene sutures. No attempt should be made to reinfuse

cardioplegic solution directly into the coronary arteries. The aortotomy is closed, air is vented through a small stab incision in the aortic root, and the aortic crossclamp is released. The lie of the coronary artery is checked, and hemostasis is assessed. The main pulmonary artery is reconstructed, including a pericardial patch to ensure that there is no tension on the anastomosis. Previous mobilization of the right and left pulmonary arteries, as well as division of the ligamentum arteriosum, further contributes to a tension-free pulmonary artery anastomosis.

Careful venting of the left heart throughout the rewarming period is just as important as during the cooling phase. When cardiac action is re-established—generally coincident with the administration of calcium—venting may be cautiously discontinued, with monitoring of left atrial pressure. Appropriate inotropic support, generally with dopamine, should already be established. If the left ventricle is unable to handle the left heart return on bypass, as indicated by a progressive increase in left atrial pressure, venting should be re-established, and arrangements should be made to assist the left ventricle. Likewise, if weaning from bypass is only possible with very high levels of inotropic support and high left atrial pressure, left ventricular assistance should be seriously considered. Remarkable improvement in left ventricular function can be observed within 48 to 72 hours.

Transpulmonary Artery Baffle (Takeuchi)[27] (Fig. 19–1)

Currently, transpulmonary artery baffle (the Takeuchi procedure) (Fig. 19–1) is rarely indicated, although it may be preferred in certain anatomic circumstances (e.g., leftward anomalous ostium). Preparatory steps are identical to those used for coronary reimplantation. Once again, the right and left pulmonary arteries should be occluded with tourniquets immediately after establishing bypass, and the left heart must be carefully vented. After clamping of the aorta, the main pulmonary artery is opened with a very short transverse incision, carefully taking into account the anticipated location of the anomalous ostium. The incision is extended leftward at either the upper or lower edge of the baffle, which will hinge at its rightward end. The baffle is made long enough and wide enough that it can be carried around the anomalous ostium without tension and provide an adequate pathway for blood to the anomalous left coronary artery. An aortopulmonary window is constructed immediately posterior to the hinge plane of the baffle. The corresponding aortic defect, also about 3 mm in diameter, is constructed, with the same caveat regarding the aortic

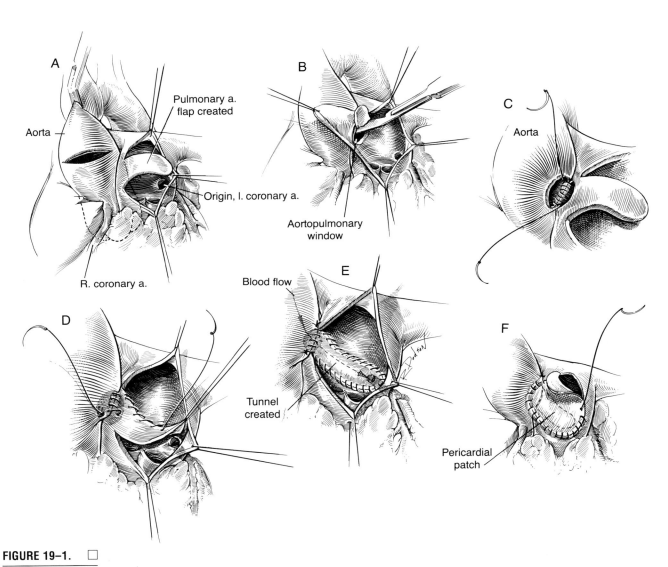

FIGURE 19–1. □

A, The first step in the Takeuchi procedure is the creation of a flap from the anterior wall of the main pulmonary artery. *B,* An aortopulmonary window is created, working through an aortotomy as well as through the previous incision in the main pulmonary artery. *C,* The aortopulmonary window is completed by suturing the aorta to the main pulmonary artery. *D,* The baffle tunnel is constructed by suturing the flap of anterior pulmonary artery wall across the posterior wall of the main pulmonary artery. *E,* Blood flow is established from the aorta through the aortopulmonary window, under the pulmonary artery baffle, and into the anomalous coronary artery. *F,* Repair is completed by closing the defect in the main pulmonary artery with a pericardial patch.

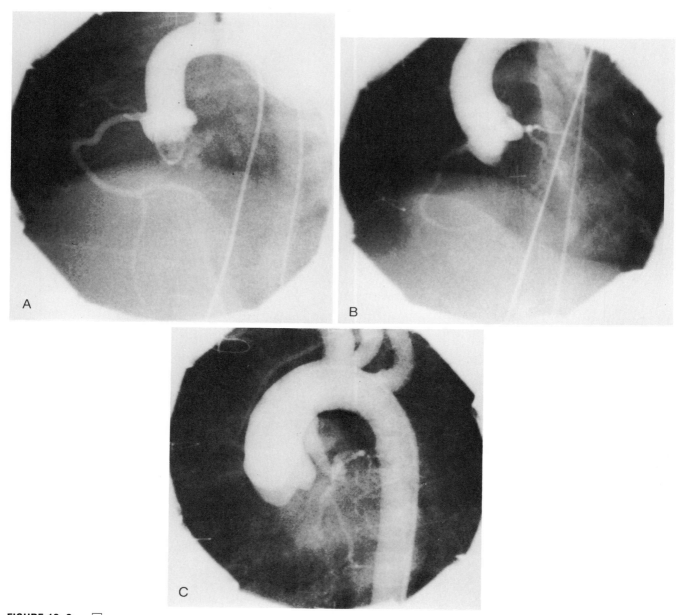

FIGURE 19–2. ☐

A, A preoperative aortogram shows early lack of filling of the anomalous left coronary artery. *B*, A postoperative aortogram after the Takeuchi procedure shows simultaneous filling of the right and left coronary arteries. *C*, A postoperative aortogram shows filling of the intrapulmonary aorta–left coronary artery baffle constructed in the Takeuchi procedure.

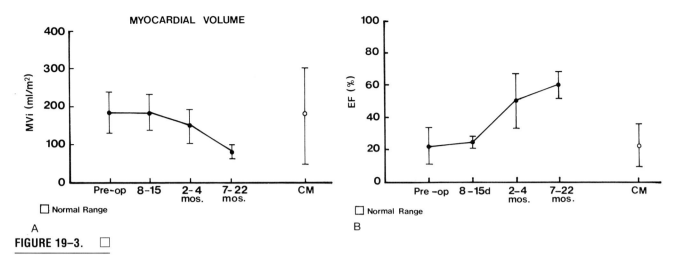

FIGURE 19–3. ☐

A, Myocardial volume indexed to body surface area is markedly increased preoperatively in patients with an anomalous left coronary artery but returns to normal by 7 to 22 months after surgery (i.e., Takeuchi procedure). *B,* Ejection fraction is markedly depressed in patients with an anomalous left coronary artery before repair by the Takeuchi procedure but returns to normal within 7 to 22 months of surgery. (From Rein AJJT, Colan SD, Parness IA, Sanders SP. Regional and global left ventricular function in infants with anomalous origin of the left coronary artery from the pulmonary trunk: Preoperative and postoperative assessment. Circulation 75:115–123, 1987.)

valve noted previously. The aorta is sutured to the pulmonary artery at the window using continuous 7-0 Prolene or polydioxanone sutures. The baffle pathway is completed by suturing the edges of the flap to the posterior wall of the main pulmonary artery. The aortotomy is closed, air is vented from the aortic root, and the aortic crossclamp is released. The pulmonary artery is reconstructed with a generous patch of glutaraldehyde-treated autologous pericardium. As with the coronary reimplantation method, careful attention is paid to left heart venting, monitoring of left atrial pressure, and inotropic support during rewarming.

RESULTS

In 1987, results achieved with the baffle procedure in 11 patients seen after 1979 were compared with the results in 11 patients who had undergone anomalous left coronary artery ligation or ostial closure at Children's Hospital in Boston (Fig. 19–2).[6] In patients who underwent the baffle procedure, there were no deaths, either early or late, over a mean follow-up period of 18.5 months (Table 19–1). In contrast, in the patients who underwent ligation or ostial closure, there were three early deaths and two late deaths. However, those with a baffle were not free from morbidity. Of seven patients recatheterized a mean of 18 months postoperatively, one was found to have an obstructed baffle (the only patient in whom left ventricular end-diastolic volume had not normalized postoperatively from a mean preoperative left ventricular end-diastolic volume of 268 ± 97 ml/m², almost four times greater than normal)

(Fig. 19–3). Aortic regurgitation developed in one patient secondary to injury of the aortic valve during creation of the aortopulmonary window; this subsequently required aortic valve replacement. Obstruction of the right ventricular outflow tract, related to the baffle, developed in two of the 11 patients, one of whom required reoperation. One patient has a baffle leak with a 1.5:1 shunt.

Our experience with coronary translocation is limited, but we are in agreement with others that this is currently the procedure of choice for ALCAPA. Vouhe and associates[30] reported the results in 22 patients less than 4 years of age who underwent coronary reimplantation; there were five early deaths and no late deaths. This group has concluded, as we have, that the mitral valve should rarely, if ever, be replaced at the initial procedure, because mitral regurgitation almost always improves after establishment of a two-coronary system. One of the six long-term surviving patients in our ligation group has required mitral valve replacement 20 months after ligation.

TABLE 19–1. ☐ MORTALITY AFTER REPAIR OF ANOMALOUS LEFT CORONARY FROM THE PULMONARY ARTERY

PROCEDURE	NO. OF PATIENTS	MORTALITY	
		Early	Late
Ligation and ostial closure	11	3	2
Takeuchi procedure	11	0	0
Ligation/coronary artery bypass grafting (saphenous vein)	1	0	0*
Thoracotomy	1	1	—
TOTAL	24	4	2

*Lost to follow-up.

SUMMARY

The regenerative capacity of immature myocardium by hyperplasia in the first months of life mandates early diagnosis and establishment of a dual coronary system for ALCAPA. Although data are limited regarding coronary artery translocation with aortic implantation, we believe this is the procedure of choice. Takeuchi's baffle procedure has resulted in low mortality rates and excellent recovery of ventricular function. Technical details to optimize myocardial protection are of paramount importance to the success of surgery for this rare anomaly.

CORONARY FISTULAE

Isolated congenital coronary artery fistulae are even rarer in our experience than anomalous left coronary artery from the pulmonary artery (ALCAPA). A review in 1989[13] reported a total of only 286 cases collected from the world literature. As in ALCAPA, surgery is potentially curative. Surgery during infancy is exceedingly rare.

PATHOLOGIC ANATOMY

Isolated fistulae arise from both the right and left coronary arteries, probably with similar frequency, but terminate much more commonly in the right heart or pulmonary artery than in the left heart. Lowe and associates[16] reported drainage to the right ventricle in 39%, to the right atrium in 33%, and to the pulmonary artery in 20%; only 2% drained to the left ventricle. In a report in 1983 from the Texas Heart Institute,[29] 58 patients with coronary artery fistulae were described. In five, the fistulae drained into the right atrium from an anomalous artery to the sinus node. In 84% of patients, there was a single fistula, while the remainder had multiple fistulae. Thirty-seven patients had coronary artery fistulae as their only anomaly, while 21 had associated lesions, including coronary artery disease in nine, mitral regurgitation in two, aortic stenosis in two, and double-outlet right ventricle, pulmonary stenosis, patent ductus arteriosus, tricuspid regurgitation, aortic stenosis with mitral regurgitation, and mitral valve prolapse each occurring in one patient.

Coronary artery fistulae are an important component of pulmonary atresia with intact ventricular septum, in which they can be associated with proximal coronary artery stenoses. In this setting, the fistulae may provide the only blood supply (derived from the hypertensive right ventricle) to a significant portion of the left ventricle. Sauer and coworkers[23] suggested that a similar situation may be present in children with mitral stenosis and aortic atresia as part of the hypoplastic left heart syndrome. Both of these conditions, including the significance of associated coronary artery fistulae, are discussed in greater detail in other chapters. Bogers and associates[5] described four patients with tetralogy of Fallot and pulmonary atresia in whom the pulmonary artery circulation was dependent on a fistula from the left main coronary artery. We also encountered this anomaly in four patients during the 1980s, always in the setting of severe hypoplasia of the true pulmonary arteries and dependency on multiple aortopulmonary collaterals.

PATHOPHYSIOLOGY

The flow of blood through the fistula into a low-pressure right heart chamber causes myocardial ischemia, both by producing a coronary steal and by imposing a volume load on the left ventricle. Patients seen after the age of 25 years are almost always symptomatic with angina, congestive heart failure, or palpitations. Shear-induced intimal damage, caused by the high flow in the coronary artery supplying the fistula, may result in premature development of atherosclerosis, as well as aneurysmal dilatation of that artery. The fact that there are acquired as well as congenital aspects of coronary artery fistulae, including the slowly progressive enlargement of fistulae with time, may be responsible for the rarity with which this anomaly is seen during infancy.

PREOPERATIVE EVALUATION AND MEDICAL THERAPY

Preoperative signs and symptoms are dependent on the volume of runoff through the fistula and are unlikely to be impressive in the infant. A continuous murmur is the classic physical finding. The electrocardiogram may be normal, although in 16 of the 58 patients reported by the Texas Heart Institute,[29] there was evidence of myocardial ischemia or recipient chamber overload (atrial or ventricular hypertrophy). Asymptomatic patients usually have a normal cardiothoracic ratio. The sensitivity of two-dimensional echocardiography with color Doppler in defining coronary artery fistulae remains to be defined. Experience in neonates with pulmonary atresia and an intact ventricular septum suggests that this should be a useful method to define coronary artery fistulae, but coronary angiography, with assessment of a left-to-right shunt by oximetric data, remains the gold standard. The details of coronary anatomy are important for designing an operation that will not place at risk a large area of viable myocardium distal to the fistula. This is particularly true of coronary fistulae found in association with pulmonary atresia with an intact ventricular septum.

There is no specific medical therapy for coronary artery fistulae other than management of congestive heart failure, which may have developed secondary to the volume load with or without associated myocardial ischemia. Such therapy should be temporary and should simply optimize the patient's condition before surgical management. Undoubtedly there is a role for interventional catheter techniques; embolization methods and indications are described in Chapter 7.

SURGICAL MANAGEMENT

History

The first report of surgical correction of a coronary artery fistula was by Biorck and Crafoord in 1947.[3] Cardiopulmonary bypass was first employed in conjunction with closure of a fistula as described in the 1959 report by Swan and coworkers.[26]

Indications

It is extremely unusual for coronary artery fistulae to be seen early in life before a significant left-to-right shunt has developed. Thus, the natural history of this lesion is not well known. Lowe and associates[16] described follow-up of one patient for 31 years before surgery was undertaken. During this time he underwent five cardiac catheterizations and progressed from being asymptomatic to having disabling angina and congestive heart failure. The presence of any symptoms or documentation of a measurable left-to-right shunt should almost certainly be an indication for surgery. However, the role of surgery for the patient who is asymptomatic and who has an unmeasurable shunt by oximetry remains to be defined.

Technique

Careful preoperative angiographic definition of the fistula, including its relationship to the coronary artery distal to the fistula, the presence of aneurysmal dilatation of the coronary artery, and the site of entry of the fistula into the heart, is essential. Several surgical options are available, as detailed in the following text.

Suture Ligation Without Cardiopulmonary Bypass

If the fistula arises very distally (e.g., from the distal acute marginal branch of the right coronary artery entering the apex of the right ventricle), it can simply be oversewn. Digital pressure on the fistula before suturing will confirm operative assessment that no myocardium is at risk and that the thrill can be readily abolished. Intraoperative echocardiography may be useful in confirming that the fistula has been obliterated.

Suture ligation has also been successfully employed when the fistula arises laterally from a main coronary trunk. Pledgetted horizontal mattress sutures can be placed under the coronary artery in the area where the thrill is localized (Fig. 19–4).

Closure of a Transcoronary Artery Aneurysm With Cardiopulmonary Bypass

If a large aneurysm is present, it is advisable to perform an aneurysmorrhaphy simultaneously with closure of the fistula. Before establishing bypass, the site of origin of the fistula should be confirmed by digital pressure. After bypass is begun, care must be taken to avoid excessive runoff through the fistula. A short period of aortic crossclamping is necessary, during which time a longitudinal incision is

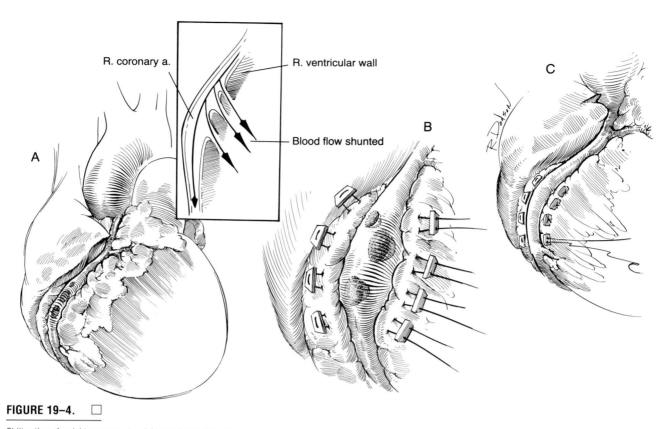

FIGURE 19–4. ☐

Obliteration of a right coronary–to–right ventricular fistula by undersewing. Cardiopulmonary bypass is not required. *A*, Fistulae arise from right coronary artery in A-V groove and pass into right ventricle. *B*, Doubly pledgetted sutures are passed under artery at site of fistulae. *C*, After tying of sutures, palpation confirms obliteration of thrill.

made in the aneurysm of the fistula. The fistula is oversewn from within the aneurysm, which is then appropriately tailored during closure (Fig. 19–5).

Transcardiac Chamber Closure With Cardiopulmonary Bypass

If an important area of myocardium is supplied distal to the origin of a fistula—particularly if external identification of the fistula is difficult or there are multiple fistulae—approach from within the appropriate cardiac chamber is indicated. Identification of the fistulous orifice can be confirmed by delivery of cardioplegic solution. Likewise, the security of the closure, generally by pledgetted horizontal mattress sutures, can be confirmed by release of the aortic crossclamp. Some prefer not to clamp the aorta, simply relying on blood flow through the fistula to identify it (Fig. 19–6).

RESULTS

Both early and late mortality should be low. Liberthson and associates[15] reported a 4% early mortal-

ity rate in a review of 173 patients. Delaying treatment until later in life can result in aneurysmal and atherosclerotic changes and can increase the risk of infarction and death.

The risk of recurrence is also extremely low. Lowe and colleagues[16] found no recurrent fistulae in 22 patients for 10 years after closure.

We have had no experience with surgery for coronary artery fistulae in infants. Experience with interventional catheter methods is described in Chapter 7.

SUMMARY

The advent of color Doppler two-dimensional echocardiography may improve our understanding of the natural history of coronary artery fistulae. With our present understanding, however, it would seem appropriate to recommend surgery for all but the smallest fistulae, as surgery can be performed with extremely low risk and is essentially curative.

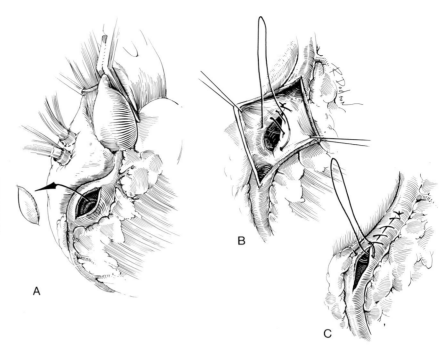

FIGURE 19–5. □

A, Approach to a right coronary–to–right ventricular fistula through a right coronary aneurysm. Part of the anterior wall of the aneurysm is excised as part of an aneurysmorrhaphy. *B*, Direct suture closure of the fistula working within the coronary aneurysm. *C*, Direct suture closure of the right coronary artery as part of an aneurysmorrhaphy.

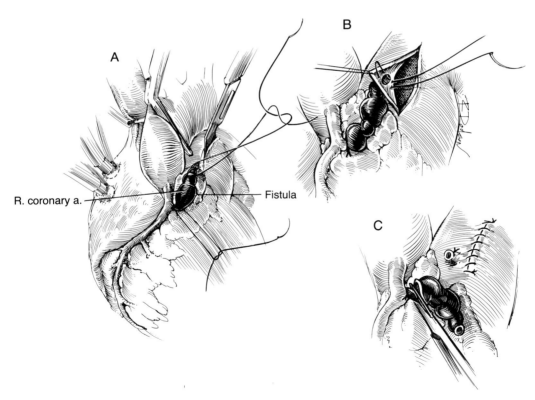

R. coronary a.

Fistula

FIGURE 19–6. □

Surgical management of a right coronary artery–to–pulmonary artery fistula. *A*, Cardiopulmonary bypass is employed. The fistula is ligated proximally; and the main pulmonary artery is opened. *B*, The entrance of the fistula into the main pulmonary artery is oversewn from within the pulmonary artery. *C*, Excision of the right coronary–to–pulmonary artery fistula.

ABERRANT LEFT CORONARY ARTERY ORIGINATING FROM THE AORTA WITH NORMAL INTRACARDIAC ANATOMY

Many anatomic variants of aberrant left coronary artery have been described. However, it would seem that an aberrant coronary artery originating from the aorta has clinical consequences only when the left main coronary artery passes between the aorta and the pulmonary artery. There are several reports of sudden death associated with exercise in patients with such anatomy.

PATHOLOGIC ANATOMY

The left main coronary artery arises as a single trunk with the right coronary artery from the anterior sinus of Valsalva. It passes posteriorly and leftward between the pulmonary artery and the aorta before dividing into the circumflex and left anterior descending arteries. Cheitlin and coworkers[7] noted that the course of the left coronary artery may be "actually incorporated in the wall of the aorta. The coronary artery and the aorta share the same media without any adventitia separating them." This is a perfect description of the "intramural coronary artery" that is occasionally encountered in association with transposition of the great arteries.

PATHOPHYSIOLOGY

Several authors[2, 7, 8, 15] have postulated that the increased cardiac output associated with exercise results in compression of the left coronary artery between the aorta and the pulmonary artery, thereby causing left ventricular ischemia. In addition, the ostium is often slit-like. Dilatation of the aorta associated with exercise may result in the slit-like ostium actually being occluded by a flap-like closure of the orifice.

PREOPERATIVE EVALUATION AND MEDICAL THERAPY

There are several reports of coronary angiography identification of an aberrant origin and course of the left main coronary artery. No medical therapy is available.

SURGICAL MANAGEMENT

History

Although anomalous origin of the left coronary artery from the aorta has been described as a benign anomaly in several reviews of coronary anatomy,[14, 20] case reports in the 1960s[2, 8] suggested that such an anomaly could be the cause of sudden death in young people. In 1974 Cheitlin and coworkers[7] described 51 patients in whom both coronary arteries arose from the same sinus of Valsalva. In 33 of these, both coronaries arose from the anterior sinus and passed between the aorta and the pulmonary artery. Nine of these patients died suddenly between the ages of 13 and 36 years; death was generally related to exercise. They also described surgery in a 14-year-old boy who had been successfully resuscitated from ventricular fibrillation. In 1974 he underwent enlargement of a slit-like orifice of the left coronary artery; others have recommended coronary artery bypass surgery for this anomaly.[15, 24]

Indications

It is highly unlikely that this very rare anomaly will be identified during infancy. In the older child or adult, surgery is justified by the high risk of sudden death.

Technical Considerations

We have had no experience with this anomaly in infants. However, the principles learned from the arterial switch procedure could likely be applied to this anomaly. In general, for intramural left coronary arteries associated with transposition, it has been possible to separate the right and left coronary ostia and to transfer the left coronary in the usual fashion, except that particularly fine sutures must be placed along one side of the button where the ostium itself abuts the edge of the button. It may be necessary to implant the left coronary relatively distally in the aorta to allow for the length of the vessel that previously ran between the aorta and pulmonary artery. As with any coronary transfer, complete mobilization is necessary to avoid kinking or other distortion. Coronary artery bypass surgery, preferably using the internal mammary artery, may be more appropriate in the older child and adult, in whom tissue elasticity and pliability are less than in the young child.

REFERENCES

1. Becker AE, Anderson RH. Pathology of Congenital Heart Disease. London, Butterworths, 1981, p 369.
2. Benson PA, Lack AR. Anomalous aortic origin of left coronary artery. Arch Pathol 86:214, 1968.
3. Biorck G, Crafoord C. Arteriovenous aneurysm on the pulmonary artery simulating patent ductus arteriosus botalli. Thorax 2:65, 1947.
4. Bland EF, White PD, Garland J. Congenital anomalies of the coronary arteries; report of an unusual case associated with cardiac hypertrophy. Am Heart J 8:787, 1933.
5. Bogers AJJC, Rohmer J, Wolsky SAE, et al. Coronary artery fistula as source of pulmonary circulation in pulmonary atresia with ventricular septal defect. Thorac Cardiovasc Surg 38:30, 1990.
6. Bunton R, Jonas RA, Lang P, et al. Anomalous origin of left coronary artery from pulmonary artery. J Thorac Cardiovasc Surg 93:103, 1987.
7. Cheitlin MD, DeCastro CM, McAllister HA. Sudden death as a complication of anomalous left coronary origin from the anterior sinus of Valsalva. Circulation 50:780, 1974.
8. Cohen LS, Shaw LD. Fatal myocardial infarction in an 11 year old boy associated with a unique coronary artery anomaly. Am J Cardiol 19:420, 1967.
9. Cottrill CM, Davis D, McMillen M, et al. Anomalous left coronary artery from the pulmonary artery: Significance of associated intracardiac defects. J Am Coll Cardiol 6:237, 1985.
10. Driscoll DJ, Nihill MR, Mullins CE, et al. Management of symptomatic infants with anomalous origin of the left coronary artery from the pulmonary artery. Am J Cardiol 47:642, 1981.
11. Edwards JE. The direction of blood flow in coronary arteries arising from the pulmonary trunk. Circulation 29:163, 1964.
12. Ihenacho HNC, Sing SP, Astley R, et al. Anomalous left coronary artery: Report of an unusual case with spontaneous remission of symptoms. Br Heart J 35:562, 1973.
13. Karagoz HY, Zorlutuna YI, Babagan KM, et al. Congenital coronary artery fistulas: Diagnostic and surgical considerations. Jpn Heart J 30:685, 1989.
14. Laurie W, Woods JD. Single coronary artery. Am Heart J 67:95, 1964.
15. Liberthson RR, Dinsmore RE, Bharati S, et al. Aberrant coronary artery origin from the aorta: Diagnosis and clinical significance. Circulation 50:774, 1974.
16. Lowe JE, Oldham HN, Sabiston DC. Surgical management of congenital coronary artery fistulas. Ann Surg 194:373, 1981.
17. Masel LF. Tetralogy of Fallot with origin of the left coronary from the right pulmonary artery. Med J Aust 1:213, 1960.
18. Menahem S, Venables AW. Anomalous left coronary artery from the pulmonary artery: A 15 year sample. Br Heart J 58:378, 1987.
19. Midgley FM, Watson DC, Scott LP, et al. Repair of anomalous origin of the left coronary artery in the infant and small child. J Am Coll Cardiol 4:1231, 1984.
20. Ogden JA. Congenital anomalies of the coronary arteries. Am J Cardiol 25:474, 1970.
21. Ortiz E, deLeval M, Somerville J. Ductus arteriosus associated with an anomalous left coronary artery arising from the pulmonary artery: Catastrophe after duct ligation. Br Heart J 55:415, 1986.
22. Rein AJJT, Colan SD, Parness IA, et al. Regional and global left ventricular function in infants with anomalous origin of the left coronary artery from the pulmonary trunk: Preoperative and postoperative assessment. Circulation 75:115, 1987.
23. Sauer U, Gittenberger-de Groot AC, Gieshauser M, et al. Coronary arteries in the hypoplastic left heart syndrome. Circulation 80(suppl I):168, 1989.
24. Scully RE (ed). Case Records of the Massachusetts General Hospital, Case 22-1989. N Engl J Med 320:1475, 1989.
25. Smith A, Arnold R, Anderson RH, et al. Anomalous origin of the left coronary artery from the pulmonary trunk. J Thorac Cardiovasc Surg 98:16, 1989.
26. Swan H, Wilson JH, Woodwark G, et al. Surgical obliteration of a coronary artery fistula to right ventricle. Arch Surg 79:820, 1959.
27. Takeuchi S, Imamura H, Katsumoto K, et al. New surgical method for repair of anomalous left coronary artery from pulmonary artery. J Thorac Cardiovasc Surg 78:7, 1979.
28. Tyrrell MJ, Duncan WJ, Hayton RC, et al. Anomalous left coronary artery from the pulmonary artery: Effect of coronary anatomy on clinical course. Angiology 38:833, 1987.
29. Urrutia-S CO, Falaschi G, Ott DA, et al. Surgical management of 56 patients with congenital coronary artery fistulas. Ann Thorac Surg 35:300, 1983.
30. Vouhe PR, Baillot-Vernant F, Trinquet F, et al. Anomalous left coronary artery from the pulmonary artery in infants. J Thorac Cardiovasc Surg 94:192, 1987.
31. Wilcox WD, Hagler DJ, Lie JT, et al. Anomalous origin of left coronary artery from pulmonary artery in association with intracardiac lesions: Report of two cases. J Thorac Cardiovasc Surg 78:12, 1979.
32. Wright NL, Baue AE, Baum S, et al. Coronary artery steal due to an anomalous left coronary artery originating from the pulmonary artery. J Thorac Cardiovasc Surg 59:461, 1980.

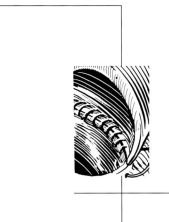

20

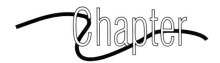

Obstruction of the Left Ventricular Outflow Tract

Impedance to ventricular ejection can occur from obstruction at various levels along the transition from the left ventricular cavity to the ascending aorta. Traditionally, these levels have been categorized as subvalvar, valvar, and supravalvar, a scheme that will be followed in this chapter. Although helpful from an organizational standpoint, this categorical approach is nevertheless somewhat simplistic when dealing with obstruction of the left ventricular outflow tract in infants, as the obstruction is commonly at more than one level in the same patient.

This chapter will consider left ventricular outflow obstruction requiring intervention in the neonatal and infancy periods and therefore will deal with only a small fraction of the patients who have this lesion. This small fraction, however, consists of those with the most severe forms of the disease. An effort will be made to give some perspective as to where the neonatal and infant forms fit into the overall spectrum of the lesion. Obstruction of the left ventricular outflow tract associated with the hypoplastic left heart syndrome, interrupted aortic arch, single ventricle with small bulboventricular foramen, and transposed or malposed great vessels will not be discussed in this chapter.

It should be emphasized that the spectrum of obstruction of the left ventricular outflow tract includes isolated valvar aortic stenosis at one end and the hypoplastic left heart syndrome at the other. Whether to consider the patient as having the hypoplastic left heart syndrome (thus requiring staged palliation for single-ventricle physiology) or as having multiple left-sided, obstructive, hypoplastic lesions but being capable of achieving a two-ventricle physiology is a complex decision and involves much more than simply considering the size of the left ventricular cavity. This issue has been addressed at Children's Hospital in Boston,[56] and the conclusions emphasize the importance of multifactorial assessment in determining the appropriateness of two-ventricle physiology in these borderline cases.

315

DEFINITION

Of the various types of obstruction of the left ventricular outflow tract, valvar aortic stenosis is the only one in which a distinct clinical entity is present in neonates and infants. The spectrum of aortic valve abnormalities represents the most common form of congenital heart disease, with the great majority of patients being asymptomatic until midlife (e.g., those with isolated bicuspid aortic valve). When aortic stenosis occurs in the neonatal or early infancy period, it is commonly referred to as *neonatal critical aortic stenosis*. This form of the lesion accounts for less than 10% of congenital aortic stenosis.[5] It usually consists of abnormalities in the number and thickness of the cusps, in commissure development, and in cross-sectional area and is accompanied by other left-sided cardiac abnormalities. These include abnormalities of the mitral valve and ventricular cavity, the subaortic region, the aortic arch, and the aortic isthmus.

MORPHOLOGY

The critically stenotic aortic valve in the neonate or infant is usually unicommissural or bicommissural, with thickened, dysmorphic, and myxomatous leaflet tissue and a reduced cross-sectional area at the valve level. In a review of 32 cases from Children's Hospital in Boston,[71] 19 (59%) of the valves had one commissure, and 13 (41%) had two. The diameter of the ventriculoarterial junction ranged from 4.5 to 8 mm (mean, 6.1 ± 1 mm). The valve tissue was dysmorphic in all cases. When patients are seen later in infancy or childhood, the incidence of bicommissural valves increases. Typically, in bicommissural valves, the two commissures are oriented in the anterior and posterior positions, with left and right leaflets. There is variable fusion of the commissures, but usually the most significant fusion is in the anterior commissure.[64, 69] Endocardial fibroelastosis is also common among neonates.[35] The left ventricle is usually markedly hypertrophied, with a smaller cavity than normal, although occasionally a dilated ventricle is encountered.

Associated lesions occurred frequently in 28 of these 32 patients (88%). Table 20–1 shows the incidence of specific lesions. The concept of concurrent, multiple left-sided lesions is an important one to appreciate with regard to neonatal obstruction of the left ventricular outflow tract. The classic description by Shone and associates[63] of the complex consisting of supramitral ring, single mitral papillary muscle, subaortic membrane, and coarctation underscores this concept. Although only a small number of neonates and infants with critical valvar aortic stenosis will have all of these associated abnormalities, many will have some associated left-sided obstructive lesions, or various degrees of hypoplasia of the left ventricle, or both.

PATHOPHYSIOLOGY AND NATURAL HISTORY

During fetal life, even critical aortic stenosis is not usually a life-threatening lesion. The obstruction to left ventricular ejection causes left ventricular hypertrophy, hypertension, and, in the most severe cases, ischemia. Left ventricular systolic and diastolic dysfunction occurs, resulting in mitral regurgitation and left atrial hypertension, with markedly reduced right-to-left flow (or possibly even left-to-right flow) across the patent foramen ovale. Increased right ventricular volume loading thus occurs, and the right ventricle maintains cardiac output via the patent ductus arteriosus. As a result, cardiac output and fetal development in general are not significantly compromised. However, the left ventricle may suffer profound injury with the mismatch between intracavitary left ventricular pressure and coronary perfusion pressure, resulting in severe left ventricular dysfunction, infarction, and subendocardial fibroelastosis. The significance of this insult is realized after the transition from fetal life to independent existence, when the left ventricle must provide the systemic cardiac output. The postnatal physiologic effects depend on the degree of left ventricular functional compromise and on the completeness of the transition from fetal to in-series circulation (i.e., on closure of the patent foramen ovale and the patent ductus arteriosus).

Patients with mild-to-moderate aortic stenosis in which left ventricular function is not compromised are physiologically normal at birth, manifesting

TABLE 20–1. □ NEONATAL CRITICAL VALVAR AORTIC STENOSIS: ASSOCIATED LESIONS (*N* = 32)

LESION	NO.	%
Patent ductus arteriosus	17	53
Coarctation	3	9
Mitral regurgitation	19	59
Hypoplastic left ventricle	9	28

only a systolic ejection murmur and electrocardiographic evidence of left ventricular hypertrophy. The transition to an in-series circulation will have no consequences. Increasingly severe stenosis will result in increasingly severe left ventricular failure, with left atrial hypertension and pulmonary hypertension. If the patent foramen ovale becomes incompetent (or if an atrial septal defect is present), left-to-right atrial level flow will occur. As long as the ductus arteriosus remains open, circulatory collapse will not occur, as the systemic perfusion will be compensated by ductal flow from the right ventricle. However, cyanosis will be present. Depending on the amount of cardiac output supplied by the left ventricle as forward flow across the aortic valve, there may be discernible differential cyanosis between the upper and lower body. When the ductus arteriosus closes, circulatory compromise develops with dyspnea and tachypnea, irritability, extreme pallor, narrowed pulse pressure, oliguria, and metabolic acidosis.

Aortic valve stenosis accounts for about 5% of congenital heart disease, with critical stenosis in neonates and infants accounting for only about 10% of those cases.[5] At Children's Hospital in Boston, 36 cases of critical aortic stenosis in the neonate or young infant were evaluated between 1982 and 1991; the condition occurs predominantly in males, with a male-to-female ratio of approximately 3:1 or 4:1.

DIAGNOSIS AND INDICATIONS FOR SURGERY

Neonates or infants with critical aortic stenosis are either reasonably well compensated with transitional cardiovascular physiology or, if the ductus arteriosus has closed, have signs of circulatory collapse as described previously. A history of poor feeding is typical in patients not identified immediately after birth. A systolic ejection murmur is usually present but may disappear if left ventricular failure progresses. In infants, the electrocardiogram typically indicates left ventricular hypertrophy and may also show right ventricular hypertrophy. The chest radiograph shows cardiomegaly and pulmonary congestion.

Echocardiography usually can confirm the specific diagnosis of valvar aortic stenosis and also can identify associated lesions and assess the status of the left ventricular myocardium with regard to contractile function and endocardial fibroelastosis.[24, 26] The gradient across the valve can be estimated relatively accurately by Doppler studies; however, the gradient may not accurately reflect the severity of stenosis when the left ventricle is not functioning

well, when left-to-right interatrial shunts are present, or when the ductus arteriosus is open. Echocardiography can also identify this lesion prenatally.[25]

Cardiac catheterization is performed routinely, both for diagnostic evaluation and for therapeutic intervention. Access is initially attempted from the umbilical artery in infants less than 72 hours old; otherwise, it is attempted from the femoral artery.[71] A critical coarctation may present difficulties with this approach, and others have reported successful access through the carotid artery.[19] Complete right and left heart catheterization is carried out to obtain the peak-to-peak systolic ejection gradient, left ventricular end-diastolic pressure, and right-sided pressures. Biplane cineangiography is used to assess aortic regurgitation, aortic annulus size, and left ventricular volume and contractility, and to help identify associated lesions. In Zeevi and co-workers' series,[71] the peak systolic ejection gradient ranged from 10 to 130 mm Hg; left ventricular end-diastolic pressure, from 8 to 28 mm Hg; and left ventricular end-diastolic volume, from 30% to 202% of normal (10.4 to 69.0 ml/m²; mean, 32 ml/m²). The angiographic ejection fraction ranged from 23% to 73% (mean, 37%). There were no cases of preintervention aortic regurgitation.

For neonates and infants, intervention is indicated to relieve the obstruction. In neonates who are in circulatory collapse, a period of hours to days may be necessary to resuscitate the patient using prostaglandin E_1 to open the ductus arteriosus before intervention is undertaken.[29] In older infants, a gradient of more than 50 mm Hg or symptoms attributable to the aortic stenosis are indications for intervention.

MANAGEMENT

Historical Perspective

In 1910, Alexis Carrel performed experimental surgery using a conduit from the apex of the left ventricle to the aorta as a means of addressing left ventricular outflow obstruction.[6] In 1912, Tuffier approached the lesion directly, performing successful transaortic digital dilatation in a young man with aortic stenosis.[68] More than 40 years passed before any additional significant advance occurred. In 1953, Larzelere and Bailey performed a closed surgical commissurotomy.[37] In 1955, Marquis and Logan performed closed surgical dilatation of a stenotic aortic valve using antegrade introduction of dilators via an incision in the left ventricular apex.[45] Inflow occlusion with open valvotomy was reported in 1956 by both Lewis and Swan and their associates.[38, 67] Also in 1956, Lillehei and colleagues performed an aortic valvotomy using cardiopulmonary bypass.[39] All of these milestones were achieved in patients well beyond infancy. In 1969, Coran and Bernhard, at Children's Hospital in Boston, reported on surgical relief of critical aortic stenosis focusing solely on neonates and infants, with cases dating back to 1960.[12]

Percutaneous balloon aortic valvotomy was described in 1984 by Lababidi and coworkers,[34] and its use specifically in infants was reported in 1985 by Rupprath and Neuhaus[58] and by Sanchez and associates.[59] Balloon valvuloplasty for neonatal critical aortic stenosis was described by Lababidi and Weinhaus in 1986.[33] At Children's Hospital in Boston, percutaneous balloon valvotomy for critical aortic stenosis in neonates and infants was begun in 1985. A comparison of surgical and percutaneous techniques reported from that institution in 1989 indicated comparable immediate and intermediate results.[71] At the present time, percutaneous balloon valvuloplasty is our procedure of choice.

Preintervention Management

Resuscitation of a neonate after circulatory collapse is often necessary.[29] The principles include administration of intravenous prostaglandin E_1 to open or maintain patency of the ductus arteriosus, pharmacologic neuromuscular blockade and mechanical ventilation, inotropic support, and use of sodium bicarbonate to reverse metabolic acidosis. Details of the resuscitative effort and the timing of intervention are similar to those described for critical aortic coarctation in the neonate (see Chapter 21).

Technique

Percutaneous Balloon Valvuloplasty. After premedication with morphine sulfate, local anesthesia (1% lidocaine [Xylocaine]) is used at the site of percutaneous vascular access. The preferred site is the umbilical artery in newborns; however, if this is not possible, or for older neonates and infants, the femoral artery is routinely used. A No. 3.2 French or a No. 4 French cutoff pigtail catheter is used for peripheral cannulation, and heparin is given (100 U per kilogram of body weight). A soft guide wire initially is passed across the aortic valve to avoid valve damage, followed by the pigtail catheter. A larger bore guide wire is then exchanged through the pigtail catheter. In neonates, a 4- to 5-mm, low-profile,

balloon dilatation catheter is then exchanged for the pigtail catheter and passed retrograde across the aortic valve. Accurate assessment of the position of the valve orifice by echocardiography, angiography, or both is important to avoid valve damage. Balloons with diameters about 90% of the diameter of the annulus are used. Balloon diameters approaching or exceeding the diameter of the annulus have caused significant aortic regurgitation in experimental procedures.[23] Careful control of inflation pressure by hand (usually 3 to 8 atm) is used to vary the actual balloon diameter. Two to four 15-second inflation-deflation cycles are performed with withdrawal of the balloon to the descending aorta between cycles. Criteria for success include initial gradient reduction, reduction in left ventricular end-diastolic pressure, mild or no valve regurgitation, and clinical improvement. In neonates, objective evidence of the result is often not immediately available either by postdilatation angiography or by hemodynamics, because the gradient may gradually increase as the ventricular function improves after dilatation.

Surgical Valvotomy. At Children's Hospital in Boston, we have not found it necessary to perform surgical aortic valvotomy in neonates or young infants since the introduction of percutaneous valvuloplasty in 1985. Before this time, our preferred approach was open valvotomy, using normothermic inflow occlusion.[28] Others have recommended open surgical valvotomy using cardiopulmonary bypass support[47] or closed surgical valvotomy via left ventricular access.[5]

Our approach involves a median sternotomy, stay sutures in the ascending aorta, and a partially occluding side-biting clamp on the aorta (Fig. 20–1). A longitudinal incision is made in the tissue sequestered by the clamp. After 5 minutes of ventilation

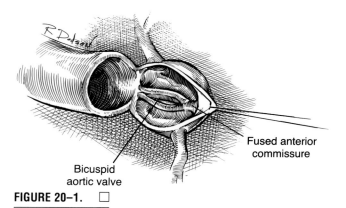

Fused anterior commissure

Bicuspid aortic valve

FIGURE 20–1. ☐

Technique for open surgical aortic valvotomy. The aortic incision is shown. Valvotomy is performed at the site of the fused commissure, but in severely deformed valves, commissures may not be identifiable.

with 100% oxygen, the cavae are occluded using fine vascular clamps, the heart is allowed to beat five or six times, and the distal ascending aorta is cross-clamped. The side-biting clamp is removed, and the valve is visualized through the longitudinal incision. A conservative valvotomy is made using a No. 11 bladed knife, preferably in the fused anterior commissure, extending the opening to within 1 to 2 mm of the annulus. Because of the dysmorphic nature of these valves, however, discrete commissures often cannot be discerned, in which case a small central valvotomy is performed. Careful attention should be given to avoid an extensive valvotomy, as the regurgitation that may develop is poorly tolerated. Resistance at the valve level is inversely proportional to the fourth power of the radius of the orifice; therefore, a seemingly conservative valvotomy will produce a satisfactory clinical result. After the valvotomy, the inferior vena caval clamp is released, allowing the heart to fill and thereby venting air from the heart and aorta via the longitudinal incision. The side-biting clamp is then replaced to encompass the aortotomy, and the distal crossclamp is removed. The superior vena caval clamp is then removed, and the heart is resuscitated. Usually the heart continues to beat through the 1- to 2-minute period in which the inflow occlusion is maintained. After stabilization the longitudinal aortotomy is repaired, and the side-biting clamp is removed.

RESULTS

Percutaneous Balloon Valvuloplasty

In 38 consecutive neonates and young infants ranging in age from 1 to 120 days (median, 9 days) who underwent balloon aortic valvuloplasty between 1984 and 1992 at Children's Hospital in Boston, there were 13 peri-interventional deaths (34%). In the 25 patients less than 30 days old, there were 12 deaths (48%). Discriminant analysis of this experience (which also included some patients who had undergone surgical valvotomy before 1985) has indicated four morphologic variables that are predictive of death after attempted relief of valvar obstruction: a left ventricular long axis–to–heart long axis ratio of less than or equal to 0.8; an indexed aortic root diameter less than or equal to 3.5 cm/m²; an indexed mitral valve area less than or equal to 4.75 cm/m²; and a left ventricular mass index of less than 35 gm/m².[71] The mortality rate was 100% in patients with two or more of these risk factors and 8% in patients with one or no risk factors. This analysis suggests that death after relief of aortic stenosis is more related to patient selection than to

the procedure per se. Underdevelopment of multiple left-sided cardiac structures is associated with increasing mortality if patients are managed as having two-ventricle physiology.

Surgical Valvotomy

From 1972 to 1984, 21 patients underwent surgical valvotomy at Children's Hospital in Boston using normothermic inflow occlusion. Nine of these were neonates, and 12 were infants.[28] (During the same period, more than 200 patients older than 12 months who had aortic valve stenosis underwent open commissurotomy using cardiopulmonary bypass.) In the group of 21 neonates and young infants, there were four hospital deaths (19%), all in patients less than 5 weeks of age. The cause of death was persistent low cardiac output. In only one patient was aortic regurgitation contributory. Six patients required reoperation during intermediate follow-up (27 months; range, 1 to 84 months). One survivor had persistent low cardiac output and underwent successful stage 1 palliation as described for the hypoplastic left heart syndrome. Another had a conduit placed between the left ventricular apex and the aorta for persistent aortic stenosis, while another required a second aortic valvotomy. Two patients underwent coarctation repair, and one underwent mitral valve replacement. Significant aortic regurgitation was not found during follow-up, and there were no intermediate-term deaths.

Of historical interest, between 1979 and 1982, nine infants (age 3 days to 13 months) underwent placement of valved conduits between the left ventricular apex and the descending aorta for various forms of aortic stenosis.[53] Although there were only two early deaths, late follow-up revealed two late deaths, as well as significant technical problems at reoperation. At the present time there are no indications for this operation at our institution.

SUMMARY

Various techniques have been used to relieve critical aortic stenosis in the neonate and young infant. These include closed transventricular surgical dilatation with dilators or balloons, percutaneous catheter dilatation, open valvotomy using inflow occlusion with or without moderate hypothermia, and open valvotomy using cardiopulmonary bypass with or without the use of cardioplegia or hypothermia. When discussing outcome, many of these reports have focused on differences among support and technique variables used to accomplish relief of the obstruction. In reality, patient selection is probably the predominant factor in determining differences among various reported series. If patients with significant underdevelopment of multiple left-sided structures are excluded—leaving only patients who can tolerate two-ventricle physiology—survival after relief of critical aortic valve stenosis, using any one of various techniques, is likely to be in the range of 80% to 90%. Further refinements in the assessment of multiple morphologic characteristics will allow more appropriate identification of patients who will be best served by the maintenance of two-ventricle cardiovascular systems.

Percutaneous balloon valvuloplasty appears to achieve acute relief of aortic valve stenosis without producing significant aortic regurgitation as effectively as open surgical techniques. At the present time, this is our procedure of choice. Further follow-up will be necessary to determine whether long-term differences between open valvotomy and closed valvuloplasty techniques will have clinical importance.

Finally, two groups have introduced refinements in open surgical valvotomy (i.e., extended commissurotomy[48] and extended aortic valvuloplasty).[27] It remains to be seen whether these techniques will offer advantages over more established surgical and percutaneous techniques.

SUBVALVAR AORTIC STENOSIS

DEFINITION

Obstruction of the left ventricular outflow tract that occurs below the aortic valve constitutes subaortic stenosis. Subaortic stenosis is a distinct clinical entity in older patients but not in neonates and infants. In these younger patients, isolated subaortic stenosis is rare and of variable etiology. In this chapter, only two-ventricle hearts with concordant ventriculoarterial connection and a normally aligned conal septum will be considered.

The most common form of subaortic obstruction of the left ventricular outflow tract—discrete fibromuscular obstruction—is rarely seen in infants. This lesion almost certainly has an embryologic basis; however, it usually remains subclinical until after the first year of life. In neonates and infants, other origins of subaortic stenosis include abnormal mitral valve attachments impinging on the left ventricular outflow tract, space-occupying lesions such as endocardial cushion remnants and tumors, and rare cases of hypertrophic cardiomyopathy. Therefore, each case of clinically significant subaortic stenosis in the neonate or infant is quite distinct, representing either a very rare lesion or an unusual variant of a more common lesion.

MORPHOLOGY

Fibromuscular Obstruction

Fibromuscular obstruction represents a spectrum ranging from a thin membrane of fibrous tissue, to a thicker fibromuscular ridge, to an elongated fibrous tunnel. It can be found anywhere in the space between the base of the anterior mitral valve leaflet and the bottom of the aortic valve leaflets. The area of aortomitral continuity may be elongated in this lesion,[57] possibly representing a substrate for later development of obstructive tissue. Although the aortic valve is usually trileaflet, the diameter of the valve may be smaller than normal. Thickening of the aortic valve cusps can occur and is thought to be acquired secondary to turbulence created by the subaortic abnormality. Associated lesions are common with fibromuscular stenosis, occurring in about one third of these patients. However, the frequency of associated lesions is inversely related to the age at presentation. Associated lesions include coarctation, interrupted aortic arch, ventricular septal defect, and atrioventricular canal defects. Subaortic stenosis is one of the four components of the complex of multiple left-sided obstructive lesions described by Shone et al.[63] In the 119 patients with fibromuscular subaortic stenosis diagnosed in infancy at Children's Hospital in Boston between 1972 and 1992, 105 (88%) had associated lesions.

Hypertrophic Cardiomyopathy

Hypertrophic cardiomyopathy is a self-descriptive term that refers to lesions with a number of different etiologies. The primary form of the disease is the most common form. It has no known stimulus and appears to follow autosomal dominant transmission.[7] Histologically, a disorganized arrangement of bizarrely shaped, hypertrophied myocytes characteristically develops in an asymmetric pattern, particularly in the ventricular septum.[42] When the hypertrophy leads to obstruction of left ventricular outflow, it has been called *idiopathic hypertrophic subaortic stenosis* (IHSS). Clinical symptoms are thought to occur in only a small portion of patients who harbor the genetic defect. The symptoms of obstruction usually develop in the second and third decades of life; rarely, they can occur in infants.[43]

The hypertrophy can occur in any portion of the left ventricle, but typically it occurs in the ventricular septum at its most basal aspect, thereby producing subaortic stenosis. It may also occur in the midportion of the septum (producing a double-chambered left ventricle or hourglass obstruction)[18] or more apically (producing cavity obliteration at this point).[62] When the hypertrophy is in the typical basal portion of the septum, it is accompanied by systolic anterior motion of the mitral anterior leaflet.[61]

In infants and neonates, hypertrophic cardiomyopathy, including asymmetric septal hypertrophy, can have origins other than the genetically transmitted primary form. A very similar lesion associated with various structural congenital heart defects can be seen in young patients.[40] In this setting the hypertrophy often seems to regress within the first several years of life.[36] Hypertrophic cardiomyopathy can also be present in approximately 30% of neonates born to mothers with insulin-dependent diabetes.[21] This also appears to be a transient lesion and regresses in the first 6 to 12 months of life. Finally, hypertrophic cardiomyopathy has been reported in infants and children after the chronic use of steroids or adrenocorticotropic hormone (ACTH).[70]

Other Causes

A number of unusual space-occupying lesions, such as endocardial cushion tissue excrescences, can cause subaortic stenosis in neonates and infants.

Various forms of subaortic obstruction of the left ventricular outflow tract have been described in patients with atrioventricular canal defects (especially those without Down syndrome)[13] and in those with partial atrioventricular canal defects.[17] The presence of an anterolateral left ventricular muscle bundle between the superior bridging leaflet and the left coronary cusp, as described by Moulaert,[49] is common in atrioventricular canal defects. Also, anterior displacement of the left atrioventricular valve, malattachment of papillary muscles or

chords, and the presence of accessory left or right atrioventricular valve tissue[3, 11, 22, 50, 60] have been described in addition to the more usual fibromuscular forms of subaortic stenosis in atrioventricular canal defects.

PATHOPHYSIOLOGY AND NATURAL HISTORY

Fibromuscular Obstruction

The basic pathophysiology induced by the various fibromuscular forms of subaortic stenosis is essentially identical to the pathophysiology of valvar aortic stenosis (i.e., there is fixed obstruction to left ventricular outflow below the level of the coronary ostia). Because fibromuscular subaortic stenosis is rarely seen in the neonatal period, the more complex pathophysiology associated with the transitional circulation described previously for neonatal critical valvar aortic stenosis is usually not encountered. The turbulence caused by subaortic stenosis can cause thickening and distortion of the aortic valve leaflets, leading to the development of aortic regurgitation.[52] Again, this occurs in older patients. Although it is not unusual for this lesion to be diagnosed in infants, it rarely requires surgical intervention in infancy. The incidence of clinically significant lesions begins to become apparent in the first few years of life and peaks in adolescence.

Hypertrophic Cardiomyopathy

The pathophysiology of obstruction in hypertrophic cardiomyopathy has been extensively studied; however, the applicability of this knowledge to infants is questionable. Although hypertrophic cardiomyopathy has been documented to be present at birth and frequently has a genetic basis, clinical manifestation of this form of subaortic stenosis is most common in adolescence and young adulthood. The genetically transmitted form of hypertrophic cardiomyopathy with obstruction in infancy has been documented but is unusual.[41]

When primary hypertrophic cardiomyopathy (i.e., that not associated with diabetes mellitus or structural congenital heart lesions) causes clinical symptoms in infancy, the natural history is unfavorable. The clinical picture is atypical compared with that in the more common older patient. Congestive heart failure is common, and right ventricular outflow obstruction is frequently present, as is obstruction of the left ventricular outflow tract. Right ventricular hypertrophy often develops, and right-to-left shunting across a patent foramen ovale may result in cyanosis. The diagnosis is often difficult to make in neonates and infants. Typically, a heart murmur is detected, and a presumptive diagnosis of structural congenital heart disease is made. Sudden death appears to be less common in symptomatic infants than in older patients; the mode of death in infants is often progressive congestive heart failure. The onset of congestive heart failure in infancy was associated with death in nine of 11 infants in one series.[43] Medical management with propranolol and calcium channel blockers has been cautiously recommended in these unusual patients.

In contrast, the natural history of hypertrophic cardiomyopathy related to maternal diabetes mellitus is more favorable, with regression occurring within the first year of life. The natural history of hypertrophic cardiomyopathy associated with structural congenital heart defects is also more favorable, with regression occurring over several years. The influence of correction of the structural heart defects on this regression has not been studied.

DIAGNOSIS AND INDICATIONS FOR SURGERY

Fibromuscular Obstruction

Symptoms related to fibromuscular forms of subaortic stenosis are similar to those caused by valvar aortic stenosis. It is difficult to distinguish between these two lesions by physical examination; prominent findings consist of a systolic ejection murmur and a peripheral pulse with a slow upstroke. Electrocardiographic findings indicate left ventricular hypertrophy, and the chest radiograph may be normal unless associated lesions are present. Two-dimensional echocardiography can identify the structural lesion quite reliably. It can also document left ventricular hypertrophy, assess left ventricular function, and identify associated lesions. Doppler studies will indicate the size of the gradient across the obstruction. Cardiac catheterization should be performed if surgical intervention is being considered. Indications for surgery in all forms of subaortic stenosis in infants are similar to those for valvar aortic stenosis (i.e., symptoms or obstructive gradients greater than 50 mm Hg). At present, the development of aortic regurgitation, even in a mild form, is an indication for surgical correction of subaortic stenosis.

Hypertrophic Cardiomyopathy

Infants with symptomatic hypertrophic cardiomyopathy usually have atypical symptoms, and therefore, the distinct physical findings associated with this lesion in older patients[20] are usually not appreciated. The typical findings of congestive heart failure will be present. The electrocardiogram in infants is more likely to show right ventricular hypertrophy, in addition to left ventricular hypertrophy, because of the increased likelihood of obstruction of the right ventricular outflow tract. The chest radiograph will show cardiomegaly and may show pulmonary congestion. Echocardiography is an important diagnostic tool, revealing the pattern of differential hypertrophy and confirming the presence or absence of associated lesions.[44] Typically, there is a small left ventricular cavity and possibly also a small right ventricular cavity. If surgical intervention is contemplated, complete right and left heart catheterization is routinely performed to assess ventricular function and the degree and level of obstruction in both ventricles, and to rule out associated lesions.

Indications for surgical intervention for symptomatic hypertrophic cardiomyopathy in infancy are not well defined because of the rarity of the lesion and the atypical presentation. The presence of intractable congestive heart failure with significant left or right outflow gradients or visual evidence of obstruction on diagnostic studies is probably an indication for surgical intervention. Congestive failure with predominantly midcavity or apical obliteration is not likely to improve after surgical intervention unless associated structural lesions are present.

MANAGEMENT

Historical Perspective

In 1956, Brock reported the surgical relief of subaortic membranous stenosis using closed transventricular dilatation.[4] This was followed by Spencer's report of surgical management using cardiopulmonary bypass in 1960.[64] Diffuse subaortic stenosis associated with aortic annular hypoplasia was addressed by Konno and co-workers[32] in 1975. Clarke and associates reported on the use of aortic root replacement combined with ventricular septoplasty, using a valved aortic allograft with coronary transfer, for diffuse subaortic stenosis in infants.[8] Cooley introduced ventricular septoplasty with preservation of the native aortic valve in 1986.[9]

Surgical Technique

Subaortic Membranous or Ridge-Like Stenosis

The cardiopulmonary bypass technique is straightforward, utilizing aortic cannulation and

OBSTRUCTION OF THE LEFT VENTRICULAR OUTFLOW TRACT □ **323**

single venous cannulation of the right atrial appendage, with moderate hypothermia, aortic cross-clamping and crystalloid cardioplegic protection (Fig. 20–2). A left ventricular vent may be placed through the right upper pulmonary vein. A transverse aortotomy is made several millimeters above the tops of the aortic valve commissures, and the aortic valve leaflets are retracted to allow direct vision of the subaortic region. Alternatively, and especially in cases in which there is some question concerning the possible need for a more extensive subaortic procedure, a longitudinal aortic incision that has the potential to be extended into the right sinus of Valsalva may be made above the aortic valve, just to the left of the right coronary ostium.

The membrane or ridge is studied in relation to the three structures that can be damaged during the resection: the aortic valve leaflets, the base of the anterior mitral leaflet, and the membranous septum, which identifies the region of the bundle of His. The fibrous curtain of normal tissue below the commissure between the right coronary and noncoronary cusps of the aortic valve makes up the portion of the central fibrous body through which the conduction system passes en route to the ventricular septum. In relation to the leaflets of the normal trileaflet aortic valve, the segment of the ring of abnormal tissue beginning below the base of

the right coronary cusp and extending clockwise to the base of the noncoronary cusp is the segment where damage to the conduction system is possible. Incision into muscle must be avoided in this area. The segment beneath the left and noncoronary cusps is the region of the base of the anterior mitral leaflet and of potential mitral valve injury. The membrane or ridge may be partially attached to the base of the aortic leaflets as well, creating the possibility of aortic valve injury at the time of resection. The abnormal tissue may form a complete ring or be crescent shaped.

Once these relationships are clarified, a small skin hook is placed in the ridge of tissue anteriorly, just beneath the base of the right coronary cusp, to stabilize the tissue. A No. 11 bladed knife is used to incise the ring radially to its muscular base at this point. The incision is then extended circumferentially in a counterclockwise direction at a depth that removes the fibromuscular ring and any septal muscle that is bulging into the left ventricular outflow tract. The absolute amount of muscular resection will depend on the size of the patient and the degree of protrusion into the outflow tract. Care must be taken, however, not to create a ventricular septal defect. As the mitral valve is approached, the depth of the incision is modified to remove only the ridge of fibrous tissue (if present) from the base of the

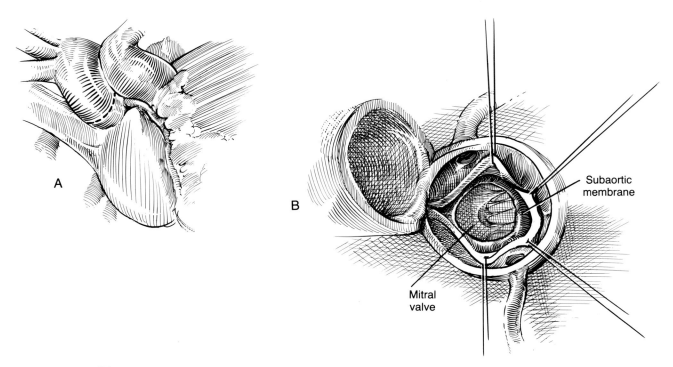

FIGURE 20–2. □

Technique for resection of discrete subaortic stenosis. *A,* Exposure is through a supravalvar aortotomy. *B,* The valve leaflets are carefully retracted. The area of conduction and the mitral valve must be avoided.

mitral valve, without damaging the valve itself. Returning to the original radial incision below the base of the right coronary cusp, the circumferential incision is continued in a clockwise direction. However, the depth of the incision is modified to avoid resection of muscle in this region, excising only the fibrous ridge. As this incision moves in a clockwise direction, the underlying septal muscle supporting the ridge tapers into the membranous septum. If the obstructing tissue is attached to the base of the aortic leaflets, careful, sharp excision must be accomplished so as not to cause a buttonhole injury to the base of the aortic valve cusps. The aortotomy is then closed with a nonabsorbable, monofilament running suture. Standard maneuvers for venting air are performed. The aortic crossclamp is removed, and the patient is rewarmed to normothermic core temperatures and separated from bypass.

In many older patients with discrete fibrous membranes, the lesion can be peeled from the underlying muscle quite effectively, without the need for sharp dissection. At the present time, it is felt that left ventricular outflow tract muscle resection should accompany the membrane removal in order to minimize recurrence. At Children's Hospital in Boston, we have used this approach successfully; however, we have not encountered any infants with lesions appropriate for this technique.

A similar exposure is used for hypertrophic cardiomyopathy with a relatively discrete subaortic stenosis. The obstructing muscle is stabilized with a skin hook beneath the base of the right aortic valve cusp, and a radial incision is made at this point. A separate radial incision is made beneath the left coronary cusp and as close to the mitral apparatus as possible. Both radial incisions are deepened into the muscle, and the wedge of muscle between the two radial incisions is then removed with a circumferential incision connecting the deepest points of the two radial incisions.

Diffuse Subaortic Stenosis With a Well-Developed Aortic Valve

The technique of ventricular septoplasty is best applied to patients with a form of fibromuscular subaortic stenosis that has morphologic characteristics between those of membranous and tunnel stenosis or to those who have hypertrophic cardiomyopathy with subaortic stenosis.

Cardiopulmonary bypass is as described for membranous subaortic stenosis, with the exception that bicaval venous cannulation is preferred, because the right side of the heart will be opened. An oblique incision is made in the infundibulum below the pulmonary valve, extending to the level of the aortic

annulus and just to the left side of the right coronary ostium (Fig. 20–3). This incision exposes the floor of the right ventricular outflow tract, which is the ventricular septum. A longitudinal incision is made in the ventricular septum and the fibrous curtain below the commissure, between the left and right coronary cusps, beginning just below the aortic valve. When making the septal incision, an incision in the aorta is sometimes helpful for visualization of the aortic valve. The septal incision is extended proximally along the subaortic left ventricular outflow tract until the most proximal aspect of the obstruction is relieved. Thickened septal muscle in the left ventricular outflow tract is then resected, taking care to avoid conduction injury. An oval patch of glutaraldehyde-treated autologous pericardium or Dacron is then used to close the defect by applying the patch to the right ventricular side of the septum using pledgetted interrupted mattress sutures. The incision in the free wall of the right ventricular outflow tract is then closed primarily if it is unobstructed. If right ventricular outflow tract obstruction is present or there is concern that iatrogenic obstruction of the right ventricular outflow tract will be created, a second patch may be used. The remainder of cardiopulmonary bypass is routine.

Tunnel Subaortic Stenosis With a Hypoplastic Aortic Valve

For tunnel subaortic stenosis with a hypoplastic aortic valve, the principles of the operation described by Konno are used (Fig. 20–4).[32] However, in infants, root replacement with an aortic or pulmonary allograft and coronary reimplantation are preferred.

The patient is prepared as in the septoplasty procedure described previously. A transverse incision is made in the free wall of the right ventricular outflow tract, and a longitudinal subaortic septal incision, as described for septoplasty, is made. The longitudinal incision is extended in a distal direction, through the aortic annulus, to the left of the right coronary ostium, and onto the ascending aorta. The coronary ostia are removed from the sinuses of Valsalva with as much surrounding tissue as possible in a manner similar to that used for coronary artery mobilization in the arterial switch operation. The aortic root, including aortic valve tissue, is then excised proximally at the level of the ventriculoarterial junction and distally at the level of the mid–ascending aorta. An appropriate-size aortic homograft is then used to reconstruct the left ventricular outflow tract, attaching the subannular margin of the valved allograft to the ventriculoarterial junction with running nonabsorbable monofilament su-

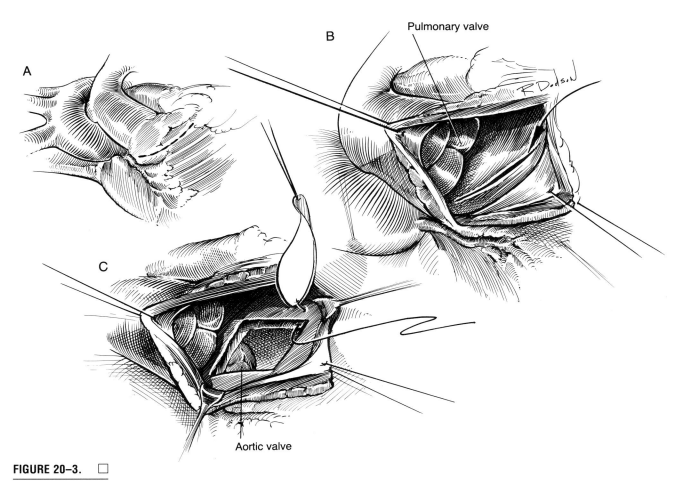

FIGURE 20–3. □

Technique for ventricular septoplasty performed for relief of subaortic stenosis. *A,* Infundibular and septal incisions are shown. *B,* The septal incision must be extended with care to ensure relief of obstruction proximally in the left ventricle. *C,* Placement of septal patch.

ture. The segment of the allograft containing the curtain of anterior mitral leaflet tissue is positioned so that it is anterior and can be used to patch the incision in the subaortic septum. Resection of obstructing muscle in the left ventricular outflow tract is also achieved as described previously for the septoplasty procedure. The coronary arteries are then transferred to the allograft, again as in the arterial switch operation. The distal anastomosis between the allograft and the ascending aorta is performed in end-to-end fashion, and the free wall infundibular incision in the right ventricle is closed with a separate patch. The remainder of the operation is conducted routinely.

RESULTS

A review of records at Children's Hospital in Boston between 1972 and 1991 revealed 119 cases in which the diagnosis of subaortic stenosis was made in infants. This is a small fraction of all patients with subaortic stenosis seen during this same period. In a great majority of these 119 cases, subaortic stenosis was either incidental to other cardiovascular lesions or was not severe enough to require surgical intervention. Only 17 of these infants (14%) required surgery for the subaortic obstruction.

A number of associated cardiovascular lesions were seen in these 119 patients, as shown in Table 20–2. (This table excludes variants of hypoplastic left heart syndrome, interrupted aortic arch, any form of transposition or malposition of the great vessels, and single-ventricle hearts.) In most of these infants, it was the associated lesions that prompted evaluation and recognition of the subaortic stenosis. This is consistent with observations made by others that subaortic stenosis is usually subclinical in infancy.

Of the 17 patients who underwent surgery for subaortic stenosis in infancy, only five had surgery addressing only the subaortic stenosis (29%). Three of these five had resection of a discrete subaortic membrane at 5, 9, and 10 months of age, respec-

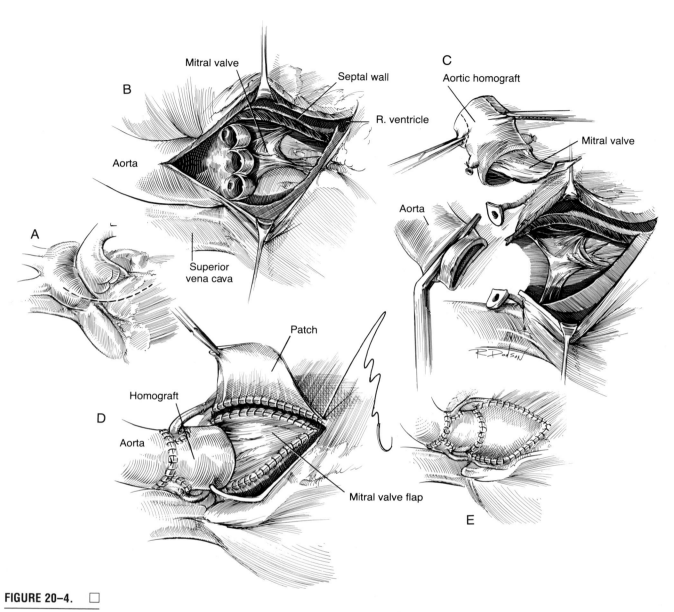

FIGURE 20–4. ☐

Aortic root replacement using aortic allograft tissue for subaortic tunnel stenosis. *A,* The incision in the infundibulum is extended onto the aorta to the left of the right coronary ostium. *B,* The ventricular septum is then incised to relieve the subaortic obstruction. *C,* After mobilization of the coronary ostia, the entire aortic root is excised. *D,* The homograft reconstruction is shown. *E,* Infundibular patch in place.

tively. All three survived, and all three also required late reoperations for recurrent subaortic stenosis. Two underwent Konno procedures at 8 and 9 years of age, and one underwent re-excision of obstructing subaortic tissue at 5 years of age. One of the other two patients initially underwent placement of a conduit from the left ventricular apex to the aorta at 1 month of age; this patient died perioperatively. The other patient initially underwent a patch septoplasty at 2 months of age for diffuse subaortic stenosis. This patient had a form of hypertrophic cardiomyopathy that later (at 2 years of age) caused significant obstruction of the right ventricular out-

flow tract, requiring further surgery. The mortality rate for patients operated on in infancy for isolated subaortic stenosis was (20%) (one of five patients). All surviving patients required reoperation.

The 12 remaining infants underwent correction of at least one other lesion simultaneously with the resection of the subaortic stenosis. Seven required repair of a ventricular septal defect, and four required mitral valve replacement. Double-chambered right ventricle, complete atrioventricular canal, and coarctation each occurred in one patient. One infant had an aortic valvotomy, and one had a mitral commissurotomy. One patient with a ventricular septal

TABLE 20–2. □ SUBAORTIC STENOSIS DIAGNOSED IN INFANCY: ASSOCIATED LESIONS (*N* = 119)

LESION	NO.	%
Ventricular septal defect	31	26
Ventricular septal defect with coarctation	22	18
Multiple left-sided lesions	20	17
Hypertrophic cardiomyopathy	16	13
Complete atrioventricular canal	7	6
Pulmonary stenosis	7	6
Abnormal mitral valve	7	6
Double-chambered right ventricle	4	3
Tetralogy of Fallot	3	3
Cor triatriatum	1	1
Polysplenia	1	1
Patent ductus arteriosus	1	1

defect underwent a Damus-Kaye-Stansel procedure with a right ventricle–to–pulmonary artery conduit.

There were four deaths in these 12 patients (33%): two in patients undergoing concomitant mitral valve replacement, one in a patient undergoing concomitant aortic valvotomy (this patient had previously undergone coarctation repair and pulmonary artery banding as a neonate), and, one in the patient with polysplenia syndrome who underwent the Damus-Kaye-Stansel procedure. Follow-up was available in all eight survivors and was complete in seven. Four (50%) have required reoperation for mitral valve problems (two of these had mitral valve procedures at the initial operation); one patient with a history of hypertrophic cardiomyopathy required surgery for new obstruction of the right ventricular outflow tract, and one had a pacemaker placed after development of complete heart block after resection of subaortic stenosis.

SUMMARY

In contrast to subaortic stenosis in older individuals, subaortic stenosis in infants is a rare and heterogeneous lesion and is frequently associated with other significant cardiovascular defects. Each case must be approached in an individual manner, as the subaortic lesion must be assessed against a backdrop of other progressing or regressing complex lesions and associations, such as Shone's complex (or variants) or hypertrophic cardiomyopathy.

SUPRAVALVAR AORTIC STENOSIS

DEFINITION

Supravalvar aortic stenosis is obstruction of the left ventricular outflow tract caused by aortic narrowing above the level of the aortic valve. Of the three major sites of obstruction of the left ventricular outflow tract discussed in this chapter, supravalvar aortic stenosis is the least common. Supravalvar aortic stenosis occurring as the primary or only obstruction to left ventricular outflow is extremely rare in infants and does not constitute a well-defined clinical entity. This lesion occurs in three forms: as part of Williams' syndrome, in a sporadic form, and in a familial form that is genetically transmitted as an autosomal dominant trait.[30] The few patients we have seen with symptomatic supravalvar aortic stenosis in infancy have had the familial form.

MORPHOLOGY

Morphologic descriptions are taken from analyses of patients seen at ages well beyond infancy and therefore may not be appropriate to the rare infant with supravalvar aortic stenosis. The "classic" description is that the lesion varies—it may be membranous, shaped like an hourglass, or diffuse.[55] The ring-like membranous and hourglass deformities occur just at the tops of the aortic valve commissures. There is intimal thickening, as well as medial disorganization and thickening, with areas of necrosis and calcification.[54] The intimal thickening may involve the edges of the aortic valve leaflets, occasionally causing stenosis of the inlet into the sinus of Valsalva, thereby causing coronary insufficiency.[14] The diffuse form of the lesion is less common and consists of a thickened aortic wall with a narrow lumen that may extend over a variable distance but may reach the aortic arch and its branches.[51] Marked thickening of the vessel wall with fibromuscular dysplasia and replacement of elastic medial tissue is present. Occasionally, the diffuse form can be associated with similar diffuse disease in the main pulmonary artery. As described by Strong and associates,[66] this extreme form of the disease is more likely to be found when the disease is clinically manifested in infancy.

Unlike in valvar and subvalvar forms of aortic stenosis, in supravalvar aortic stenosis, the coronary arteries usually are exposed to high pressure, and degenerative coronary changes are accelerated.[51] Multiple peripheral pulmonary artery stenoses are commonly associated with supravalvar stenosis in patients who have Williams' syndrome, as well as in those with the familial and sporadic forms.[2] Peripheral systemic arterial stenoses can also be found occasionally.

PATHOPHYSIOLOGY AND NATURAL HISTORY

As with other forms of obstruction of the left ventricular outflow tract, the basic physiologic derangement is a pressure gradient between the left ventricle and aorta that stimulates left ventricular hypertrophy. In supravalvar aortic stenosis, the coronary arteries are generally proximal to the obstruction and therefore are exposed to the same pressure as the left ventricular cavity in systole.

The natural history is that newborns and infants rarely develop clinical obstruction. However, when it does occur, it is usually in the familial form.[14, 16] Patients typically have progressive obstruction beginning in the first and second decades. Sudden death is common in untreated patients with severe obstruction, as in other forms of progressive obstruction of the left ventricular outflow tract, possibly because of the combination of left ventricular hypertrophy and accelerated sclerotic changes in the coronary arteries. In Williams' syndrome, the general tendency over time is for supravalvar aortic stenosis to progress and peripheral pulmonary stenosis to gradually regress.

DIAGNOSIS AND INDICATIONS FOR SURGERY

In infants, a history of familial involvement, the presence of idiopathic infantile hypercalcemia, or the stigmata of Williams' syndrome should suggest the possibility of supravalvar aortic stenosis. Cardiovascular signs and symptoms of obstruction are similar to those already described for other forms of obstruction of the left ventricular outflow tract. The electrocardiogram and chest radiograph do not provide any specific information regarding the site of obstruction, although right ventricular hypertrophy on the electrocardiogram may suggest concomitant pulmonary obstruction. Two-dimensional echocardiography and Doppler studies can define the supravalvar narrowing and indicate the size of the gradient. Cardiac catheterization, with contrast arteriography of the aorta and pulmonary arteries, is always indicated to document the supravalvar anatomy, determine gradients, evaluate inflow to the coronary arteries, and evaluate peripheral arteries, including the visceral arteries, in both the systemic and pulmonary artery vascular beds.

Indications for surgery are symptoms referable to the obstruction, a documented gradient greater than 50 mm Hg, or evidence of coronary obstruction.

MANAGEMENT

Historical Perspective

Both McGoon and Starr and their associates[46, 65] reported independent series of patch enlargement for localized supravalvar aortic stenosis in 1961. In 1976, Keane and coworkers reported on a series of 18 patients who underwent operation at Children's Hospital in Boston,[31] with the first procedure performed in 1956. A major conceptual and therapeutic advance was made in 1976 when Doty and colleagues described the extended aortoplasty technique for this lesion.[15] Both Bernhard and Cooley and their collaborators[1, 10] reported different techniques for placing valved conduits from the left ventricle to the aorta for treatment of the diffuse form of this lesion in 1975. Neither of these techniques is presently recommended.

Surgical Technique

Discrete Supravalvar Aortic Stenosis

Cardiopulmonary bypass is begun by cannulation of the distal ascending aorta and the right atrial appendage in standard fashion (Fig. 20–5). For discrete supravalvar aortic stenosis, moderate hypothermia with aortic crossclamping and crystalloid cardioplegic protection is used. A longitudinal incision in the ascending aorta is extended distally to the level of the aortic crossclamp and proximally, as an inverted Y, into both the noncoronary and right coronary sinuses of Valsalva. The bifurcation point of the Y incision should begin well above the area of discrete narrowing. The limb of the incision into the right coronary sinus is made to the left of the right coronary ostium. A tube graft of either expanded PTFE or Dacron, equal in diameter to the normal ascending aorta, is tailored to the rough configuration of the inverted Y to reconstruct the aorta, using a running monofilament suture technique. Before placing the patch, the obstructing ridge of abnormal tissue is excised without compromising the integrity of the aortic wall. This excision includes the tissue

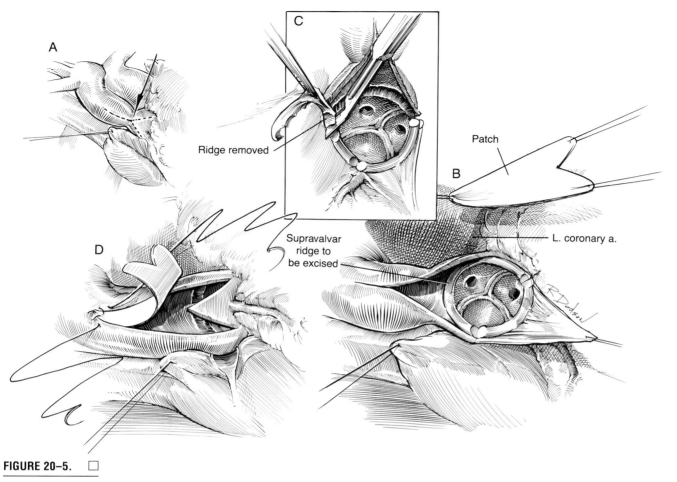

FIGURE 20–5. □

Surgical technique for repair of discrete supravalvar aortic stenosis. Inverted Y incision and patch repair. *A*, Initial incision. *B*, Exposure of ridge and valve. *C*, Resection of ridge from left cusp. *D*, Placement of patch straddling the right coronary ostium.

in the left coronary sinus as well. Occasionally it may be necessary to place a separate diamond-shaped patch into the left sinus if this remains markedly deformed or obstructed.

Careful assessment of the orifices of the sinuses of Valsalva should be made. If obstruction to flow into the sinuses is a reality or a concern after resection of the ridge, careful release of the cusps may also be necessary, with care taken not to compromise the suspensory apparatus of the leaflets at the tips of the commissures.

Diffuse Supravalvar Aortic Stenosis

Repair of diffuse supravalvar aortic stenosis is carried out using deep hypothermic circulatory arrest. Care must be taken when cannulating the markedly thickened ascending aorta, especially in infants. During the cooling phase of cardiopulmonary bypass, the arch vessels and aorta are dis-

sected well beyond the areas of suspected stenosis. It may be difficult to determine the limits of the narrowing, because the aorta is typically uniformly small externally, and the marked mural thickening is variable, thereby diminishing the value of external inspection. Careful study of the preoperative aortogram is most helpful in making this judgment. When deep hypothermia is achieved, cardioplegic solution is administered, the arch vessels are temporarily occluded, and circulatory arrest is induced. The same incision is used as for discrete supravalvar aortic stenosis; however, it is extended as far distally as necessary along the undersurface of the aortic arch to relieve all of the obstruction. It may be necessary to extend this incision well onto the transverse or distal aortic arch. The width of the patch should be tailored so that the reconstructed aorta is at least of normal caliber. After the reconstruction, an intraluminal pressure tracing should be obtained during catheter withdrawal from the

TABLE 20–3. ☐ SUPRAVALVAR AORTIC STENOSIS DIAGNOSED IN INFANCY: ASSOCIATED LESIONS (*N* = 16)

LESION	NO.	%
Valvar aortic stenosis	6	38
Pulmonary stenosis	6	38
Ventricular septal defect	5	31
Williams' syndrome	2	13
Coarctation	1	6
Total anomalous pulmonary venous connection	1	6
Polysplenia	1	6

descending aorta to the ascending aorta to document relief of the obstruction.

RESULTS

From 1972 to 1991, 109 cases of supravalvar aortic stenosis were diagnosed at Children's Hospital in Boston. Seventy-nine (72%) of these were familial or sporadic cases, and 30 (28%) were associated with Williams' syndrome. Only 16 of these 109 patients (15%) were diagnosed in infancy, and only two of the 16 had Williams' syndrome. The 16 infants had a high incidence of associated lesions (Table 20–3): six had associated valvar aortic stenosis, six had some form of pulmonary stenosis, five had ventricular septal defects, one had coarctation, and one had total anomalous pulmonary venous connection. In only two of the 16 infants was the supravalvar aortic stenosis severe enough to require surgery in infancy; both died perioperatively. One of these underwent repair of severe coarctation and a large perimembranous ventricular septal defect, using cardiopulmonary bypass. Early postoperative cardiac catheterization was necessary and revealed a supravalvar hourglass obstruction (not secondary to cannulation). At a second operation at 16 days of life, a diamond-shaped patch was used to alleviate the obstruction; however, this very ill neonate could not be weaned from cardiopulmonary bypass. The other patient clearly had a familial form of supravalvar aortic stenosis, with several immediate family members manifesting similar lesions. She had heart failure at 6 months of age, and a diagnosis of diffuse supravalvar aortic stenosis and central diffuse supravalvar pulmonary stenosis was made. At 8 months of age, she underwent supravalvar patch repair of her ascending aorta, along with intraoperative balloon dilatation of the main pulmonary artery and its branches. Both great vessels were noted to be markedly thickened at the time of the operation. The patient could not be weaned from bypass, and postmortem examination revealed a poor result of the balloon dilatation in the pulmonary arteries

and residual obstruction in the proximal transverse aortic arch just distal to the patch.

SUMMARY

It is uncommon to diagnose supravalvar aortic stenosis in infants, and obstruction severe enough to require surgical intervention is rare. Familial forms of this lesion (not Williams' syndrome), with diffuse and severe disease, appear more likely to occur in infants and pose a very difficult management problem. At present, based on a very small experience with this rare lesion, we feel that aggressive surgical patching of both great vessels, to relieve all obstruction, should be attempted in infants.

REFERENCES

1. Bernhard WF, Porier V, La Farge CG. Relief of congenital obstruction to left ventricular outflow with a ventricular-aortic prosthesis. J Thorac Cardiovasc Surg 69:223, 1975.
2. Beuren AJ, Schulze C, Eberle P, et al. The syndrome of supravalvular aortic stenosis, peripheral pulmonary stenosis, mental retardation and similar facial appearance. Am J Cardiol 13:471, 1964.
3. Bjork VO, Hultquist G, Lodin H. Subaortic stenosis produced by an abnormally placed anterior mitral leaflet. J Thorac Cardiovasc Surg 41:659, 1961.
4. Brock R. Aortic subvalvar stenosis. A report of 5 cases diagnosed during life. Guy's Hosp Rep 105:391, 1956.
5. Brown JW, Stevens LS, Holly S, et al. Surgical spectrum of aortic stenosis in children: A thirty-year experience with 257 children. Ann Thorac Surg 45:393, 1988.
6. Carrel A. On the experimental surgery of the thoracic aorta and the heart. Ann Surg 52:83, 1910.
7. Clark CE, Henry WL, Epstein SE. Familial prevalence and genetic transmission of idiopathic hypertrophic subaortic stenosis. N Engl J Med 289:709, 1973.
8. Clarke DR. Extended aortic root replacement for treatment of left ventricular outflow tract obstruction. J Cardiovasc Surg 2:121, 1978.
9. Cooley DA, Garret JT. Septoplasty for left ventricular outflow obstruction without aortic valve replacement: A new technique. Ann Thorac Surg 42:445, 1986.
10. Cooley DA, Norman JC, Mullins CE, et al. Left ventricle to abdominal aorta conduit for relief of aortic stenosis. Cardiovasc Dis 2:376, 1975.
11. Cooperberg P, Hazell S, Ashmore PG. Parachute accessory anterior mitral valve leaflet causing left ventricular outflow tract obstruction. Circulation 53:908, 1976.
12. Coran AG, Bernhard WF. The surgical management of valvular aortic stenosis during infancy. J Thorac Cardiovasc Surg 58:401, 1969.
13. DeBiase L, Di Common V, Ballerini L, et al. Prevalence of left-sided obstructive lesions in patients with atrioventricular canal without Down's syndrome. J Thorac Cardiovasc Surg 91:467, 1986.
14. Denie JJ, Verheugt AP. Supravalvular aortic stenosis. Repair by extended aortoplasty. J Thorac Cardiovasc Surg 74:362, 1977.
15. Doty DB, Polansky DB, Jenson CB. Supravalvular aortic stenosis. Repair by extended aortoplasty. J Thorac Cardiovasc Surg 74:362, 1977.
16. Downing BF. Congenital aortic stenosis. Clinical aspects and surgical treatment. Circulation 14:188, 1956.

17. Draulans-Noe HA, Wenink AC. Anterolateral muscle bundle of the left ventricle in atrioventricular septal defect: Left ventricular outflow tract and subaortic stenosis. Pediatr Cardiol 12:83, 1991.

18. Falicov RE, Resnekov L. Mid-ventricular obstruction in hypertrophic obstructive cardiomyopathy. New diagnostic and therapeutic challenge. Br Heart J 39:701, 1977.

19. Fischer DR, Ettedgui JA, Park SC, et al. Carotid artery approach for balloon dilation of aortic valve stenosis in the neonate: A preliminary report. J Am Coll Cardiol 15:1633, 1990.

20. Goodwin JF. Hypertrophic cardiomyopathy: A disease in search of its own identity. Editorial. Am J Cardiol 45:177, 1980.

21. Gutgesell HP, Mullins CE, Gillette PC, et al. Transient hypertrophic subaortic stenosis in infants of diabetic mothers. J Pediatr 89:120, 1976.

22. Hatem J, Sade RM, Taylor A, et al. Supernumerary mitral valve producing subaortic stenosis. Chest 79:483, 1981.

23. Helgason H, Keane JF, Fellows KE, et al. Balloon dilation of the aortic valve: Studies in normal lambs and in children with aortic stenosis. J Am Coll Cardiol 9:816, 1987.

24. Hofstetter R, Zeike B, Messmer BJ, et al. Echocardiographic evaluation of systolic left-ventricular function in infants with critical aortic stenosis before and after aortic valvotomy. Thorac Cardiovasc Surg 38:236, 1990.

25. Huhta JC, Carpenter RJ Jr, Moise KJ Jr, et al. Prenatal diagnosis and postnatal management of critical aortic stenosis. Circulation 75:573, 1987.

26. Huhta JC, Latson LA, Gutgesell HP, et al. Echocardiography in the diagnosis and management of symptomatic aortic valve stenosis in infants. Circulation 70:438, 1984.

27. Ilbawi MN, DeLeon SY, Wilson WR Jr, et al. Extended aortic valvuloplasty: A new approach for the management of congenital valvar aortic stenosis. Ann Thorac Surg 52:663, 1991.

28. Jonas RA, Castaneda AR, Freed MD. Normothermic caval inflow occlusion. J Thorac Cardiovasc Surg 89:780, 1985.

29. Jonas RA, Lang P, Mayer JE, et al. The importance of prostaglandin E1 in resuscitation of the neonate with critical aortic stenosis. J Thorac Cardiovasc Surg 89:314, 1985.

30. Kahler RL, Braunwald E, Plauth WH Jr, et al. Familial congenital heart disease. Am J Med 40:384, 1966.

31. Keane JF, Fellows KE, La Farge G, et al. The surgical management of discrete and diffuse supravalvar aortic stenosis. Circulation 54:112, 1976.

32. Konno S, Imai Y, Iida Y, et al. A new method for prosthetic valve replacement in congenital aortic stenosis associated with hypoplasia of the aortic valve ring. J Thorac Cardiovasc Surg 70:909, 1975.

33. Lababidi Z, Weinhaus L. Successful balloon valvuloplasty for neonatal critical aortic stenosis. Am Heart J 112:913, 1986.

34. Lababidi Z, Wu JR, Walls TJ. Percutaneous balloon aortic valvuloplasty: Results in 23 patients. Am J Cardiol 53:194, 1984.

35. Lakier JB, Lewis AB, Heymann MA, et al. Isolated aortic stenosis in the neonate. Natural history and hemodynamic considerations. Circulation 50:801, 1974.

36. Larter WE, Allen HD, Sahn DJ, et al. The asymmetrically hypertrophied septum. Further differentiation of its causes. Circulation 53:19, 1976.

37. Larzelere HB, Bailey CP. Aortic commissurotomy. J Thorac Surg 26:31, 1953.

38. Lewis FJ, Shumway NE, Niazi SA. Aortic valvulotomy under direct vision during hypothermia. J Thorac Cardiovasc Surg 32:481, 1956.

39. Lillehei CW, Gott VL, Varco RL. Direct vision correction of calcific aortic stenosis by means of pump-oxygenator and retrograde coronary sinus perfusion. Dis Chest 30:123, 1956.

40. Maron BJ, Edwards JE, Ferrans VJ, et al. Congenital heart malformations associated with disproportionate ventricular septal thickening. Circulation 52:926, 1975.

41. Maron BJ, Edwards JE, Henry WL, et al. Asymmetric septal hypertrophy (ASH) in infancy. Circulation 50:809, 1974.

42. Maron BJ, Roberts WC. Quantitative analysis of cardiac muscle cell disorganization in the ventricular septum of patients with hypertrophic cardiomyopathy. Circulation 59:689, 1979.

43. Maron BJ, Tajik AJ, Ruttenberg HD, et al. Hypertrophic cardiomyopathy in infants: Clinical features and natural history. Circulation 65:7, 1982.

44. Maron BJ, Wolfson JK, Cirjo E, et al. Relation of electrocardiographic abnormalities and patterns of left ventricular hypertrophy identified by 2-dimensional echocardiography in patients with hypertrophic cardiomyopathy. Am J Cardiol 51:189, 1983.

45. Marquis RM, Logan A. Congenital aortic stenosis and its surgical treatment. Br Heart J 17:373, 1955.

46. McGoon DC, Mankin HT, Vlad P, et al. The surgical treatment of supravalvular aortic stenosis. J Thorac Cardiovasc Surg 41:125, 1961.

47. Messina LM, Turley K, Stanger P, et al. Successful aortic valvotomy for severe congenital valvular aortic stenosis in the newborn infant. J Thorac Cardiovasc Surg 88:92, 1984.

48. Messmer BJ, Hofstetter R, von Bernuth G. Surgery for critical congenital aortic stenosis during the first three months of life. Eur J Cardiothorac Surg 5:378, 1991.

49. Moulaert AJ, Oppenheimer-Dekker A. Anterolateral muscle bundle of the left ventricle, bulboventricular flange and subaortic stenosis. Am J Cardiol 37:78, 1976.

50. Nanton MA, Belcourt CL, Gillis DA, et al. Left ventricular outflow tract obstruction owing to accessory endocardial cushion tissue. J Thorac Cardiovasc Surg 78:537, 1979.

51. Neufeld HN, Wagenvoort CA, Ongley PA, et al. Hypoplasia of ascending aorta. An unusual form of supravalvular aortic stenosis with special reference to localized coronary arterial hypertension. Am J Cardiol 10:746, 1962.

52. Newfeld EA, Muster AJ, Paul MH, et al. Discrete subvalvular aortic stenosis in childhood. Study of 51 patients. Am J Cardiol 38:53, 1976.

53. Norwood WI, Lang P, Castaneda AR, et al. Management of infants with left ventricular outflow obstruction by conduit interposition between the ventricular apex and thoracic aorta. J Thorac Cardiovasc Surg 86:771, 1983.

54. Perou M. Congenital supravalvular aortic stenosis. Arch Pathol 71:453, 1961.

55. Peterson TA, Todd DB, Edwards JE. Supra valvular aortic stenosis. J Thorac Cardiovasc Surg 50:73, 1965.

56. Rhodes LA, Colan SD, Perry SB, et al. Predictors of survival in neonates with critical aortic stenosis. Circulation 84:2325, 1991.

57. Rosenquist GC, Clark EB, McAllister HA, et al. Increased mitral-aortic separation in discrete subaortic stenosis. Circulation 60:70, 1979.

58. Rupprath G, Neuhaus KL. Percutaneous balloon valvuloplasty for aortic valve stenosis in infancy. Am J Cardiol 55:1655, 1985.

59. Sanchez GR, Metha AV, Ewing LL, et al. Successful percutaneous balloon valvuloplasty of the aortic valve in an infant. Pediatric Cardiol 6:103, 1985.

60. Sellers RD, Lillehei CW, Edwards JE. Subaortic stenosis caused by anomalies of the atrioventricular valves. J Thorac Cardiovasc Surg 48:289, 1964.

61. Shah PM, Taylor RD, Wong M. Abnormal mitral valve coaptation in hypertrophic obstructive cardiomyopathy. Proposed role in systolic anterior motion of mitral valve. Am J Cardiol 48:258, 1981.

62. Sheikhzadeh A, Ghabussi P. A case of asymmetrical apical hypertrophy which is a form of hypertrophic nonobstructive cardiomyopathy with giant negative T waves. Jpn Heart J 23:843, 1982.

63. Shone JD, Sellers RD, Anderson RL, et al. The developmental complex of parachute mitral valve, supravalvular ring of left atrium, subaortic stenosis, and coarctation of aorta. Am J Cardiol 11:714, 1963.

64. Spencer FC, Neill CA, Sank L, et al. Anatomical variations in 46 patients with congenital aortic stenosis. Am Surg 26:204, 1960.

65. Starr A, Dotter C, Griswold H. Supravalvular aortic stenosis: Diagnosis and treatment. J Thorac Cardiovasc Surg 41:134, 1961.

66. Strong WB, Perrin E, Liebman J, Silvert DR. Systemic and pulmonary artery dysplasia associated with unexpected death in infancy. J Pediatr 77:233, 1970.

67. Swan H, Kortz A. Direct vision trans-aortic approach to the aortic valve during hypothermia: Experimental observations and report of a successful clinical case. Ann Surg 144:205, 1956.

68. Tuffier T. Etat actuel de la chirugie intrathoracique. Transactions of the International Congress of Medicine, London, 1913, Section VII, Surgery, pp 247–327.

69. Van Praagh R, Bano-Rodrigo A, Smolinsky A, et al. Anatomical variations in congenital valvar, subvalvar and supravalvar aortic stenosis: A study of 64 post-mortem cases. In Takahashi M (ed). Challenge in the Treatment of Congenital Cardiac Anomalies. New York, Futura Publishing, 1986, pp 13–41.

70. Werner JC, Sicard RE, Hansent TW, et al. Hypertrophic cardiomyopathy associated with dexamethasone therapy for bronchopulmonary dysplasia. J Pediatr 120:286, 1992.

71. Zeevi B, Keane JF, Castaneda AR, et al. Neonatal critical valvar aortic stenosis. A comparison of surgical and balloon dilation therapy. Circulation 80:831, 1989.

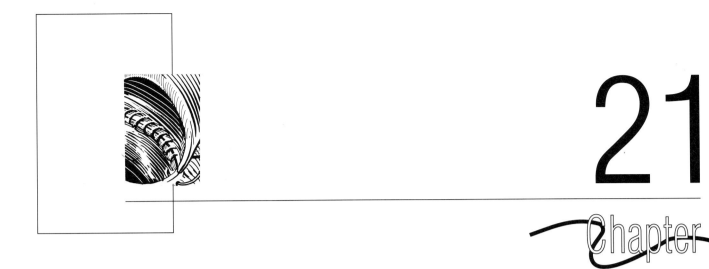

21

Chapter

Aortic Coarctation

Coarctation of the aorta is a narrowing of the lumen of the aorta, but this simple definition belies the deceptively complex nature of the lesion. This complexity is underscored by the following issues and controversies:

1. Variability in coarctation morphology;
2. Associated lesions;
3. The numerous reparative techniques available;
4. Differences between neonatal, infant, and older patients;
5. Use of prostaglandin E_1 in the preoperative management;
6. Uncertainty regarding the criteria used to assess the quality of surgical repair in both short- and long-term follow-up; and
7. Poor understanding of the etiology and physiology of systemic hypertension after surgical repair.

These issues and controversies will be addressed in this chapter as they pertain to neonates and infants who undergo isolated coarctation repair. Certain associated lesions will be considered, including patent ductus arteriosus, tubular hypoplasia of the isthmus or aortic arch, and more remote lesions that are not surgically addressed at the time of the coarctation repair (for example, bicuspid aortic valve, patent foramen ovale or atrial septal defect, and various types and sizes of ventricular septal defect).

Coarctation of the aorta is commonly associated with other complex congenital cardiovascular lesions. In some of these, the coarctation is addressed surgically as part of the repair of a more complex

lesion (for example, hypoplastic left heart syndrome, the Taussig-Bing anomaly, complex transposition with tricuspid atresia, single ventricle with subaortic stenosis, and coarctation with certain types of large ventricular septal defect). These situations will not be addressed specifically in this chapter but will be discussed in the chapters dealing with the individual lesions. Unusual forms of obstruction of the aorta related to Takayasu's arteritis or other forms of aortitis, the aortic narrowing in Williams' syndrome, and rare cases of discrete coarctation of the aorta distant from the aortic isthmus (i.e., either in the transverse aortic arch or in the abdominal aorta) will not be discussed.

ANATOMY

Developmental Considerations

Classically, coarctation of the aorta has been divided into infantile and adult forms (Fig. 21–1). Although there is some merit to this distinction, both types exist along a spectrum, are interrelated, and may share common etiologies in fetal life. Some weighted combination of two embryologic factors will cause aortic obstruction at or near the isthmus; these are not mutually exclusive and may actually influence each other. One is underdevelopment or hypoplasia of the aortic arch or isthmus. If this is present, tubular hypoplasia will be prominent, pos-

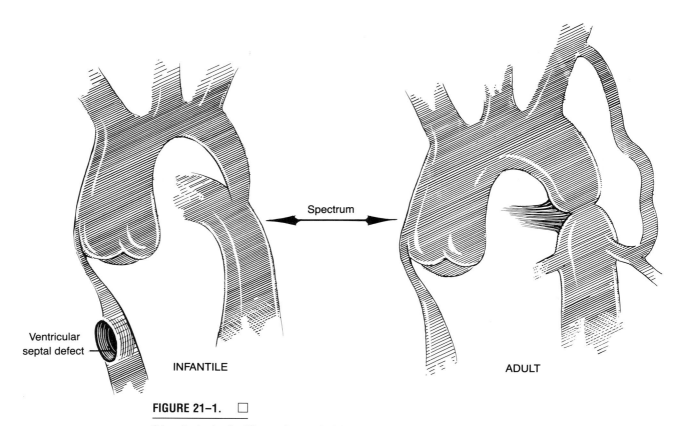

Ventricular septal defect

INFANTILE

Spectrum

ADULT

FIGURE 21–1. ☐

Schematic showing the differences between the infantile (left) and adult (right) forms of coarctation.

sibly without a discrete coarctation. The second factor is the presence of ectopic ductal tissue in the aorta at the aortic insertion of the ductus. Theoretically, this anomaly alone can result in aortic coarctation as ductal tissue constricts after birth. A prominent, discrete, coarctation shelf without associated proximal tubular hypoplasia or associated intracardiac lesions will result. If both mechanisms are operative, there will be a discrete coarctation associated with proximal tubular hypoplasia.

Ectopic ductal tissue in the aorta seems to occur only when fetal ductal flow is in the right-to-left (normal) direction. It is not clear whether excessive ductal flow (i.e., caused by associated intracardiac lesions) influences this process. Interestingly, a similar mechanism may be responsible for the stenosis of the left pulmonary artery associated with cardiac lesions that result in predominantly left-to-right intrauterine ductal flow.

The prevailing theory regarding the etiology of underdevelopment (hypoplasia) of the arch and isthmus is that it is promoted by proximal cardiac lesions that limit antegrade flow into the ascending aorta in utero.[33, 59] The amount of flow across the distal aortic arch and isthmus is thought to be an important determinant of growth of these vascular

structures. The proximal lesion may be either an obstruction within the left side of the heart, an inadequate patent foramen ovale, or an interventricular defect that encourages the left ventricle to eject through the defect rather than the aorta. A combination of both of these defects may occur also. As a result, the balance of total fetal cardiac output provided by the left and right ventricles is disrupted, with a greater percentage of cardiac output passing through the right ventricle. This results in increased flow through the fetal patent ductus arteriosus (derived from the right ventricle) and less flow across the aortic isthmus (derived from the left ventricle). A variable amount of right ventricular output via the patent ductus arteriosus may also supply vascular beds to the upper body by retrograde flow through the isthmus. This contrasts with the normal fetal state in which the flow to the lower body is made up of antegrade flow across the aortic isthmus (10% to 15% of total cardiac output derived from the left ventricle) and ductal flow (50% to 60% of total cardiac output derived from right ventricular output).

In the mildest form of coarctation, fetal flow patterns may have been normal. However, ectopic ductal tissue may be present in the aorta beyond the ductal insertion. After birth, ductal constriction may result in aortic constriction opposite the ductal insertion. This contraductal shelf in the periductal aorta may result in the typical "adult" coarctation with a discrete shelf-like obstruction at the ligamentum arteriosum.[32]

Mild-to-moderate disruption of intrauterine flow, with or without ectopic ductal tissue, can explain more moderate forms of aortic coarctation. The ductal flow may be bifurcated by a contraductal shelf in a manner analogous to the bifurcation of the abdominal aorta. Therefore, some ductal flow may reach the left subclavian artery.[50] Vascular capacitance characteristics in the systemic and pulmonary arterial beds may result in phasic changes in the direction of blood flow at the isthmus during systole and diastole. The distal aortic arch and isthmus may be moderately hypoplastic, and a discrete coarctation may be present. The aorta may grow correspondingly, resulting in mild or moderate tubular hypoplasia in addition to the discrete coarctation shelf.

If the disruption of normal fetal flow patterns is severe, marked tubular hypoplasia of the isthmus, the distal aortic arch, or both, may occur. After birth the area will represent an inadequate conduit for the entire cardiac output to the lower part of the body. Such a patient will be brought to the hospital in the neonatal period with ductus-dependent cardiac output to the lower body or with cardiovascular collapse if the patent ductus arteriosus closes before the lesion is recognized. Interrupted aortic arch, discussed in Chapter 22, may represent a more profound flow-related lack of aortic growth at either the distal arch or the isthmus. Alternatively, interruption may be the result of similar degrees of flow-related influences, beginning at an earlier developmental stage.

This flow-related theory of vascular development[59] is supported by the types of lesions commonly associated with aortic coarctation (all of which may limit left ventricular output or encourage diversion of left ventricular output to the right ventricle in utero)[2]: isolated ventricular septal defect (35% incidence with coarctation), sometimes with posterior malalignment of the conal septum and subaortic stenosis; bicuspid aortic valve; various forms of supravalvar, valvar, and subvalvar mitral stenosis; aortic atresia; and complex single-ventricle anatomy with subaortic stenosis.

Morphologic Features

The isolated discrete coarctation (with or without bicuspid aortic valve) is a common form of aortic coarctation when the diagnosis is made in older children and adolescents; however, it becomes progressively less common as patients are seen earlier in life. This is logical, as associated lesions and severe tubular hypoplasia of the arch cause earlier symptomatology and therefore present in infancy. In the older infant with isolated coarctation, the external appearance of the aorta may reflect the shelf-like coarctation with a waist or hourglass narrowing similar to that seen in older patients. Prominent collateral intercostal arteries are usually not present, although some increase in the size of these vessels is often detectable. Modest post-stenotic dilatation of the upper descending aorta may be present; however, the degenerative findings in older patients—saccular aneurysm formation, intimal erosion and dissection, and marked disruption of elastic tissue—are not prominent. Thickened and infolded aortic media, hypertrophied intima, and fibrosis are present microscopically at the coarcted shelf, with the shelf itself being most prominent directly opposite the ligamentum arteriosum. The shelf tapers as it moves circumferentially, finally becoming absent at the site of insertion of the ligamentum.

In the neonate the external appearance is dominated by the apparent continuity of the large patent ductus arteriosus and the descending aorta, contrasting with the hypoplastic isthmus and arch. A contraductal shelf is often present but may be less prominent than in older patients because of the proximal hypoplasia. Microscopically, ductal cells may be found in the periductal aortic wall.[32]

Degenerative changes in the aorta and compensatory changes (e.g., aneurysm formation, collateral vessel formation) are not prominent in neonates and infants. Tubular hypoplasia of the distal aortic arch and isthmus is common. The criterion for defining hypoplasia of the proximal arch (i.e., between the innominate artery and left carotid artery) is a diameter less than 60% of that of the ascending aorta; the criterion for hypoplasia of the distal arch (i.e., between the left carotid artery and left subclavian artery) is a diameter less than 50% of the ascending aorta; and the criterion for isthmic hypoplasia (i.e., between the left subclavian artery and the ductus insertion) is a diameter less than 40% of the ascending aorta.[52]

Associated Lesions

The frequency of associated lesions is inversely proportional to the age at presentation. According to one study, major associated lesions are present in 85% of neonates who have aortic coarctation and in about 50% of infants.[64] In the neonate there often is

TABLE 21–1. □ ASSOCIATED LESIONS IN 138 PATIENTS UNDERGOING ISOLATED COARCTATION REPAIR (JANUARY 1984 TO JANUARY 1992)

LESION	NO.	%
Patent ductus arteriosus	88	64
Patent foramen ovale/atrial septal defect	76	55
Ventricular septal defect	76	55
Bicommissural aortic valve	60	43
Hypoplastic arch	35	25
Aortic stenosis	35	25
Hypoplastic left ventricle/Shone's syndrome	23	17

hypoplasia of the distal arch or isthmus that can vary from mild to severe. Patent ductus arteriosus is considered part of the lesion complex in neonates, as is tubular hypoplasia of more proximal segments. An atrial-level communication, either a small secundum atrial septal defect or an incompetent patent foramen ovale, is also common. Two other general categories of associated cardiovascular lesions occur frequently with neonatal and infant coarctation. These are left-sided obstructive lesions (aortic stenosis or atresia, bicuspid aortic valve, subaortic stenosis, Shone's syndrome) and lesions with abnormal interventricular or great vessel communications (ventricular septal defect [VSD], either isolated or in combination with transposition or double-outlet right ventricle; aortopulmonary window). Coarctation of the aorta associated with right-sided obstructive lesions is extremely rare.

Table 21–1 shows the associated lesions in the 138 neonates and infants undergoing repair for isolated coarctation at the Children's Hospital in Boston between January 1984 and December 1991. This analysis excludes patients with coarctation and complex associated cardiovascular lesions in which simultaneous cardiac procedures were performed other than ligation of a patent ductus arteriosus.

Even in patients undergoing only isolated coarctation repair, associated lesions were more common in neonates than in infants. Patent ductus arteriosus was present in 79% of neonates and 28% of infants; VSD in 62% of neonates and 40% of infants; hypoplasia of the arch in 30% of neonates and 15% of infants; and atrial-level left-to-right shunts (patent foramen ovale/atrial septal defect [PFO/ASD]) in 67% of neonates and 28% of infants. Additionally, all of the cases of hypoplastic left ventricle/Shone's complex occurred in neonates, and all four cases of severe aortic stenosis occurred in neonates.

Depressed left ventricular contractility was documented in 35 cases, 29 in neonates and six in infants. Left ventricular hypertrophy was a consistent finding in all patients.

Table 21–2 lists a number of the features of the

VSDs found in this group of patients. Seventy-six of the 138 patients had VSDs. Large septal defects are under-represented, as a number of these were repaired along with the coarctation as a single-stage repair, thereby removing this group from this present analysis.

PATHOPHYSIOLOGY AND NATURAL HISTORY

As can be appreciated from the discussion of etiology, aortic coarctation, especially in infancy, is a challenging physiologic lesion. At first glance the lesion is simply an obstruction in the conduit that provides blood flow to the lower half of the body, implying a straightforward obstructive alteration to the normal physiology. However, a number of factors combine to make aortic coarctation an extremely complex physiologic problem.

After birth the pathophysiology of aortic coarctation depends on three variables; the degree of obstruction, the status of the ductus arteriosus, and the presence of associated intracardiac lesions. The simplest physiologic case consists of an isolated coarctation causing mild or moderate obstruction and associated with a closed ductus. This results in proximal systemic hypertension, left ventricular hypertrophy without left ventricular failure, and a pressure gradient between the upper and lower extremities. As collateral vessels develop over time, the gradient may become reduced or even disappear. This physiologic milieu is well tolerated by the patient, who may remain asymptomatic for many years until complications related to left ventricular hypertrophy, degenerative aortic changes, or chronic systemic hypertension occur.

If the obstruction is more severe, the patient may manifest signs of left ventricular failure with depressed left ventricular contractility, dilatation, mi-

TABLE 21–2. □ VSD IN 138 ISOLATED COARCTATION REPAIRS (N = 76)

CHARACTERISTIC	NO.
Age	
Neonates	60
Infants	16
Size of VSD	
Small	25
Moderate	18
Large	24
Unknown	9
VSD Type	
Perimembranous	30
Muscular	31
Atrioventricular canal	8
Malalignment	7

VSD, Ventricular septal defect.

tral valve insufficiency, and elevated left ventricular end-diastolic and atrial pressure, with subsequent potential for left-to-right atrial level shunting through an atrial septal defect or stretched incompetent patent foramen ovale. Signs of severe hypoperfusion to organs distal to the coarctation will be prominent and may be manifested by metabolic acidemia; oliguria; gut ischemia; and cold, constricted extremities.

If the ductus arteriosus is open, severe hypoperfusion of the lower body is avoided, because the right ventricular output provides lower body perfusion via the ductus. However, a pressure gradient between the upper and lower extremities is usually still present, as the reduced pulmonary afterload, and also some degree of ductal constriction, result in a lower blood pressure in the lower half of the body. In addition, a difference between oxygen saturations in the upper and lower parts of the body is also present when right ventricular output contributes significantly to lower body perfusion. Immediately after birth, the presence of a patent ductus arteriosus and relatively high pulmonary vascular resistance may make detection of even very severe aortic coarctation somewhat difficult if it is not suspected. The likelihood of acute left ventricular decompensation will depend on the acuteness of ductal closure. If this occurs rapidly, the neonate's left ventricle will not respond favorably to the rapidly increased afterload, and lower body hypoperfusion cannot be counteracted.[27] More gradual ductal closure (allowing time for left ventricular hypertrophy to develop and collateralization to form) may be responsible for the less urgent presentation of the many patients with isolated severe aortic coarctation.

In the more complex anatomic forms with associated intracardiac defects, the pathophysiology may be even more complicated. Commonly a VSD is present. When this is the case and patent ductus arteriosus is present, the findings just after birth may be even more subtle than when the ventricular septum is intact. Pulmonary artery pressures are more likely to remain elevated for more prolonged periods; therefore, upper body–to–lower body pressure gradients are less likely to be present. The left-to-right ventricular-level shunt also increases pulmonary artery, and therefore descending aortic, oxygen saturations. However, the tendency for both pulmonary vascular resistance to drop and the patent ductus arteriosus to close in the setting of the elevated systemic vascular resistance found with coarctation results in severe hypoperfusion of the lower body and also in a markedly increased left-to-right ventricular-level shunt shortly after birth. In this setting left ventricular failure occurs from volume overload rather than from elevated afterload, as in the case of coarctation with an intact ventricular septum. Patients with both significant coarctation and a significant VSD almost always become severely symptomatic in the neonatal or early infancy periods.

In contrast to patients with coarctation and VSD, in whom the basic physiology is aortic obstruction and left-to-right intracardiac shunting, patients with more complex intracardiac lesions may have the additional pathophysiologic component of the mixing of oxygenated and unoxygenated blood. This may reduce the oxygen supply to the myocardium and brain. The cyanosis also makes it more likely that a diagnosis will be made before ductal closure occurs.

A particularly difficult group of associated defects are those consisting of multiple left-sided obstructive or hypoplastic lesions. These may exist in mild form, being of little physiologic consequence, or they may be numerous and severe, in which case the affected patient should be considered to have either some variant of Shone's complex or a form of the hypoplastic left heart syndrome. Whether to treat such patients as though they have two-ventricle or one-ventricle hearts is a difficult question. This problem is addressed in more detail in Chapter 23.

In the New England region, coarctation of the aorta is found in slightly more than 5% of cases of congenital heart disease.[24] The natural history depends on the severity of the coarctation and on associated lesions. If the coarctation is isolated, a very small fraction of patients will have severe left heart failure, severe hypoperfusion of the lower body, or both, in the neonatal period. This small group of patients would likely die without some form of surgical or medical intervention. However, about 85% of patients with isolated coarctation survive to the end of the first decade, only to succumb at an accelerated pace relative to the normal population, mainly because of the various complications associated with sustained systemic hypertension and degenerative aortic changes.[10]

In contrast, major associated lesions combined with aortic coarctation may result in a much less favorable natural history. Neonatal presentation is often precipitated by cardiovascular collapse from a closed or closing patent ductus arteriosus or by congestive heart failure from a combination of aortic coarctation with an associated isolated VSD or more complex intracardiac disease. Interestingly, the natural history is influenced mostly by the physiology resulting from a combination of the systemic obstruction of the coarctation associated with an unrestricted left-to-right intracardiac shunt. In the great majority of such patients, severe heart failure will develop in the neonatal and early infancy period, regardless of whether the associated lesion is simply an unrestrictive VSD or a much more complex lesion (e.g., tricuspid atresia with transposition).[41]

The logical extension of this natural history is that most neonates and infants with coarctation and severe symptomatology have associated cardiovascular lesions. This has been proven in multiple reports and in our own experience.

DIAGNOSIS AND INDICATIONS FOR SURGERY

In mild-to-moderate isolated coarctation, the infant may be asymptomatic and well developed. Physical examination will be most notable for systemic hypertension, often a gradient between the upper and lower extremity blood pressures, and a systolic murmur heard best in the interscapular region. Collateral vessels have been shown to be present in early infancy, and these may be developed in the older infant to such a degree that the pressure gradient is reduced, and no murmur is present. The electrocardiogram may show left ventricular hypertrophy. The chest radiograph may show mild cardiomegaly or be unremarkable. Echocardiography is very useful for the infant with mild or moderate coarctation, confirming and characterizing the coarctation by imaging and giving an estimate of the hemodynamic gradient by Doppler flow signals. In addition, associated cardiovascular lesions can be identified with accuracy. If physical examination and echocardiography confirm a coarctation in an asymptomatic infant, it is not necessary to perform cardiac catheterization. In patients with significant collateral development, pressure gradients are a poor indication of the severity of the coarctation, and a firm diagnosis can be made only by more specific imaging of the aortic isthmus. Echocardiography may be adequate; however, the coarctation can be visualized with excellent resolution using magnetic resonance imaging. Computerized tomography scanning and aortography can accomplish this also. Using any of these modalities, an evident decrease in luminal diameter approaching 50% at the site of coarctation indicates a significant lesion requiring repair. A resting gradient of 20 mm Hg or more is also an indication for surgery. However, the exact timing of intervention is controversial for the asymptomatic, healthy-appearing infant.

The presentation of the symptomatic neonate or infant with coarctation is dramatic. After birth, a relatively asymptomatic period of days to weeks is followed by a precipitous decompensation as the ductus arteriosus closes and the coarctation remodels. Cardiovascular collapse quickly develops, with hypotension, tachycardia, tachypnea, and pulselessness in the lower body; in the most severely ill patients, pulses in the upper body become weakened or thready secondary to left ventricular failure. Obtundation, anuria, and metabolic acidosis can develop in hours.

The chest radiograph shows significant cardiomegaly, and the electrocardiogram shows sinus tachycardia and biventricular hypertrophy. Echocardiography will confirm the diagnosis, and associated intracardiac lesions should be suspected. It is likely that either complex intracardiac disease will be detected or a moderate-to-large VSD will be found. In the unusual case in which significant structural heart disease is not present, left ventricular dysfunction, with dilatation and reduced contractility, and a distended left atrium with left-to-right shunting across an incompetent patent foramen ovale, will be found.

Prompt resuscitation followed by a period of stabilization ranging from hours to days, depending on the degree of physiologic insult, will be necessary before the infant is ready for surgical correction of the aortic coarctation. Isolated coarctation repair is performed if no major intracardiac structural defects are present or if a restrictive VSD is present. If a large VSD exists, the decision regarding surgical management is complicated. Occasionally a VSD that was judged to be small or moderate (restrictive) is found to be more significant after isolated coarctation repair. If significant heart failure persists, the patient should be returned promptly to the operating room for closure of the septal defect.

When coarctation is found with more complex intracardiac disease, the procedure will largely be dictated by the intracardiac lesion. In general, lesions in which normal, two-ventricle physiology can be restored are completely repaired at the time of coarctation repair, whereas various palliative procedures are performed for lesions with obligatory, single-ventricle physiology. These lesions and their association with coarctation are discussed in the chapters dealing primarily with the individual complex intracardiac problem.

SURGICAL MANAGEMENT

Historical Perspective

Two reports of successful surgical repair of aortic coarctation appeared independently in 1945, one by Gross from Children's Hospital in Boston and the other by Crafoord and Nylin.[16, 28] Although Crafoord's actual clinical procedure (October 1944) preceded that of Gross (June 1945) by a number of months, the clinical work of Gross was the culmination of years of careful experimental work in animals demonstrating the efficacy of aortic resection with end-to-end aortic anastomoses.[30] Experimental work by Blalock and Park, using the transected subclavian artery as a conduit to the postcoarctation site,[6] also was eventually applied clinically. Concerns about circumferential anastomotic growth and recoarctation stimulated the development of patch aortoplasty and isthmusplasty by Vosschulte[73] in 1961 and the subclavian flap aortoplasty procedure by Waldhausen and Nahrwold in 1966.[74] Tube grafts of either allograft[29] or synthetic material[51] were also introduced for patients in whom the other techniques were not advisable.

Initially, clinical applications of many of the early techniques were performed in older patients. The first coarctation repair in an infant was reported by Calodney and Carson in 1950; however, the infant died.[8] Neonatal repair was reported by Mustard and associates in 1955.[53]

Later, technical modifications were developed, including the extended resection and anastomosis technique[54] and the subclavian flap aortoplasty, which maintain distal subclavian perfusion.[19, 48]

The original recommendation of Gross was that elective repair be performed at approximately 10 years of age. This was based on the argument that the normal aorta has reached about 50% of its adult diameter at this age and that resection and anastomosis will establish a lumen 50% as large or larger than the eventual adult aorta, even if no further growth of the anastomosis occurred. This would obviate the need for reoperation. However, this is no longer considered the optimal form of management of asymptomatic coarctation. First, circumferential anastomoses can, and do, grow. Second, repair can be performed more safely and with greater technical ease much earlier in life, before marked collateral formation, aortic degeneration, aneurysm formation, and decreased tissue elasticity have developed. Third, chronic postoperative systemic hypertension is a significant problem in patients with repaired coarctation, and this may be related to prolonged periods of preoperative upper body hypertension and the resetting of baroreceptor mechanisms.[3, 9, 18, 65] Other studies suggest that postoperative hypertension is related to age at repair.[45, 75] These reasons, coupled with the technical experience gained in constructing aortic anastomoses in neonates and infants with other lesions, have influenced most surgeons to electively repair coarctation at a much earlier age. For some time this recommended age was 3 to 5 years. However, more recently, at Children's Hospital in Boston, elective repair has been

advocated at 3 to 6 months of age, or at the time of diagnosis if the coarctation is discovered after this age. Delaying elective repair until the age of 3 months is recommended because ductal remodeling in early infancy may theoretically compromise the result if it is performed earlier, as in the case of emergency neonatal coarctation repair. At this early age, ductal remnants may be retained in the anastomotic suture line, inhibiting normal growth. By 3 to 6 months of age, however, true ductal remodeling has stabilized, allowing reliable reconstruction. Although this has not been proven, it is hoped that early elective repair will also reduce the problem of chronic systemic hypertension postoperatively. It should be emphasized, however, that late hypertension after coarctation repair is poorly understood. Abnormalities in tone in peripheral vascular beds, in the left ventricular kinetic state, and in baroreceptor sensitivity have all been documented independent of the presence of residual stenosis.[11, 26, 34]

General Management Principles

The use of prostaglandin E_1 is routine in neonates who are in extremis secondary to coarctation. In the majority of cases, this is to ensure ductal patency and thereby support lower body circulation by the right ventricle; however, in some cases, even if the duct is closed, relaxation of the aortic end of the ductus, without actually opening the entire ductal lumen, may partially relieve the obstruction of the coarctation, improving the patient's condition. The application of prostaglandin E_1 to reopen the ductus arteriosus has been a major therapeutic advance in treating this lesion, changing the clinical setting from one of a truly urgent operative procedure in a severely compromised patient to a controlled operation in the stabilized patient. Prostaglandin E_1 is the most important, but not the only, component of resuscitation. Other principles of resuscitation include pharmacologic paralysis, mechanical ventilation, inotropic support, sodium bicarbonate supplementation, and intravenous nutrition and diuretic therapy once the infant has been stabilized. If an intracardiac shunt is present, pulmonary vascular resistance should be controlled to reduce the shunt volume, using low levels of inspired oxygen while keeping arterial PCO_2 at about 50 mm Hg once the metabolic acidosis has been resolved. Recovery of all major organ systems before operation is the goal of this resuscitative effort. After the resuscitation period, the infant is prepared for surgery.

Before placing the patient in the right lateral decubitus position, a right radial artery line is placed. Especially in the case of complex obstructions, another arterial line (in a lower extremity or the umbilical artery) is ideal for assessing the gradient after repair. At the very least a pulse oximeter and sphygmomanometer should be placed on the lower extremity. Ambient temperature in the operating room should be carefully controlled, and a heating-cooling blanket used such that core body temperature is carefully manipulated to approximately 35°C. Spinal cord ischemia is rare in neonates and infants but has been reported when core temperature is elevated at the time of aortic clamping.[17]

With the exception of repairs performed using cardiopulmonary bypass, surgical exposure is accomplished using a left posterolateral thoracotomy through the third or fourth intercostal space. The upper lobe of the left lung is retracted anteriorly and inferiorly. The positions of the phrenic and vagus nerves are noted, and the pleural reflection overlying the aortic isthmus is opened and extended superiorly well onto the left subclavian artery and inferiorly to the level of the second pair of intercostal arteries below the coarctation. The ductus arteriosus is exposed to the pericardial reflection, and the position of the recurrent laryngeal nerve is noted. The dissection plane should remain just superficial to the aortic adventitia to avoid injury to the thoracic duct and other major lymphatic vessels. If intercostal or other small arteries are present above the anticipated level of placement of the distal aortic crossclamp, it is necessary to control these vessels just before the crossclamp is applied. In small infants this can be done effectively, without taking up critical space, by using small metal clips placed gently on these vessels several millimeters from their aortic origin. However, some members of our group prefer tourniquets. At completion of the repair, these clips can be removed from the intercostal vessels atraumatically.

Depending on the technique of repair and the morphology of the aortic arch, it may be necessary to extend the dissection to the level of the left carotid artery or even to the base of the innominate artery. This dissection must accomplish thorough mobilization of the proximal and distal arch so that the aorta can be crossclamped at this level. Particular care should be taken not to injure the thoracic duct when the distal arch is dissected.

Suture material may be important with regard to anastomotic growth. When tissue-to-tissue anastomoses are performed, 6-0 polydioxanone is used in neonates and infants. If a polytetrafluoroethylene (PTFE) patch or conduit is used in the reconstruction, PTFE suture (Gore-Tex) may be considered for hemostatic reasons. If pericardium or other nonviable material is used, polypropylene suture is the best choice.

The physiology of aortic clamping and ductal ligation in the neonate should be clearly understood. The exact physiology will depend on whether the coarctation is isolated or accompanied by intracardiac defects that allow left-to-right shunting. If the ventricular septum is intact, clamping presents an acute afterload to the left ventricle, not only by completely clamping the coarctation, but also by clamping the left subclavian artery and possibly the left carotid artery as well. If acute left ventricular decompensation occurs, the patent foramen ovale may become incompetent, reducing obligatory preload but not changing afterload. Acute increases in left ventricular wall tension and ischemia may occur, leading to decreased contractility and possibly ventricular fibrillation. Inotropic support may ameliorate acute left ventricular decompensation; however, the arrythmogenic potential of inotropic agents should be considered. If a ventricular-level shunt is present along with the coarctation, aortic clamping and ductal ligation will not result in an acute increase in left ventricular afterload. The presence of a nonrestrictive interventricular communication will allow the left ventricle to decompress across the VSD to the pulmonary circulation; therefore, an increase in left ventricular wall tension is avoided. However, the physiologic derangement may be just as severe, as systemic output is reduced to the degree that pulmonary blood flow is increased. Rapid development of lactic acidosis from profound systemic underperfusion can occur in spite of preserved left ventricular function. In this case, high doses of inotropic agents are not likely to be beneficial and in fact may further increase systemic resistance, thereby further increasing the left-to-right shunt. Careful attention to ventilation, avoiding both hyperventilation and high inspired oxygen, may help counter the left-to-right shunt by elevating pulmonary vascular resistance.

After the repair the distal clamp is released first to remove air from the lumen through the suture line. This is followed by gradual removal of the proximal clamp while noting the drop in proximal arterial blood pressure. Controlled release of the proximal clamp can prevent transient but profound hypotension at the point of maximal myocardial stress. Immediately after clamp removal, "washout" of lactic acid from lower body hypoperfusion can occur, and reduced systemic vascular resistance is present. Careful attention should be given to these transient aberrations; however, active pharmacologic treatment (administration of sodium bicarbonate or afterload augmentation) is not usually indicated.

After stabilization of hemodynamics after clamp removal, an intraluminal catheter pullback gradient across the anastomosis documents the adequacy of the reconstruction. The goal of the procedure is to have no detectable gradient. If a gradient is measured, a judgment should be made as to whether the reconstruction is flawed and can be revised to eliminate the gradient. If so, the revision should be undertaken at the same operation after allowing for a period of spinal chord perfusion. However, if the reconstruction is judged to be flawless but arch morphology is such that a pullback gradient of no more than 20 mm Hg is present, the reconstruction should be accepted. If the gradient is greater than 20 mm Hg, even if the anastomosis itself cannot be improved, serious consideration should be given to performing a more radical reconstruction.

At the conclusion of the procedure a continuous polypropylene suture is used to reapproximate the cut edges of the mediastinal pleura over the reconstruction. A drainage tube is placed in the thoracic cavity, and routine closure of the thoracotomy is carried out.

Choice of Procedure

Although all of the historically described techniques may have a place in certain circumstances, three methods have currently emerged as the techniques of choice for routine coarctation repair: the subclavian flap aortoplasty (and modifications), the resection-and-anastomosis techniques (and modifications), and the synthetic patch aortoplasty. Each technique has its advantages and disadvantages.

The advantages of the subclavian flap aortoplasty include exclusive use of all-natural tissue, avoidance of tension on the suture line, less overall dissection, and no circumferential scar. Disadvantages include interruption of blood flow to the left arm and potential growth alteration,[44, 66, 68, 72] retention of abnormal ductal tissue, inability to easily address proximal tubular hypoplasia, and the potential for the late formation of an aneurysm.[46]

The resection-and-anastomosis technique and its modifications (extended) have the great advantages of completely removing the ductal tissue in the pericoarctation region[37] and addressing proximal tubular hypoplasia. More recent developments, such as the principles of microvascular technique; the availability of absorbable suture material; and experience with surgery on great vessels, which has been derived from other procedures (the arterial switch operation), currently make this approach even more attractive. The major disadvantages of the resection approach include the potential for tension on the suture line, a greater degree of technical difficulty,

more extensive dissection, and the presence of a circumferential scar.

The advantages of the patch aortoplasty are similar to those of the subclavian flap aortoplasty, except that even less dissection is needed, and the left arm perfusion is not interrupted. Minimal dissection requirements and the rapid clamp times possible with this technique (usually 5 to 8 minutes) offered a significant advantage for this method of repair in the preprostaglandin era, when the neonate was often brought to the operating room in extremis with a closed or closing ductus arteriosus. The introduction of prostaglandin E_1 has completely altered the physiologic condition of these infants, making these advantages less compelling. The disadvantages of the synthetic patch aortoplasty include retention of ductal tissue, the presence of foreign material, and an extensively documented incidence of aneurysm formation in the retained natural tissue opposite the patch.[5, 13, 30, 31, 35, 47, 57]

The various advantages and disadvantages of all of these techniques must be measured in terms of outcome as judged by mortality, recurrent or residual gradients, and technique-related complications (aneurysm, nerve injury, chylothorax, left arm dysfunction, paraplegia, and bleeding). At the present time, no clear objective distinction can be made between them in spite of a large body of clinical experience. There are a number of reasons for this. First, since the introduction of prostaglandin E_1, mortality related to isolated coarctation in infancy has become very low regardless of the technique used, making it an insensitive measure of success. Second, other than a probable higher incidence of aneurysm formation using synthetic patch aortoplasty and a present (but low) incidence of arm dysfunction using the standard subclavian flap aortoplasty, other unfavorable occurrences are low and probably comparable among the three techniques. Thus the major criterion for distinguishing among the types of repair is the incidence of residual or recurrent coarctation. However, there is no consensus as to the most appropriate criteria for defining residual or recurrent coarctation. A resting gradient of 20 mm Hg is the most common criterion used, although both greater and lesser resting thresholds have been advocated. Various exercise-related changes in hemodynamics, ranging from measured pressure gradients, to echocardiographic flow signals, to more sophisticated analyses of changes in pulse waves (pulsatile index) and Doppler spectrum analysis in the descending aorta, have been offered as other methods for assessing residual or recurrent stenosis.[7, 15, 23, 36, 71] Other variables, in addition to the criteria used for defining stenosis (such as reports that variably include only neonates, neonates and infants less than 3 months of age, or infants up to 1 year old) and reports that extend over varying time periods (before and after the introduction of prostaglandin E_1), make it impossible to objectively determine the most effective technique. With all of these variables, in the final analysis it is possible to find a study in the literature that supports any bias one chooses.[4, 14, 22, 38–40, 42, 49, 62, 63, 67, 69, 70]

Our own analysis of neonates undergoing coarctation repair between 1972 and 1984 failed to identify any technique as clearly superior, although this study is subject to some of the same concerns mentioned earlier.[76] Studies that rigidly advocate one technical approach are misguided. The variability in morphology and physiology argue strongly that each case should be assessed individually and the most appropriate surgical technique applied. The following discussion outlines the logic that we use in approaching aortic coarctation.

At the present time we believe that either routine or extended resection and anastomosis is the most appropriate procedure for a large number of neonates and infants with isolated aortic coarctation. The other techniques are used, less frequently, in relatively specific circumstances, which will be discussed. We defend this approach with several lines of reasoning. First, the routine use of prostaglandins allows surgery to be performed in stable patients. This allows the necessary time at surgery for careful and extensive mobilization of both the arch and the distal aorta, which is required for the resection procedures, so that tension can routinely be avoided. Second, in our extensive experience with the neonatal arterial switch operation for transposition (see Chapter 26), the circumferential suture line has proven to grow quite well using absorbable running sutures, suggesting that the circumferential suture line at the distal arch will grow equally as well if proper care is taken to resect all ductal tissue and resect or bypass all hypoplastic tissue. Third, there is a certain compelling logic in the concept that excluding all of the abnormal tissue from the periductal aorta will minimize the likelihood of recurrent obstruction.

Although this approach seems applicable in a large number of cases, flexibility nevertheless must be emphasized, and the full repertoire of techniques should be considered when the resection-and-anastomosis technique is not considered optimal.

When coarctation is associated with certain types of large VSDs, the approach is via a median sternotomy, using cardiopulmonary bypass and circulatory arrest, similar to the approach used for interrupted aortic arch (see Chapter 22). The arch can be reconstructed primarily, as in interrupted aortic arch; otherwise, if there is a very elongated segment of

tubular hypoplasia, a glutaraldehyde-treated autologous pericardial patch applied to the undersurface of the arch and extending beyond the coarctation site (as in the initial aspect of the distal arch reconstruction in the hypoplastic left heart syndrome) (see Chapter 23) may be the best approach.

Another situation we have seen on several occasions is the presence of a discrete coarctation with a significantly hypoplastic distal arch and isthmus in combination with a spectrum of aortic arch variants best described as the "bovine" innominate trunk (i.e., the left carotid artery arises either very close to, or as a branch of, the innominate artery). This may result in a technically difficult, if not impossible, exposure via a left thoracotomy, as it may not be possible to place the upper aortic clamp proximal to the entire hypoplastic segment without seriously compromising flow to the innominate artery during clamping. Variations in the bovine trunk do exist in which the clamp can be placed proximal to the hypoplasia without compromising the innominate inflow; however, when there is no continuity of the left carotid origin with the aorta itself (i.e., the left carotid is a discrete branch off the innominate), especially in a small infant, clamp placement may be impossible. In this case it may be best to approach this lesion via a median sternotomy, using cardiopulmonary bypass and deep hypothermic circulatory arrest (as in interrupted aortic arch) with either advancement of the descending aorta to the distal part of the ascending aorta or patching of the undersurface of the arch and isthmus as described previously.

Another anatomic variant, also best approached with flexibility, is coarctation with significant hypoplasia of the isthmus and distal arch and an elongated distal arch. An extended resection-and-anastomosis approach may be possible; however, the elongated segment of hypoplastic distal arch may present a problem with suture line tension even if extensive mobilization is carried out. In this case the left subclavian artery may be used as a flap, in retrograde fashion, to augment the top of the distal arch between the left carotid and left subclavian arteries. This enlarges the hypoplastic distal arch very effectively. The isthmus and the discrete coarctation are then resected, and the descending aorta is anastomosed end to end to the proximal segment, which consists of the augmented tube made up of tissue from both the arch and the left subclavian artery.

Specific indications for standard subclavian flap aortoplasty, patch aortoplasty, and conduit reconstruction are discussed below under "Specific Techniques."

Specific Techniques

Resection and Anastomosis

Resection and anastomosis is our preferred technique for discrete coarctation of the aorta without significant tubular hypoplasia of the proximal arch (Fig. 21–2). The distal arch, left subclavian artery, isthmus, ductus arteriosus, and descending aorta are dissected, and a curved, side-biting vascular clamp of appropriate size is used to crossclamp the distal aortic arch, including the left subclavian artery. An angled, vascular crossclamp is used to crossclamp the descending aorta approximately 1.5 cm below the insertion of the ductus, also using the clamp to control intercostal arteries if possible. Intercostals may need to be individually controlled as mentioned previously. The ductus arteriosus is then ligated with a polypropylene fixation suture.

The aorta is transected at the level of the ductus. Ductal tissue is carefully trimmed from the proximal and distal edges of the aorta. It may be necessary to resect the proximal tissue more aggressively, even though all ductal tissue has been removed, to augment the proximal circumference if any isthmic hypoplasia is present. The distal end often presents a somewhat different problem. Usually the circumference of the distal stoma is quite adequate without aggressive resection of tissue; however, there is much more uncertainty about leaving retained ductal tissue. Objective assessment of the completeness of ductal resection is usually lacking; however, careful attention to the appearance of the endothelial surface and the integrity of the vascular musculature can often help. The surgeon should approach the distal aorta aggressively, because suture line tension is usually not a problem with standard end-to-end anastomosis. The anastomosis itself is begun at the point of the aortic circumference farthest from the surgeon, completing sequentially the posterior and then the anterior aspect of the suture line.

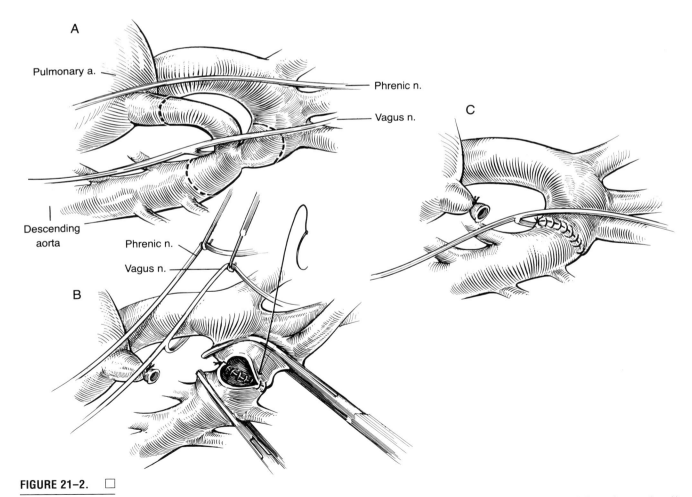

FIGURE 21–2. ☐

A, Discrete aortic coarctation in an infant with a small ductus arteriosus or ligamentum arteriosum, seen via left thoracotomy exposure. *B*, Repair technique using resection with end-to-end anastomosis. *C*, Complete repair.

Extended Resection and Anastomosis

Some prefer an extended resection and anastomosis when significant tubular hypoplasia is present in the isthmus or the distal or proximal portions of the arch (Fig. 21–3). Proximal mobilization to the level of the base of the innominate artery is mandatory, and more extensive mobilization of the distal part of the aorta (to the level of the third or even fourth set of intercostal arteries) is also carried out. The ductus arteriosus and the descending aorta are otherwise managed as described previously. The upper curved aortic crossclamp is placed as proximally as possible, usually at the level of the undersurface of the arch and opposite the origin of the innominate artery, while documenting unobstructed forward flow to the innominate artery by pulse oximetry or a radial arterial line. This clamp will also isolate the left carotid and subclavian arteries as well. After placement of both proximal and distal clamps and ligation of the ductus arteriosus, the reconstruction proceeds. Some members of our group begin by ligating the hypoplastic isthmus just above the coarctated site with a polypropylene fixation suture. The descending aorta is then transected at the ductal insertion and prepared as in the standard technique described previously. A longitudinal incision is made in the undersurface of the aortic arch and extended proximal to the hypoplastic segment. If the distal arch is hypoplastic, this incision must extend to the level of the base of the left carotid artery, while if the proximal arch is also hypoplastic, it must extend to the base of the innominate artery. This incision must also be made long enough to create a circumference at least as large as that of the descending aorta. Others in our group prepare the undersurface of the arch by transecting the isthmus and filletting open the arch from the transection site proximally to beyond the hypoplastic segment. An end-to-side anastomosis of the descending aorta to the undersurface of the arch is then performed, using the same suture technique used for the standard procedure. Tension at the anastomosis is a much more real possibility with the extended procedure, emphasizing the need for aggressive proximal and distal mobilization.

Reverse Subclavian Flap Aortoplasty

Some prefer the reverse subclavian flap aortoplasty technique when there is any significant hypoplasia of the proximal or distal arch, while others reserve this technique for significant distal arch hypoplasia combined with an elongated arch in which the extended resection-and-anastomosis technique may produce unacceptable tension on the suture line (Fig. 21–4).

After mobilizing the arch as previously described, the left subclavian artery is divided peripherally, just before it branches. The arch is exposed to the level of the proximal arch, including a 5-mm length of the proximal part of the left carotid. The proximal curved clamp is placed between the innominate and left carotid arteries so that the carotid itself is included. The distal clamp is placed across the isthmus, allowing continued perfusion of the lower body via the ductus arteriosus if it is open. A longitudinal incision is made in the roof of the distal arch and extended proximally onto the base of the left carotid artery and distally onto the left subclavian artery, creating the subclavian flap. This flap is then turned back proximally onto the incision in the roof of the arch and the left carotid artery base to augment the distal arch lumen. After this the ductus arteriosus is ligated, and the distal clamp is moved to its standard position on the descending aorta. The discrete coarctation and isthmus are reconstructed as in the standard resection-and-anastomosis procedure. This combined technique provides relief of obstruction at the distal arch and at the isthmus and coarctation site, without creating tension on the suture line.

Standard Subclavian Flap Aortoplasty

In our opinion there are only a few morphologic or physiologic circumstances in which the standard subclavian flap aortoplasty is preferred over resection and anastomosis as the initial procedure. When previous coarctation or other aortic surgery has been performed and extensive scarring is present, this approach may be beneficial in that circumferential mobilization is not necessary. Also, in neonates in whom it is desirable that the ductus arteriosus be preserved (borderline small left ventricle), this approach may be considered.[69]

The proximal clamp is placed across the distal arch between the left carotid and subclavian arteries after ligating the left subclavian artery peripherally (Fig. 21–5). A longitudinal incision is made in the posterior aspect of the divided subclavian artery and extended distally across the junction of the subclavian artery and the aorta, the isthmus, and the coarctation site and onto the descending aorta. The discrete coarcted shelf, if prominent, is then carefully excised, taking care not to disrupt the aortic media. The resulting subclavian flap is then turned down to augment the isthmus and coarctation site, using running suture. To minimize late aneurysm formation, careful attention should be given to avoiding aggressive resection of the intimal shelf and unnecessary ballooning of the patch. These

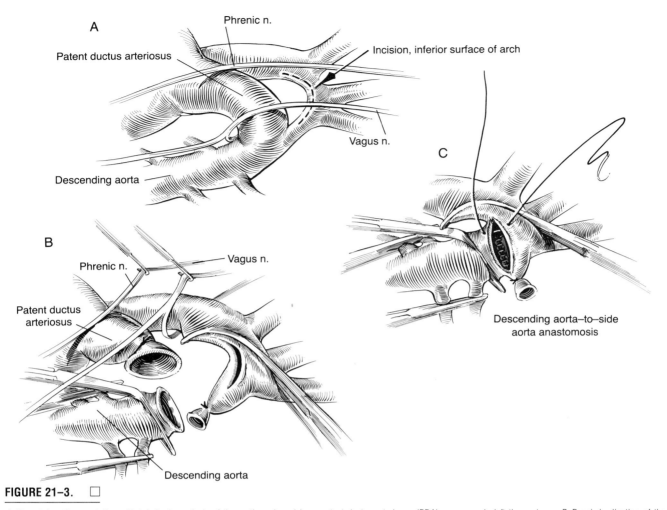

A
Phrenic n.
Patent ductus arteriosus
Incision, inferior surface of arch
Vagus n.
Descending aorta

C
Descending aorta–to–side
aorta anastomosis

B
Phrenic n.
Vagus n.
Patent ductus
arteriosus
Descending aorta

FIGURE 21–3. □

A, Neonatal aortic coarctation with tubular hypoplasia of the aortic arch and large patent ductus arteriosus (PDA) exposure via left thoracotomy. *B,* Repair by ligation of the isthmus and ductus arteriosus, resection of the discrete coarctation, and advancement of the descending aorta to the undersurface of the aortic arch.

same issues are discussed in more detail in the next section.

Patch Aortoplasty

In our opinion, patch aortoplasty is indicated only for specific situations. These include cases of discrete recoarctation that do not respond to balloon dilatation, some cases of diffuse hypoplasia with an elongated arch, and the rare infant who is in extremis because of inability to reopen the ductus with prostaglandin E_1 and in whom speed is of utmost importance.

Minimal noncircumferential dissection of the isthmus is all that is necessary (Fig. 21–6). After ligation of the ductus or ligamentum, a single, appropriate-size, side-biting curved clamp can be used to isolate the aorta from the base of the left subclavian artery to beyond the coarctation. A longitudinal incision is made opposite the ductal insertion and extended proximally onto the base of the left subclavian artery and distally well beyond the coarctation itself. If a discrete shelf is present, it may be cautiously resected, avoiding injury to the media of the aorta. An oval synthetic patch is created such that the resulting lumen at the most narrow point will be at least as large as the descending thoracic aorta. The patch is applied with a continuous suture. Because formation of an aneurysm opposite the patch is a real concern, steps should be taken to avoid this problem. Although the mechanism of aneurysm formation is not completely understood, a number of factors that may predispose to it have been suggested. These include excessive resection of the intimal shelf,[21] retention of abnormal aortic tissue,[1] excessive bulging of the patch itself,[20] and intensification of the pulse wave at the native tissue opposite the patch owing to inelasticity of the prosthetic material.[55] Although none of these potential mechanisms has been definitely proven, the empiric obser-

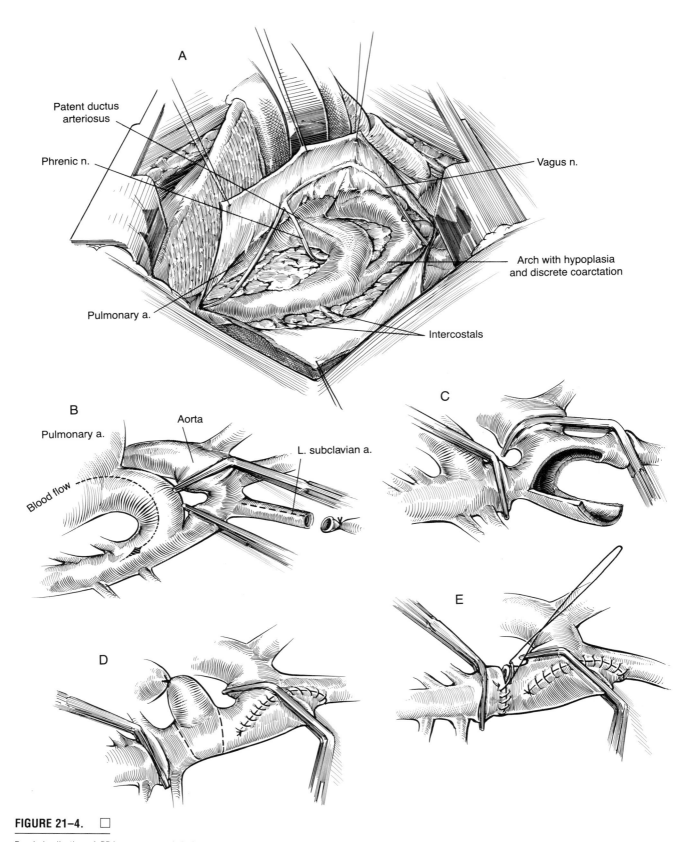

FIGURE 21–4. □

Repair by ligation of PDA, a reverse subclavian artery flap, resection of the discrete coarctation, and end-to-end anastomosis. *A,* Exposure. *B,* Initial clamp placement. *C,* Incision of distal arch, subclavian artery, and carotid artery. *D,* Reverse subclavian reconstruction completed and clamps readjusted. *E,* Resection of isthmus and discrete coarctation and end-to-end anastomosis.

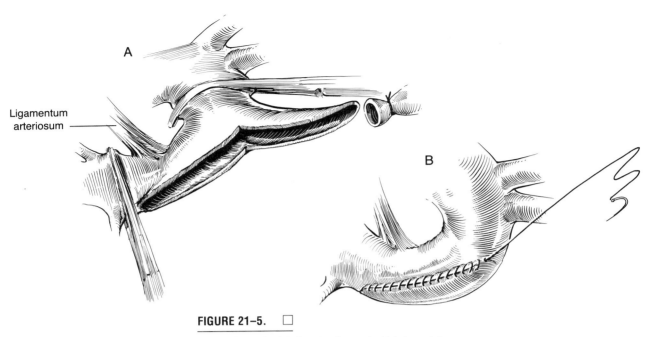

FIGURE 21–5. □

A and *B*, Standard subclavian artery flap repair of infant coarctation.

Ligamentum arteriosum

vation of the development of aneurysms is undisputed. It would seem reasonable to avoid excessive resection of the shelf and to tailor the patch to minimize ballooning. These same principles apply to the subclavian flap aortoplasty as well. These maneuvers, along with control of chronic hypertension, may reduce aortic wall stress opposite the patch, thereby minimizing the elastin fiber disruption and

disintegration found in the walls of these aneurysms.[5, 20, 31]

Conduit Reconstruction

In the present era conduit reconstruction should be used rarely and only as a last resort (e.g., when an unacceptable gradient is present after initial re-

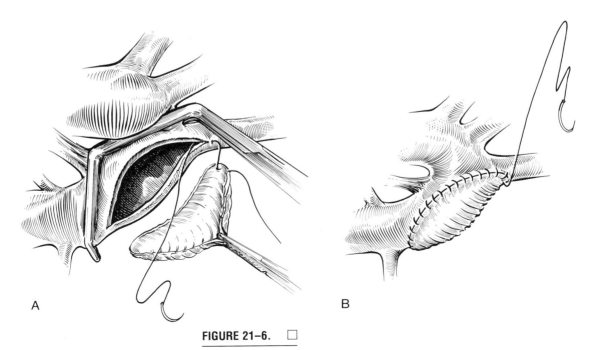

FIGURE 21–6. □

A and *B*, Patch aortoplasty repair of infant coarctation.

construction using one of the other techniques and when no other method of revision is judged likely to be successful). In the neonate or small infant, a 6-mm diameter PTFE tube is attached to the arch in end-to-side fashion, proximal to the segment of hypoplasia. The distal anastomosis is created end to end to the descending aorta after the distal part of the aorta is prepared in the usual way, as described previously. Alternatively, the distal anastomosis may be end to side as well. Continuous suture technique is used. In reoperative situations, tube grafts can also be placed via a median sternotomy or right thoracotomy, with the approach determined by practical considerations.

Postoperative Care

Systemic hypertension in the early postoperative period is not unusual after coarctation repair in neonates and infants. This paradoxic hypertension is thought to be due to imbalances in sympathetic discharge, baroreceptor activity, and the renin-angiotensin system.[58] Evidence suggests that paradoxic hypertension may be avoided if coarctation is relieved by balloon dilatation rather than by surgery.[12] However, we do not recommend this technique for native coarctation. A review of the collective experience from nine centers regarding balloon dilatation for native coarctation revealed an aneurysm rate of about 12%.[56]

Hypertension can be treated effectively with a continuous intravenous infusion of sodium nitroprusside. Others have recommended beta blockers, beginning before surgery.[25] The threshold for treating hypertension is somewhat arbitrary. In neonates and infants we consistently treat any patient whose systolic blood pressure is greater than 120 mm Hg. If there is concern regarding the security of the anastomosis, this threshold is lowered. Postoperative hypertension may be relatively transient, lasting hours to days, or it may be more sustained. About 30% of neonates and infants are discharged from the hospital taking an afterload-reducing agent such as captopril. This can often be discontinued within several months; however, definitive long-term conclusions regarding the incidence of chronic hypertension after adequate repair of neonatal coarctation is not available.

The postcoarctation syndrome of intestinal ischemia secondary to splanchnic vasospasm is not a well-recognized entity in neonates and infants in our experience. Postoperative hemorrhage is also rare; however, bleeding at the suture line can be exacerbated by uncontrolled systemic hypertension.

Chylothorax is an unusual but well-recognized complication of coarctation repair in infants. This most often responds within 5 to 10 days to conservative therapy consisting of continuous tube drainage and a diet restricting fat intake to only medium-chain triglycerides. Rarely, a patient must undergo an exploratory thoracotomy for control of the lymphatic injury. Primary control of the injury is preferred to ligation of the thoracic duct.

In uncomplicated coarctation repair, the thoracotomy drainage tube can be removed within 24 to 48 hours after surgery.

It is not unusual for repaired infants to be discharged taking digoxin and some form of diuretic until left ventricular mass, compliance, and systolic function return to normal. These medications become even more necessary if remaining cardiovascular lesions, such as a moderate-size VSD, are present.

If recurrent coarctation develops, it usually becomes manifest in infants and neonates within 1 year after the initial operation.[61] This observation fits with the hypothesis that remodeling of retained ductal tissue plays a prominent role in recoarctation. Management of recoarctation involves reoperation or balloon dilatation. We prefer balloon dilatation if the recoarctation occurs more than 2 months after the initial repair.[43, 62] Others have also reported success with this approach.

RESULTS

At Children's Hospital in Boston, a review of the surgical experience from January 1984 through December 1991 was undertaken of patients who underwent repair of isolated aortic coarctation (or repair with ligation of the patent ductus arteriosus) during the first year of life. Of the 138 patients, 98 (71%) were neonates, 17 (12%) were infants between 1 and 3 months old; 10 (7%) were between 4 and 6 months old; and 13 (9%) were between 7 and 12 months of age. Table 21–3 summarizes the total cases and mortality. Of the 14 neonatal deaths, 12 were in patients with one or more associated left-sided obstructive or hypoplastic lesions (Table 21–4). Many of these patients had a diagnosis of Shone's complex or moderate forms of the hypoplas-

TABLE 21–3. □ ISOLATED INFANT COARCTATION REPAIR, 1984 TO 1992

AGE AT REPAIR	NO. OF CASES	NO. OF DEATHS (%)
<1 mo	98	14 (14)
1–12 mo	40	0 (0)
TOTAL	138	14 (10)

TABLE 21–4. □ LESIONS ASSOCIATED WITH DEATHS IN
NEONATES UNDERGOING ISOLATED COARCTATION REPAIR (*N* = 14)

ASSOCIATED LESIONS	NO.
Various left-sided obstructive lesions	12
Congenital diaphragmatic hernia on extracorporeal membrane oxygenation	1
VSD, unroofed coronary sinus syndrome	1

VSD, Ventricular septal defect.

tic left heart syndrome and were judged to have a better prognosis with an attempted two-ventricle repair. For example, one of these 12 had a moderate variant of the hypoplastic left heart syndrome. Coarctation repair was attempted at 7 days of age. The patient was unable to be weaned from the ventilator and died at 1 month of age at the time of surgical conversion to stage 1 hypoplastic left heart physiology. A second patient underwent coarctation repair at 8 days of age with a known moderate-size VSD and significant valvar aortic stenosis. Persistent postoperative congestive heart failure 1 week after surgery precipitated cardiac catheterization to evaluate the aortic valve and ventricular septal defect. The patient died during the cardiac catheterization. In all, 58 patients in this series had significant associated left-sided obstructive or hypoplastic lesions, with 12 deaths (21%).

The other two deaths occurred in patients without left-sided lesions. One had coarctation repair at 10 days of age after undergoing surgery to correct a large left diaphragmatic hernia. After the diaphragmatic hernia repair, the patient was placed on extracorporeal membrane oxygenation (ECMO) and underwent the coarctation repair while on ECMO. The second patient had an associated VSD and unroofed coronary sinus syndrome and died at 3 months of age of a preventable complication in the intensive care unit after closure of the septal defect and atrial repair. All 14 deaths occurred in patients who underwent coarctation repair during the neonatal period; nine of the 14 deaths occurred in the hospital.

Intermediate-term follow-up was available in 98 of the 129 hospital survivors, with a mean follow-up time of 1.75 years. There were five additional deaths associated with subsequent cardiac procedures not directly related to the coarctation itself.

At Children's Hospital in Boston, our technical approach to coarctation has evolved. In the 1984–1985 period, only one patient underwent resection with anastomosis; most patients received either a standard subclavian flap aortoplasty or patch aortoplasty. In 1986 all three of these techniques were used frequently. From 1987 to the present, resection with anastomosis was the preferred method of re-

pair. Recently, standard patch aortoplasty and the standard subclavian flap aortoplasty have not been used. However, retrograde subclavian flap aortoplasty combined with resection and anastomosis has been used in a number of patients who had hypoplasia of the arch, and extended resection and anastomosis has been used more liberally when moderate or severe hypoplasia is present.

Deaths occurred in patients receiving patch aortoplasty, standard subclavian flap aortoplasty, and resection and anastomosis. None of the deaths could be attributed to the technique itself. There were 12 second interventions for a residual or recurrent aortic coarctation (12/138, or 9%). All of these were in patients who had initial neonatal repairs, with a mean age of 9.5 days at the time of original repair. In neonates the reintervention rate was 12/98, or 12%.

Reintervention was by operation in four early recurrences (after 17, 24, 30, and 60 days) and three later recurrences (after 6 months, 2 years, and 3 years) and by balloon dilatation in five (one at 2 months, two at 3 months, two at 1 year). This experience is consistent with that of others who have found that recurrence after neonatal coarctation repair most commonly occurs within the first year.[61] Recurrences were present in patients who initially received standard subclavian flap aortoplasty, patch aortoplasty, and resection. An additional seven recurrent coarctations (less than 20 mm Hg resting gradient) were identified at follow-up, but these patients did not undergo reintervention.

A total of 27 patients with associated VSD were not able to be managed without reintervention to close the defect (27/76, or 36%). Twenty of these 27 were neonates at the time of the initial repair. The timing of subsequent VSD closure ranged from 2 days to 10 months after coarctation repair. In only 16 of these 27 cases was the VSD judged to be large before the coarctation repair. Therefore, 16 of the 24 patients (67%) with known large VSDs required subsequent closure. (It must be emphasized that a group of neonates and infants with coarctation and associated large VSDs who underwent single-stage repair of both lesions is not included in this analysis. Of the 43 patients with known small or moderate defects, 11 (26%) required reintervention to address the septal defect. If malalignment and complete atrioventricular canal ventricular septal defects are excluded from the group with large defects, leaving only large muscular and membranous ventricular defects, then seven of 15 (47%) required subsequent closure. A total of six pulmonary artery bands were placed for isolated VSD, all before 1987. Six required closure, while one closed spontaneously.

SUMMARY

Aortic coarctation, especially in neonates and infants, is a deceptively complex lesion. Mortality rates, residual or recurrent coarctation rates, and complication rates do not provide definitive information on which to base recommendations for exclusive use of any of the various methods of repair. Each technique has advantages and disadvantages, some theoretical and others practical. Familiarity with the various techniques and awareness of the specific advantages and disadvantages of each, coupled with a clear understanding of the individual patient's morphology and physiologic status, allows the surgeon to make the best possible decision regarding the timing and technique of surgery. The most important principle is that the surgeon not take an intellectually rigid approach.

At the present time we believe that some form of resection with anastomosis is the procedure of choice under the following conditions: the patient is physiologically stable when taken to the operating room, and there is the potential for complete resection of ductal tissue and anastomosis proximal to all significant tubular hypoplasia without producing tension on the suture line. As discussed in this chapter, the availability of prostaglandin E$_1$, the development of absorbable suture material, the attractive concept of completely removing the abnormal tissue from the aortic lumen, and the experience gained from other procedures (e.g., arterial switch operation) demonstrating that circumferential tension-free aortic suture lines invariably grow normally when normal tissue is involved, all support this approach. If these criteria cannot be met with confidence, another repair technique should be chosen, based on specific morphologic and physiologic considerations.

Recommendations regarding the timing of coarctation repair cannot be made with certainty. At the present time we believe that elective coarctation repair is best performed at 3 to 6 months of age and repair in symptomatic patients should be undertaken at the time of diagnosis.

Assessment and management of the patient with coarctation and VSD remain problematic. At Children's Hospital in Boston, we recommend single-stage repair of both lesions via a median sternotomy, using cardiopulmonary bypass if the VSD is large and unlikely to close spontaneously. In the patient with a muscular or perimembranous defect, significant reduction in size and even spontaneous closure are not uncommon, even if the defect is large at the time initial imaging studies are made. In neonates it is often difficult to accurately characterize the physiologic significance of the VSD preoper-

atively because of the patency of the ductus arteriosus. We recommend repair of the coarctation alone in this situation, with a low threshold for subsequent early repair of the ventricular defect. Pulmonary artery banding is used only for patients who cannot be repaired (i.e., inaccessible or multiple VSDs). Further efforts directed at defining physiologic and morphologic characteristics that can better predict those VSDs that are likely to close or be restrictive are needed.

Mortality after coarctation repair in patients without associated defects or with an isolated VSD is rare. In our experience, mortality is almost exclusively limited to patients with variants of Shone's complex or borderline forms of the hypoplastic left heart syndrome, suggesting that mortality is related mostly to inappropriate selection of patients rather than to technically related issues. The problem of deciding when a patient with multiple left-sided lesions is better managed as a single-ventricle patient is addressed in more detail in Chapter 15.

REFERENCES

1. Ala-Kulju K, Jarvinen A, Maamies T, et al. Late aneurysms after patch aortoplasty for coarctation of the aorta in adults. Thorac Cardiovasc Surg 31:301, 1983.
2. Becker AE, Becker MJ, Edwards JE. Anomalies associated with coarctation of the aorta. Particular reference to infancy. Circulation 41:1067, 1970.
3. Beekman RH, Katz BP, Moorehead-Steffens C, et al. Altered baroreceptor function in children with systolic hypertension after coarctation repair. Am J Cardiol 52:112, 1983.
4. Beekman RH, Rocchini AP, Behrendt DM, et al. Long-term outcome after repair of coarctation in infancy: Subclavian angioplasty does not reduce the need for reoperation. J Am Coll Cardiol 8:1406, 1986.
5. Bergdahl L, Ljungqvist A. Long-term results after repair of coarctation of the aorta by patch grafting. J Thorac Cardiovasc Surg 80:177, 1980.
6. Blalock A, Park EA. Surgical treatment of experimental coarctation (atresia) of aorta. Ann Surg 119:445, 1944.
7. Bone GE, Ammons D. Characterization of experimental arterial stenosis by numerate analysis of the Doppler velocity waveform. Surg Forum 29:208, 1978.
8. Calodney MM, Carson MJ. Coarctation of the aorta in early infancy. J Pediatr 37:46, 1950.
9. Campbell DB, Waldhausen JA, Pierce WS, et al. Should elective repair of coarctation of the aorta be done in infancy? J Thorac Cardiovasc Surg 88:929, 1984.
10. Campbell M. Natural history of coarctation of the aorta. Br Heart J 32:633, 1970.
11. Carpenter MA, Dammann JF, Watson DD, et al. Left ventricular hyperkinesis at rest and during exercise in normotensive patients 2 to 27 years after coarctation repair. J Am Coll Cardiol 6:879, 1985.
12. Choy M, Rocchini AP, Beekman RH, et al. Paradoxical hypertension after repair of coarctation of the aorta in children: Balloon angioplasty versus surgical repair. Circulation 75:1186, 1987.
13. Clarkson PM, Brandt PWT, Barratt-Boyes BG, et al. Prosthetic repair of coarctation of the aorta with particular reference to Dacron onlay patch grafts and late aneurysm formation. Am J Cardiol 56:342, 1985.
14. Cobanoglu A, Teply JF, Grunkemeir GL, et al. Coarctation of

the aorta in patients younger than three months: A critique of the subclavian flap operation. J Thorac Cardiovasc Surg 89:128, 1985.

15. Connor TM, Baker WP. A comparison of coarctation resection and patch angioplasty using postexercise blood pressure measurements. Circulation 64:567, 1981.

16. Crafoord C, Nylin G. Congenital coarctation of the aorta and its surgical treatment. J Thorac Surg 37:46, 1950.

17. Crawford FA, Sade RM. Spinal cord injury associated with hyperthermia during aortic coarctation repair. J Thorac Cardiovasc Surg 87:616, 1984.

18. Daniels SR, James FW, Loggie JM, et al. Correlates of resting and maximal exercise systolic blood pressure after repair of coarctation of the aorta: A multivariable analysis. Am Heart J 113:349, 1987.

19. De Mendonca JT, Carvalho MR, Costa RK, et al. Coarctation of the aorta. A new surgical technique. J Thorac Cardiovasc Surg 90:445, 1985.

20. Del Nido PJ, Williams WG, Wilson GJ, et al. Synthetic patch angioplasty for repair of coarctation of the aorta. Experience with aneurysm formation. Circulation 74(suppl I):32, 1986.

21. DeSanto A, Bills RG, King H, et al. Pathogenesis of aneurysm formation opposite prosthetic patches used for coarctation repair. J Thorac Cardiovasc Surg 94:720, 1987.

22. Fenchel G, Steil E, Seybold-Epting W, et al. Repair of symptomatic aortic coarctation in the first three months of life. Early and late results after resection and end-to-end anastomosis and subclavian flap angioplasty. J Cardiovasc Surg 29:257, 1988.

23. Freed M, Rocchini A, Rosenthal A, et al. Exercise-induced hypertension after surgical repair of coarctation of the aorta. Am J Cardiol 42:253, 1979.

24. Fyler DC. Report of the New England regional infant cardiac program. Pediatrics 64(suppl):432, 1980.

25. Gidding SS, Rocchini AP, Beekman R, et al. Therapeutic effect of propranolol on paradoxical hypertension after repair of coarctation of the aorta. N Engl J Med 312:1224, 1985.

26. Gidding SS, Rocchini AP, Moorehead C, et al. Increased forearm vascular reactivity in patients with hypertension after repair of coarctation. Circulation 71:495, 1985.

27. Graham TP Jr, Atwood GF, Boerth RC, et al. Right and left heart size and function in infants with symptomatic coarctation. Circulation 56:641, 1988.

28. Gross RE. Surgical correction for coarctation of the aorta. Surgery 18:673, 1945.

29. Gross RE. Treatment of certain aortic coarctations by homologous grafts. Ann Surg 134:753, 1951.

30. Gross RE, Hufnagel CA. Coarctation of the aorta. Experimental studies regarding its surgical correction. N Engl J Med 233:287, 1945.

31. Hehrlein FW, Mulch J, Rautenberg HW, et al. Incidence and pathogenesis of late aneurysms after patch graft aortoplasty for coarctation. J Thorac Cardiovasc Surg 92:226, 1986.

32. Ho SY, Anderson RH. Coarctation, tubular hypoplasia, and the ductus arteriosus. Histological study of 35 specimens. Br Heart J 41:268, 1979.

33. Hutchins GM. Coarctation of the aorta explained as a branch point of the ductus arteriosus. Am J Pathol 63:203, 1971.

34. Igler FO, Boerboom LE, Werner PH, et al. Coarctation of the aorta and baroreceptor resetting. A study of carotid baroreceptor stimulus-response characteristics before and after surgical repair in the dog. Circ Res 48:365, 1981.

35. John CN, Cartmill TB, Johnson DC, et al. Report of four cases of aneurysm complicating patch aortoplasty for repair of coarctation of the aorta. Aust NZ J Surg 59:748, 1989.

36. Johnston KW, Kassam M, Cobbold RSC. Relationship between Doppler pulsatility index and direct femoral pressure measurements in the diagnosis of aortoiliac occlusive disease. Ultrasound Med Biol 9:271, 1983.

37. Jonas RA. Coarctation: Do we need to resect ductal tissue? Ann Thorac Surg 52:604, 1991.

38. Kopf GS, Hellenbrand W, Kleinman C, et al. Repair of aortic coarctation in the first three months of life: Immediate and long-term results. Ann Thorac Surg 41:425, 1986.

39. Kron IL, Flanagan TL, Rheuban KS, et al. Incidence and risk

40. Ladusans EJ, Campalani G, Parsons JM, et al. Recurrence of aortic coarctation following repair by re-implantation of the subclavian artery. Int J Cardiol 23:321, 1989.

41. Lang HT Jr, Nadas AS. Coarctation of the aorta with congestive heart failure in infancy—medical treatment. Pediatrics 17:45, 1956.

42. Levin SE, Milner S, Colsen P, et al. Patch graft aortoplasty for repair of coarctation of the aorta in infants under 1 year of age. S Afr Med J 28:535, 1983.

43. Lock JE, Bass JL, Amplatz K, et al. Balloon dilation angioplasty of aortic coarctations in infants and children. Circulation 68:109, 1983.

44. Lodge FA, Lamberti JJ, Goodman AH, et al. Vascular consequences of subclavian artery transection for the treatment of congenital heart disease. J Thorac Cardiovasc Surg 86:18, 1983.

45. Markel H, Rocchini AP, Beekman RH, et al. Exercise-induced hypertension after repair of coarctation of the aorta: Arm versus leg exercise. J Am Coll Cardiol 8:165, 1986.

46. Martin MM, Beekman RH, Rocchini AP, et al. Aortic aneurysms after subclavian angioplasty repair of coarctation of the aorta. Am J Cardiol 61:951, 1988.

47. McGoldrick JP, Brown IW, Ross DN. Coarctation of the aorta: Late aneurysm formation with Dacron onlay patch grafting. Ann Thorac Surg 45:89, 1988.

48. Meier MA, Lucchese FA, Jazbik W, et al. A new technique for repair of aortic coarctation. Subclavian flap aortoplasty with preservation of arterial blood flow to the left arm. J Thorac Cardiovasc Surg 92:1005, 1986.

49. Metzdorff MT, Cobanoglu A, Grunkemeir GL, et al. Influence of age at operation on late results with subclavian flap aortoplasty. J Thorac Cardiovasc Surg 89:235, 1985.

50. Moffat DB. Pre- and postnatal changes in the left subclavian artery and their possible relationship to coarctation of the aorta. Acta Anat 43:346, 1960.

51. Morris GC, Cooley DA, DeBakey ME, et al. Coarctation of the aorta with particular emphasis upon improved techniques of surgical repair. J Thorac Cardiovasc Surg 40:705, 1960.

52. Moulaert AJ, Bruins CC, Oppenheimer-Dekker A. Anomalies of the aortic arch and ventricular septal defects. Circulation 52:1011, 1976.

53. Mustard WT, Rower RD, Keith JD, et al. Coarctation of the aorta with special reference to the first year of life. Ann Surg 141:249, 1955.

54. Olansman S, Shapiro AJ, Schiller MS, et al. Extended aortic arch anastomosis for repair of coarctation in infancy. Circulation 74(suppl III):37, 1986.

55. Olsson P, Soderlund S, Dubiel WT, et al. Patch grafts or tubular grafts in the repair of coarctation of the aorta. Scand J Thorac Cardiovasc Surg 10:139, 1976.

56. Rao PS, Chopra PS. Role of balloon angioplasty in the treatment of aortic coarctation. Ann Thorac Surg 52:621, 1991.

57. Rheuban KS, Gutgesell HP, Carpenter MA, et al. Aortic aneurysm after patch angioplasty for aortic isthmic coarctation in childhood. Am J Cardiol 58:178, 1986.

58. Rocchini AP, Rosenthal A, Barger AC, et al. Pathogenesis of paradoxical hypertension after coarctation resection. Circulation 54:382, 1976.

59. Rudolph AM, Heymann MA, Spitznas U. Haemodynamic considerations in the development of narrowing of the aorta. Am J Cardiol 30:514, 1972.

60. Sahn DJ, Allen HD, McDonald G, et al. Real-time cross-sectional echocardiographic diagnosis of coarctation of the aorta. Circulation 56:762, 1977.

61. Sanchez GR, Balsara RK, Dunn JM, et al. Recurrent obstruction after subclavian flap repair of coarctation of the aorta in infants. Can it be predicted or prevented? J Thorac Cardiovasc Surg 91:738, 1986.

62. Saul JP, Keane JF, Fellows KE, et al. Balloon dilation angioplasty of postoperative aortic obstructions. Am J Cardiol 59:943, 1987.

63. Sciolaro C, Copeland J, Cork R, et al. Long-term follow-up

comparing subclavian flap angioplasty to resection with modified oblique end-to-end anastomosis. J Thorac Cardiovasc Surg 101:1, 1991.

64. Shinebourne EA, Tam ASY, Elseed AM, et al. Coarctation of the aorta in infancy and childhood. Br Heart J 38:375, 1976.

65. Simsolo R, Grunfeld B, Gimenez M, et al. Long-term systemic hypertension in children after successful repair of coarctation of the aorta. Am Heart J 115:1268, 1988.

66. Skovranek J, Goetzova J, Samanek M. Changes in muscle blood flow and development of the arm following the Blalock-Taussig anastomosis. Cardiology 61:131, 1975.

67. Smith RT Jr, Sade RM, Riopel DA, et al. Stress testing for comparison of synthetic patch aortoplasty with resection and end to end anastomosis for repair of coarctation in childhood. J Am Coll Cardiol 4:765, 1984.

68. Todd PJ, Dangerfield PH, Hamilton DI, et al. Late effects on the left upper limb of subclavian flap aortoplasty. J Thorac Cardiovasc Surg 85:678, 1983.

69. Ungerleider RM. Is there a role for prosthetic patch aortoplasty in the repair of coarctation? Ann Thorac Surg 52:601, 1991.

70. van Son JA, Daniels O, Vincent JG, et al. Appraisal of resection and end-to-end anastomosis for repair of coarctation of the aorta in infancy: Preference for resection. Ann Thorac Surg 48:496, 1989.

71. Van Son JAM, van Asten WNJC, van Lier HJJ, et al. A comparison of coarctation resection flap angioplasty using ultrasonographically monitored postocclusive reactive hyperemia. J Thorac Cardiovasc Surg 100:817, 1990.

72. Van Son JAM, van Asten WNJC, van Lier HJJ, et al. Detrimental sequelae on the hemodynamics of the upper left limb after subclavian flap angioplasty in infancy. Circulation 81:996, 1990.

73. Vosschulte K. Surgical correction of coarctation of the aorta by an "isthmusplastic" operation. Thorax 16:338, 1961.

74. Waldhausen JA, Nahrwold DL. Repair of coarctation of the aorta with a subclavian flap. J Thorac Cardiovasc Surg 51:532, 1966.

75. Williams WG, Shindo G, Trusler GA, et al. Results of repair of coarctation of the aorta during infancy. J Thorac Cardiovasc Surg 79:603, 1980.

76. Ziemer G, Jonas RA, Perry SB, et al. Surgery for coarctation of the aorta in the neonate. Circulation 74(suppl I): I-25, 1986.

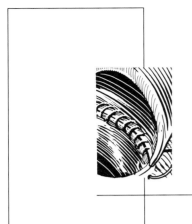

22

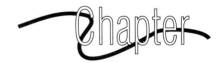

Interrupted Aortic Arch

Interrupted aortic arch (IAA) is the archetype of complex congenital cardiac anomalies that, before the advent of prostaglandin E_1 (PGE_1) carried an extremely high mortality rate during the neonatal period. Not surprisingly, various simple palliative surgical procedures have emerged in an attempt to minimize this high mortality. Through the 1980s, as knowledge increased regarding the preoperative resuscitation of these children, there was an impressive decline in the mortality rate. By the end of the decade, one-stage repair, including direct anastomosis of the arch, emerged as the procedure of choice in most specialized centers. This chapter will focus on the typical complex of IAA with ventricular septal defect (VSD). IAA associated with other complex intracardiac lesions (e.g., truncus arteriosus) will be discussed in detail in the chapters dealing with those intracardiac lesions.

PATHOLOGIC ANATOMY

The arch of the aorta is described as three segments (Fig. 22–1). The proximal component extends from the takeoff of the innominate artery to the left common carotid artery. The distal component extends from the left common carotid artery to the takeoff of the left subclavian artery. The segment of aorta that connects the distal aortic arch to the juxtaductal region of the descending aorta is termed the *isthmus*. These segments have various embryo-

logic origins. The proximal arch is derived from the aortic sac, the distal arch from the fourth embryonic arch, and the isthmus from the junction of the sixth embryonic arch (ductus) with the left dorsal aorta and the fourth embryonic arch. This complex com-

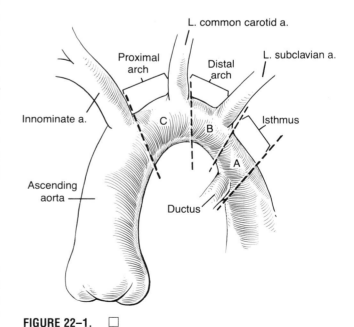

FIGURE 22–1. ☐

The aortic arch is described in three segments: the proximal arch, between the innominate artery and the left common carotid artery; the distal arch, between the left common carotid artery and the left subclavian artery; and the isthmus, which connects the arch to the proximal descending aorta. The classification by Celoria and Patton[2] into interrupted arch types A, B, and C is indicated.

TABLE 22–1. □ TYPE OF INTERRUPTED AORTIC ARCH

ASSOCIATED CARDIAC ANOMALIES	TOTAL NO. OF PATIENTS	TYPE A		TYPE B		TYPE C	
		No. of Patients	Percentage of 20	No. of Patients	Percentage of 49	No. of Patients	Percentage of 2
VSD (isolated)	44	7	35	35	71	2	100
Single ventricle	8	5	25	3	6	—	—
Truncus arteriosus	7	2	10	5	10	—	—
DORV	5	2	10	3	6	—	—
TGA + VSD	2	2	10	—	—	—	—
Complete AV canal	2	1	5	1	2	—	—
DOLV	1	—	—	1	2	—	—
Isolated ventricular inversion + VSD	1	1	5	—	—	—	—
None (PDA present)	1	—	—	1	2	—	—
TOTAL	71	20	100	49	100	2	100

AV, Atrioventricular; DOLV, double-outlet left ventricle; DORV, double-outlet right ventricle; PDA, patent ductus arteriosus; TGA, transposition of the great arteries; VSD, ventricular septal defect.

posite of segments introduces a risk of developmental anomalies in the form of interruptions at the various junction points.

A useful classification of IAA was introduced by Celoria and Patton in 1959.[2] Type A interruption occurs at the level of the isthmus. Not uncommonly it is seen in a milder form in which a fibrous chord connects across the interruption, even though there is no luminal continuity. This has been termed *aortic arch atresia* and generally presents less of a surgical challenge than does a long-segment discontinuity.

Type B interruption occurs between the left common carotid artery and the left subclavian artery. It is the most common type, occurring in between 55% and 69% of cases in various series. Importantly, type B interruption is often associated with an aberrant origin of the right subclavian artery from the descending aorta. In this subtype, more flow must pass through the ductus arteriosus during fetal development and less flow through the left ventricular outflow tract and ascending aorta than with the usual type B interruption (i.e., with normal origin of the right subclavian from the innominate artery). This developmental difference may have implications regarding the risk of left ventricular outflow tract obstruction (LVOTO).

Type C interruption occurs between the innominate artery and the left common carotid. It is extremely rare, having been described in less than 4% of cases in most large clinical and pathologic series.

ASSOCIATED ANOMALIES

Isolated IAA is exceedingly rare. In fact, of necessity there must be an associated anomaly, such as a patent ductus (PDA), to supply blood to the descending aorta and thereby permit survival, even in utero. Apart from PDA, a single conoventricular VSD is the most common associated anomaly (Table 22–1). In the unusual case of an intact ventricular septum, a search should be made for an aortopulmonary window. Frequently, there is posterior malalignment of the conal septum relative to the ventricular septum that contributes to obstruction of the left ventricular outflow tract. It is tempting to ascribe the downstream interruption to this more proximal obstruction, but there are other constituents that can potentially contribute to obstruction of the left ventricular outflow tract.[6] The aortic annulus itself may be hypoplastic. Frequently, the aortic valve is bicuspid, and there may be commissural fusion. Opposite the septum there may be a prominent bundle of muscle that extends from the anterolateral papillary muscle into the outflow tract, the so-called muscle of Moulaert (Fig. 22–2). A fibrous membrane in the left ventricular outflow tract is almost never seen in the neonate with IAA.

Another anomaly commonly associated with IAA is an atrial septal defect. Usually, this is in the form of a stretched patent foramen ovale. Perhaps this defect results from the left-to-right shunt that occurs during in utero development because of the left-sided obstruction resulting from the interruption itself, as well as the associated obstruction of the left ventricular outflow tract, although the presence of a nonrestrictive VSD would argue against this.

Other anomalies seen in association with IAA are listed in Table 22–1. Eleven per cent of these patients have various forms of single ventricle, and 10% have associated truncus arteriosus.

PATHOPHYSIOLOGY

For the patient with the most common form of IAA (i.e., with an associated PDA and conoventric-

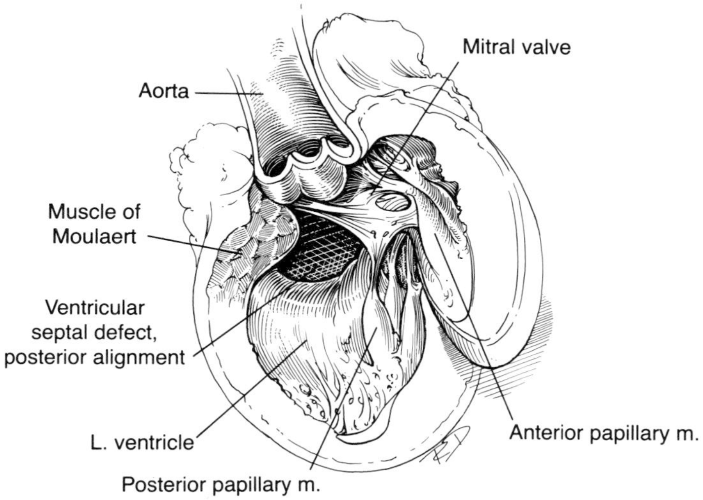

FIGURE 22-2. ☐

Morphologic factors contributing to obstruction of the left ventricular outflow tract with an interrupted aortic arch include posterior malalignment of the conal septum relative to the ventricular septum, hypoplasia of the aortic annulus, a bicuspid aortic valve, and a prominent muscle of Moulaert.

ular VSD), there may be little suspicion of serious heart disease during the early neonatal period until ductal closure begins. If this occurs abruptly or is not recognized rapidly, the child will soon become profoundly acidotic and anuric as perfusion of the lower body becomes entirely dependent on collateral communication between the two separate aortic systems. The distribution of palpable pulses depends on the anatomic subtype. For example, with type B IAA, the pulse in the right arm remains palpable when the left arm and femoral pulses become impalpable secondary to ductal closure. Ischemic injury to the liver is reflected in a marked elevation of hepatic enzymes (serum glutamic-oxaloacetic transaminase [SGOT] and lactate dehydrogenase [LDH]), and ischemic injury to the gut may be followed by evidence of necrotizing enterocolitis (e.g., bloody stools). Renal injury can be quantitated to some extent by the elevation observed in serum creatinine levels.

Ultimately, a severe degree of systemic acidosis (prolonged pH less than 7.0) results in injury to all tissues of the body, including the brain and the heart itself. The child may have seizures and become flaccid and poorly responsive. Myocardial injury becomes apparent from decreased contractility (demonstrated by two-dimensional echocardiography) and the low cardiac output state, despite normalization of other parameters. Because pulmonary blood flow is preserved during ductal closure, it is rare to see evidence of pulmonary insufficiency, although the child will hyperventilate in an attempt to compensate for the metabolic acidosis.

Occasionally, the ductus does not close during the neonatal period, and the diagnosis may be delayed for several weeks. As pulmonary resistance falls, there will be an increasing left-to-right shunt, and the child will show evidence of congestive heart failure, including failure to thrive.

PREOPERATIVE EVALUATION

Diagnosis of Interrupted Aortic Arch

Anatomy

Currently, an accurate anatomic diagnosis can be made using echocardiography alone. This is an important advantage to the critically ill neonate, because the additional insult of an invasive cardiac catheterization can be avoided. In addition to localizing the site of the interruption, the echocardiographer should provide the following information:

1. The distance between the discontinuous aortic segments should be measured.
2. The narrowest dimension of the left ventricular outflow tract (generally related to posterior displacement of the conal septum), the diameter of the aortic annulus, and the diameter of the ascending aorta should also be measured. It is unusual for the segments of the arch that are present to be so hypoplastic that they cause hemodynamic compromise.
3. The features of associated anomalies must be carefully defined. For example, the location of an associated VSD should be defined in relation to its margins. The conal septum is often severely hypoplastic, rendering approach to the superior margin of the defect through the tricuspid valve difficult. Additional VSDs are rare.

Hemodynamic Assessment

Because the diagnosis is generally made when ductal patency has been re-established using PGE$_1$, pressure data are of little use in formulating a plan for surgical management. The issue that most commonly arises concerns the adequacy of the left ventricular outflow tract. Attempts to quantitate the degree of obstruction by measuring a pressure gradient are hampered by a lack of information regarding the amount of flow passing through this area. The VSD is almost always nonrestrictive. There is no evidence that multiple VSDs are more accurately identified by angiography than by color flow Doppler echocardiography.

MEDICAL AND INTERVENTIONAL MANAGEMENT

The introduction of PGE$_1$ in 1976 revolutionized the management of IAA. Before this time, which also predated the introduction of two-dimensional echocardiography, it was necessary to manage acidotic neonates symptomatically as they underwent emergency cardiac catheterization and were then rushed from the catheterization laboratory to the operating room. PGE$_1$ must be infused through a secure intravenous line. If ductal patency does not become apparent in any neonate less than 1 week old within 1 hour after the administration of PGE$_1$, it should be assumed, until proven otherwise, that there is a dosage error or a technical problem with delivery of the medication into the central blood stream. Establishing ductal patency represents just the first step in medically resuscitating the neonate with IAA. Because the lower half of the body is dependent on perfusion through the ductus and because blood in the ductus has the choice of passing into the pulmonary circulation or the systemic circulation, it is important that pulmonary resistance be maximized. This can be achieved by avoiding a high level of inspired oxygen (usually room air is appropriate) and by avoiding respiratory alkalosis through hyperventilation. In fact, control of ventilation is best accomplished by intubating the neonate, sedating him or her with a fentanyl infusion, and inducing paralysis with pancuronium. A peak inspiratory pressure and ventilatory rate that will achieve a PCO$_2$ level of 40 to 50 mm Hg should be selected. Metabolic acidosis must be aggressively treated with boluses of sodium bicarbonate. Because myocardial function is likely to be depressed when the child is first seen and because it may be necessary for the heart to handle a moderate volume load (depending on the success with which pulmonary resistance is maintained), an inotropic agent such as dopamine is almost routinely employed. Dopamine has the added advantage of maximizing renal perfusion in this context of an ischemic renal insult. It is not uncommon to persist with medical resuscitation for 2 to 3 days before surgery is undertaken. It is very unusual for a child to be taken to the operating room with any acid-base, renal, or hepatic abnormalities.

SURGICAL MANAGEMENT
History

IAA was first described by Steidele in 1778.[12] In 1959, Celoria and Patton reported their anatomic classification, as described previously.[2] Successful surgical repair was first accomplished by Samson in 1955 in a patient with a short-segment type A IAA.[8] A direct anastomosis was possible. However, the associated VSDs were not closed at the time of the arch repair. One-stage repair was first reported by Barratt-Boyes and associates.[1] In this procedure, arch continuity was established using a synthetic conduit. One-stage repair, including direct anastomosis of the arch, was first described by Trusler and Izukawa in 1975.[13] IAA carried an extremely high mortality risk until the introduction of PGE$_1$ by Elliott et al. in 1975.[3] Over the ensuing 5 to 10 years, it became apparent that careful resuscitation of the neonate before proceeding to surgery (often maintained for several days) produced a dramatic improvement in surgical outcome.[4]

Indications for Surgery

Because the presence of IAA is incompatible with life unless ductal patency is maintained (generally with PGE$_1$), the diagnosis alone is the indication for surgery. Surgery should be undertaken as soon as complete metabolic resuscitation has been achieved using the techniques described previously.

Surgical Techniques

IAA With VSD

The ideal method of surgical management remains controversial. Palliative options, still used in many centers, include application of a pulmonary artery band during the neonatal period with closure of the associated VSD at some time beyond infancy, but usually before 5 years of age. Arch continuity can be achieved by insertion of a synthetic conduit rather than by direct anastomosis.[9] Both of these palliative options are generally undertaken by working through a left thoracotomy, although some surgeons prefer to use a combined thoracotomy and sternotomy approach for placement of an ascending-to-descending aortic conduit. Our preference is to undertake one-stage repair during the neonatal period, including a direct anastomosis of the arch.[11]

During transportation to the operating room and while preparing and positioning the child, it is important to scrupulously maintain the management principles which were employed during the resuscitation over the preceding few days in the intensive care unit. In particular, a high level of inspired oxygen and hyperventilation must be avoided. In addition to the usual monitoring equipment, careful consideration must be given to the monitoring of arterial pressure. It is preferable to be able to measure blood pressure both above and below the forthcoming anastomosis. Often this is achieved by placement of a right radial arterial line (unless an aberrant right subclavian artery is present) in addition to an umbilical arterial line. Not only does this allow the physician to immediately assess any pressure gradient across the anastomosis, but it also enables the adequacy of perfusion of the separate upper and lower body circulations to be assessed during the cooling phase, when the patient is on cardiopulmonary bypass.

Approach is via a median sternotomy alone. If a thymus is present, it is largely excised. Pericardium is not usually harvested. Accurate arterial cannulation is an essential key to the success of the procedure. Although a single arterial cannula will ultimately achieve complete cooling, we believe that cannulation of both the ascending aorta and pulmonary artery optimizes tissue perfusion, particularly of the brain and heart, in the critical early phase of cooling when all organs are still warm. Generally a No. 8 French arterial cannula is used for the ascending aorta. As indicated by Figure 22–3, this cannula should be inserted in the right lateral aspect of the ascending aorta, opposite the anticipated location of the anastomosis. This decreases the chance that either retrograde flow to the coronary arteries or antegrade flow to the brain will be compromised. The second arterial cannula is connected to the arterial tubing by a Y connector and is in-

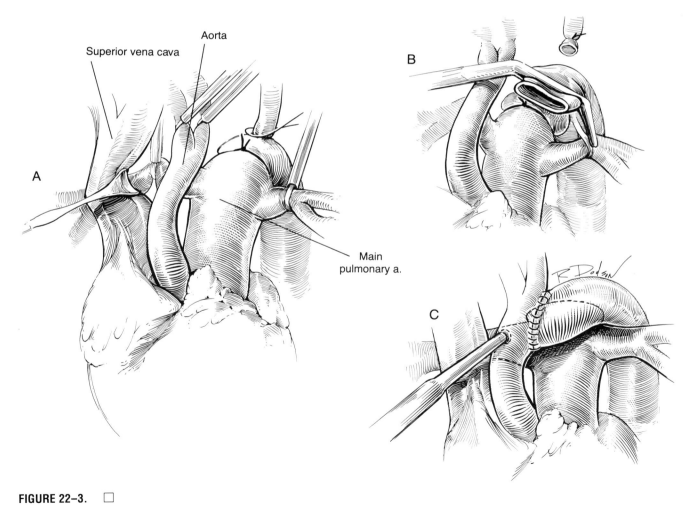

FIGURE 22–3. □

Depiction of the technique for repair by direct anastomosis of interrupted arch type B. *A,* Tourniquets control the branch pulmonary arteries during core cooling. During circulatory arrest, tourniquets control the carotid arteries to prevent cerebral air embolism. *B,* Following wide mobilization of the ascending and descending aorta, including division of the left subclavian artery, if necessary, in addition to the ductus arteriosus, the descending aorta is approximated to the ascending aorta with a C-clamp. *C,* The completed arch anastomosis. Note the precise positioning of the arterial cannula opposite the middle of the anastomosis.

serted in the anterior surface of the main pulmonary artery. Immediately after beginning bypass, it is necessary to tighten tourniquets around the right and left pulmonary arteries so that flow will be entirely directed through the ductus arteriosus to the descending aorta. (PGE_1 infusion must be continued during the cooling phase of cardiopulmonary bypass.) Venous cannulation is routine, with a single straight cannula in the right atrium.

During cooling, the ascending aorta and its branches are thoroughly mobilized. The ductus and descending aorta are also mobilized to minimize tension on the anastomosis. If an aberrant right subclavian artery is present, it should be ligated and divided at its origin from the descending aorta to improve mobility of the distal aortic segment. Also, in a type B interruption (Fig. 22–3), it is often useful to divide the left subclavian artery to further minimize anastomotic tension as well as to simplify the anastomosis, thereby decreasing the risk of bleeding and stenosis. When both rectal and tympanic temperatures are less than 18°C, bypass is ceased. Tourniquets are tightened around the innominate and left common carotid arteries, and the pulmonary artery tourniquets are removed. Cardioplegic solution is infused through a sidearm on the ascending arterial cannula connector. This same sidearm can be used to monitor ascending aortic pressure during the early postbypass phase. Both arterial cannulae are then removed, along with the venous cannula.

The ductus is ligated and divided at its junction with the descending aorta. Any residual ductal tissue is excised from the descending aorta. A C-clamp applied across the descending aorta helps to draw it to the level of the anastomosis, which then can be performed with the opposing tissues under no tension. The anastomosis should be situated on the ascending aorta, where tension will be minimized. Although many surgeons believe that this requires the site of the anastomosis to be partially on the left common carotid artery, we generally prefer it to be completely on the ascending aorta. The anastomosis will be exactly opposite the site of the ascending aortic cannulation. Absorbable polydioxanone 6-0 continuous suture may be used, although there is no evidence that the use of this suture results in a lower incidence of anastomotic stenosis. Many surgeons continue to prefer polypropylene suture. Its lesser tissue drag distributes tension more evenly throughout the suture line, which appears to enhance hemostasis.

The approach to the VSD will depend on the preoperative echocardiographic assessment. When there is extreme hypoplasia of the conal septum, the best approach is via a transverse incision in the proximal main pulmonary artery, immediately distal to the pulmonary valve. At the superior margin, sutures are passed through the pulmonary annulus, with the pledgets lying above the pulmonary valve leaflets in the sinus of Valsalva. If the conal septum is well developed, the VSD is approached through the right atrium.

A decision should be made preoperatively regarding the need to close an atrial septal defect. If there is any doubt, the atrial septum should be examined through a short right atrial incision. Because of the poor left-sided compliance that often persists for some time postoperatively, even a small atrial septal defect can result in a large left-to-right shunt.

One arterial cannula is carefully reinserted (in the ascending aorta only) for rewarming after filling the heart with saline to exclude air. Routine monitoring lines (i.e., a left atrial, pulmonary artery, and right atrial line) are placed during rewarming. Separation from the bypass and early postoperative management should be uncomplicated, as a biventricular repair has been achieved. If problems are encountered, a residual VSD or anastomotic stenosis must be excluded. It is unusual for obstruction of the left ventricular outflow tract to result in hemodynamic compromise early after surgery.

IAA With VSD and Severe Obstruction of the Left Ventricular Outflow Tract

Very occasionally, obstruction of the left ventricular outflow tract may be sufficiently severe to justify a radical alternative procedure.[14] Although some have believed it necessary to employ such a procedure relatively frequently, we did not employ it at all in 37 patients with IAA from 1974 to 1987.[11] The principle employed is analogous to that in the Damus-Stansel-Kaye procedure described for transposition (see Chapter 26). Left ventricular output is directed through the VSD by a baffle patch to the pulmonary artery. The main pulmonary artery is divided proximal to its bifurcation. The proximal divided main pulmonary artery is anastomosed to the side of the ascending aorta. A conduit (preferably an aortic or pulmonary homograft) is placed between the right ventricle and the distal divided main pulmonary artery.

Although this procedure is corrective in the sense that biventricular physiology is achieved, it is not truly corrective in that it does not incorporate growth potential. Variations on this theme have included an interim palliative procedure analogous to the Norwood procedure.[5] When two ventricles are present, such an approach is difficult to justify, as it introduces all of the difficult postoperative management problems observed in the management of the hypoplastic left heart syndrome (see Chapter 23).

Recent data from the Congenital Heart Surgeons Society suggest that these procedures are rarely, if ever, indicated (Kirklin J. W., personal communication, August, 1993).

IAA With Other Anomalies

The general principle should be applied that if two ventricles are present, a biventricular repair incorporating growth potential should be undertaken whenever possible. For example, the child with transposition of the great arteries, VSD, and interrupted arch should undergo an arterial switch procedure with VSD closure and direct anastomosis of the arch. Although this complex procedure requires a long crossclamp time, it is generally well tolerated as long as an accurate repair is achieved. In fact, transfer of the aorta posteriorly, as part of the arterial switch, helps to reduce tension on the anastomosis of the arch. Similarly, in a child with truncus arteriosus and IAA, the large size of the truncus decreases the difficulty with which aortic cannulation is achieved when compared with such difficulty in a child with simple IAA, where the ascending aorta is often hypoplastic. Only single arterial cannulation is required for the cooling phase.

Management of the child with a single functional ventricle and IAA remains a significant challenge, presenting many of the same problems experienced with management of the hypoplastic left heart syndrome. Frequently, there is significant obstruction within the single ventricle, often in the form of an obstructive bulboventricular foramen. This must be either bypassed, using a pulmonary-to-aortic anastomosis (Damus-Stansel-Kaye or Norwood procedure), or relieved by enlargement of the bulboventricular foramen. Residual obstruction of the arch is poorly tolerated with either a shunt-dependent circulation (after a pulmonary-to-aortic anastomosis) or with a pulmonary artery band if bulboventricular foramen enlargement is undertaken. Such obstruction will result in excessive pulmonary flow unless such flow is severely restricted. This becomes a highly labile situation.

POSTOPERATIVE MANAGEMENT

After biventricular repair of simple IAA with VSD, postoperative management should be routine. Failure to progress appropriately (i.e., minimal inotrope requirement within 24 to 48 hours and satisfactory progress toward extubation within 3 to 4 days, depending largely on preoperative status)

should stimulate an aggressive search for residual hemodynamic lesions. A residual VSD can be excluded by oxygen saturation data collected with the pulmonary artery line on the first postoperative morning. An anastomotic gradient should have been excluded both intraoperatively and in the early postoperative period by appropriate blood pressure determinations. Echocardiography—and, if there is any doubt, cardiac catheterization—can exclude significant obstruction of the left ventricular outflow tract. A left-to-right shunt at the atrial level should also be excluded. If an important residual hemodynamic lesion is identified, the child should be expeditiously returned to the operating room for correction of the problem.

RESULTS OF SURGERY

Figure 22–4 illustrates the dramatic improvement in both early and late results of surgery for IAA with VSD performed at Children's Hospital in Boston from 1974 to 1987.[11] In 1974 the risk of death within 2 weeks of surgery was greater than 50%, but by 1987 this risk had dropped to less than 10%. There were many changes in the management of neonates during this time that may have contributed to this improvement. The importance of complete preoperative resuscitation, for example, is illustrated in Figure 22–5. This effect is apparent for children with complex associated anomalies such as single ventricle and truncus arteriosus, as well as for patients with VSD as the only associated anomaly. This 1988 analysis did not conclusively demonstrate that one-stage repair during the neonatal period or direct anastomosis of the arch, rather than

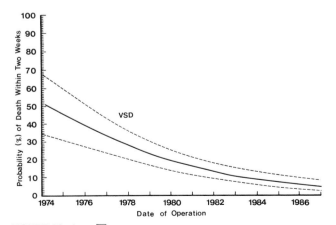

FIGURE 22–4. ☐

Probability of death within 2 weeks of repair of an interrupted aortic arch with a ventricular septal defect (VSD) as the only associated anomaly, according to year of operation at Children's Hospital, Boston, from 1974 to 1987.

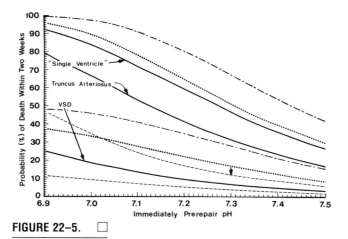

FIGURE 22–5. ☐

Probability of death within 2 weeks of surgery for patients with a single ventricle, truncus arteriosus, and VSD in assocation with interrupted aortic arch relative to the arterial pH sampled immediately before surgery at Children's Hospital, Boston, from 1974 to 1987. The important influence of complete preoperative resuscitation is demonstrated; 70% confidence intervals are shown.

placement of a conduit, contributed to the reduction in mortality.

COMPLICATIONS OF SURGERY

Early Complications

Potential technical complications were enumerated in the section, "Postoperative Management." In addition, bleeding can be troublesome. Bleeding is more likely if the arch anastomosis is performed under excessive tension, which is usually the result of inadequate mobilization of the ascending and descending aorta. Extreme friability of tissue also contributes to the risk of bleeding. Friability can result from severe preoperative acidosis but is also apparent if ductal tissue is incorporated in the anastomosis. Presumably, including ductal tissue also increases the risk of late anastomotic stenosis. As with all neonatal surgery, hemostasis must be accelerated by appropriate use of blood replacement, with truly fresh blood representing the optimal choice. In the absence of fresh blood, judicious (but nevertheless aggressive) transfusion of concentrated factors, including cryoprecipitate as well as platelet concentrates, is indicated.

The left recurrent laryngeal and phrenic nerves are both at risk during repair of IAA. In our experience, phrenic nerve injury was particularly frequent after placement of an ascending-to-descending aortic synthetic conduit, despite meticulous care of the nerve itself. Direct compression of the nerve by the synthetic material may be the cause of this problem.

Phrenic nerve palsy has been seen rarely after direct anastomosis of the arch.

Late Complications

Pressure Gradient Across the Arch. Ultimately all patients who have a tube graft inserted during the neonatal period will have obstruction (defined as a pressure gradient greater than 30 mm Hg) across the graft related to somatic growth alone. In addition, synthetic grafts have a variable rate of accumulation of a pseudointima, which may accelerate the rate of obstruction. The actuarial freedom from obstruction of the tube graft was 55% at 5 years. In contrast, patients who underwent direct anastomosis of the arch were more likely to have obstruction early, with only 40% having less than a 30–mm Hg gradient within 18 months of surgery (Fig. 22–6).[11] Balloon dilatation can successfully relieve such gradients in the majority of children who have a direct anastomosis,[10] whereas conduit replacement is inevitable for those with conduits. More recent data from Children's Hospital, Boston, as well as from the Congenital Heart Surgeons Society have revealed that the risk of late arch obstruction following direct anastomosis has decreased substantially since 1987.

Obstruction of the Left Ventricular Outflow Tract. Although obstruction of the left ventricular outflow tract is rarely sufficiently severe to justify an alteration in surgical strategy at the time of the neonatal reparative procedure, it is, by contrast, not uncommon for surgical intervention to be required for LVOTO occurring late postoperatively.[6] Of 33 patients who underwent repair of a conoventricular VSD as the only associated anomaly with IAA, only

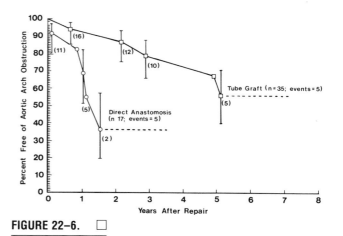

FIGURE 22–6. ☐

Actuarial freedom from aortic arch obstruction (defined as a gradient greater than 30 mm) after repair of an interrupted aortic arch by interposition of a tube graft or by direct anastomosis at Children's Hospital, Boston, from 1974 to 1987.

58% were free of evident obstruction of the left ventricular outflow tract (defined as a gradient greater than 40 mm Hg) 3 years after operation (Fig. 22–7). The morphology of LVOTO with IAA varies, and therefore, surgical management also varies according to the specific circumstances. In some cases it is possible to resect the posteriorly deviated conal septum, working through the aortic valve. An aortic valvotomy may also be required if there is valvar stenosis. If there is annular hypoplasia and a longer tunnel subaortic stenosis, our approach is to perform an annular enlarging procedure such as the extended aortic root replacement, using an aortic allograft with either an anterior incision into the ventricular septum (for very severe stenosis) or a posterior incision into the anterior leaflet of the mitral valve (when stenosis is less severe). Alternative procedures that have been used in the past include the Konno procedure[7] and the use of a conduit from the left ventricular apex to the descending aorta.

DiGeorge's Syndrome. Absence or severe hypoplasia of the thymus was common in our series of patients with IAA but was limited to patients with type B interruption. Comprehensive testing of lymphocyte function was undertaken in only a small number of patients, so no definite inferences can be drawn regarding the incidence of the full-blown DiGeorge syndrome. Although a large calcium requirement is often seen during the early postoperative period, it is rarely necessary for children to receive oral calcium supplements when they leave the hospital. This is fortunate, as these supplements are often poorly tolerated. Occasionally, vitamin D supplements are useful to maintain serum calcium levels during the first few postoperative weeks. We are not aware of any serious problems with immune function in long-term survivors of IAA surgery, although it must be recognized that there were very few survivors before the early 1980s.

Left Bronchial Obstruction. The left main bronchus usually passes under the arch of the aorta. If a direct anastomosis is performed without adequate mobilization, a bowstring effect over the left main bronchus may result. This is manifested by air trapping in the left lung with hyperexpansion, as seen on the plain chest radiograph. The diagnosis can be confirmed by bronchoscopy along with a computed tomographic or magnetic resonance imaging scan. Surgical management may entail placement of an ascending-to-descending aortic conduit after division of the arch. With adequate initial mobilization of the ascending and descending aorta, this should almost never be necessary.

SUMMARY

PGE$_1$ has revolutionized the management of IAA. Complete resuscitation should be maintained over several days, if necessary, before surgery is undertaken. Direct anastomosis of the arch with closure of the VSD is the preferred surgical approach at Children's Hospital in Boston. Although this procedure is physiologically corrective, it should not be viewed as fully corrective because of the high incidence of significant late obstruction of the left ventricular outflow tract. Such obstruction may respond to a simple surgical intervention such as subaortic resection, but in some cases an extensive procedure is necessary to enlarge the left ventricular outflow tract. Procedures to enlarge or bypass the subaortic arch at the time of the initial surgical procedure are rarely, if ever, indicated.

REFERENCES

1. Barratt-Boyes BG, Nicholls TT, Brandt PWT, et al. Aortic arch interruption associated with patent ductus arteriosus, ventricular septal defect and total anomalous pulmonary venous connection. J Thorac Cardiovasc Surg 63:367, 1972.
2. Celoria GC, Patton RB. Congenital absence of the aortic arch. Am Heart J 58:407, 1959.
3. Elliott RB, Starling MB, Neutze JM. Medical management of the ductus. Lancet 1:140, 1975.
4. Freed MD, Keane JF, Van Praagh R, et al. Coarctation of the aorta with congenital mitral regurgitation. Circulation 49:1175, 1974.
5. Ilbawi MN, Idriss FS, Deleon SY, et al. Surgical management of patients with interrupted aortic arch and severe subaortic stenosis. Ann Thorac Surg 45:174, 1988.
6. Jonas RA, Sell JE, Van Praagh R, et al. Left ventricular outflow obstruction associated with interrupted aortic arch and ventricular septal defect. In Crupi G, Parenzan L, Anderson RH (eds). Perspectives in Pediatric Cardiology. New York, Futura, 1989, pp 61–65.
7. Konno S, Imai Y, Lida Y, et al. A new method for prosthetic valve replacement in congenital aortic stenosis associated

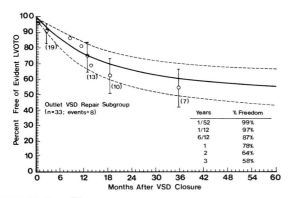

FIGURE 22–7. □

Actuarial freedom from obstruction of the left ventricular outflow tract (defined as a gradient greater than 40 mm) after repair of an interrupted aortic arch with conoventricular VSD at Children's Hospital, Boston, from 1974 to 1987.

with hypoplasia of the aortic valve ring. J Thorac Cardiovasc Surg 70:909, 1975.

8. Merrill DL, Webster CA, Samson PC. Congenital absence of the aortic isthmus. J Thorac Surg 33:311, 1957.

9. Norwood WI, Lang P, Castaneda AR, et al. Reparative operations for interrupted aortic arch with ventricular septal defect. J Thorac Cardiovasc Surg 86:837, 1983.

10. Saul JP, Keane JF, Fellows KE, et al. Balloon dilation angioplasty of postoperative aortic obstructions. Am J Cardiol 59:943, 1987.

11. Sell JE, Jonas RA, Mayer JE, et al. The results of a surgical program for interrupted aortic arch. J Thorac Cardiovasc Surg 96:864, 1988.

12. Steidele RJ. Samml Chir u Med Beob, Vienna, 2:114, 1778.

13. Trusler GA, Izukawa T. Interrupted aortic arch and ventricular septal defect. Direct repair through a median sternotomy incision in a 13-day-old infant. J Thorac Cardiovasc Surg 69:126, 1975.

14. Yasui H, Kado H, Nakano E, et al. Primary repair of interrupted aortic arch with severe aortic stenosis in neonates. J Thorac Cardiovasc Surg 93:539, 1987.

Hypoplastic Left Heart Syndrome

The term *hypoplastic left heart syndrome* (HLHS) is used to describe a wide spectrum of congenital heart anomalies with various degrees of hypoplasia of the structures of the left side of the heart. At the milder end of this continuum, there is little to distinguish the child with HLHS from the child with critical neonatal aortic valve stenosis. At the severe end of the spectrum, however, there is complete absence of the left ventricle, and the aortic arch may be severely hypoplastic or even interrupted. Children with HLHS continue to present a serious challenge to cardiac surgeons, cardiologists, and neonatologists. Although some have questioned the concentration of expensive resources for the relatively small number of patients involved, it has become clear that efforts to improve the outlook for this subgroup of patients have resulted in important advances in the management of many other groups of congenital heart patients, particularly those with other forms of single ventricle. Children with this syndrome have spurred advances in echocardiographic diagnosis, including in utero diagnosis and intervention; they have presented the paradigm for early postnatal resuscitation of the acidotic neonate with a closing ductus; they have demonstrated that neonates can survive complex nonreparative surgical procedures; they have fundamentally changed the management of all children with a single ventricle, who are pursuing the Fontan pathway through more widespread application of intermediate procedures such as the bidirectional cavopulmonary

(Glenn) shunt and the development of the fenestrated Fontan procedure; and they have been the primary focus for the introduction of neonatal heart transplant programs.

PATHOLOGIC ANATOMY

As is implicit in the name, HLHS involves various degrees of underdevelopment of left heart structures. The mitral valve may be stenotic or atretic, as may the aortic valve. Therefore, HLHS can be subcategorized into four anatomic subtypes based on the morphology of the left heart valve is: (1) aortic and mitral stenosis, (2) aortic and mitral atresia, (3) aortic atresia and mitral stenosis, and (4) aortic stenosis and mitral atresia. Figure 23–1 depicts the frequency of these subtypes among 78 consecutive patients with the HLHS who underwent surgery between 1983 and 1991. Aortic atresia tends to be associated with a more severe degree of hypoplasia of the ascending aorta than does aortic stenosis. Typically, the ascending aorta in a neonate with the aortic atresia form of this syndrome is 2.5 mm in diameter, whereas in the neonate with aortic stenosis as part of the syndrome, the ascending aorta often is 4 to 5 mm in diameter. The ascending aorta is often narrowest at its junction with the arch of the aorta and innominate artery, although it may be equally narrow at the sinotubular ridge, where it

Hypoplastic Left Heart Syndrome
1983–1991 (N=78)
Anatomic Subtype

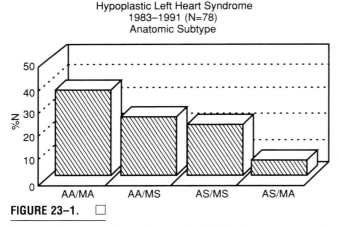

FIGURE 23–1. ☐

Frequency of anatomic subtypes of the hypoplastic left heart syndrome among 78 patients undergoing stage 1 palliation between 1983 and 1991. AA = aortic atresia; AS = aortic stenosis; MA = mitral atresia; MS = mitral stenosis.

joins the small sinuses of Valsalva. The wall of the ascending aorta is usually thin and fragile.

The arch of the aorta is hypoplastic to various degrees and may be interrupted. The diameter of the proximal arch is usually similar to that of the distal arch, usually between 3 and 5 mm. A coarctation shelf is present opposite the junction of the ductus with the proximal descending aorta in at least 80% of patients (Fig. 23–2). The ductus itself is large, often close to 10 mm in diameter. It is a direct extension of the main pulmonary artery, which is even larger (11 to 15 mm in diameter, and occasionally even larger). The right pulmonary artery arises very proximally from the main pulmonary artery, usually within 2 to 3 mm of the tops of the commissures of the pulmonary valve. It emerges from the posterior and rightward aspect of the main pulmonary artery. It is our impression that both pulmonary artery branches are smaller in HLHS than in similar anomalies with a single ventricle and systemic outflow tract obstruction (e.g., tricuspid atresia with transposed great arteries and severe subaortic stenosis). The left pulmonary artery arises from the posterior and leftward aspect of the main pulmonary artery some distance from the takeoff of the right pulmonary artery. It runs parallel to the ductus and immediately adjacent to it for some distance. It often appears to be slightly smaller than the right pulmonary artery. The hypoplasia of the pulmonary artery branches may be a consequence of decreased in utero pulmonary blood flow, which is itself a consequence of the left-sided obstruction.

The left atrium is usually smaller than normal; this is exacerbated by the leftward displacement of the septum primum, which is often heavily muscularized. Occasionally the foramen ovale is severely restrictive. The left atrium may have a thickened and fibrotic endocardium analogous to that seen in endocardial fibroelastosis. Occasionally this process can extend into the pulmonary veins, resulting in an obliterative, generalized stenosis of these veins. There is also generally increased muscularization of the walls of the pulmonary veins.

Associated Cardiac Anomalies

A number of observed associated cardiac anomalies are of surgical relevance, particularly if a reconstructive approach is to be followed. A ventricular septal defect is often associated with normal or near-normal size of the left ventricle, despite the presence of aortic atresia. This introduces the feasibility of biventricular repair in the neonate.

Structural abnormalities of the tricuspid and pulmonary valves have been seen but appear to be rare. A bicuspid pulmonary valve was seen in 4% of 54 specimens reviewed by Hawkins and Doty.[26] Cleft tricuspid valve and tricuspid and pulmonary valve dysplasia were also seen in 4%. Very rare associated cardiac anomalies include total anomalous pulmonary venous connection, coronary sinus atresia, common pulmonary vein atresia, complete atrioventricular canal defect, quadricuspid pulmonary valve,

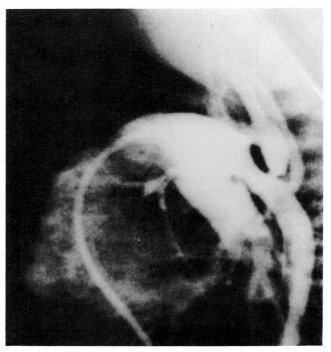

FIGURE 23–2. ☐

A coarctation of the aorta is present opposite the insertion of the ductus arteriosus in 80% of patients with the hypoplastic left heart syndrome.

double-orifice tricuspid valve, and interrupted aortic arch.[26]

Sauer and coworkers[56] reported that the coronary arteries were stenotic in more than 50% of patients in the subgroup with aortic atresia and mitral stenosis. By contrast, coronary artery anomalies were rarely seen in patients with aortic atresia and mitral atresa.

Associated Extracardiac Anomalies, Including Chromosomal Anomalies

In 1988, in a review of 83 autopsies of patients with HLHS at the Children's Hospital of Philadelphia, Natowicz et al.[47] reported that nine had underlying chromosomal abnormalities, four had single gene defects, and 10 had one or more major extracardiac anomalies without an identifiable chromosomal disorder. Overall, 28% had genetic disorders, major extracardiac anomalies, or both. Chromosomal abnormalities included Turner's syndrome and trisomies 18, 13, and 21. Anomalies not associated with chromosomal defects included diaphragmatic hernia, hypospadias, and omphalocele. In a separate report from the same group in 1990,[23] congenital brain anomalies associated with HLHS were reviewed. The authors found that, overall, 29% of the 41 autopsies revealed either a major or minor central nervous system abnormality. Seventeen percent had specific recognizable patterns of malformations such as agenesis of the corpus callosum. Twenty-seven percent were found to have microcephaly, defined as brain weight at autopsy more than two standard deviations below the mean for age. The absence of dysmorphic physical features did not preclude overt or subtle central nervous system malformations.

PATHOPHYSIOLOGY

Before birth there is probably less pulmonary blood flow than is usual for the fetal circulation because of the obstruction to egress of blood from the pulmonary circulation. Right ventricular output is directed across the ductus, where it can pass antegrade down the descending aorta or retrograde around the aortic arch to the head vessels and the ascending aorta, which functions as a single coronary artery. After birth there is an immediate reduction in pulmonary vascular resistance, which reduces the proportion of right ventricular output passing to the systemic circulation. If the ductus remains patent, the child's continuing viability will be dependent on a reasonable balance between pulmonary and systemic vascular resistance.

Several pathologic studies have documented an increase in pulmonary arteriolar smooth muscle in neonates with HLHS.[46, 57, 58] This muscle is likely to be very sensitive to changes in the inspired oxygen concentration and the arteriolar pH. Thus, exposure of the neonate to supplemental oxygen or mechanical ventilation, thereby lowering the pH and P_{CO_2}, is likely to adversely shift the balance of pulmonary and systemic flow in favor of excessive pulmonary flow. This tendency to excessive pulmonary blood flow and inadequate systemic flow will be further exacerbated by even partial closure of the ductus. Complete closure of the ductus is clearly incompatible with life.

PREOPERATIVE EVALUATION

Clinical Presentation

Without intervention, HLHS is almost always fatal in the first weeks, if not the first days, of life, although there are occasional exceptions.[20] In 1992 we examined a 9-year-old child in China who had aortic atresia as part of HLHS.

Generally, a child with this syndrome has a history of respiratory distress within the first 24 to 48 hours of life, usually while still in the newborn nursery. A mild degree of cyanosis may be noted. Prompt referral to a pediatric cardiologist should result in a rapid echocardiographic diagnosis of HLHS. The child can then be safely transported to a center specializing in neonatal and infant cardiac surgery while receiving a prostaglandin E_1 infusion; supplemental oxygen should be avoided. Many transport teams prefer to electively intubate such children because of the risk of apnea induced by the prostaglandin. Facilities must be available to ventilate the child with room air when the child is intubated.

Currently HLHS is being increasingly diagnosed in utero at 16 to 20 weeks' gestation by ultrasonography. This allows complete counseling of the parents, hopefully by both surgical and cardiology personnel involved in the management of such children and familiar with the most current results; the fetal ultrasonography team may not be in a position to answer more detailed inquiries posed by the parents. Prenatal diagnosis allows for expeditious transfer of the child to the tertiary care facility immediately after birth. Preferably the obstetric care should be undertaken in a facility immediately adjacent to the pediatric center.[16]

Occasionally children are discharged from the

nursery without any suspicion of congenital heart disease. This may be the result of insufficiently careful assessment of the child before discharge, but it may also be the result of continuing patency of the ductus and a spontaneously appropriate balance of pulmonary and systemic vascular resistance, resulting in a balance of pulmonary and systemic blood flow. Although at this point the child is free of the risk of exposure to supplemental oxygen (which frequently results in deterioration while the child is in the hospital), there is a risk that the ductus will close precipitously or when the child is at a location geographically remote from medical attention. Under such circumstances the child is likely to develop serious metabolic acidosis and may be in a state of profound shock with cardiovascular collapse by the time the diagnosis is made and treatment with prostaglandin is begun. There may be multiple organ failure secondary to this acidotic insult, resulting in seizures, renal failure, hepatic failure, and depressed ventricular function.[24] The reversibility of these various organ deficits will depend on both the severity of the acidosis and its duration.

Very occasionally the foramen ovale is severely restrictive to left-to-right flow, thereby limiting pulmonary blood flow to the point where the child is profoundly cyanotic from the moment of birth. In these circumstances the child will maintain adequate systemic blood flow initially, but metabolic acidosis will eventually develop secondary to the severe degree of hypoxia. This situation cannot be palliated medically.

Diagnosis of HLHS

The diagnosis of HLHS is being made with increasing frequency by prenatal ultrasound. In many cases the diagnosis can be made confidently by 16 to 18 weeks of gestation. In a series of 6000 high-risk pregnancies reviewed by Allan and coworkers,[2] the diagnosis of HLHS was not missed once. Prenatal ultrasound is likely to provide fascinating new information regarding the normal development and natural history of the fetus with HLHS. In one case report, Allan[2] described identification of a dilated, poorly contractile left ventricle at 22 weeks of gestation. By 32 weeks the ventricle had not grown since the first study and had become hypoplastic and densely echogenic. Clearly the ability to diagnose this anomaly early in gestation invites prenatal intervention, either in the form of echocardiographically guided balloon dilatation of the aortic valve, as reported by Maxwell and associates,[40] or by surgical means.

The diagnosis of HLHS after birth is also primarily an echocardiographic one. The physical findings of a slightly cyanotic neonate in respiratory distress, with a variable degree of general circulatory collapse, are nonspecific. Likewise, the appearance on the chest radiograph of a slightly enlarged heart with congested lung fields does not help to distinguish this anomaly from many others. The electrocardiogram will show dominant right ventricular forces, as it does in any neonate. Echocardiography will generally provide excellent definition of the relevant features, including the annular diameters of the mitral and aortic valves, left ventricular volume, and any associated left-sided anomalies. The investment of the aortic arch with the prominent thymus in the neonate usually guarantees excellent definition of this area, which may not be as clearly seen in an older infant or child. It is usually possible to define whether a shelf or coarctation is present opposite the insertion of the ductus; this is encountered in 80% of neonates with this anomaly. In fact, none of the morphologic features of HLHS is of particular importance to the surgeon in terms of planning the exact surgical strategy, as both a transplant or a reconstructive approach are relatively generic operations, regardless of the individual anatomy. What is of importance is to be sure that the child does in fact have HLHS rather than a severe degree of critical aortic valve stenosis. The only possible exception to this is the assessment of the diameter of the ascending aorta, which may influence the surgical team to choose a transplant rather than a reconstructive approach (see later discussion).

The avoidance of cardiac catheterization when diagnosing the sick neonate with HLHS has been an important advance since the 1980s. Previously, to define the aortic arch it was necessary to pass a catheter either through or close to the ductus. This could result in injury to the ductus, with a subsequent need for emergency surgery if ductal patency was compromised. The osmotic load of angiographic dye was a further insult to the neonate, who may have already had compromised renal function. In addition, there were the general stresses inherent in any cardiac catheterization procedure (e.g., heat loss, blood loss, and the catecholamine response to the stress of the procedure). Therefore, except in unusual circumstances, catheterization is avoided, and the diagnosis is based primarily on the echocardiogram.

Differentiation of HLHS From Critical Aortic Valve Stenosis

The problem of distinguishing HLHS from critical stenosis of the neonatal aortic valve represents the major diagnostic challenge with this spectrum of anomalies. Several reports have examined this issue. Ludman and colleagues[38] found that the diameter of the mitral valve annulus was the single most distinctive variable. Because of the considerable overlap among patients with respect to the various measured indices, they concluded that the diagnosis of HLHS should not be based on any single echocardiographic feature. Karl and associates[32] reported a high mortality rate of 31% for infants managed with surgery as though they had critical aortic valve stenosis (i.e., pursuing a biventricular approach by performing a surgical valvotomy). This high mortality rate almost certainly can be partially attributed to the inclusion of a number of children who would have been more correctly categorized as having HLHS. From this experience, Karl et al. concluded that a biventricular approach should not be pursued if the cardiac apex is not formed by the left ventricle or if the dimensions of the aortic annulus, ascending aorta, mitral valve, or left ventricular cavity are less than 60% of the mean for body weight.

Leung and coworkers[36] examined 20 heart specimens and reviewed the clinical course of 20 patients with critical aortic valve stenosis. From a comparison of survivors and nonsurvivors of open valvotomy, they concluded that a biventricular approach was not justified if the left ventricle was small (i.e., with an echocardiographic inflow dimension of <25 mm), if the ventriculoaortic junction was <5 mm, or if the mitral annulus was <9 mm. At Children's Hospital in Boston, Rhodes and associates[53] employed discriminant analysis to determine which of several echocardiographically measured left heart structures were independent predictors of survival after valvotomy for neonatal critical aortic stenosis. It was possible to predict outcome after a biventricular approach with 95% accuracy based on mitral valve area (<4.75 cm^2/m^2), long-axis dimension of the left ventricle relative to the long-axis dimension of the heart (<0.8), diameter of the aortic root (<3.5 cm/m^2), and left venticular mass (<35 gm/m^2). Left ventricular volume was not found to have a statistically significant relationship to outcome in this study (in contrast to previous practice at this institution, where a left ventricular end-diastolic volume of 20 ml/m^2 was used to determine suitability for valvotomy).

MEDICAL MANAGEMENT OF THE NEONATE WITH HLHS

The fundamental principle applied to the medical management of children with HLHS is that surgery should not be undertaken until the child is essen-tially normal with respect to all organ systems other than the cardiorespiratory system itself. Failure to achieve this goal will almost certainly cause any surgical endeavor to fail. This is particularly true when a palliative reconstructive procedure is to be performed, although it will certainly also influence the outcome after heart transplantation. The child undergoing a stage 1 reconstructive procedure undergoes an extensive operation, including exposure to the deleterious effects of cardiopulmonary bypass and deep hypothermic circulatory arrest, without any resultant fundamental improvement in circulation. The only change in hemodynamics after the first stage of palliative reconstruction is a possible reduction in volume load in the child who has low pulmonary vascular resistance preoperatively, including no restriction at the level of the foramen ovale.

Transport to a Tertiary Center

The medical management by the referral obstetric hospital and the transport team is an essential key to the ultimate outcome for the child. Early infusion of prostaglandin is currently practiced at most referral centers before definitive diagnosis is made, in the same way that antibiotics are begun before a diagnosis of sepsis is confirmed. Supplemental oxygen must be avoided. Medical management has been greatly simplified with the advent of reliable pulse oximeters. In fact, these instruments, which did not become widely available until approximately 1985, have improved the management of children with HLHS throughout all phases of their treatment. Metabolic acidosis must be aggressively treated with an infusion of sodium bicarbonate or with tromethamine (THAM) if the sodium level becomes dangerously elevated. If the child continues to have poorly palpable pulses or if the blood pressure measured by an umbilical arterial line is low, a careful check should be made to ensure that the prostaglandin is being delivered into the blood stream. Usually an umbilical venous line with excellent blood return is the safest venous access at this stage. If the team is sure that the prostaglandin is being delivered at an adequate dose (initially 0.1 μg/kg/min), consideration should be given to supporting the child with a dopamine infusion, beginning at a dose of 5 μg/kg/min up to 20 μg/kg/min.

Children who have suffered a serious insult should be intubated before transport. This is often appropriate for any child receiving prostaglandin who may become apneic in the confined area of a transport vehicle, where intubation will be hazardous. Elective intubation before transport should be seriously considered for all patients. The general principles of neonatal resuscitation and transport, such as maintenance of adequate body temperature and blood glucose levels, should be carefully adhered to. Note, however, that a mild degree of hypothermia may be protective to the central nervous system exposed to an ischemic insult, and hyperthermia is deleterious under such circumstances; therefore, overly aggressive rewarming should be avoided. Likewise, there is evidence that hyperglycemia in mature animals exacerbates ischemic brain injury, although whether this applies in neonates is not clear. Nevertheless, it would seem wise to avoid very high levels of blood glucose.

Resuscitation in the Cardiac Intensive Care Unit

It is important that the child be managed preoperatively in an intensive care unit specializing in neonatal and infant cardiology and cardiac surgery. Cardiologists, cardiac surgeons, and intensive care specialists should be aware of the child's arrival at the hospital so that they can collaborate in the child's resuscitation. Clear lines of communication are essential so that discussion can ensue regarding such issues as whether to pursue a univentricular or biventricular approach (balloon valvotomy in the catheterization laboratory or surgical valvotomy in the operating room), the role of transplantation, the timing of surgery, the need and timing of ancillary interventions (balloon dilatation of a restrictive atrial septal defect), and, perhaps, the decision to withhold medical or surgical therapy for the child who has been severely compromised or who has such serious associated anomalies that the consensus among all parties, including the child's parents, is that only supportive measures should be given.

Counseling the Child's Parents

Prenatal diagnosis is undoubtedly of great benefit to the child with HLHS in that obstetric services can be provided close to a cardiac center, and the supportive measures previously outlined can be initiated expeditiously, including the immediate infusion of prostaglandin. In addition, there is an important psychological advantage to the prospective parents, who can prepare themselves logistically, intellectually, and emotionally for the hurdles that may lie ahead for them and that can be explained in detail several months before the delivery. When the diagnosis is made after delivery—particularly if the child has been at home for some time and rec-

ognition of the child's deteriorating status may have been delayed—great care must be taken by the hospital team in carefully counseling the parents regarding the challenges ahead for the infant and the family as a whole. For many families, support groups are of great help, particularly after the child has left the hospital and the parents are faced with the prospect of future hospital visits, cardiac catheterizations, and surgery. Meeting children who are attending school and leading normal lives after completion of surgical treatment is a great emotional boost to parents who may be anticipating caring for a child who is chronically incapacitated.

Specific Measures in the Intensive Care Unit

As described in Chapter 5, the key to management of the child with HLHS in the intensive care unit is to achieve a balance between systemic and pulmonary blood flow by manipulation of pulmonary and systemic vascular resistances. The only agent that has specifically opposite effects on systemic and pulmonary resistance is oxygen. Success in manipulating the balance of blood flow can be assessed by observing arterial blood gases. Assuming there is no forward flow through the aortic valve (aortic atresia), and assuming adequate cardiac output, an arterial oxygen saturation of 80% will generally signify that pulmonary blood flow is not grossly excessive. In most children this level is achieved by ventilation with room air (FiO_2, 0.21). We have had no personal experience with the use of inspired oxygen concentrations less than room air or with supplemental carbon dioxide, but such strategies are currently being investigated at several centers. Deliberate induction of respiratory acidosis (PCO_2 >40 mm) does introduce the risk that the child's pH will become dangerously acidotic if the resultant increase in pulmonary vascular resistance fails to correct any metabolic acidosis that may be present (i.e., by increasing systemic blood flow).

Other details of management in the intensive care unit are identical to those described for management of the child by the transport team. Prostaglandin must be delivered by a secure line. It is usually possible to decrease the dose to 0.05 μg/kg/min when ductal patency has been confirmed by echocardiography. Low doses of dopamine (<5 μg/kg/min) are often infused to improve cardiac output and to particularly improve renal blood flow. If there is unconjugated hyperbilirubinemia, the child is given appropriate phototherapy. Sepsis is aggressively sought by blood culture as well as by culture of urine and tracheal aspirate. Careful attention must be paid to nutritional support. If it is clear that the child has not suffered a serious insult, enteral feedings by nasogastric tube are to be preferred. However, enteral feedings, particularly if high-caloric-density formula is used, introduce the risk of necrotizing enterocolitis if there has been an ischemic intestinal insult. Detection of heme-positive stools should result in immediate cessation of enteral feeding and initiation of antibiotics and parenteral feeding.

Timing of Surgery

The average duration of resuscitation for neonates with HLHS admitted to Children's Hospital in Boston is 2 to 3 days. Occasionally there may be factors that result in a need for surgery sooner than this, although more commonly there are factors that result in a greater delay of surgery. The child who, at several days of age, has signs of very high pulmonary blood flow despite a widely patent ductus and who cannot be controlled by the measures described earlier to increase pulmonary vascular resistance, should undergo surgery within 12 to 24 hours of confirmation of the diagnosis by echocardiography. The child who is severely hypoxic because of a restrictive foramen ovale may require an urgent surgical atrial septectomy as part of the stage 1 palliative procedure. In these circumstances, however, there is concern that pulmonary vascular resistance will be markedly elevated, resulting in the need for a large shunt at the time of surgery. If pulmonary vascular resistance falls, the child will develop congestive failure within a few days because of excessive pulmonary blood flow. The preferred approach is to undertake decompression of the hypertensive left atrium in the catheterization laboratory several days before the surgical procedure. A simple Rashkind balloon septostomy is rarely effective because the atrial septum is so heavily muscularized. Blade septostomy is hazardous in these patients, because the left atrium is small. A safer approach is Brockenbrough puncture of the atrial septum followed by balloon dilatation of the resultant septal defect.

For the typical child with mild elevation of serum creatinine and urea levels and abnormal liver function test results and in whom pulmonary blood flow can be controlled without great difficulty, the supportive measures previously outlined should be continued until all indices of organ function have returned to normal. Although some centers have recommended routine balloon septostomy so that pulmonary vascular resistance will be as low as possible at the time of surgery, this has not been our practice at Children's Hospital in Boston. Not only

does the catheter procedure itself carry significant risk, but there is also a chance that grossly excessive pulmonary blood flow will develop, resulting in the need for relatively urgent surgery. Nevertheless, there is certainly a "gray area" in which pulmonary vascular resistance that is elevated preoperatively (in part related to a restrictive foramen ovale) would be better dealt with preoperatively.

THE RECONSTRUCTIVE APPROACH IN THE MANAGEMENT OF HLHS

History

There are a multitude of articles in the surgical literature describing various ingenious procedures that could enable survival of the neonate without a continuing requirement for prostaglandin. For example, in 1970 Cayler and colleagues[14] described an anastomosis between the right pulmonary artery and ascending aorta with the placement of bilateral pulmonary artery bands. In a follow-up report,[13] this patient was said to be symptom free at 3 years of age. No report of a successful Fontan operation was published. Between 1977 and 1981, a number of authors, including Doty, Levitsky, Behrendt, Norwood, and their respective coworkers,[7, 19, 37, 48] described multiple modifications of possible surgical procedures. While there were a few short-term survivors, there were no reports of a successful stage 1 procedure leading to a successful Fontan procedure until Norwood and co-workers' report in 1983.[49] The child described in that report, who underwent his Fontan procedure in 1982, was still alive in 1992. Many of the alternative procedures to Norwood's first-stage operation suffer from inherent impediments to the successful development of a low-risk Fontan candidate. For example, banding of the main pulmonary artery distal to a conduit taken from the proximal main pulmonary artery fails to take into account the very short distance between the tops of the commissures of the pulmonary valve and the takeoff of the right pulmonary artery. Distortion of the right pulmonary artery takeoff will almost certainly ensue if the child survives the procedure. Procedures including an incision in the right ventricle will result in some deterioration in ventricular function. Many proposed procedures fail to take into account the restrictive nature of the aortic arch or the common occurrence of a coarctation. Procedures incorporating a synthetic conduit fail to incorporate growth potential.

Indications for Surgery

Because this anomaly is uniformly fatal without surgery, it is currently our practice to offer surgery to any child with HLHS who comes to Children's Hospital in Boston, as long as the following contraindications do not apply. Prematurity (gestational age less than approximately 34 weeks) and low birth weight (<2000 gm) are generally though not absolutely considered to be contraindications to surgery because of a uniformly unsuccessful outcome when surgery has been attempted for such children in the past. Likewise, serious chromosomal anomalies or serious extracardiac anomalies represent contraindications,[23, 47] although in our experience, these have been exceedingly rare reasons for not undertaking surgery. Severe tricuspid or pulmonary regurgitation is an occasional contraindication to surgery, as is severe right ventricular dysfunction. Ventricular dysfunction is often present at the time of presentation, particularly if the child is still acidotic or is recovering from a recent acidotic insult. Ventricular function should be reassessed when the child has had a chance to be fully resuscitated, including a return to normal of all metabolic parameters, such as urea and creatinine levels, and liver function test results. Occasionally a child does not recover from the initial insult and lapses into progressive renal or hepatic failure in spite of satisfactory cardiac output and appropriate distribution of blood flow between the pulmonary and systemic circulations. In our opinion, in the majority of cases, a failure to recover from the initial insult should also represent a contraindication to heart transplantation as well as to reconstruction. In contrast, significant tricuspid or pulmonary regurgitation and isolated ventricular dysfunction represent contraindications only to reconstruction. Children with any of these problems should be fully assessed for possible heart transplantation after a complete discussion with the parents.

Although some centers may still consider no intervention appropriate for any child with HLHS, we consider such an approach to be both ethically and logically inconsistent. There are many other congenital heart anomalies that carry a prognosis that is just as bad if not worse; these include other forms of single ventricle with systemic outflow obstruction, single ventricle with heterotaxia, critical neonatal Ebstein's anomaly, and even severe forms of pulmonary atresia with an intact ventricular septum. For some reason these anomalies are generally accepted as being part of a wide spectrum, and treatment is almost never withheld for those at the more mild end of the spectrum. We maintain that a similar philosophy should hold for children with HLHS.

Technical Considerations in Stage 1 Palliative Reconstruction

General Aims. The goals of the first-stage reconstructive procedure for HLHS are identical to those of any palliative procedure that is preparatory to an ultimate Fontan operation. Ventricular function must be preserved by avoiding a pressure load (reconstructed aortic arch gradient) or excessive volume load (excessive pulmonary blood flow—e.g., a shunt that is too large), minimizing pulmonary vascular resistance (avoiding excessive pulmonary blood flow or pulmonary venous obstruction by a restrictive atrial septal defect), and maintaining optimal pulmonary artery growth. In the absence of structural abnormalities of the tricuspid valve, this approach will also preserve tricuspid valve function by avoiding ventricular dilatation associated with excessive volume work by the ventricle.

Current Technique of First-Stage Palliation. At present, the operative procedure in use at Children's Hospital in Boston is fundamentally the same as that described by Norwood et al. in their 1983 report (Fig. 23–3).[49] However, attention to fine points of technique can mean the difference between a low-risk candidate for a Fontan operation and a nonsurvivor of the first stage. Meticulous coordination and communication between the anesthesia and surgical teams is an essential ingredient for the success of the procedure.[25] Inappropriate ventilatory, anesthetic, and inotropic manipulations substantially increase the risk of early mortality for this procedure.

The child is transported to the operating room while receiving room air ventilation with a view to maintaining carbon dioxide levels close to normocarbia. Hyperventilation at this time is a common error and must be avoided. Monitoring of arterial pressure is continued, using the umbilical arterial line as pulse oximetry is maintained. Central venous access is avoided at this time, as two atrial catheters will be placed by the surgical team during the procedure. Anesthesia is induced and maintained with a high-dose fentanyl technique, using pancuronium to accomplish muscle paralysis. A urinary catheter is placed, and electrocardiographic monitoring is continued. The child is allowed to cool spontaneously somewhat during this phase related to the low ambient air temperature of the operating room.

Approach is through a median sternotomy. The thymus is almost completely excised to allow access to the aortic arch and head vessels. A tourniquet is applied around the right pulmonary artery; this may be tightened before bypass to increase pulmonary vascular resistance and improve systemic per-

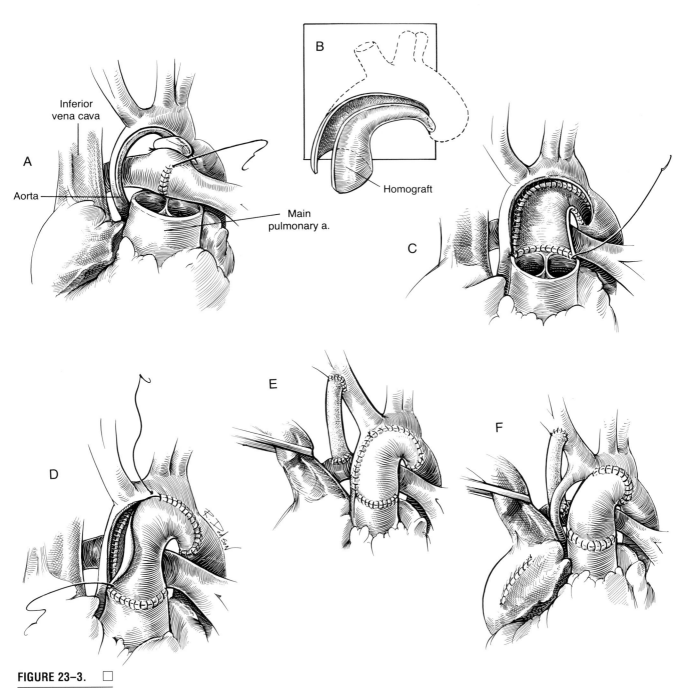

FIGURE 23–3. □

Current techniques for first-stage palliation of the hypoplastic left heart syndrome. *A,* Incisions used for the procedure, incorporating a cuff of arterial wall allograft. The distal divided main pulmonary artery may be closed by direct suture or with a patch. *B,* Dimensions of the cuff of the arterial wall allograft. *C,* The arterial wall allograft is used to supplement the anastomosis between the proximal divided main pulmonary artery and the ascending aorta, aortic arch, and proximal descending aorta. *D, E,* The procedure is completed by an atrial septectomy and a 3.5-mm modified right Blalock shunt. *F,* When the ascending aorta is particularly small, an alternative procedure involves placement of a complete tube of arterial allograft. The tiny ascending aorta may be left in situ, as indicated, or implanted into the side of the neoaorta.

fusion. After heparinization, the arterial cannula is placed in the main pulmonary artery and the venous cannula in the right atrium. Immediately after commencing bypass with a flow rate of 150 ml/kg/min, a tourniquet is placed around the left pulmonary artery and tightened. Tourniquets are loosely applied around the common carotid arteries, and the ascending aorta, ductus, and aortic arch are dissected free. When the child has been cooled to a rectal temperature of less than 18°C, at which time tympanic membrane temperature will be 15°C or less, bypass is ceased, and the child's blood is drained into the reservoir. The carotid artery tourniquets are tightened, and the pulmonary artery tourniquets are removed. Both cannulae are removed. No attempt is made to infuse cardioplegic solution directly into the tiny ascending aorta because of the risk of injury to that vessel. Some centers infuse it into the main pulmonary artery with temporary occlusion of the descending aorta and the arch vessels.

Optimizing Pulmonary Artery and Aortic Arch Development. The ductus is ligated distally at its aortic end. Ligation close to the left pulmonary artery takeoff may increase the risk of stenosis at that point, as residual ductal tissue fibroses. The main pulmonary artery is divided, carefully avoiding an incision very close to the right pulmonary artery takeoff, which may become the source of a central pulmonary artery stenosis. The distal portion of the divided main pulmonary artery can often be closed by direct suture because of the redundant nature of the large main pulmonary artery, although some routinely use a pericardial patch to close the distal portion. The ductus is divided at its junction with the descending aorta. The resulting aortotomy is extended at least 5 mm distally (more if the isthmus and juxtaductal area are severely hypoplastic). Proximally, the arch and ascending aorta are filleted open to the level of the division of the main pulmonary artery (see Fig. 23–3A). An anastomosis is fashioned between the proximal portion of the divided main pulmonary artery and the filleted aorta with a supplementary cuff of homograft arterial wall (see Fig. 23–3B,C).[29] It is important that this neoaorta is not redundant and that it does not create a bowstring effect over the left pulmonary artery, which will be compressed between the neoaorta and the left main bronchus (Fig. 23–4). These aims are best achieved by conceptualizing the more distal component of the homograft patch as a patch plasty for the distal part of the arch and proximal part of the descending aorta, while the more proximal component of the patch will create a tube that should be a little smaller in diameter than the original main pulmonary artery. Careful consid-

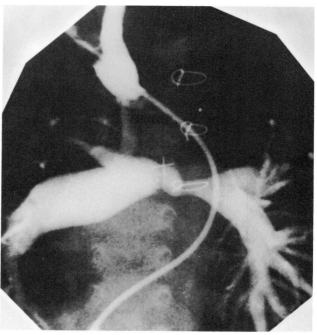

FIGURE 23–4. ☐

Care must be taken to ensure that the reconstructed neoaorta does not cause central pulmonary artery stenosis. This may result from the bowstring effect of an improperly shaped neoaorta or from posterior compression by an excessively large neoaorta.

eration must be given to the distensibility of the homograft tissue,[31] as well as to the contribution to the neoaorta by the original ascending aorta. An excessively large proximal neoaorta will compress the area around the pulmonary artery bifurcation, resulting in a central stenosis.

Avoiding Coronary Artery Compromise. Great care must be taken to avoid obstructing flow to the coronary arteries when anastomosing the small ascending aorta to the proximal portion of the pulmonary artery. A marking suture placed on the pulmonary artery while that vessel is distended is often useful to indicate placement of the anastomosis. At least three interrupted sutures are placed at the apex of the ascending aortotomy. In children in whom the ascending aorta is particularly small (2 mm or less), we have, on occasion, divided the ascending aorta and implanted it end to side into a complete tube of homograft.

Atrial Septectomy. The septum primum must be completely excised from the base of the foramen ovale down to the level of the inferior vena cava. Partial excision or simple incision, as practiced in the past, frequently led to later restriction at the atrial septal level.[50] The septectomy can be performed through a very short incision low in the right atrial free wall or through the venous cannulation site in the right atrial appendage.

Shunts. We and others have used a number of

different types of shunt.[29, 55] Our current preference is a modified right Blalock shunt with either a 3.5-mm shunt from the distal innominate artery or proximal subclavian artery, or a 4-mm shunt from the subclavian artery to the pulmonary artery (see Fig. 23–3E).

Many factors enter into the selection of appropriate shunt size and site. For example, a judgment must be made as to the child's probable pulmonary vascular resistance, including consideration of the contribution of the atrial septum to total pulmonary resistance that will be eliminated by the septectomy. The size and length of the innominate and right subclavian arteries must also be taken into consideration. Finally, there are important differences among surgeons in the construction of the shunt anastomoses. For example, it is currently Norwood's preference to use a 4-mm central shunt, but at Children's Hospital in Boston, we believe that a 4-mm central shunt provides excessive pulmonary blood flow. We currently avoid central shunts because of the greater difficulty of control and takedown of such shunts at the time of Fontan surgery. In addition we have found that there is a tendency for differential growth in the cephalocaudal plane between the aorta and the pulmonary arteries, resulting in a central tenting effect on the pulmonary arteries. Nevertheless, the central shunt does result in more uniform development of the left pulmonary artery relative to the right pulmonary artery, just as hypothesized when this shunt was originally proposed as an alternative to the Blalock shunt.[29]

Discontinuation of Cardiopulmonary Bypass. The Blalock shunt may be constructed when bypass has been re-established after deep hypothermic circulatory arrest and when the appropriate vessels have been controlled with clamps. Care must be taken to avoid compression of the ascending aorta, particularly when it has a very small diameter. During rewarming to normothermia, before adequate cardiac action is regained, the shunt is controlled with a vascular clamp. A dopamine infusion is routinely employed at the time of discontinuation of bypass. This is administered via a catheter inserted through a pursestring suture into what is, at this point, a common atrium. The same catheter is used to monitor the filling pressure of the ventricle. At least 5 minutes before bypass is discontinued, the clamp on the shunt is released. A 5- to 10-mm decrease in arterial pressure should be observed, confirming satisfactory shunt anastomoses. Ventilation is begun at this time, and the filling pressure within the atrium is increased by the perfusionist so that the heart is ejecting relatively vigorously. Frequent arrhythmias at this stage, particularly

when associated with discoloration of the ventricle, usually indicate coronary insufficiency. Reliable saturation sensing by a pulse oximeter must be established, once pulsatile flow is present, before the patient is weaned from bypass. Pulmonary vascular resistance is often elevated for the first 15 to 30 minutes after weaning from bypass, and thus it is often necessary to aggressively hyperventilate the child during this time. The oxygen saturation may be as low as 50% to 60% during this period, but as long as adequate cardiac output appears to be maintained, these low saturations should be tolerated. If very low saturations persist or if ventricular function appears to be impaired, it will be necessary to revise the shunt. This is simply done by recommencing bypass and controlling the subclavian and innominate arteries with a C-clamp. The proximal anastomosis is moved more proximally onto the innominate artery. Of course, low arterial oxygen saturation may also represent inadequate cardiac output, in which case shunt revision would clearly be contraindicated. Only by careful observation of the chronologic sequence of the failure to wean from bypass can the primary cause of the low-output state be established. A sufficiently severe degree of hypoxia ultimately will always lead to myocardial failure, even when the myocardium itself, when well oxygenated, has excellent reserve.

The child who is weaned from bypass with a high oxygen saturation (>85% to 90%) is likely to have excessive pulmonary blood flow, which may be associated with hypotension and the development of metabolic acidosis. However, it is important to consider that a high oxygen saturation may be the result of some forward flow through an open aortic valve in the patient with aortic stenosis and mitral stenosis. It may also be a reflection of excellent cardiac output with low oxygen extraction. Residual aortic arch obstruction will also be reflected in high oxygen saturation, as blood will be selectively directed into the shunt, which arises proximal to the obstruction. If residual arch obstruction is suspected, it can be easily ruled out by measurement of the neoaortic root pressure relative to umbilical arterial pressure. Placement of both a pulse oximeter probe and a blood pressure cuff on a lower extremity is particularly important in the patient who does not have an umbilical arterial line. Detection of arterial pulsation by a pulse oximeter probe on the foot is often a useful indicator of at least adequate cardiac output. If it becomes clear that the problem is simply one of excessive shunt size, the shunt can be narrowed by running a polytetrafluoroethylene (PTFE) suture line along one edge of the graft and producing a gently tapered, hourglass-shaped stenosis.

Closure of the Chest. If there is any doubt as to the child's stability, the sternum should not be approximated. Chest tubes should be carefully placed where there is no possibility that they will impinge on the myocardium or the reconstructed vessels in the superior mediastinum. An elliptic Silastic sheet should be sutured accurately to the skin edges and povidone-iodine ointment applied to the skin–Silastic interface.

Intensive Care Management after Stage 1 Reconstruction

The intensive care management of the child with a palliated "in-parallel" circulation is described in Chapter 5. Because of the frequently observed wide fluctuations in the balance of systemic and pulmonary blood flow, meticulous fine tuning of ventilatory and other manipulations on a minute-to-minute basis is often necessary. After 24 to 48 hours, there usually is gradual stabilization. At this time consideration can be given to discontinuing the infusion of fentanyl and muscle relaxant that has been maintained until this time. Since introducing a policy of continued anesthesia for the first 24 to 48 hours in the intensive care unit, the number of sudden, unexpected events (such as collapse after endotracheal tube suctioning) has dramatically decreased. This is most likely due to the decrease in pulmonary vasoreactivity seen with fentanyl infusion.[28]

Inotropic support must be used cautiously in the early postoperative period. In particular, high doses of epinephrine are poorly tolerated and are often associated with continuing metabolic acidosis. As with the child who has metabolic acidosis preoperatively, sodium bicarbonate should be employed, even if the acidosis is mild. Amrinone is a preferable inotropic agent to epinephrine for the patient in whom dopamine appears insufficient to meet inotropic requirements. As always, a continuing need for inotropic support must stimulate a careful exclusion of remediable causes of low output, such as persistent aortic arch obstruction. Echocardiography has not been particularly reliable in establishing this diagnosis, being neither very sensitive nor very specific. This may be related in part to the removal of the thymus that previously invested this area, as well as to the introduction of air into the mediastinum and to foreign objects, such as chest tubes, that can cause acoustic shadowing. In addition, pressure of the echo transducer on the chest wall may be poorly tolerated in a patient soon after surgery. In fact, it is wise to think of a postoperative echocardiogram as an invasive procedure. If there is reasonable sus-

picion of a residual hemodynamic problem, the child should be taken to the cardiac catheterization laboratory and studied to exclude arch obstruction, shunt or pulmonary artery distortion, or residual obstruction at the atrial septal level. In addition, measurement of the ratio of systemic-to-pulmonary blood flow is useful information.

It is not uncommon for the child to remain in a mild to moderate degree of congestive heart failure in the early days to weeks postoperatively. This may necessitate continuing medical support in the hospital. The average duration of hospitalization at Children's Hospital in Boston after stage 1 surgery is 19 days, 1 week to 10 days of which are spent in the intensive care unit. Establishing adequate intake of formula by mouth is often the limiting factor in determining the time of discharge. Rarely, it is necessary to place a gastrostomy tube. Failure to establish adequate feeding or continued ventilator dependence beyond the time frame described should stimulate exclusion of hemodynamic causes of compromised circulation. The most common problem developing during this time is obstruction of the aortic arch caused by remodeling and fibrosis of the periductal area. This area is notoriously poorly visualized by echocardiography. Therefore, as in the very early postoperative period, serious consideration should be given to studying the child by cardiac catheterization. Clearly, if the distal reconstructed area appears angiographically narrow, even though there may be a relatively minor gradient (e.g., 15 to 20 mm Hg), some intervention should be undertaken. Whether this consists of surgery or balloon dilatation will depend on the time elapsed since surgery and the particular preferences of the cardiologists and surgeons involved.

Follow-Up After Stage 1 Surgery

The principles of follow-up after stage 1 palliation for HLHS are identical to those applied to any child with single-ventricle physiology in whom a Fontan procedure is anticipated. Specifically, careful attention should be directed toward optimal pulmonary artery development, maintenance of ventricular function, and maintenance of low pulmonary vascular resistance, including absence of restriction at the level of the atrial septal defect. A high index of suspicion for the various problems frequently seen in patients undergoing stage 1 surgery will clearly aid early detection of similar problems. All patients should be catheterized by 6 months of age; this recommendation is quite independent of clinical progress. A child may be feeding and growing well and yet have very severe stenosis in the area of the central pulmonary artery bifurcation. The lack of sensitivity of postoperative echocardiography to the various problems observed in the first 6 months after stage 1 surgery is an additional reason catheterization should not be postponed beyond this age. Nevertheless, this is not to say that echocardiography should not be used as a screening tool early in the first 6 months of life. Clear demonstration of a problem developing in either the aortic arch or the pulmonary artery is an indication for earlier catheterization.

Obvious symptomatic indications for earlier investigation are the development of severe cyanosis or persistent signs of congestive heart failure, especially difficulty with feeding and failure to thrive.

Intermediate-Step Surgery: Bidirectional Cavopulmonary (Glenn) Shunt

The fundamental physiologic problem with the first-stage procedure, as currently performed, is the decrease in pulmonary resistance observed in the hours, days, weeks, and months after surgery. In addition, pulmonary resistance is likely to be temporarily elevated at the time of surgery because of the general deleterious effects of cardiopulmonary bypass and circulatory arrest. Therefore, a systemic-to-pulmonary artery shunt that is of adequate size to enable the child to separate from bypass without failing from the effects of hypoxia will be too large within weeks of surgery, if not earlier. To some extent this problem will be countered by the growth of the child, but if the child is in a relatively severe degree of congestive failure related to the large shunt, there may be very slow somatic growth. One option available to decrease the volume load on the ventricle is to convert the systemic-to-pulmonary artery shunt to a cavopulmonary shunt.[11] Attempts to perform a cavopulmonary shunt in the first weeks of life have been unsuccessful because of severe hypoxia, not because of excessively high superior vena caval pressures. However, cavopulmonary shunt procedures have been successfully performed in infants between 3 and 4 months of age, although there may be a higher incidence of pleural effusions, which are very rarely seen in older infants and children.

If the 6-month catheterization demonstrates a problem, such as distortion of the central pulmonary artery, that is likely to compromise development of the left pulmonary artery, the intervention undertaken should be a bidirectional cavopulmonary shunt with an associated pulmonary arterioplasty. Other indications for application of the cavopulmonary shunt have included the need for aortic arch reconstruction; the need for atrial septal defect enlargement; early outgrowth of the Blalock shunt, resulting in unacceptably low oxygen saturation (<75%); and the development of tricuspid regurgitation or right ventricular dysfunction secondary to excessive volume load on the ventricle. One other problem that is emerging as a possible long-term risk after the first-stage procedure is the development of regurgitation of the neoaortic valve (i.e., the original morphologic pulmonary valve). This finding, per se, is not a current indication to proceed to a bidirectional cavopulmonary shunt.

Occasionally a decision is made not to perform surgery after the 6-month catheterization, but in such cases, when the child returns for additional assessment at 12 to 18 months of age and immediately before a planned Fontan operation, multiple risk factors are often identified. There may be moderate depression of ventricular function, moderate hypoplasia of the pulmonary arteries, and moderate elevation of pulmonary vascular resistance (e.g., 2.5 U/m^2). Although in the past this child may have been managed with a bidirectional cavopulmonary shunt, our current preference would be to proceed directly to a fenestrated Fontan procedure. In older children the cavopulmonary shunt tends to be applied to those children who require extensive additional surgery concomitantly with the cavopulmonary shunt. Adding an ancillary procedure to a fenestrated Fontan procedure will increase the bypass and crossclamp time, as well as the general complexity of the procedure.

Technique. The approach is through a reoperative median sternotomy (Fig. 23–5). The arterial cannula is placed in the neoaorta. Generally the child will be large enough to withstand the procedure on continuous bypass. Although it is possible to undertake the procedure without bypass at all by introducing a bypass shunt between the superior vena cava and right atrium, this method is not recommended so that cerebral protection[24] and surgical outcome can be optimized as a result of the improved exposure afforded by cardiopulmonary bypass. A straight venous cannula is placed in the right atrium and a small, metal-tipped, right-angled cannula in the innominate vein. This latter cannula should be small enough to allow flow around it so that both right and left upper body venous return is adequately drained. Immediately after beginning bypass, the Blalock shunt, which has already been dissected free, is ligated. During cooling the azygos vein is dissected free, doubly ligated, and divided. The procedure can be done with the heart beating at a temperature of 30°C. The superior vena cava is divided between clamps some distance above the atriocaval junction, well clear of the sinoatrial node

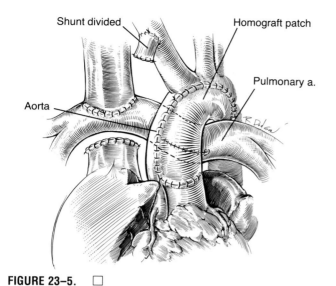

FIGURE 23–5. ☐

Technique of a bidirectional Glenn shunt. The divided right superior vena cava has been anastomosed at the previous site of the distal anastomosis of the modified right Blalock shunt. The cardiac end of the divided superior vena cava may also be anastomosed to the right pulmonary artery, with the internal orifice being closed with a Gore-Tex patch.

area. An end-to-side anastomosis is fashioned between the cephalic end of the divided superior vena cava and a longitudinal arteriotomy in the right pulmonary artery. This is usually the site of the previous Blalock distal anastomosis, which can be extended a few millimeters to the left and right, taking care not to compromise the right upper lobe branch. Continuous, absorbable polydioxanone suture is used for the anastomosis. The greater tissue drag of this suture material is an advantage when compared with polypropylene, as the risk of narrowing the anastomosis by a pursestring effect is decreased. Nevertheless, it may still be useful to place several interrupted sutures across the anterior layer of the anastomosis.

Although the cardiac end of the divided superior vena cava can be simply oversewn (which has the advantage that the atrium does not need to be opened), another approach is to open the right atrium after applying a tourniquet around the cannula in the inferior vena cava. The cardiac end of the divided superior vena cava is anastomosed to the pulmonary artery. A small patch of pericardium or PTFE is sutured around the internal orifice of the superior vena cava. This step is preparatory for a subsequent Fontan procedure. It undoubtedly benefits the sinus node and its arterial supply, as the anastomosis is kept some distance superior to the atriocaval junction.

Ancillary Procedures. The most commonly performed procedure in conjunction with the bidirectional cavopulmonary shunt at the Children's Hos-

pital in Boston is a patch arterioplasty of the central pulmonary artery area. Because this area often lies directly posterior to the neoaorta, it is usually best to divide the neoaorta so that the patch can be extended to the left pulmonary artery bifurcation. Biologic tissues, including autologous pericardium or homograft pulmonary arterial wall, are the preferred patch materials, although PTFE has also been applied with success in this situation. Dacron is best avoided because of the intense fibrotic reaction that is often seen after its use.

If the neoaortic arch must be reconstructed, this is most safely done from the sternotomy approach under conditions of circulatory arrest. However, with distal extension of the initial patch into the descending aorta and balloon dilatation, this procedure is rarely required. Previous experience with a closed surgical procedure employing a side-biting clamp on the stenotic area (much as for a coarctation repair) revealed that this approach carried significant risk. In addition, the opportunity to convert the arterial shunt to a venous shunt is lost.

Weaning From Bypass. In contrast to the postoperative course for the neonate who has undergone a stage 1 procedure in which ventilatory manipulations are essential to the success of the procedure, the early postbypass course of children after a bidirectional cavopulmonary shunt is remarkably benign. As long as ventricular function was no more than mildly to moderately depressed preoperatively, there was satisfactory myocardial protection intraoperatively, the pulmonary arteries have been adequately repaired, and pulmonary resistance is not severely elevated, the child can be expected to be weaned from bypass with an arterial saturation of approximately 80% to 85%. Increasing cardiac output with a dopamine infusion will serve to further improve the arterial oxygen saturation.

Superior vena caval pressure can be temporarily monitored in the operating room by introducing a catheter into the innominate vein through the cannulation site previously used for the venous cannula. It is extremely unusual for this pressure to be severely elevated (>18 mm Hg) as long as the conditions described earlier have been met. It is preferable to avoid a longer term indwelling catheter in the superior vena cava because of a high risk that thrombi will form at the tip of the catheter, particularly if the catheter is used for parenteral hyperalimentation. Therefore, the catheter is removed from the innominate vein and is replaced in the right atrium through the other venous cannulation site.

Early Postoperative Management. It is usually possible to extubate the child within 12 to 18 hours of surgery. Postoperative management is usually entirely routine. Support with low doses of dopamine (<5 μg/kg/min) is often employed. The head of the bed may be elevated to encourage venous drainage from the upper body. Chest tubes can be removed within 24 hours of surgery in the majority of children. The incidence of long-standing pleural effusions has been remarkably low, particularly when one considers that the children selected for this procedure have been considered to have too many risk factors to proceed directly to a Fontan procedure.

Follow-Up. Like early postoperative management, later postoperative management after a cavopulmonary shunt is routine. The main issues in follow-up continue to be the same principles pursued as part of follow-up after the first-stage procedure. However, because the volume load of the systemic-to-pulmonary artery shunt has been eliminated by the new shunt, at this point there is less urgency to proceed to the fenestrated Fontan procedure. At Children's Hospital in Boston, we have arbitrarily selected 9 months without symptoms as the required interval before cardiac catheterization is repeated. Assuming that the hemodynamic and anatomic findings are satisfactory, the child will proceed to a fenestrated Fontan procedure approximately 1 year after the bidirectional cavopulmonary shunt, at an age of 18 months to 2 years.

Occasionally, cyanosis will become excessive after the cavopulmonary shunt. At cardiac catheterization it may be possible to demonstrate venovenous collateral vessels that are decompressing the superior vena caval venous system into the inferior vena caval system. Such venous collateral vessels can be closed in the catheterization laboratory using embolization coils.

Fenestrated Fontan Procedure for HLHS

Preoperative assessment of the child before the fenestrated Fontan stage of the reconstructive procedure for HLHS is no different than the assessment of any child who is being considered for a Fontan operation. The primary considerations are the size and uniformity of the central pulmonary arteries, the pulmonary vascular resistance, the contractility and compliance of the right ventricle, the presence of tricuspid regurgitation, and the presence of stable sinus rhythm. Age is not a consideration, as long as the child is at least 9 months old. Although the Fontan operation has certainly been successfully undertaken at younger ages and although, with future developments and refinements, the age for elective surgery may well move earlier into infancy, at present a child who requires surgery before 9 months of age because of symptoms (e.g.,

worsening cyanosis because of a small shunt) is more likely to be managed with a bidirectional cavopulmonary shunt than a fenestrated Fontan procedure.

Absolute Contraindications. With carefully planned palliative surgery and close monitoring in the brief interval period during infancy, there are few children in whom a fenestrated Fontan procedure is absolutely contraindicated. Children who are unsuitable for this procedure, either with or without a preliminary bidirectional cavopulmonary shunt, are likely to have undergone multiple palliative procedures in a misguided attempt to postpone the Fontan operation.[43] Any attempt to increase pulmonary blood flow by placing an additional systemic-to-pulmonary artery shunt in the child who has become cyanotic after the first-stage procedure is almost always unwise.

At the current point of evolution of the intermediate bidirectional cavopulmonary shunt and of the fenestrated Fontan operation itself, it is difficult to confidently specify guidelines regarding contraindication to a fenestrated Fontan operation. This is discussed in greater detail in Chapter 15. In summary, any individual major risk factor, if present as an isolated factor, must be present to at least a moderate to severe degree to absolutely contraindicate a fenestrated Fontan operation. Clearly, however, the greater the number of risk factors that are present, the more stringent are the requirements regarding each individual risk factor.

Technical Considerations. As stated in the introduction to this chapter, the particular needs of the child with HLHS have been responsible for many of the changes in the general management of the child with single-ventricle physiology. Nowhere has this been more true than in the technical modifications of the Fontan procedure that have occurred since the mid-1980s as large numbers of survivors of the first-stage procedure presented for their Fontan operation.

Cavopulmonary Anastomosis. In their landmark paper introducing the clinical reality of a successful Fontan operation, Fontan and Baudet connected the right atrium to the pulmonary arteries, in part using a valved homograft conduit routed anteriorly in the mediastinum.[22] As the serious disadvantages of even minor gradients across this conduit became clear, it also became obvious that conduits of any sort should be avoided in these children because of growth and the inherent tendency of any conduit to ultimately become obstructed.[21] A technique described by Bjork and associates[8] avoided a conduit but still placed the atrio–right ventricular correction anteriorly in the mediastinum, where it was susceptible to compression by the sternum. An important advance by Kreutzer and coworkers[34] was to introduce a posteriorly placed atriopulmonary anastomosis, although this location threatened the integrity of the sinus node artery, and when adhesions were present and obscured the location of the right coronary artery, it was often technically difficult to achieve a widely open anastomosis. In February 1986, we changed the technique to a double cavopulmonary anastomosis as part of the Fontan operation for HLHS.[30] The child in whom this technique was used was the third long-term survivor of the reconstructive procedure at Children's Hospital in Boston, there having been no other survivors after the initial two patients reported by Norwood in 1983. This child continued to do well 6 years after this procedure.

Lateral Cavopulmonary Baffle. One of the original premises regarding the Fontan operation was that pulsatile assistance from the right atrium was essential to the success of the procedure. In their report of 1984 describing direct diversion of all caval return into the pulmonary arteries in the subgroup of patients with heterotaxia and azygos continuation of the interrupted inferior vena cava to the superior vena cava, Kawashima and associates[33] conclusively demonstrated that atrial pulsatility was not, in fact, a necessary condition for a successful Fontan operation. This led several investigators[30, 52] to remodel the systemic and pulmonary venous pathways constructed as part of the Fontan operation. Although separation of pulmonary and systemic venous blood could be easily achieved in the patient with tricuspid atresia by simply closing the atrial septal defect, a baffle of some sort was required in the patient with atresia or stenosis of the left atrioventricular valve. At the time, when it was believed that the right atrium should be as large as possible to contribute pulsatility, this baffle was placed obliquely within the right atrium, with the suture line passing around the atrial septal defect and tricuspid annulus. While this was not critical in the patient with two atrioventricular valves, it did become critical in the patient with atresia of the left atrioventricular valve, where the entire pulmonary venous return must pass through the atrial septal defect and tricuspid valve. Increasing pressure in the right atrium led to a bowing of this oblique baffle into the septal defect, the tricuspid valve, or both, resulting in pulmonary venous obstruction. Thus a vicious cycle was easily set up in which even a minor degree of systemic venous obstruction resulted in worsening of pulmonary venous obstruction and, therefore, systemic venous hypertension. Children who did survive this procedure were often hospitalized for many weeks because of persistent drainage of pleural effusions. It is also likely that their ultimate exercise tolerance will be limited by this same phenomenon. The solution to this problem was the creation of a lateral tunnel along the right atrial free wall that could not expand into the pulmonary venous pathway.[30] There are additional advantages to this style of baffle as demonstrated by deLeval and coworkers in a series of hydrodynamic studies.[18] They showed that there was likely to be less energy loss through the reduction in turbulence created by the interposition of a large reservoir, such as the atrium, in the cavopulmonary pathway. In addition, simple application of Laplace's law will reveal that the very much smaller radius of curvature of the systemic venous pathway created by the lateral tunnel, relative to the radius of the entire right atrium, will result in considerably lower stress in the atrial wall. Theoretically, this will reduce the incidence of supraventricular arrhythmias, which have complicated the late postoperative course of a significant percentage of Fontan patients, particularly those with higher right atrial pressures. Finally, it is possible that high right atrial wall stress contributes to the secretion of atrial natriuretic factor, although at present the exact clinical significance of elevated atrial natriuretic factor in these patients is unknown.

Baffle Fenestration. The importance of maintaining patency of the foramen ovale after repair of tetralogy of Fallot has been recognized at Children's Hospital in Boston for many years.[12] During the early postoperative period, when right ventricular function is likely to be compromised, a patent foramen ovale allows right-to-left shunting at the atrial level, thereby maintaining cardiac output and decompressing the systemic venous system at the expense of a mild degree of oxygen desaturation, which is well tolerated by the infant. As right ventricular function improves, the right-to-left shunt decreases. The fenestrated Fontan procedure is an application of this principle. An important reason for the delay in incorporating this principle into the Fontan operation was the common observation by those caring for patients after a standard Fontan procedure that a right-to-left shunt appeared to be poorly tolerated. In fact, this observation was made in patients who were often desperately ill and were in a profound low-output state at the time of catheterization. The very low venous saturations that were present did indeed cause important arterial desaturation in patients with very low cardiac output. However, in retrospect this was an effect, not a cause, of the low-output state. The other development that stimulated the application of the fenestration principle was the clinical application of devices delivered by catheter to close atrial septal defects. Although Laks and coworkers had described an adjustable atrial septal defect device,[35] this method carried some risk of infection and necessitated intervention in the early postoperative period. The approach of fenestration closure some weeks or months after surgery allows careful hemodynamic assessment of the advisability of permanent closure by undertaking temporary balloon occlusion first.

The details of the surgical technique of the fenestrated Fontan operation, including indications for takedown to a bidirectional cavopulmonary shunt and indications and technique of fenestration closure, are described in detail in Chapter 15.

Results of the Reconstructive Approach

Early Results. In 1986[29] we described 25 neonates who had undergone various modifications of the first-stage reconstructive procedure at Children's Hospital in Boston between 1984 and mid-1985. There were six early deaths, for an early mortality rate of 24%. Of these, one was a premature neonate weighing less than 2 kg and two were neonates who could not be adequately resuscitated with prostaglandin and who received cardiac massage immediately before emergency surgery. Early death was related to excessive pulmonary blood flow in two patients and to a possible coronary embolus in one. There were four late deaths, for a total mortality rate of 40%. In an update of our experience with HLHS, including the previously reported 25 patients, 78 patients underwent first-stage reconstruction between 1984 and 1991, with 32 early deaths, for an early mortality rate of 41%. The causes of early death are shown in Table 23–1.

Only two other centers have reported on a significant series of patients who have undergone first-

TABLE 23–1. ☐ PROBABLE PRIMARY CAUSE OF HOSPITAL DEATH AFTER FIRST-STAGE RECONSTRUCTIVE SURGERY FOR HYPOPLASTIC LEFT HEART SYNDROME

CAUSE	NO. OF PATIENTS
Coronary insufficiency	6
Preoperative insult	5
Sudden/unknown	3
Sepsis	3
Hypoxia	2
Prematurity	2
Neoaortic arch obstruction	2
Renal failure	2
Persistent acidosis	1
Hepatic failure	1
Right ventricle dysfunction	1
Hemorrhage	1
Pleural effusion	1
Rupture of neoaorta	1
Shunt obstruction	1

stage reconstruction. In 1988 Pigott and associates[51] described 104 consecutive neonates who underwent surgery between 1985 and 1987. The early mortality rate was 29%, while the total mortality rate was 39%. The authors concluded that future improvement in the mortality rate would most likely result from refined management of intensive care problems as well as surgical improvements.

In 1990 Meliones and colleagues[42] described 57 neonates who had undergone first-stage palliation between 1983 and 1989. There were 31 early deaths for an early mortality rate of 54%. There were 14 late deaths, for a total mortality rate of 79%. The authors suggested that more aggressive perioperative support, for example with extracorporeal membrane oxygenation, might improve the results of first-stage surgery. They also recommended careful ongoing comparison of the results of neonatal heart transplantation with the results of the reconstructive procedure.

Intermediate Follow-Up After First-Stage Reconstruction. Analysis is currently being undertaken of the longer term results in 78 patients operated on by one of the authors between 1984 and 1991. This shows that, similar to the experience reported by Murdison and Meliones and their respective colleagues,[42, 44] there is substantial attrition in the first 2 years after surgery, and patients then stabilize. The early mortality rate was 41%, with an actuarial survival rate at 1 year of 43% and at 2 years of 28%. The 5-year actuarial survival rate was 17%. In interpreting these results, it is important to recognize that this period encompasses the development of the various modifications of the Fontan procedure that are currently employed on a routine basis, resulting in dramatic improvement in mortality risk for that procedure, as well as recognition of the advantages of incorporating the bidirectional cavopulmonary shunt as an intermediate step for high-risk candidates. These developments were in response to the excessively high mortality rate demonstrated by the actuarial survival curve just described. Nevertheless, the survival curve shows a high rate of attrition in the first months after the first-stage procedure; this high rate will not be improved by modifications to the subsequent procedures. Therefore, we are attempting to identify predictors of poor outcome using multivariate analysis.

The preliminary analysis suggests that long-term survival is markedly better for patients who have aortic and mitral stenosis than for patients who have aortic and mitral atresia. Those who have aortic atresia and mitral stenosis have an intermediate level of survival relative to the other two groups, in contrast to the findings of Sauer and associates,[56] who suggested that survival would be worse in this subgroup because of the frequency of coronary artery anomalies. Analysis of early mortality, however, suggests that the subgroup with aortic atresia and mitral stenosis may be more at risk for early death. In the preliminary analysis, attrition in the first 2 years after first-stage surgery also appeared to be related to the diameter of the ascending aorta. Patients who had an ascending aortic diameter of less than 2 mm (rare) had a higher rate of attrition than children with an ascending aortic diameter of between 2 and 4 mm (common) or a diameter greater than 4 mm. It is possible that these findings are a reflection of the disadvantages of procedures in which a complete tube graft (either prosthetic or homograft) has been employed, requiring blood to pass retrograde down the full length of the ascending aorta to the coronary arteries. Such methods were not employed in the series reported by Murdison and colleagues.[44] However, if the high rate of attrition of patients with aortic and mitral atresia, and with particularly small ascending aortas, is independent of the surgical method of first-stage reconstruction, this would suggest that this small subgroup might be more appropriately treated with heart transplantation than with reconstruction.

Late Complications After First-Stage Reconstruction. Several studies have been reported by investigators from Children's Hospital of Philadelphia examining such issues as the fate of the pulmonary valve when exposed to systemic pressure after first-stage reconstruction and the significance of tricuspid regurgitation.[17] Color Doppler was used to examine the pulmonary (neoaortic) valve in 45 survivors of pulmonary artery–to–ascending aorta anastomosis a mean of 202 days postoperatively. Of 37 patients with HLHS, nine (24%) had mild regurgitation and one (3%) had moderate regurgitation. Seven of 11 patients imaged more than 12 months postoperatively had regurgitation. The authors concluded that pulmonary regurgitation should not be considered a contraindication to a Fontan operation, although close follow-up is clearly warranted, as the long-term implications remain unknown.[17]

Tricuspid regurgitation was followed serially in 100 patients undergoing first-stage reconstruction. Preoperatively, 37% of the patients had mild regurgitation, 13% had moderate regurgitation, and 3% had severe regurgitation. In the first 2 postoperative years, most patients demonstrated no significant change in the degree of tricuspid regurgitation when the postoperative echocardiogram was compared with the preoperative echocardiogram. However, in patients with moderate or severe tricuspid regurgitation preoperatively, survival was significantly reduced when compared with that in patients who had no or mild regurgitation.

An analysis of pulmonary artery configuration after first-stage surgery in 28 patients was reported by Alboliras and associates.[1] Fourteen patients had undergone Blalock shunts, and 14 had undergone central shunts. Approximately 3 weeks after surgery, patients with Blalock shunts showed a decrease in the diameter of all pulmonary artery segments except the distal right pulmonary artery, while patients with central shunts showed a decrease in the diameter of all pulmonary artery segments. Similar findings persisted in 19 of the 28 patients who were examined 6 months after the first study. At 6 months the diameter of the pulmonary arteries after a Blalock shunt ranged from 3.8 mm in the distal left pulmonary artery to 6.3 mm in the distal right pulmonary artery. In the central shunt group, the distal left pulmonary artery diameter was 4.4 mm, and the distal right pulmonary artery diameter was 5.0 mm. Thus, although the central shunt results in more uniform development of the pulmonary arteries, the absolute dimensions of the pulmonary arteries remain relatively small. It has been our subjective impression that children with a more severe degree of HLHS are more likely to have smaller pulmonary arteries, perhaps related to restriction of fetal pulmonary blood flow. This is in contrast to children with tricuspid atresia, transposed great arteries, and a restrictive ventricular septal defect who may also undergo first-stage reconstruction, who presumably have not had restriction to fetal pulmonary blood flow, and whose pulmonary arteries at surgery appear relatively larger.

Results of the Fontan Operation for HLHS. In 1991 Mayer and coworkers at Children's Hospital in Boston[41] reported on the factors that were associated with a marked reduction in mortality rate for patients with single-ventricle physiology who underwent a Fontan operation, including patients with HLHS. Between 1984 and 1990, 225 patients underwent Fontan operations for anomalies other than tricuspid atresia. The operation failed (death or takedown) in 30 of the 225 patients (13%). Results improved significantly over the period of the study, with failure rates of 6.5% and 3%, respectively, in the last 2 years of the study, when 31% of the patients were <3 years of age. Multivariate analysis showed that pulmonary artery distortion was a powerful predictor of a failed operation ($P = .0003$). For patients with left atrioventricular valve atresia or stenosis, the technique of atrial partitioning was the most important predictor of outcome when one excluded cardiopulmonary bypass duration. Seventeen of these patients had undergone first-stage reconstruction for HLHS, with an overall failure rate of 41%, which is remarkably similar to the 42% failure rate reported by Chang and coworkers from Philadelphia over approximately the same time period.[15] Since the introduction of the bidirectional cavopulmonary shunt in 1988 and the fenestrated Fontan procedure in 1989, there has been one death in 57 children waiting to undergo the second-stage procedure for HLHS.

In 1991 Chang and colleagues[15] reported the results of surgery in 50 patients who had undergone modified Fontan procedures after first-stage palliative reconstructive surgery at Children's Hospital of Philadelphia. These patients represented the long-term survivors of a group of 200 patients who had undergone their first-stage operation between 1985 and 1989, with a 33% early mortality rate. There were an additional nine patients who underwent an intermediate bidirectional cavopulmonary shunt (hemi-Fontan), six of whom subsequently underwent a successful Fontan procedure. There were eight early deaths (defined as death <30 days after operation) in the 50 Fontan candidates, with an additional 13 late deaths, giving an overall mortality rate of 42%. Univariate comparison of survivors and nonsurvivors suggested to the authors that important tricuspid regurgitation was the only possible predictor of poor outcome. They did not find that elevated pulmonary vascular resistance (>4 U/m^2) or pulmonary artery distortion was predictive of outcome. Bridges and associates[10] had previously reported from Philadelphia that small pulmonary artery size was not a predictor of outcome after a Fontan procedure. However, it must be remembered that the pulmonary artery size was measured on preoperative angiography, and extensive pulmonary artery reconstruction may have made these measurements invalid.

The frequency of risk factors for the Fontan procedure in the series reported by Chang and colleagues (10 patients had pulmonary vascular resistance >4 U/m^2, five had right ventricular end-diastolic pressure >12 mm, and eight had pulmonary artery distortion) suggests that application of either an intermediate procedure, such as a bidirectional cavopulmonary shunt, or the fenestrated Fontan procedure is likely to result in a substantial improvement in mortality in the future, as has been observed at Children's Hospital in Boston since the introduction of these modifications.

Aortic Atresia With a Normal Left Ventricle

There is a small subgroup of patients with aortic atresia and normal-size left ventricles who may be considered to be part of the spectrum of HLHS. In approximately 4% to 7% of infants with aortic atresia, there is an associated ventricular septal defect and a normal-size mitral valve.[54] This suggests the possibility of physiologic correction, either in one stage during the neonatal period or as a staged procedure. In 1989 we described four consecutive neonates with this anomaly who underwent one-stage correction, with one death.[3]

Surgical Method of One-Stage Correction. The preliminary phases of this operation are similar to those described previously for the palliative, reconstructive, stage 1 neonatal procedure. Deep hypothermic circulatory arrest is employed. The proximal part of the main pulmonary artery is divided (Fig. 23–6A), and an anastomosis is fashioned between the proximal main pulmonary artery and the ascending aorta, aortic arch, and proximal descending aorta. Working through an incision in the right ventricular infundibulum, the ventricular septal defect is closed so as to baffle left ventricular outflow to the pulmonary artery and thence to the aorta. A homograft conduit between the right ventricle and the distal divided main pulmonary artery completes the repair (Fig. 23–6B). Because a biventricular, "in-series" circulation has been achieved (Fig. 23–6C), weaning from bypass and postoperative management do not involve the delicate manipulations required after the palliative first-stage procedure.

THE TRANSPLANT PATHWAY FOR HLHS

General Philosphy

There are a number of underlying concerns regarding the very long-term outlook for children who traverse the reconstructive pathway. Many consider the long-term experience with the Mustard and Senning operations persuasive evidence that long-term function of the right ventricle as a systemic ventricle will be inadequate, particularly when it must function without the assistance of a pulmonary ventricle. Tricuspid valve function has also been demonstrated to deteriorate when exposed to systemic pressure work, both in patients corrected by atrial level repairs for D-transposition and in those with congenitally corrected transposition. The studies of Chin and coworkers[17] also bring into question the long-term function of the pulmonary valve as a systemic valve after anastomosis of the proximal pulmonary artery to the ascending aorta. The first-stage reconstructive procedure described by Norwood[49] is a technically demanding procedure, more so because it must be performed in the limited time available using deep hypothermic circulatory arrest. Highly skilled anesthesiologists and nurses and intensive care support are essential to achieve even the modest early results that have been re-

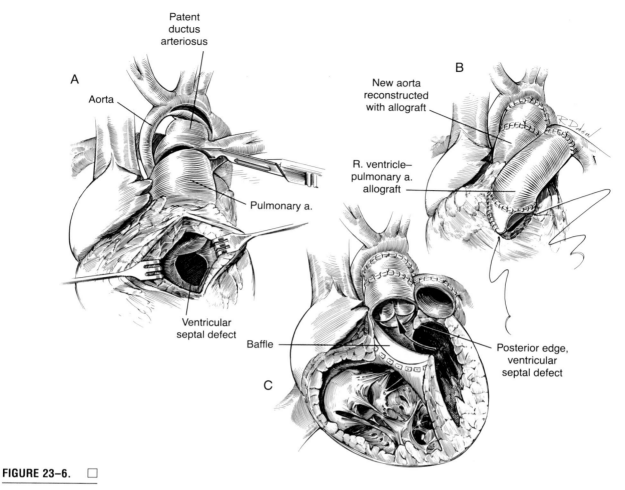

FIGURE 23–6. □

A, Typical anatomic features of aortic atresia with a normal left ventricle, including a tiny ascending aorta, a large pulmonary artery with a patent ductus arteriosus, a coarctation, and a posterior malalignment ventricular septal defect. The incisions used for the repair are noted. *B,* At completion of the repair, continuity between the proximal main pulmonary artery and the aorta and between the right ventricle and distal pulmonary arteries has been achieved with homograft conduits. *C,* The left ventricular outflow has been baffled through the ventricular septal defect to the pulmonary valve. (Redrawn from Austin EH, Jonas RA, Mayer JE, et al. Aortic atresia with normal left ventricle: Single stage repair in the neonate. J Thorac Cardiovasc Surg 97:392, 1989.)

ported. In fact, many centers attempting the reconstructive pathway have had unacceptably high mortality rates. In 1986 Sade and associates[55] described the results presented at a symposium on HLHS. In centers that treated more than 35 patients, there was a 53% mortality rate, while in centers treating less than 16 patients, the mortality rate was 91%. The authors concluded that further efforts should be focused on heart transplantation, as well as on continuing to improve results of the reconstructive approach.

The pioneering work, both clinically and experimentally, in neonatal heart transplantation for HLHS has been led by Bailey and coworkers at Loma Linda University.[5] The first successful human allograft heart transplant in a neonate with HLHS took place in 1985, 6 years after the first long-term successful reconstructive procedure by Norwood et al.[49] In comparing the results of these two approaches, it is important to bear in mind that the long-term follow-up of the reconstructive approach is now almost twice as long as that of neonatal transplantation. The technique of heart transplantation is described in Chapter 30.

Results

Early Results. The results of transplantation at Children's Hospital are described in Chapter 30. In 1990 Bailey and Gundry[6] reported the results of heart transplantation in 28 neonates and young infants with HLHS between 1985 and 1989. There were five perioperative deaths, for an early mortality rate of 18%. Of the last 19 consecutive patients, there were 17 survivors (89%). Although they reported that during 1988, 22 of 26 patients registered for heart transplantation received transplants, other centers, including our own, have had a considerably higher interim mortality rate. Long-term palliation (weeks) with prostaglandin E_1 is associated with progressive signs of congestive heart failure as pulmonary vascular resistance decreases with age and becomes more resistant to the measures employed to maximize systemic perfusion and pulmonary vascular resistance. Attempts have been made to increase pulmonary resistance on a longer term basis using hypoxic and hypercarbic gas mixtures (S. Gundry, personal communication, 1991). One study[27] has identified important histologic pulmonary vascular changes, including necrotizing vasculitis associated with lung infarcts, after prolonged prostaglandin E_1 treatment. It is possible that many of the patients who are compromised by severe preoperative insults or tricuspid regurgitation and right ventricular dysfunction and who are likely to be the patients who will die over the first months after a reconstructive operation, are the same patients who are unable to survive the 1- to 2-month waiting period required to locate a donor or who are not listed for transplantation because it is anticipated that such survival is not likely.

In their 1988 report, Mavroudis and coworkers[39] described 16 infants who were evaluated for heart transplantation; 14 of these had HLHS. Eight of the 16 families who were offered transplantation refused. In the remaining eight patients, there were three deaths during the interim period while attempts were made to locate a donor. In-house retrieval was used in the five transplant procedures that were undertaken, with one perioperative death. Death was related to pretransplant donor heart dysfunction and size discrepancy.

Coronary Artery Disease. Patients in the Chicago report[4] have undergone comprehensive yearly cardiac catheterization, and selective coronary angiography has been performed 12 times in eight patients. Coronary artery disease was not identified in any of these studies. However, of concern was the finding of early coronary artery disease with intimal proliferation at autopsy of a child who died at 13 months from acute rejection.

In a report by Braunlin and associates,[9] coronary artery disease was specifically sought in nine children with a mean age of 11 years (range, 0.5 to 16 years) who had survived more than 1 year after heart transplantation. Three of the nine had mild disease at 1 year, and four of eight surviving patients had mild disease at 2 years. In two patients, mild coronary artery disease progressed to severe coronary artery disease 3 years after transplantation. The authors concluded that although the incidence of rejection had been decreased by the use of a triple immunosupressive regimen, this had not been associated with a decreased incidence of coronary artery disease, which might limit the long-term survival of pediatric patients after heart transplantation.

Lymphoma. As yet, there are only anecdotal reports regarding the risk of lymphoma and other neoplastic conditions after infant heart transplantation. This and the other serious long-term consequences of immunosuppression, such as hypertension and renal failure, merit close attention in the coming years.

SUMMARY

Although there has been great progress in the management of HLHS since the early 1980s, many issues remain to be resolved. Clearly, heart transplantation can result in an impressive intermediate-term survival rate, with an excellent quality of life for the majority of survivors. However, it is unlikely, with current ethical determinations of brain death, that the supply of allograft donors would be adequate to satisfy the demand generated if all infants born with HLHS were to receive transplants. There are also doubts regarding the very long-term implications of the intermediate-term findings of coronary artery disease and the other sequelae of long-term immunosuppression.

The reconstructive approach has provided an excellent quality of life for many children, although there are continuing concerns regarding the very long-term performance of the right ventricle, tricuspid valve, and pulmonary valve. Perhaps a reasonable compromise is to identify the subgroup of patients who are not likely to do well with the reconstructive approach and to reserve the limited resource of small donor hearts for this subgroup. This assumes that a widening disparity does not develop over time between the sequelae of long-term immunosuppression and the disadvantages of a systemic right ventricle unsupported by a pulmonary ventricle. Until these issues are resolved, the neonate with HLHS presents a disturbing challenge to those entrusted with the management of congenital heart disease.

REFERENCES

1. Alboliras ET, Chin AJ, Barber G, et al. Pulmonary artery configuration after palliative operations for hypoplastic left heart syndrome. J Thorac Cardiovasc Surg 97:878, 1989.
2. Allan LD, Sharland G, Tynan MJ. The natural history of hypoplastic left heart syndrome. Int J Cardiol 25:341, 1989.
3. Austin EH, Jonas RA, Mayer JE, et al. Aortic atresia with normal left ventricle: Single stage repair in the neonate. J Thorac Cardiovasc Surg 97:392, 1989.

4. Backer CL, Zales VR, Harrison HL, et al. Intermediate term results of infant orthotopic cardiac transplantation from two centers. J Thorac Cardiovasc Surg 101:826, 1991.

5. Bailey L, Concepcion W, Shattuck H, et al. Method of heart transplantation for treatment of hypoplastic left heart syndrome. J Thorac Cardiovasc Surg 92:1, 1986.

6. Bailey LL, Gundry SR. Hypoplastic left heart syndrome. Pediatr Clin North Am 37:137, 1990.

7. Behrendt DM, Rocchini A. An operation for the hypoplastic left heart syndrome: Preliminary report. Ann Thorac Surg 32:284, 1981.

8. Bjork VO, Olin CL, Bjarke BB, et al. Right atrial-right ventricular anastomosis for correction of tricuspid atresia. J Thorac Cardiovasc Surg 77:452, 1979.

9. Braunlin EA, Hunter DW, Olivari MT, et al. Coronary artery disease in pediatric cardiac transplant patients undergoing triple-drug immunosuppression. Circulation 82(suppl III):III-1985, 1990.

10. Bridges ND, Farrell PE, Pigott JD, et al. Pulmonary artery index: A nonpredictor of operative survival in patients undergoing modified Fontan repair. Circulation 80(suppl I):I-216, 1989.

11. Bridges ND, Jonas RA, Mayer JE, et al. Bidirectional cavopulmonary anastomosis as interim palliation for high risk Fontan candidates. Circulation 82(suppl IV):IV-170, 1990.

12. Castaneda AR, Jonas RA, Mayer JE, et al. Repair of tetralogy of Fallot in infancy. In Doyle EF, Engle MA, Gersony WN, et al (eds). Pediatric Cardiology/Proceedings of the 2nd World Congress. New York, Springer-Verlag, 1985.

13. Cayler GG. Hypoplastic left heart syndrome. Letter. Am J Cardiol 30:450, 1972.

14. Cayler GG, Smeloff EA, Miller GE. Surgical palliation of hypoplastic left side of the heart. N Engl J Med 282:780, 1970.

15. Chang AC, Farrell PE, Murdison KA, et al. Hypoplastic left heart syndrome: Hemodynamic and angiographic assessment after initial reconstructive surgery and relevance to modified Fontan procedure. J Am Coll Cardiol 17:1143, 1991.

16. Chang AC, Huhta JC, Yoon GY, et al. Diagnosis, transport, and outcome in fetuses with left ventricular outflow tract obstruction. J Thorac Cardiovasc Surg 102:841, 1991.

17. Chin AJ, Barber G, Helton JG, et al. Fate of the pulmonic valve after proximal pulmonary artery–to–ascending aorta anastomosis for aortic outflow obstruction. Am J Cardiol 62:435, 1988.

18. deLeval MR, Kilner P, Gewillig M, et al. Total cavopulmonary connection: A logical alternative to atriopulmonary connection for complex Fontan operations. J Thorac Cardiovasc Surg 96:682, 1988.

19. Doty DB, Knott HW. Hypoplastic left heart syndrome. J Thorac Cardiovasc Surg 74:624, 1977.

20. Ehrlich M, Bierman FZ, Ellis K, et al. Hypoplastic left heart syndrome: Report of a unique survivor. J Am Coll Cardiol 7:361, 1986.

21. Fernandez G, Costa F, Naftel DC, et al. Prevalence of reoperation for pathway obstruction after Fontan operation. Ann Thorac Surg 48:654, 1989.

22. Fontan F, Baudet E. Surgical repair of tricuspid atresia. Thorax 26:240, 1971.

23. Glauser TA, Rorke LB, Weinberg PM, et al. Congenital brain anomalies associated with the hypoplastic left heart syndrome. Pediatrics 85:984, 1990.

24. Glauser TA, Rorke LB, Weinberg PM, et al. Acquired neuropathologic lesions associated with the hypoplastic left heart syndrome. Pediatrics 85:991, 1990.

25. Hansen DD, Hickey PR. Anesthesia for hypoplastic left heart syndrome. Use of high dose fentanyl in 30 neonates. Anesth Analg 65:127, 1986.

26. Hawkins JA, Doty DB. Aortic atresia: Morphologic characteristics affecting survival and operative palliation. J Thorac Cardiovasc Surg 88:620, 1984.

27. Heffelfinger S, Hawkins EP, Nihill M, et al. Pulmonary vascular changes associated with prolonged E_1 treatment. Pediatr Pathol 7:165, 1987.

28. Hickey PR, Hansen DD, Wessel DL, et al. Pulmonary and systemic hemodynamic response to fentanyl in infants. Anesth Analg 64:483, 1985.

29. Jonas RA, Lang P, Hansen D, et al. First stage palliation of hypoplastic left heart syndrome: The importance of coarctation and shunt size. J Thorac Cardiovasc Surg 92:6, 1986.

30. Jonas RA, Castaneda AR. Modified Fontan procedure: Atrial baffle and systemic venous to pulmonary artery anastomotic techniques. J Cardiac Surg 3:91, 1988.

31. Kadoba K, Armiger LC, Sawatari K, et al. Mechanical durability of pulmonary allograft conduits at systemic pressure. J Thorac Cardiovasc Surg. 105:132–141, 1993.

32. Karl TR, Sano S, Brawn WJ, et al. Critical aortic stenosis in the first month of life: Surgical results in 26 infants. Ann Thorac Surg 50:105, 1990.

33. Kawashima Y, Kitamura S, Matsuda H, et al. Total cavopulmonary shunt operation in complex cardiac anomalies. J Thorac Cardiovasc Surg 87:74, 1984.

34. Kreutzer G, Galindez E, Bono H, et al. An operation for the correction of tricuspid atresia. J Thorac Cardiovasc Surg 66:613, 1973.

35. Laks H, Pearl JM, Haas G, et al. Partial Fontan: Advantages of an adjustable interatrial communication. Ann Thorac Surg 52:1084, 1991.

36. Leung MP, McKay R, Smith A, et al. Critical aortic stenosis in early infancy. J Thorac Cardiovasc Surg 101:526, 1991.

37. Levitsky S, van der Horst RL, Hastreiter AR, et al. Surgical palliation in aortic atresia. J Thorac Cardiovasc Surg 79:456, 1980.

38. Ludman P, Foale R, Alexander N, et al. Cross sectional echocardiographic identification of hypoplastic left heart syndrome and differentiation from other causes of right ventricular overload. Br Heart J 63:355, 1990.

39. Mavroudis C, Harrison H, Klein JB, et al. Infant orthotopic cardiac transplantation. J Thorac Cardiovasc Surg 96:912, 1988.

40. Maxwell D, Allan L, Tynan MJ. Balloon dilatation of the aortic valve in the fetus: A report of two cases. Br Heart J 65:256, 1991.

41. Mayer JE, Bridges ND, Lock JE, et al. Factors associated with marked reduction in mortality for Fontan operations in patients with single ventricle. J Thorac Cardiovasc Surg. 103:44, 1992.

42. Meliones JN, Snider AR, Bove EL, et al. Longitudinal results after first-stage palliation for hypoplastic left heart syndrome. Circulation 82(suppl IV):IV-151, 1990.

43. Mietus-Snyder M, Lang P, Mayer JE, et al. Childhood systemic-pulmonary shunts: Subsequent suitability for Fontan operations. Circulation 76:1139, 1987.

44. Murdison KA, Baffa JM, Farrell PE, et al. Hypoplastic left heart syndrome. Outcome after initial reconstruction and before modified Fontan procedure. Circulation 82(suppl IV):IV-199, 1990.

45. Murphy JD, Sands BL, Norwood WI, et al. Intraoperative balloon angioplasty of aortic coarctation in infants with hypoplastic left heart syndrome. Am J Cardiol 59:949, 1987.

46. Naeye RL. Perinatal vascular changes associated with underdevelopment of the left heart. Chest 41:287, 1962.

47. Natowicz M, Chatten J, Clancy R, et al. Genetic disorders and major extracardiac anomalies with hypoplastic left heart syndrome. Pediatrics 82:698, 1988.

48. Norwood WI, Kirklin JK, Sanders SP. Hypoplastic left heart syndrome: Experience with palliative surgery. Am J Cardiol 45:87, 1980.

49. Norwood WI, Lang P, Hansen DD. Physiologic repair of aortic atresia–hypoplastic left heart syndrome. N Engl J Med 308:23, 1983.

50. Perry SB, Lang P, Keane JF, et al. Creation and maintenance of an adequate interatrial communication in patients with left atrioventricular valve atresia or stenosis. Am J Cardiol 58:622, 1986.

51. Pigott JD, Murphy JD, Barber G, et al. Palliative reconstructive surgery for hypoplastic left heart syndrome. Ann Thorac Surg 45:122, 1988.

52. Puga FJ, Chiavarelli M, Hagler DJ. Modifications of the Fontan operation applicable to patients with left atrioventricular

valve atresia or single atrioventricular valve. Circulation 76(suppl III):III-52, 1987.

53. Rhodes LA, Colan SD, Perry SB, et al. Predictors of survival in neonates with critical aortic stenosis. Circulation 84:2325, 1991.

54. Roberts WC, Perry LW, Chandra RS, et al. Aortic valve atresia: A new classification based on necropsy study of 73 cases. Am J Cardiol 37:753, 1976.

55. Sade RM, Crawford FA, Fyfe DA. Symposium on hypoplastic left heart syndrome. J Thorac Cardiovasc Surg 91:937, 1986.

56. Sauer U, Gittenberger-deGroot AC, Geishauser M, et al. Coronary arteries in the hypoplastic left heart syndrome. Circulation 80(suppl I):I-168, 1989.

57. Shone JD, Edwards JE. Mitral atresia associated with pulmonary venous anomalies. Br Heart J 26:241, 1964.

58. Wagenvort CA, Edwards JE. The pulmonary arterial tree in aortic atresia with intact ventricular septum. Lab Invest 10:924, 1961.

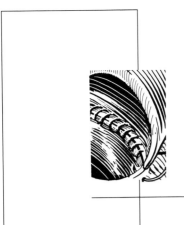

24

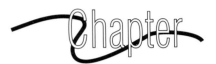

Pediatric Valve Replacement

EMPHASIS ON VALVULOPLASTY TECHNIQUES

The palliative nature of valve replacement in both adults and children has become widely appreciated since the 1980s. There is evidence that mitral valve replacement is more likely to interfere importantly with ventricular function (both early and late after the procedure) than are valvuloplasty methods.[12,13,22] Valvuloplasty preserves the normal subvalvar apparatus, which is important for both valve function and ventricular function. In the past, complete atrioventricular canal repair was often followed by the need for mitral valve replacement.[5] With a better understanding of valvuloplasty methods, as well as a better understanding of the complex anatomy of the atrioventricular valves in this anomaly, the need for mitral valve replacement has declined dramatically since the 1980s.[17] Valvuloplasty methods are also being used more frequently than valve replacement for other anomalies such as Ebstein's anomaly and aortic regurgitation associated with a ventricular septal defect.

BIOLOGIC VALVES

Allografts

The history of the development of allografts as conduits was described in Chapter 6. The aortic valve was first implanted as an allograft orthotopic valve replacement in 1962 by both Barratt-Boyes[2] and Ross.[26] The excellent hemodynamic characteristics of this valve were soon confirmed. In addition, there appeared to be virtually no risk of thromboembolism, even in the absence of anticoagulants. Freedom from a need for anticoagulants during early childhood and through the child-bearing years was an obvious advantage. The valve was also silent, and in many countries it could be obtained without great logistic difficulty at a reasonable cost for harvesting and processing. Like any biologic material that is not wholly viable, there is eventual tissue deterioration resulting in failure of the valve leaflets, usually adjacent to the hinge areas. Barratt-Boyes and coworkers reported the rate of freedom from significant valve incompetence to be 78% at 10 years.[3] O'Brien and associates reported a 100% rate of freedom from valve failure owing to tissue deterioration at 10 years in 192 valves that were stored by cryopreservation.[24]

Since the sudden increase in interest in allograft aortic valve replacement in the United States that began in the mid-1980s, regional organ banks have had difficulty coping with the demand. This has been particularly true with respect to small pediatric sizes. Studies at Children's Hospital in Boston[15] have confirmed satisfactory structural integrity of allografts collected up to 48 hours after donor death, which means that collection no longer needs to be confined to brain-dead, heart-beating organ donors in whom sterile collection is undertaken in the operating room as part of a multiple-organ harvest. Extending collection to cadaver hearts may help to improve the availability of valves in pediatric sizes.

The pulmonary allograft has been used with increasing frequency in more recent years, initially because of the shortage of aortic allografts. Although the pulmonary allograft is a satisfactory substitute for the patient's own pulmonary valve, it is probably not advisable to use it as an aortic valve replacement. This is particularly true if the physician is considering aortic root replacement with the pulmonary root and valve.[16]

Various attempts have been made over the years to use allograft valves as atrioventricular valve replacements.[10, 30] The mitral valve, including the papillary muscles, has been used as an implant but has generally failed because of shortening and fibrosis of the subvalvar support apparatus. Aortic allograft valves have been mounted on a stent and placed in the mitral position but have soon failed, because in the absence of glutaraldehyde treatment, allograft tissue is not strong enough to withstand the stresses resulting from stent mounting. In addition, the normal aortic valve must withstand only aortic diastolic pressure, whereas the mitral valve must withstand left ventricular systolic pressure.

Autograft Pulmonary Valves

In 1967 Ross described the use of the patient's own pulmonary valve as an aortic valve replacement.[27] The original aortic valve and aortic root are completely excised, the pulmonary root is inserted into the aortic position, and the coronary arteries are implanted into the pulmonary autograft. The right ventricular outflow tract must be reconstructed, generally using a pulmonary allograft. The autograft has the important advantage that it will grow when used in small children, although the pulmonary allograft that must be used for right ventricular reconstruction presumably does not grow and must be replaced in time. Gerosa and associates[9] have updated the results of this method, which appear very encouraging, although there is a disappointing high incidence of bacterial endocarditis in the autografts. This is surprising in view of the known viability of the autograft and the excellent hemodynamic characteristics.

Bioprosthetic Valves

Many varieties of bioprosthetic valves have been marketed since the 1970s. The most popular have been porcine aortic valves treated with glutaralde-

hyde to cross-link collagen, followed by mounting of the valve in a plastic or metal stent. Also popular for a time were pericardial xenograft valves; these are no longer widely used because of early tissue failure. Unfortunately, bioprosthetic valves are uniformly unsuitable for pediatric implantation because of the accelerated calcification that occurs.[8, 28] The exact mechanism is not clear, although it is related in part to the accelerated calcium metabolism of children, who are in the process of ossifying cartilage.[20, 29] It appears that after 20 to 25 years of age, accelerated calcification is less of a problem. The other factor contributing to the rapid calcification of bioprostheses is glutaraldehyde treatment. It may be possible to decrease glutaraldehyde-induced calcification by the use of detergent agents such as diphosphonates.[21] Slow-release systems have been incorporated into the sewing rings and stents of prototype bioprostheses.

SYNTHETIC VALVES

The first widely used synthetic valve, the caged ball design typified by the Starr-Edwards valve (currently still available), generally is not suitable for pediatric use. This is a high-profile valve which, when placed in the mitral position, projects into the left ventricular outflow tract.[4] In the small aortic root, it is likely to have very poor hemodynamics, as blood must pass between the ball and the ascending aortic wall. The Bjork-Shiley tilting-disk valve was successfully applied for many years as a pediatric aortic or mitral valve replacement.[1, 14] The valve had a low profile and could be rotated within its sewing ring, which was an important advantage. In small infant and neonatal hearts, there is often only one position where the disk occluder will move completely freely. The Bjork-Shiley valve was removed from the market in the United States in 1988 because of a small but important incidence of outlet strut fracture.

Since the removal of the Bjork-Shiley valve from the market, the St. Jude Medical valve has been the valve of first choice for pediatric implantation. This bileaflet valve has excellent hemodynamic characteristics, although it is inferior to the aortic allograft.[7] With its use the incidence of thromboembolism is small but persistent, in spite of careful control with anticoagulants (which is certainly recommended, using sodium warfarin (Coumadin) for both aortic and mitral valve replacement). The inability to rotate the valve within the sewing ring is an important disadvantage of this valve; this has been addressed by the alternative Carbomedics valve. In other respects, the Carbomedics valve is very similar to the St. Jude valve, although a range of sewing ring thicknesses is available, which is useful for very small children. We have had no experience with the only other two disk valves available in the United States, the Medtronic-Hall valve and the Omniscience valve, which are similar in concept to the Bjork-Shiley valve.

SIZES OF VALVES FOR INFANT VALVE REPLACEMENT

One advantage of the aortic allograft, in addition to those already described, is that, in theory, it is available in an infinite range of sizes, with the internal diameter ranging from approximately 6 to 25 mm. In practice, however, because of the large demand for pediatric-size allografts to be used as conduits, it is currently very difficult to obtain an allograft aortic valve of a specific size from the various organ and tissue banks or commercial allograft preparation companies in the United States.

The Bjork-Shiley valve was previously manufactured to a minimum annular diameter of 17 mm. This was the most commonly used valve in a series of 25 infant mitral valve replacements at Children's Hospital in Boston from 1973 to 1987 (Fig. 24–1).[18] The minimum size of the St. Jude valve is 19 mm. It has the additional disadvantage that the valve cannot be rotated, and clearance must be achieved for two leaflets rather than one. The Carbomedics company has introduced modifications in the sewing ring of their 19-mm prosthesis. By using a very thin sewing ring, this valve can be reclassified as a 16- or 18-mm valve, although the hemodynamic performance is the same as that for the 19-mm valve, as the same leaflets are employed. The very thin sewing ring does not mold as well to the irregular contours of the infant heart, so the risk of paravalvular leak may be increased using this valve. Furthermore, the leaflets of the Carbomedics valve pro-

ject farther from the valve housing than those of the St. Jude valve.

INDICATIONS FOR VALVE REPLACEMENT

Aortic Valve Replacement in Infants

Replacement of the aortic valve is rarely indicated during infancy. More common is the need for replacement of the semilunar valve (truncal valve) in truncus arteriosus because of severe neonatal truncal valve regurgitation or, occasionally, mixed stenosis and regurgitation.[11] Because the truncal valve is usually large and is positioned directly over a ventricular septal defect, replacement is technically straightforward. Replacement can be undertaken with a prosthetic valve and a Konno operation or as an aortic root replacement, using an aortic allograft with reimplantation of the coronary arteries. Details of the technique are given in Chapter 17.

Hypoplasia of the aortic valve and the left ventricular outflow tract is commonly encountered in neonates, usually as part of the hypoplastic left heart syndrome. If it is sufficiently severe to warrant intervention other than simple balloon valvotomy for valvar stenosis, there is usually such severe associated hypoplasia of the left ventricle and mitral valve that a procedure to enlarge the left ventricular outflow tract, including aortic valve replacement, is not likely to be indicated. Instead, a first-stage palliative procedure for the hypoplastic left heart syndrome should be undertaken with the intent to ultimately perform a Fontan procedure. A study by Rhodes and associates has furthered our insight into the use of a one- or two-ventricle approach in this setting.[25]

In the rare case in which aortic valve replacement is indicated for the neonate with a small left ventricular outflow tract, this may be best accomplished with a pulmonary autograft.[9] An incision into the ventricular septum (as for an extended aortic root replacement) should also be made, with the resulting ventricular septal defect closed with a synthetic patch. Alternatively, an aortic allograft can be placed as for the extended aortic root replacement.[23] Technical details are given in Chapter 20.

Aortic regurgitation owing to prolapse of the cusp secondary to a ventricular septal defect is more an acquired than a true congenital anomaly and, as such, is almost never encountered during the first year of life. Aortic valve replacement is almost never indicated in early childhood because of the success of valvuloplasty techniques, as well as the prophylactic effect of closing ventricular septal defects

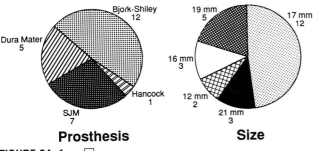

FIGURE 24–1. □

Valve types and valve sizes used for mitral valve replacement (MVR) in infants at Children's Hospital, Boston, between 1973 and 1987. SJM = St. Jude Medical valve.

either early in life or at the first hint of progressive cusp prolapse or regurgitation.

Pulmonary Valve Replacement in Infants

Although some have suggested that replacement of the pulmonary valve should be part of the routine management of tetralogy of Fallot in infants, we have not found it necessary to take this approach. Late pulmonary valve replacement, even many years after transannular patch repair of tetralogy in infants, has been exceedingly rare. In view of the current shortage of allografts, we firmly believe that small allografts should not be used in the routine reconstruction of the right ventricular outflow tract in infants with tetralogy of Fallot. The one exception to this is the rare situation of tetralogy of Fallot with absence of the pulmonary valve. These children have aneurysmal dilatation of the pulmonary artery tree, which often causes important compression of the airways. Repair should include closure of the ventricular septal defect, plication of the enormous central pulmonary arteries, and insertion of a small pulmonary allograft in the orthotopic position.

Tricuspid Valve Replacement in Infants

The management of Ebstein's anomaly has been discussed in detail in Chapter 16. Tricuspid valve replacement is virtually never indicated for this anomaly during infancy. If the child is severely compromised during the neonatal period, it is unlikely that right ventricular function will be adequate to sustain sufficient output, even if the tricuspid valve is totally competent. In these circumstances, complete closure of the valve with a patch and placement of a systemic-to-pulmonary (Blalock) shunt is indicated. In the older infant, valvuloplasty methods should be aggressively pursued before resorting to valve replacement.

An Ebstein-like malformation of the left-sided tricuspid valve is commonly seen as part of {S,L,L} (congenitally corrected) transposition. Occasionally, severe regurgitation of this valve is seen during the neonatal period, but it is usually associated with hypoplasia of the systemic right ventricle itself or its outflow tract. If this is the case, the only possible approach, other than heart transplantation, is a Norwood operation like that used for the hypoplastic left heart syndrome. In older infants and children, tricuspid regurgitation is exacerbated by the development of complete heart block, which is often secondary to surgical intervention, e.g., closure of a ventricular septal defect. This closure can also cause

further distortion of the Ebstein-like left atrioventricular valve and, by itself, exacerbate tricuspid regurgitation. For all of these reasons, the Fontan operation currently is being more widely applied for this anomaly than it was in the past.

Common Atrioventricular Valve Replacement: Single Ventricle

Patients with heterotaxia (situs ambiguus), particularly with associated asplenia, are likely to have a single right ventricle and a very large common atrioventricular valve. Particularly if there is a large volume load on the ventricle (for example, if a large shunt has been placed), there may be progressive regurgitation of the atrioventricular valve secondary to ventricular dilatation and the intrinsic abnormalities of this large valve. Replacement of this common atrioventricular valve is often followed by severe ventricular dysfunction and should be undertaken only when regurgitation is progressive and severe and cannot be improved by valvuloplasty methods. Careful consideration should be given to proceeding directly to heart transplantation rather than replacing the common atrioventricular valve.

Mitral Valve Replacement in Infants

Mitral valve replacement is by far the most common valve replacement indicated during infancy; nevertheless, it is rarely performed and currently is becoming even less frequent. Of 25 mitral valve replacements in infants between 1973 and 1987 at Children's Hospital in Boston, five were for congenital mitral stenosis, and 20 were for mitral regurgitation, most commonly after repair of a complete atrioventicular canal defect.[18] The need for mitral valve replacement after atrioventricular canal repair has decreased from an incidence of 16.7% (nine of 54) between 1973 and 1982 to 3.3% (three of 90) between 1982 and 1987 (Fig. 24–2).

Of the five patients with congenital mitral stenosis, two had a mitral arcade, two had supramitral stenosing rings associated with severe hypoplasia of the mitral valve annulus, and one had a parachute mitral valve. Of the 20 patients with mitral regurgitation, nine had previously undergone repair of complete atrioventricular canal defects, and three had had repair of incomplete atrioventricular canal defects. Of the eight patients with non–atrioventricular canal mitral regurgitation, four had similar valve abnormalities, which included dysplastic and retracted leaflets, thick and short chordae tendinae, obliterated interchordal spaces, and hypertrophied

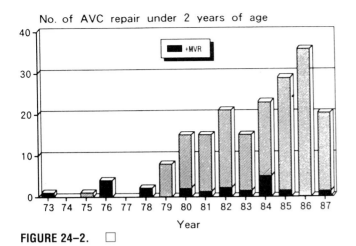

No. of AVC repair under 2 years of age

FIGURE 24–2. □

Number of cases at Children's Hospital, Boston, of surgical repair of atrioventricular canal (AVC) per year including the incidence of need for MVR.

and calcified papillary muscles. Of the other four, one had a cleft mitral valve with an idiopathic left atrial aneurysm, one had a prolapsed mitral valve with myxomatous degeneration associated with Marfan's syndrome, one had a vegetative lesion of the mitral valve caused by acute streptococcal bacterial endocarditis, and the youngest patient (2 days old) had immature and deficient valve tissue with three hypertrophied papillary muscles.

Clinical Status and Catheterization Data

Uncontrollable congestive heart failure is the usual indication for valve replacement. Of the 25 mitral valve replacements in infants at Children's Hospital in Boston before 1987,[18] 13 were performed on an emergency basis. The mean pulmonary-to-systemic pressure ratio was 0.7 ± 0.26. The mean transmitral valve gradient in the mitral stenotic patients was 14.0 ± 4.3 mm Hg. Left atrial mean pressure for the group with mitral regurgitation was 18.6 ± 8.5 mm Hg. For the patients who required emergency mitral valve replacement, the left atrial mean pressure was 23.5 ± 8.0 mm Hg, whereas it was 13.6 ± 5.6 mm Hg in the nonemergency group.

TECHNIQUE OF MITRAL VALVE INSERTION IN INFANTS

Approach is by a median sternotomy. Core cooling and circulatory arrest are generally employed in smaller infants (<7 to 8 kg). The mitral valve is exposed through a vertical incision in the atrial septum. In general, in these small patients it is neces-

sary to totally excise the entire mitral valve, including the subvalvar apparatus. It is important not to force too large a prosthesis into the true annulus, as this almost certainly contributes to a high incidence of complete heart block. If the annulus is smaller than the smallest prosthesis available, the prosthesis should be inserted in a true supra-annular position.

Supra-Annular Mitral Valve Replacement

Standard everting, horizontal, pledgetted mattress sutures are used for supra-annular mitral valve replacement (Fig. 24–3). Posteriorly the sutures are placed as close as possible to the inferior right and left pulmonary veins, between the veins and the true annulus, without compromising these veins. Anteriorly sutures are passed through the atrial septum with the pledgets lying on the right atrial aspect of the septum. If an atrioventricular canal repair has been performed previously, sutures are passed through the pericardial patch. The valve lies above the level of the coronary sinus, which should decrease the risk of complete heart block. The valve should be carefully checked for complete freedom of movement of the disk and if necessary (and if the valve design allows), the valve is rotated to a point where the greatest clearance from adjacent tissue is achieved. It is usually necessary to close the atrial septum with a patch of pericardium or polytetrafluoroethylene (PTFE). Before completion of the suture line on the atrial septal patch, the left heart is filled with saline, and air is vented through the cardioplegic infusion site in the ascending aorta.

Conduits From the Left Atrium to the Left Ventricle

One other option that has been reported for the difficult situation of congenital mitral stenosis in which hypoplasia of both the valve annulus and the left atrium does not permit an orthotopic valve replacement is the placement of a conduit from the left atrium to the left ventricle. In 1980 Laks and coworkers[19] described placement of a 12-mm porcine-valved Dacron conduit from the left atrium to the apex of the left ventricle in an 8-week-old male. Although the child was discharged from the hospital, he died 8 months postoperatively. Corno and associates[6] described a similar operation in a 3-year-old. We have successfully performed the same procedure in an 11-month-old child with mitral stenosis and a hypoplastic left ventricle. Interestingly, an

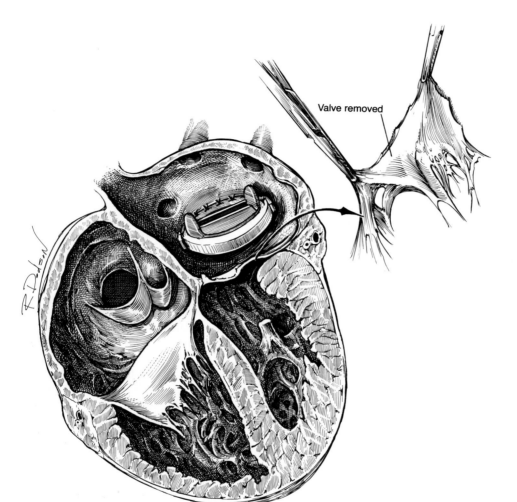

Valve removed

FIGURE 24–3. ☐

The technique for supra-annular MVR involves positioning the prosthesis entirely within the left atrium and immediately apical relative to the inferior pulmonary veins.

allograft aortic conduit was used. Postoperatively the child remained ventilator dependent and, at catheterization, was found to have what was essentially a ventricular aneurysm because of systolic dilatation of the allograft. The child was returned to the operating room, where the allograft was wrapped with Dacron. Subsequently the child was weaned from the ventilator and continues to do well after 4 years of follow-up. Nevertheless, in view of the well-recognized long-term problems with conduits, as well as the disadvantage of an apical left ventricular incision, this option should rarely, if ever, be used. Supra-annular valve replacement should be applicable in almost all cases in which this procedure might otherwise be contemplated.

RESULTS OF MITRAL VALVE REPLACEMENT IN INFANTS

Early Mortality

Nine of the 25 infants receiving mitral valve prostheses between 1973 and 1987 at Children's Hospital in Boston died within 30 days of surgery; seven had atrioventricular canal defects, one had Marfan's syndrome, and one had congenital mitral regurgitation. There were no deaths in the group with mitral stenosis. Six of the nine early deaths occurred among the 13 patients who underwent emergency surgery. In the six patients who received tissue valves, there were five deaths. There were no deaths in the seven patients operated on between 1983 and 1987 (Fig. 24–4).

Causes of Early Death. Obstruction of the left ventricular outflow tract was the cause of death in four patients who had received high-profile bioprosthetic dura mater valves. Other causes were *Candida* sepsis in one, pulmonary hypertension in one, and low cardiac output in two. In one infant, death was sudden and unexplained.

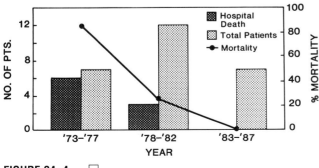

FIGURE 24–4. ☐

Hospital deaths at Children's Hospital, Boston, after MVR during infancy according to year of operation.

Postoperative Course and Complications

Three of the four patients with supra-annular mitral valve replacement had uneventful postoperative courses. One patient had temporary persistence of elevated pulmonary vascular resistance, despite absence of a significant transprosthetic gradient proved at catheterization. Pulmonary resistance was less than one third of systemic resistance within 2 weeks of surgery.

Of the 25 patients, permanent complete heart block occurred in four (16%), all of whom subsequently died. In one patient, a mild paravalvar leak developed, and three patients had important septic complications.

Anticoagulation. All surviving patients except one who received a tissue valve were placed on a regimen of sodium warfarin (Coumadin), with the aim of maintaining prothrombin time between 1.5 and 2.0 times the control value. There were no serious bleeding complications and no confirmed major episodes of thromboembolism. One patient, who was found to have a prolonged prothrombin time on routine testing, was given cryoprecipitate, which caused valve thrombosis. This was successfully managed by replacement of the prosthesis.

Follow-up. The 16 survivors were followed for a mean of 49 months. Two patients were lost to follow-up at 24 and 35 months. There were five late deaths, four of which occurred in patients 2 months to 2 years after atrioventricular canal repair. Three of these four deaths occurred during infectious illnesses. The fifth patient died at elective replacement of the prosthesis from sudden electromechanical dissociation.

The actuarial survival rates for all patients at 1 and 5 years after surgery were 52% and 43%, respectively. Actuarial survival rates for survivors of the original surgery for mitral valve replacement were 81% and 68%, respectively.

Repeated Mitral Valve Replacement. Of the 16 survivors, nine required another mitral valve replacement 5 to 69 months (mean, 30 months) after the original mitral valve replacement, giving an actuarial rate of freedom from repeated mitral valve replacement at 3 years of 45% (Fig. 24–5).

Indications for a second mitral valve replacement were acute pulmonary edema (two patients) and congestive heart failure (seven patients). One of the acute pulmonary edema patients (described previously) had acute circulatory collapse resulting from a thrombosed prosthesis after transfusion of cryoprecipitate. The other patient with pulmonary edema, who was symptomatic for several days before the second mitral valve replacement, was found to have extensive pannus ingrowth over the sewing

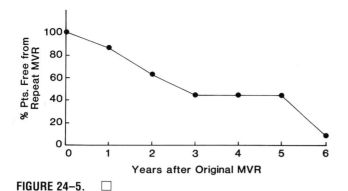

FIGURE 24–5. ☐

Acturial freedom from repeat MVR in 16 hospital survivors of MVR in infancy.

ring of the prosthesis. In the seven patients with congestive heart failure, symptoms developed gradually, and at the second valve replacement, all had exuberant pannus over the left atrial aspect of the prosthesis. However, disk motion was not impaired.

Mean body weight of the patients doubled from 5.5 ± 1.1 kg at the original mitral valve replacement to 11.0 ± 4.0 kg at the time of the second mitral valve replacement. Two patients underwent replacement of a 17-mm Bjork-Shiley valve with another 17-mm Bjork-Shiley valve, whereas the patient with a 16-mm dura mater valve received a 17-mm Bjork-Shiley valve. In five patients a valve two sizes larger, and in one patient a valve three sizes larger, than the original prosthesis was inserted (Fig. 24–6).

Three of the four patients with supra-annular mitral valve replacement required another mitral valve replacement 5 months, 11 months, and 6 years, respectively, after the initial valve replacement. In one patient the new valve was repositioned

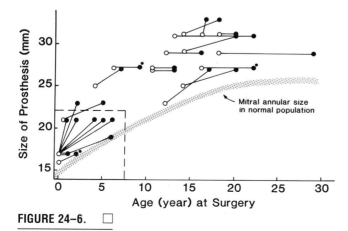

FIGURE 24–6. ☐

Increment in valve size achieved at repeat MVR in 37 children, including 10 patients who were 1 year old or younger (within dashed rectangle signifying the infant group) at the time of initial MVR. Asterisks indicate operative deaths at repeat MVR.

supra-annularly, while in the other two patients the annuli had widened sufficiently to accept a 17-mm Bjork-Shiley valve and a 21-mm St. Jude Medical valve. The fourth patient with a supra-annular mitral valve replacement was doing well at follow-up 14 months after the operation. An additional patient with a 17-mm Bjork-Shiley valve placed twice in the annular position had a 19-mm St. Jude Medical valve placed supra-annularly at a third operation.

One patient who had an atrioventricular canal defect repaired and a 16-mm dura mater valve inserted died at the second mitral valve replacement because of *Salmonella* sepsis. In one other patient, complete heart block developed at the second mitral valve replacement, and a permanent pacemaker was implanted.

SUMMARY

Although further refinement of valvuloplasty methods should continue to decrease the need for valve replacement, there will continue to be a small need for infant valve replacement, particularly in the mitral position, for severe congenital deformity. Supra-annular positioning of synthetic prostheses appears to be associated with satisfactory intermediate-term results. The risks of anticoagulants appear to be small in this population. Continuing refinement of small prostheses for the pediatric population should be encouraged. Allograft and autograft valves appear to be the valves of choice for truncal and aortic valve replacement.

REFERENCES

1. Attie F, Lopez-Soriano F, Ovseyvitz J, et al. Late results of mitral valve replacement with the Bjork-Shiley prosthesis in children under 16 years of age. J Thorac Cardiovasc Surg 91:754, 1986.
2. Barratt-Boyes BG. Homograft aortic valve replacement in aortic incompetence and stenosis. Thorax 19:131, 1965.
3. Barratt-Boyes BG, Roche AHG, Subramanyan R, et al. Long-term follow-up on patients with the antibiotic-sterilized aortic homograft valve inserted freehand in the aortic position. Circulation 75:768, 1987.
4. Castaneda AR, Anderson RC, Edwards JE. Congenital mitral stenosis resulting from anomalous arcade and obstructing papillary muscles: Report of correction by use of ball valve prosthesis. Am J Cardiol 24:237, 1969.
5. Castaneda AR, Nicoloff DM, Moller JH, et al. Surgical correction of complete atrioventricular canal utilizing ball-valve replacement of the mitral valve. J Thorac Cardiovasc Surg 62:926, 1971.
6. Corno A, Giannico S, Leibovich S, et al. The hypoplastic mitral valve. J Thorac Cardiovasc Surg 91:848, 1986.
7. Emery RW, Nicoloff DM. St. Jude Medical cardiac valve prosthesis. J Thorac Cardiovasc Surg 78:269, 1979.
8. Geha AS, Laks H, Stansel HC, et al. Late failure of porcine

valve heterografts in children. J Thorac Cardiovasc Surg 78:351, 1979.

9. Gerosa G, McKay R, Ross DN. Replacement of the aortic valve or root with a pulmonary autograft in children. Ann Thorac Surg 51:424, 1991.

10. Gianelly RE, Angell WW, Stinson E, et al. Homograft replacement of the mitral valve. Circulation 38:664, 1968.

11. Hanley FL, Heinemann MK, Jonas RA, et al. Neonatal repair of truncus arteriosus. J Thorac Cardiovasc Surg 55:1049, 1993.

12. Harpole DH, Rankin JS, Wolfe WG, et al. Effects of standard mitral valve replacement on left ventricular function. Ann Thorac Surg 49:866, 1990.

13. Hennein HA, Swain JA, McIntosh CL, et al. Comparative assessment of chordal preservation versus chordal resection during mitral valve replacement. J Thorac Cardiovasc Surg 99:828, 1990.

14. Iyer KS, Reddy S, Rao M, et al. Valve replacement in children under twenty years of age: Experience with the Bjork-Shiley prosthesis. J Thorac Cardiovasc Surg 88:217, 1984.

15. Kadoba K, Armiger L, Sawatari K, et al. The influence of time from donor death to graft harvest on conduit function of cryopreserved aortic allografts in lambs. Circulation 84(suppl III):100, 1991.

16. Kadoba K, Armiger LC, Sawatari K, et al. Mechanical durability of pulmonary allograft conduits at systemic pressure. J Thorac Cardiovasc Surg 105:132, 1993.

17. Kadoba K, Jonas RA. Replacement of the left atrioventricular valve after repair of atrioventricular septal defect. Cardiol Young 1:383, 1991.

18. Kadoba K, Jonas RA, Mayer JE, et al. Mitral valve replacement in the first year of life. J Thorac Cardiovasc Surg 100:762, 1990.

19. Laks H, Hellenbrand WE, Kleinman C, et al. Left atrial–left ventricular conduit for relief of congenital mitral stenosis in infancy. J Thorac Cardiovasc Surg 80:782, 1980.

20. Levy RJ, Schoen FJ, Levy JT, et al. Biologic determinants of dystrophic calcification and osteocalcin deposition in glutaraldehyde-preserved porcine aortic valve leaflets implanted subcutaneously in rats. Am J Pathol 113:143, 1983.

21. Levy RJ, Wolfrum J, Schoen FJ, et al. Inhibition of calcification of bioprosthetic heart valves by local controlled-release diphosphonate. Science 12:190, 1985.

22. Lillehei CW, Levy MJ, Bonnabeau RC. Mitral valve replacement with preservation of papillary muscles and chordae tendineae. J Thorac Cardiovasc Surg 47:532, 1964.

23. McKowen RL, Campbell DN, Woelfel F, et al. Extended aortic root replacement with aortic allografts. J Thorac Cardiovasc Surg 93:366, 1987.

24. O'Brien MF, Stafford EG, Gardner MAH, et al. A comparison of aortic valve replacement with viable cryopreserved and fresh allograft valves, with a note on chromosomal studies. J Thorac Cardiovasc Surg 94:812, 1987.

25. Rhodes LA, Colan SD, Perry SB, et al. Predictors of survival in neonates with critical aortic stenosis. Circulation 84:2325, 1991.

26. Ross DN. Homograft replacement of the aortic valve. Lancet 2:487, 1962.

27. Ross DN. Replacement of aortic and mitral valves with a pulmonary autograft. Lancet 2:956, 1967.

28. Sanders SP, Levy RJ, Freed MD, et al. Use of Hancock porcine xenografts in children and adolescents. Am J Cardiol 46:429, 1980.

29. Schoen FJ, Levy RJ. Bioprosthetic heart valve failure: Pathology and pathogenesis. Cardiol Clin 2:717, 1984.

30. Sievers HH, Lange PE, Yankah AC, et al. Allogeneous transplantation of the mitral valve. An open question. Thorac Cardiovasc Surg 33:227, 1985.

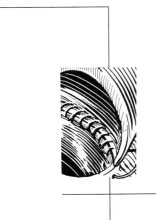

25

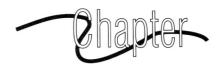

Vascular Rings, Slings, and Tracheal Anomalies

A study of the development of the mediastinal great vessels, including the aortic arch and descending thoracic aorta, is a fascinating exercise in embryology.[5, 21] The multiple paired branchial arches and paired dorsal aortae generally (but not always) fuse and resorb in a predictable sequence to result in the usual left aortic arch and left descending aorta. Failure of resorption will result in any one of a number of vascular rings or a pulmonary artery sling, which, from a cardiovascular point of view, are generally quite benign. However, their tendency to constrict the trachea, the esophagus, or both, may result in important obstructive symptoms, thereby necessitating divison of the ring or relocation of the sling.

VASCULAR RINGS

PATHOLOGIC ANANTOMY

Embryology

The paired (right and left) dorsal aortae are present in the embryo by approximately the 21st day of intrauterine life (Fig. 25–1). Subsequently, the first to sixth branchial arches form, each with its own aortic arch, and communicate with the aortic sac. The first and second arches contribute to minor facial arteries, while the third arches form the carotid arteries. The left fourth arch forms the distal aortic arch and aortic isthmus from the origin of the left common carotid artery to the origin of the descending thoracic aorta, which itself represents a persistence of the left dorsal aorta. Proximally, septation of the conotruncus produces the ascending aorta, which joins with the fourth left arch. The right dorsal aorta ultimately contributes to the right subclavian artery but otherwise resorbs.[22]

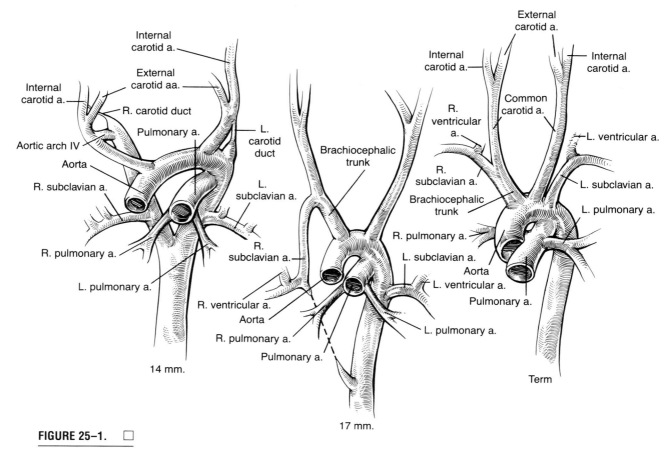

FIGURE 25–1. ☐

The formation of the normal aorta is a process of fusion and segmental resorption of the paired first to sixth branchial arches with the paired dorsal aortae.

Dominant Right Aortic Arch

By far the majority of vascular rings consist of a dominant right arch. The surgical relevance of this fact, as will be discussed later, is that almost all vascular rings are most conveniently approached through a left thoracotomy.

Double Aortic Arch. As the name implies, this anomaly consists of two aortic arches, an anterior and leftward arch and a posterior and rightward arch (Fig. 25–2). Generally the descending aorta is left sided although it may be right sided or in the midline. The right arch is generally dominant and gives rise to the right common carotid and right subclavian arteries either as an innominate artery or as two separate vessels. The left arch gives rise to the left common carotid and left subclavian arteries. It may be hypoplastic or atretic beyond the origin of either the left common carotid or left subclavian artery, being little more than a fibrous cord. In the latter case, the fibrous cord joins the descending aorta, where it emerges from behind the esophagus to become the left descending aorta near the insertion of the ligamentum arteriosum. This anom-

aly represents persistence of the right dorsal aorta. Note that the right recurrent laryngeal nerve must pass around the right aortic arch, rather than being in its usual location around the right subclavian artery.

Right Aortic Arch, Aberrant Left Subclavian Artery, and Left Ligamentum. There is a right aortic arch that gives off, in sequence, the left common carotid, the right common carotid, the right subclavian, and the left subclavian arteries. The left subclavian passes behind the esophagus and then gives rise to the ligamentum arteriosum, which passes anteriorly to connect to the left pulmonary artery, thereby completing the vascular ring. This anomaly represents persistence of the right fourth aortic arch with resorption of the left fourth aortic arch.

Right Aortic Arch, Mirror-Image Branching, and Retroesophageal Ligamentum. There is a right aortic arch that gives off, in sequence, the left innominate artery (left common carotid with left subclavian), the right common carotid, and the right subclavian artery. The final branch, often arising from a prominent ductus diverticulum, is a ligamen-

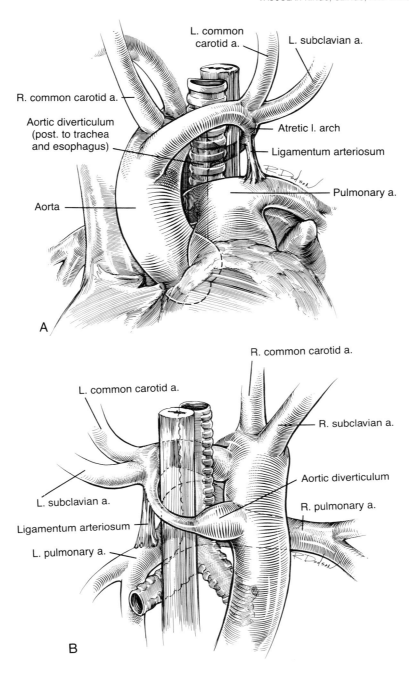

FIGURE 25–2. □

The most common double aortic arch consists of a dominant right posterior aortic arch with a hypoplastic or atretic left anterior arch. The ligamentum arteriosum contributes to secondary tracheoesophageal compression and should be divided along with the left anterior arch. *A*, anterior view; *B*, posterior view.

tum that passes leftward, behind the esophagus, and then anteriorly to attach to the left pulmonary artery. This anomaly also represents persistence of the fourth right aortic arch with resorption of the fourth left aortic arch. A short segment of the distal end of the left fourth arch persists as an aortic diverticulum, which gives rise to the ligamentum.

Note that the aortic diverticulum has been reported as the site of origin of aortic dissection. Also note that when there is mirror image branching, if the ligamentum arteriosum arises from the innominate artery to pass to the origin of the left pulmonary artery, this does not result in a vascular ring (Fig. 25–3).

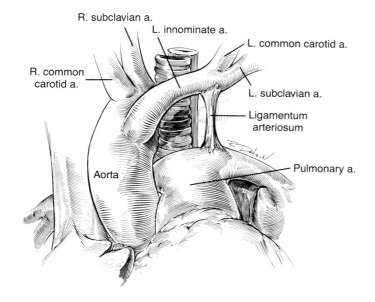

FIGURE 25–3. ☐

When there is a right aortic arch with mirror image branching and the ligamentum arteriosum arises from the innominate or left subclavian artery, no vascular ring is formed.

Dominant Left Aortic Arch

A dominant left aortic arch is extremely rare but should be recognized, because the best approach for surgical division is through a right thoracotomy.[15]

Left Aortic Arch, Mirror-Image Branching, Right Descending Aorta, and Atretic Right Aortic Arch. With this rare form of vascular ring (Fig. 25–4), the arch vessels arise normally from the normal-size left aortic arch. The right arch is atretic.

Left Aortic Arch, Right Descending Aorta, and Right-Sided Ligamentum Arteriosum to Right Pulmonary Artery. The reported branching sequence from the left aortic arch is the right common carotid, left common carotid, left subclavian, and, finally, right subclavian as a fourth branch from the proximal descending aorta (Fig. 25–5).

PATHOPHYSIOLOGY

Vascular rings, in contrast to a pulmonary artery sling, encircle both the esophagus and trachea and, therefore, may result in obstructive symptoms of both. Nevertheless, the mere presence of a ring does not guarantee that there will be compression; indeed, rings may remain asymptomatic for life and not require any intervention.

If compression is severe, the child is seen in the neonatal period with stridor or even respiratory distress, although the latter is rare. In the first months of life feeding may be slow. As the child progresses to solids, there is increasing difficulty with feeding. Reflux and respiratory infections are common. Vas-

cular obstruction of both aortic arches must be exceedingly rare.[20] At Children's Hospital in Boston, we have managed one such child in whom coarctations were present in each of her two aortic arches; this was in a setting of Shone's syndrome.

PREOPERATIVE EVALUATION AND MEDICAL MANAGEMENT

Preoperative Studies

Many studies are available for assessing the child with a vascular ring. Careful consideration should be given to the cost effectiveness of various studies before embarking on multiple imaging tests.

Barium Swallow. A simple barium swallow, combined with an echocardiogram to exclude intracardiac anomalies, should suffice for most children suspected of having a vascular ring. Unlike the pulmonary artery sling, which produces an anterior indentation of the esophagus, vascular rings invariably produce a posterior indentation. An experienced radiologist can usually distinguish a double arch from the retroesophageal subclavian or ligament, based on the angulation of the esophageal impression.[17]

Echocardiography. The aortic arch is usually invested by thymus in the neonate and young infant, so in this age group it is generally possible to accurately determine the anatomy of a vascular ring, particularly when imaging is combined with color flow Doppler. Although there is acoustic shadowing as a result of air in the trachea, transesophageal echocardiography allows accurate imaging in

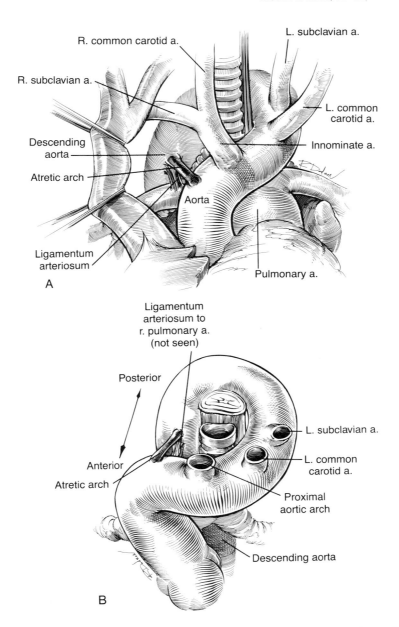

FIGURE 25–4. □

In the rare case in which the left aortic arch is dominant and the right arch is atretic as part of a vascular ring, the surgical approach should be via a right thoracotomy. *A*, anterior view; *B*, view from above.

this area when it is combined with transthoracic imaging. Echocardiography alone will not be able to reveal the presence of an atretic segment of aortic arch, but the general contours of the arch and branches in the context of an esophageal impression after a barium swallow will almost always allow accurate diagnosis.

Computed Tomography, Magnetic Resonance Imaging, and Digital Subtraction Angiography. These expensive studies are rarely necessary. In addition, computed tomography (CT) scanning and digital subtraction angiography (DSA) involve exposure to radiation and the risk of intravenous contrast dye. The authors have found CT scanning and magnetic resonance imaging (MRI) to be particularly useful when assessing the site and severity (particularly the length) of congenital tracheal stenoses in the planning of tracheal resection and reconstructive procedures,[10, 12] but this is almost never necessary for first-time management of a vascular ring.

Bronchoscopy. The same comments made for the CT scan and MRI also apply to bronchoscopy: it is expensive, involves additional risks, and although

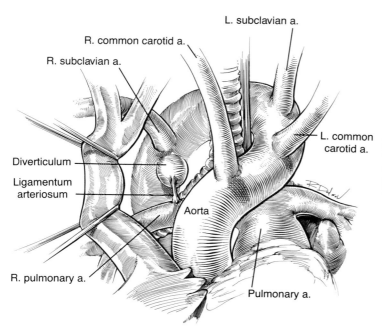

R. common carotid a.

R. subclavian a.

L. subclavian a.

L. common carotid a.

Diverticulum

Ligamentum arteriosum

Aorta

R. pulmonary a.

Pulmonary a.

FIGURE 25–5. ☐

A right thoracotomy is necessary for correction of the rare case of a dominant left arch with a right descending aorta and a right-sided ligamentum arteriosum passing to the right pulmonary artery.

it is not useful for a simple vascular ring, it is an essential part of the workup for congenital tracheal stenosis.

Aortography. Expensive, invasive, and carrying additional risk for the patient, aortography is rarely justified for the diagnosis of a vascular ring. In addition, if there is an atretic segment, such a study may not be diagnostic.

Medical Management

The general philosophy at present is that if either respiratory or dysphagic symptoms are present, surgical division of the ring is indicated. If the child is asymptomatic, surgery may be deferred. Preoperatively the child should be given maximal nutritional support as well as general respiratory care, including chest physiotherapy and appropriate treatment of respiratory infection. Surgery should not be unduly delayed because of the presence of a respiratory infection, as division of the ring, which allows more adequate clearing of respiratory secretions, is the most effective treatment of infection.

SURGICAL MANAGEMENT

History

The surgical management of double aortic arch was pioneered by Gross at Children's Hospital in Boston in 1945,[9] the same year that he undertook

the first surgical procedure in the United States for coarctation and 7 years after his first operation for patent ductus arteriosus. Gross and Ware subsequently described surgical management of the various other forms of vascular ring.[8] The diagnosis of vascular ring by careful interpretation of the plain chest radiograph and barium swallow was described at about the same time by Neuhauser, also at Children's Hospital in Boston.[17]

Indications for Surgery

The presence of symptoms is an indication for surgery. Symptoms may include stridor, wheezing, frequent respiratory infections, dysphagia, reflux, and failure to thrive. Very mild symptoms appearing for the first time in the older infant may improve with time as the child grows, in which case it may be possible to defer surgery.[7] Nevertheless, because the risks of surgery are extremely small, it is rare that a symptomatic child should not undergo surgery.

Technique of Surgery

Preoperative studies must not only establish the presence of a vascular ring, but also confirm that the optimal approach will be through a left thoracotomy, which will be true in more than 95% of cases. If a double aortic arch is present, it is important to be aware preoperatively which of the arches is dominant.[15] In the majority of cases, it will be the right aortic arch. Nevertheless, in cases of a double arch it is useful to place pulse oximeter probes on both hands and one foot so that temporary occlusion of the arch branches will allow confirmation of the anatomy. Furthermore, blood pressure cuffs placed on one leg and both arms will confirm the absence of a pressure gradient when the intended point of division of the double arch is temporarily occluded. Because the point of division will be the narrowest segment of the ring, there should be no pressure gradient with occlusion.

The child is placed in a full right lateral decubitus position, and a left posterolateral thoracotomy is performed. The chest is entered through the fourth intercostal space, and the left lung is retracted anteriorly. Palpation in the area of the ring will reveal a taut, ligamentous structure in the case of a ring with an atretic left arch. If a double arch is present, it is generally visible to some degree through the mediastinal pleura. The vagus nerve, giving off the left recurrent laryngeal nerve (which then passes around the ligamentum arteriosum), is a useful landmark. The mediastinal pleura is reflected in the area of the left arch and ligamentum. Test occlusions of the arch vessels may be performed at this time to confirm the anatomy. The segment to be divided, if patent, should be controlled with clamps. After division the vessel ends are oversewn with a continuous Prolene suture. If the segment to be divided is clearly atretic, it suffices to doubly ligate the cord and divide it. After division the ends generally retract briskly, indicating the tension with which the ring has been surrounding the esophagus and trachea. In all cases the ligamentum arteriosum should also be divided. There may be additional fibrous strands passing across the esophagus, and these should be divided. Final palpation in the area should reveal complete relief of the taut band that was present previously. The mediastinal pleura is approximated, a single chest tube is placed, and the thoracotomy is closed in a routine fashion, using absorbable pericostal suture together with absorbable suture to the muscle layers, with subcutaneous and subcuticular absorbable suture completing wound closure.

In the rare case requiring approach through a right thoracotomy, the same principles are applied. The right recurrent laryngeal nerve will pass around the right-sided ligamentum arteriosum and should be carefully visualized and preserved.

In 1993, Dr. Burke started to use video-assisted thoracoscopic management of vascular rings at Children's Hospital, Boston. This will most likely soon become the routine approach to the vascular ring.

POSTOPERATIVE MANAGEMENT

In the young infant with severe respiratory symptoms, there is likely to be an element of tracheomalacia associated with the long-standing compression by the ring during in utero development. Therefore, it should be anticipated that all respiratory symptoms will not be immediately relieved; in fact it may be several months before the child is free of stridor. However, there should be complete and immediate relief of any difficulty with feeding.

RESULTS OF SURGERY

In the absence of intracardiac or other extracardiac anomalies, surgery for vascular ring carries essentially no risk of mortality.

PULMONARY ARTERY SLING

PATHOLOGIC ANATOMY

The left pulmonary artery arises from the right pulmonary artery and passes leftward between the trachea and esophagus (Fig. 25–6). The ligamentum arteriosum passes posteriorly to the aorta from the point of origin of the right pulmonary artery from the main pulmonary artery, effectively creating a vascular ring surrounding the trachea but not the esophagus.

Associated Tracheal Anomalies

Approximately 50% of patients with a pulmonary artery sling have complete tracheal rings—that is, the posterior membranous component of the trachea is absent, and the tracheal cartilages, rather than being U shaped, are O shaped.[3, 24] The presence of complete rings does not imply that important stenosis necessarily will be present, although the trachea is often narrower than normal. The complete rings may be localized to the region where the sling

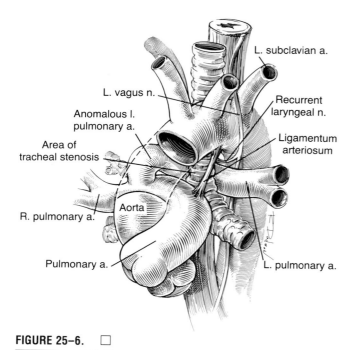

FIGURE 25–6. ☐

Anatomy of a pulmonary artery sling. The left pulmonary artery (often hypoplastic) arises from the distal right pulmonary artery and passes leftward between the trachea and esophagus. The ligamentum arteriosum arises from the junction of the main pulmonary artery and the right pulmonary artery and passes posteriorly to the undersurface of the aortic arch, thereby contributing to what is effectively a vascular ring.

passes around the trachea, although often they extend for the entire length of the trachea.

In the area where the sling passes around the trachea, there is likely to be tracheal compression resulting in important functional stenosis, even if there is not an underlying anatomic stenosis. At Children's Hospital in Boston, we recently managed a child with a pulmonary artery sling in which the sling passed around the trachea *above* a very high "pig bronchus" (bronchus suis is an association of pulmonary artery sling). Interestingly, there was a tight, localized stenosis consisting of complete rings *below* the pig bronchus and extending to the carina, although the sling lay entirely above this area.

The left pulmonary artery is often relatively hypoplastic and considerably smaller than the right pulmonary artery, which appears larger than normal—virtually a direct extension of the main pulmonary artery. The small size of the left pulmonary artery may help to explain the high incidence of anastomotic problems that have been observed in the past with attempts to reimplant it.[4, 19]

PATHOPHYSIOLOGY

Respiratory symptoms predominate because of the direct tracheal compression, with or without

congenital tracheal stenosis, and are essentially the same respiratory symptoms as those described for vascular rings. Symptoms of esophageal compression are rarely present.

PREOPERATIVE EVALUATION AND MEDICAL MANAGEMENT

Definition of the vascular anatomy may be made in the same fashion as described for vascular rings. However, unlike vascular rings, which produce a posterior indentation of the esophagus evident on barium swallow, pulmonary artery slings produce an anterior esophageal indentation, which can also be demonstrated on barium swallow. Echocardiography can usually confirm the vascular anatomy.

Assessment of the Trachea

Because of the high incidence of tracheal anomalies other than simple compression by the sling, it is important to undertake a complete assessment of the trachea. This should include bronchoscopy (recorded on videotape) and at least one other mode of imaging to delineate the severity and extent of tracheal stenosis. We generally prefer CT scan assessment of the trachea, although the role of MRI is currently being defined. The CT scan allows accurate quantitation of the tracheal luminal diameter and area at various levels and demonstrates the presence of complete rings, which will also have been noted at bronchoscopy. Bronchography can produce spectacular imaging of tracheal stenoses but is generally reserved for children who are also undergoing angiography for definition of vascular anatomy, if this is not clear from echocardiography alone, or for definition of associated cardiac problems.

Medical Management

General supportive respiratory care should be given before proceeding to surgery. As described for vascular rings, respiratory infection may be difficult to clear completely before surgery because of the difficulty in adequately clearing secretions.

SURGICAL MANAGEMENT

History

In 1954 Potts and associates[18] described the approach to a pulmonary artery sling using a left thoracotomy with division of the left pulmonary artery, followed by translocation anterior to the trachea and reimplantation. Potts performed reimplantation at the original site of origin of the left pulmonary artery, but Hiller and Maclean, in 1957,[11] using the same operation, performed reimplantation into the side of the main pulmonary artery. In this early report of what was to become the traditional operation for pulmonary artery sling, these authors also reported for the first time the complication that was to be commonly seen: namely, occlusion of the left pulmonary artery demonstrated by postoperative angiography. In 1956 Wittenborg and coworkers[23] at Children's Hospital in Boston described the diagnosis of pulmonary artery sling by the appearance of an anterior indentation of the esophagus on the radiograph after a barium swallow.

Mustard and colleagues recognized the importance of the ligamentum arteriosum in effectively completing a vascular ring as part of this anomaly, and in 1962[16] they described simple division of the ligament as management of a pulmonary artery sling. This operation has not been widely practiced.

Repair of a pulmonary artery sling through a median sternotomy with reimplantation of the left pulmonary artery (i.e., while the patient is on cardiopulmonary bypass) was described in 1985 by Kirklin and Barratt-Boyes.[14] None of the techniques described up to that time had dealt directly with the associated tracheal stenosis that was often present. These operations were based on the premise that the problem was primarily one of tracheal compression; although this was true in some cases, it was certainly not universally true. Although primary repair of the tracheal anomaly had been suggested previously, it had not been attempted because of

fear of early and late tracheal anastomotic problems in the infant. Improved cardiopulmonary bypass techniques (which allowed cumbersome airway intubation techniques to be avoided); improved sutures, such as absorbable monofilament polydioxanone; and greater familiarity with microvascular techniques have decreased the risk of tracheal anastomosis in the infant. We initially reported the successful application of cardiopulmonary bypass, tracheal resection, and anastomosis in a 2.6-kg neonate with very severe congenital tracheal stenosis[2] and have subsequently undertaken similar tracheal resections for a wide variety of tracheal problems in 15 infants since the late 1980s.[10, 12] Success with this technique led us, in 1989, to apply tracheal resection as an integral part of the repair of pulmonary artery sling when the sling is associated with important localized tracheal stenosis.[13]

Indications for Surgery

Because pulmonary artery sling is a rare entity, its natural history remains poorly defined. Therefore, surgery currently is reserved for children who have respiratory symptoms referable to the sling. Preoperative studies must indicate whether there is simple compression stenosis of the carinal region, which may be relieved by translocation of the left pulmonary artery; localized anatomic stenosis of the trachea (generally associated with complete tracheal rings in this area), which is best dealt with by tracheal resection and anterior translocation of the left pulmonary artery; or, finally, diffuse severe narrowing of the trachea related to complete tracheal rings, which may necessitate an extensive tracheoplasty procedure in addition to relocation of the left pulmonary artery.[1]

Technical Considerations

Division and Reimplantation of the Left Pulmonary Artery. Although the traditional approach has been through a left thoracotomy, we currently prefer to undertake a median sternotomy and use cardiopulmonary bypass (Fig. 25–7). If cardiopulmonary bypass should be avoided, then the traditional approach is used. When using the left thoracotomy approach, it is important to dissect as much length as possible of the proximal left pulmonary artery so as to minimize tension on the anastomosis. A side-biting clamp is applied to the side of the main pulmonary artery at a site that will minimize tension and distortion of the anastomosis. Because the left pulmonary artery has previously been located

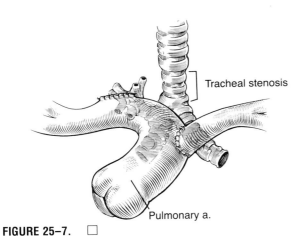

FIGURE 25–7. □

Traditional management of a pulmonary artery sling has consisted of division of the left pulmonary artery and reanastomosis of the left pulmonary artery to the side of the main pulmonary artery in front of the trachea. However, this technique does not deal with associated tracheal stenosis.

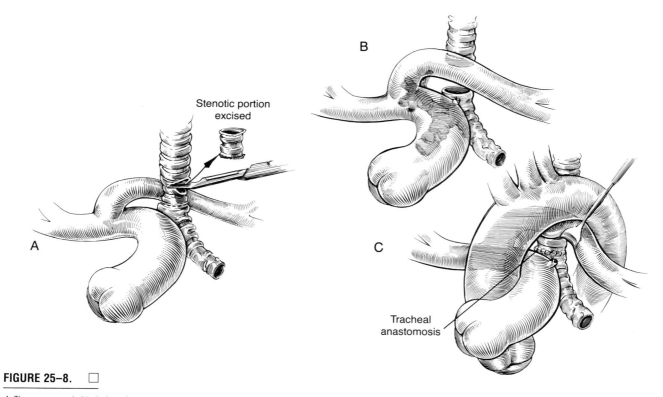

Stenotic portion
excised

FIGURE 25–8. ☐

A, The recommended technique for surgical management of a pulmonary artery sling associated with localized tracheal stenosis involves tracheal resection on cardiopulmonary bypass. *B*, The left pulmonary artery is translocated anteriorly following tracheal resection. *C*, A direct tracheal anastomosis is fashioned using continuous polydioxanone suture.

Tracheal
anastomosis

posterior to hilar structures and at this point must be brought anterior to the bronchus, there is a tendency for the anastomosis to be under quite a bit of tension, no doubt explaining the high rate of occlusion described in a number of series.[4]

The approach through a median sternotomy has the advantage of allowing complete mobilization of the main and right pulmonary arteries as well as of the left pulmonary artery, thereby decreasing tension on the anastomosis. Furthermore, a side-biting clamp does not have to be applied for the anastomosis, because cardiopulmonary bypass is employed. The left pulmonary artery can be carefully and completely mobilized where it passes around the trachea, allowing maximal length for reimplantation. Care must be taken when dissecting posterior to the trachea, particularly when complete rings are not present, as there may be an intimate association between the left pulmonary artery and the membranous component of the trachea. When complete tracheal rings are present, the dissection is easier, and it is likely that this segment of trachea will be excised. The anastomosis is constructed with continuous 6–0 or 7–0 polydioxanone or Prolene sutures. Cardiopulmonary bypass should be undertaken with an ascending aortic arterial cannula and

a single straight venous cannula in the right atrium. A nearly full-flow perfusion rate is used, with the heart beating throughout the procedure at a systemic temperature of 32°C to 34°C.

Tracheal Resection and Anastomosis With Relocation of the Left Pulmonary Artery. The approach[13] is exactly as described for reimplantation of the left pulmonary artery through a median sternotomy, including the use of cardiopulmonary bypass with a single venous cannula and with the heart beating at a systemic temperature of 32°C to 34°C (Fig. 25–8). The aorta is retracted to the left. The main pulmonary artery is traced to the origin of the left pulmonary artery, which is then dissected free where it passes behind the trachea. The stenotic segment of trachea, as defined by preoperative studies, is dissected free. The trachea is divided transversely through the center of the stenotic segment. The left pulmonary artery is brought forward between the two ends of the divided trachea. Serial sections are taken of the two ends of the trachea until a satisfactory luminal area is found; this is usually no farther than three to four tracheal rings. This amount of resection allows anastomosis with little tension. (In a case of congenital tracheal stenosis, we resected almost 50% of the trachea, which necessitated anastomosis under considerable tension; nevertheless, satisfactory healing was observed.) In fact, it is important not to compromise the amount of resection, thereby leaving important residual stenosis because of concern regarding reanastomosis. The tracheal anastomosis is undertaken with a continuous 5–0 or 6–0 polydioxanone suture. (A laboratory study in growing sheep at Children's Hospital in Boston suggested that continuous polydioxanone suture results in a greater luminal area at a tracheal anastomosis than the previously recommended technique using interrupted polyglactin [Vicryl] sutures.)[6] This is a simple anastomosis because of the absence of tubes through the anastomotic area, the absence of clamps, and the strength of the tracheal cartilages. In fact, the presence of complete tracheal rings simplifies the anastomosis because of their strength. If a membranous component is present posteriorly in the trachea, great care must be taken in this area, with the tension being absorbed by suture bites through cartilage. When the anastomosis has been completed, the trachea is pressurized to 40 cm H$_2$O to test for air leaks. The anastomosis is then wrapped with a flap of pedicled autologous pericardium, generally based on the right side of the pericardium, anterior to the right phrenic nerve.

The lie of the left pulmonary artery in its new location should be carefully observed. Because it arises more distally than normal, there is some risk of kinking at its origin. In two of six patients with pulmonary artery sling who underwent tracheal resection, we reimplanted the left pulmonary artery more proximally into the main pulmonary artery. In one case this was related to the fact that the child had absence of the right lung with a marked mediastinal shift to the right.

Very-Long-Segment Tracheal Reconstruction With Reimplantation of the Left Pulmonary Artery. Although we have not encountered this anomaly, others have described stenosis of a very long segment of the trachea, usually related to the presence of complete tracheal rings over the entire length of the trachea, in association with a pulmonary artery sling.[1] It is important to recognize that the presence of complete tracheal rings per se is not an indication for surgical intervention in that area of the trachea. Generally, stenosis of the trachea in a young infant does not become critical until the minimal diameter is between 1.5 and 2 mm. Although there is a direct relationship between the length of the stenotic segment and airway resistance, the relationship to luminal diameter is to the fourth power, so this should be the overriding factor in determining need for surgical intervention. The natural history for most airway problems, such as

tracheomalacia and minimal compression from a vascular ring, is for improvement with age. For all these reasons, these authors have not found it necessary to intervene surgically for very-long-segment tracheal stenosis.

Several surgical methods have been described, including a posteriorly placed longitudinal incision with direct suturing to the anterior wall of the esophagus, as well as an anterior longitudinal incision with placement of a longitudinal rib cartilage graft (as is commonly applied for reconstruction of subglottic stenosis). The largest series has been described by Backer and associates,[1] who used a longitudinal incision placed anteriorly along the full length of the trachea, with the child on cardiopulmonary bypass. An autologous pericardial patch is sutured into this anterior defect. The pulmonary artery sling is managed by division of the origin of the left pulmonary artery, with implantation into the main pulmonary artery. The child is ventilated for at least 2 weeks, with the endotracheal tube functioning as a stent.

RESULTS OF SURGERY

Since the late 1980s six children have undergone surgery at Children's Hospital in Boston for pulmonary artery sling. Tracheal resection and pulmonary artery translocation were employed in five of these electively referred patients. There was one death, in a neonate with absence of the right lung and other extracardiac anomalies.

REFERENCES

1. Backer CL, Idriss FS, Holinger LD, et al. Pulmonary artery sling: Results of surgical repair in infancy. J Thorac Cardiovasc Surg 103:683, 1992.
2. Benca JF, Hickey PR, Dornbusch JN, et al. Ventilatory management assisted by cardiopulmonary bypass for distal tracheal reconstruction in a neonate. Anesthesiology 68:270, 1988.
3. Berdon WE, Baker DH, Wung JT, et al. Complete cartilage ring tracheal stenosis associated with anomalous left pulmonary artery: The ring-sling complex. Radiology 152:47, 1984.
4. Castaneda AR. Pulmonary artery sling. Ann Thorac Surg 28:210, 1979.
5. Edwards JE. Anomalies of the derivatives of the aortic arch syndrome. Med Clin North Am July 32:925, 1948.
6. Freidman E, Perez-Atayde A, Silvera M, et al. Growth of tracheal anastomoses in lambs: Comparison of PDS and Vicryl suture and interrupted and continuous techniques. J Thorac Cardiovasc Surg 100:188, 1990.
7. Godtfredsen J, Wennerold A, Efsen F, et al. Natural history of vascular ring with clinical manifestations. A follow-up study of 11 unoperated cases. Scand J Thorac Cardiovasc Surg 11:75, 1977.
8. Gross RE, Ware PF. The surgical significance of aortic arch anomalies. Surg Gynecol Obstet 83:435, 1946.

9. Gross RE. Surgical relief for tracheal obstruction from a vascular ring. N Engl J Med 233:586, 1945.

10. Healy GB, Schuster SR, Jonas RA, et al. Correction of segmental tracheal stenosis in children. Ann Otol Rhinol Laryngol 97:444, 1988.

11. Hiller HG, Maclean AD. Pulmonary artery ring. Acta Radiol 48:434, 1957.

12. Jonas RA. Invited letter concerning: Tracheal operations in infancy. J Thorac Cardiovasc Surg 100:316, 1990.

13. Jonas RA, Spevak PJ, McGill T, et al. Pulmonary artery sling: Primary repair by tracheal resection in infancy. J Thorac Cardiovasc Surg 97:548, 1989.

14. Kirklin JW, Barratt-Boyes BG. Cardiac Surgery. New York, John Wiley & Sons, 1986.

15. McFaul R, Millard P, Nowicki E. Vascular rings necessitating right thoracotomy. J Thorac Cardiovasc Surg 82:306, 1981.

16. Mustard WT, Trimble AW, Trusler GA. Mediastinal vascular anomalies causing tracheal and esophageal compression and obstruction in childhood. Can Med Assoc J 87:1301, 1962.

17. Neuhauser EBD. The roentgen diagnosis of double aortic arch and other anomalies of the great vessels. AJR 56:1, 1946.

18. Potts WJ, Holinger PH, Rosenblum AH. Anomalous left pulmonary artery causing obstruction to right main bronchus. Report of a case. JAMA 155:1409, 1954.

19. Sade RM, Rosenthal AM, Fellows K, et al. Pulmonary artery sling. J Thorac Cardiovasc Surg 69:333, 1975.

20. Singer ST, Fellows KE, Jonas RA. Double aortic arch with bilateral coarctations. Am J Cardiol 61:196, 1988.

21. Stewart J, Kincaid O, Edwards J. An Atlas of Vascular Rings and Related Malformations of the Aortic Arch System. Springfield, IL, Charles C Thomas, 1964, pp 3–155.

22. Van Mierop LHS. Diseases—congenital anomalies. In Netter FH (ed). The CIBA Collection of Medical Illustrations. Vol 5. New York, Ciba Pharmaceutical, 1969, pp 160–163.

23. Wittenborg MH, Tantiwongse T, Rosenberg BF. Anomalous course of left pulmonary artery with respiratory obstruction. Radiology 67:339, 1956.

24. Wolman IJ. Congenital stenosis of the trachea. Am J Dis Child 61:1263, 1941.

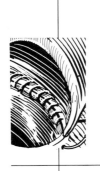

26

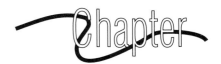

D-Transposition of the Great Arteries

D-Transposition of the great arteries, first described by Baillie in 1797,[6] is a condition in which the atria and the ventricles are concordant, while the ventricular-arterial relationship is discordant. Therefore, the aorta arises anteriorly from the right ventricle, while the pulmonary artery arises posteriorly from the left ventricle. Van Praagh and coworkers[48] introduced the terms *concordant* and *discordant connections* and also *D-transposition of the great arteries* (D-TGA); this nomenclature will be used throughout this chapter. Surgically relevant associated defects, such as ventricular septal defects (VSDs) and anomalies of the left ventricular outflow tract (LVOT), will also be discussed. Forms of transposition with atrioventricular discordance (L-transposition) and forms that include a severely hypoplastic ventricle (which precludes construction of a two-ventricle physiology) will not be discussed in this chapter.

ANATOMY

An earlier hypothesis concerning the faulty embryogenesis of D-TGA attributed the defect to a lack of spiraling of the aortopulmonary septum which caused the aorta to remain anterior and to connect with the right ventricle while the pulmonary artery remained posterior and connected with the left ventricle. Presently a more widely accepted hypothesis proposed by the Van Praaghs[47] suggests that transposition of the great arteries (TGA) results from ab-

normalities in the differential rates of growth of the subpulmonary and subaortic conal musculature. In most cases of D-TGA, there is a well-developed conus underneath the aorta and essentially no conus underneath the pulmonary artery, which leads to aorto-mitral discontinuity and pulmonary-mitral continuity. This is the reverse of the normal situation. Thus, the subaortic conus displaces the developing aorta anteriorly, relating it to the right ventricle. In normally related great arteries, the subpulmonary conus displaces the pulmonary valve anteriorly and to the left, while the aortic valve is displaced posteriorly and to the right.

D-Transposition With an Intact Ventricular Septum

In D-TGA with an intact ventricular septum (IVS) the right ventricle generally has a subaortic conus or infundibulum. In rare instances (less than 5%) there is no subaortic conus; in this case, the aorta tends to be more anterior and to the left with respect to the pulmonary artery. Much less commonly the aorta is posterior to the main pulmonary artery.

The left ventricle almost never has a subpulmonary conus; consequently there is pulmonary-to-mitral fibrous continuity.

Commonly the aorta and the pulmonary artery are of equal size, with the aorta anterior and to the right and the pulmonary artery posterior and to the left. In D-TGA with an IVS the coronaries tend to be of the more common varieties; that is, the left coronary artery arises from the left coronary sinus, giving off the anterior descending and circumflex coronary arteries, and the right coronary artery originates from the right coronary sinus (type 1), or the circumflex coronary artery may arise from the right coronary artery (type 2). Other more complex coronary artery patterns, such as single coronary arteries, inverted coronary arteries, or intramural coronary arteries, can occur but are less common than in D-TGA with a VSD. Also, additional left-sided obstructive lesions, such as coarctation of the aorta or interrupted aortic arch, are less common than they are in D-TGA with a VSD.

D-Transposition With a Ventricular Septal Defect

A hemodynamically significant VSD is present in less than 25% of patients with D-TGA. All the different types of VSDs, as described in Chapter 11, can occur in D-TGA (i.e., paramembranous (with or without malalignment), muscular, subaortic, subarterial, atrioventricular canal type, and multiple).

Semilunar Valves

The aortic and pulmonary valves are morphologically and histologically indistinguishable at birth.[27] However, distinct histologic and microscopic changes, presumably secondary to the differences in pulmonary artery and systemic pressures, occur postnatally in the normal heart, resulting in a thin delicate pulmonary valve with decreased collagen and elastic tissue compared with the normal aortic valve. This difference may become significant whenever surgical techniques are applied that rely on the anatomic pulmonary valve to function as a systemic semilunar (neoaortic) valve. In these settings, regurgitation of the anatomic pulmonary valve becomes the physiologic equivalent of aortic regurgitation.

D-Transposition With Obstruction of the Left Ventricular Outflow Tract

Left ventricular outflow tract obstruction (LVOTO) is present in less than 10% of patients with D-TGA and an IVS. The most common form of LVOTO is the dynamic form, in which the obstruction is caused by leftward displacement of the ventricular septum owing to the fact that right ventric-

ular pressure exceeds left ventricular pressure, although the obstruction is often accentuated by abnormal systolic motion of the anterior mitral leaflet. Organic LVOTO is more common in patients with D-TGA and a VSD. Posterior malalignment of the conal septum may produce long-segment tunnel-like narrowing. Abnormalities of the atrioventricular valves, with excrescences of accessory tissue causing LVOTO, are also more common in D-TGA with a VSD. Multiple areas of obstruction (dynamic and fixed) may coexist in the same patient. Coarctation of the aorta, hypoplasia of the aortic arch, and also interrupted aortic arch, albeit rarer (<5%), are sufficiently common to warrant mention.

In a series of 470 consecutive cases of D-TGA treated surgically at Children's Hospital in Boston, 62 patients had either abnormalities of the LVOT or other left-sided obstructions detected by echocardiography or at catheterization.[53] Nine patients had stenosis of the native pulmonary valve. One of these had a trileaflet pulmonary valve with a severely hypoplastic left anterior cusp. In three the trileaflet valve was nodular and thickened, and in five the pulmonary valve was bicommissural. Seven patients had fixed subpulmonary obstruction (in five this was due to excrescences of endocardial cushion tissue), and in two of these there was a subpulmonary membrane. Two patients with D-TGA and ventricular defects had abnormalities of the mitral valve causing LVOTO. One had a cleft mitral valve with trivial regurgitation and abnormal chordal attachments to the ventricular septum. The other had straddling of the mitral valve with chordae attaching to a papillary muscle group located at the infundibular free wall.

Twenty-four patients had coarctation of the aorta without hypoplasia of the aortic arch, while 14 patients had such coarctation with hypoplasia of the aortic arch. Six had interruption of the aortic arch. In 38 of these 44 patients there was a coexisting VSD.

The Coronary Artery Pattern in D-Transposition

In D-Transposition the origins and distribution of the coronary arteries are considerably more variable than they are in congenital heart defects associated with normally related great arteries. Because a successful arterial switch operation requires transfer of the coronary arteries to the neoaorta without narrowing or distortion, these coronary artery variations have become important considerations in the management of patients with D-TGA.

A number of classifications of coronary anatomy

in D-TGA have been proposed. Many investigators favor abbreviated nomenclatures with letters and numbers. We prefer a descriptive terminology, influenced by Gittenberger-DeGroot et al.,[23] that has been modified somewhat (Fig. 26–1). In more than 99% of the cases, the two sinuses of Valsalva in the aortic root, which face the pulmonary artery, give rise to the coronary arteries; these are termed the *facing sinuses*. When the great vessels are directly side by side, the facing sinuses lie anteriorly and posteriorly, with the noncoronary sinus facing rightward. When (in the usual case) the aorta is anterior and rightward, the aortic facing sinuses are leftward/anterior and rightward/posterior. The descriptive pattern shown in the upper panel of Figure 26–1 represents the image as seen both on the echocardiographic short-axis view and the angiographic "laid back" (extreme caudal angulation) anteroposterior aortogram. In the remainder of Figure 26–1, the coronary artery patterns are depicted as seen by the surgeon in the operating room.

The most common pattern in D-TGA (68%) is a left main coronary artery, originating from the leftward/anterior facing sinus, that gives rise to the left anterior descending and circumflex coronary arteries, with the right coronary artery arising from the rightward/posterior facing sinus. Not infrequently, there is no circumflex coronary artery, but instead there are several branches of the left coronary to supply the lateral and posterior portions of the left ventricle. The next most common pattern (20%) is one in which the circumflex coronary artery arises as a branch from the right coronary artery (right/posterior facing sinus) and passes behind the pulmonary artery to supply the left atrioventricular groove. In this situation, the left anterior descending coronary arises separately from the leftward/anterior facing sinus. These two coronary patterns account for almost 90% of the variability in D-TGA. Other types of coronary artery patterns include a single right (rightward/posterior) coronary artery (4.5%), a single left (leftward/anterior) coronary artery (1.5%), inverted coronary arteries (3%), and intramural coronary arteries (2%). In the cases of intramural coronary arteries, the ostia of the coronaries are commonly juxtacommissural, and there may be two separate ostia within the right sinus or a single ostium that gives rise to the right and left coronaries.

As has been pointed out by Gittenberger-DeGroot, the coronary arteries tend to follow the shortest pathway to reach the desired distribution. Thus, when the great vessels are of the usual interrelationship (anterior and rightward aorta), the more common varieties of coronary arteries are seen. When the great vessels are more side by side, the

right coronary and left anterior descending coronary tend to arise from the anterior sinus, while the circumflex coronary, supplying the posterior portion of the heart, arises from the posterior sinus. Abnormal coronary artery patterns are seen most commonly in patients with less common interrelationships of the great vessels and in patients who have an associated VSD.

PATHOPHYSIOLOGY AND NATURAL HISTORY

If not treated, more than 50% of patients with D-TGA and an IVS die during the first months of life. Few survive beyond 6 months; 90% of untreated patients will die by the age of 1 year. Therefore, treatment, whether palliative or corrective, is necessary shortly after birth. In D-TGA the pulmonary and systemic circulations are parallel rather than in series, and life is sustained exclusively through connections between the two circuits. The presence of a large atrial communication, either natural or secondary to surgical atrial septectomy or balloon atrial septostomy, affords excellent palliation early in life. However, only approximately 50% of patients with atrial defects will survive beyond 2 years of age.

Hemodynamic abnormalities in D-TGA are greatly influenced by the location, number, and size of communications among the atria, the ventricles, and the great arteries as well as by the presence and severity of LVOTO.

The principal factors that determine arterial oxygen saturation in D-TGA include the size and number of communications between the pulmonary and systemic circuits (and, consequently, the ratio between pulmonary and systemic flow, or the absolute pulmonary blood flow). Rosenthal and Fyler[40] demonstrated many years ago that when both pulmonary and systemic flow are increased by hemodilution, systemic oxygen saturation does not change significantly. In general, flow in the pulmonary circuit is much higher than normal because of the communications mentioned and the lower pulmonary vascular resistance. Therefore, systemic oxygen saturation is more dependent on the *effective* pulmonary and systemic flows—that is, the amount of desaturated blood from the systemic circuit that crosses into the pulmonary circuit for oxygenation (effective pulmonary blood flow [EPBF]) and the amount of pulmonary blood returning to the systemic circuit to contribute to gas exchange at the capillary level (effective systemic blood flow [ESBF]). The volume of EPBF and ESBF must be equal (intercirculatory mixing) or all of the blood

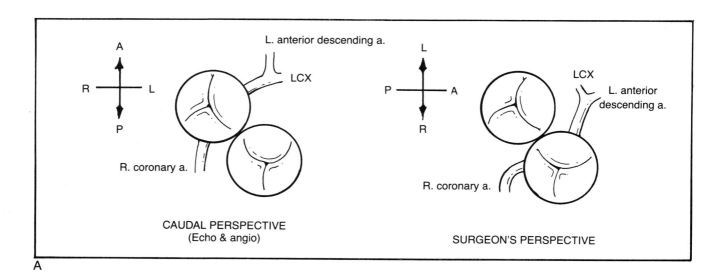

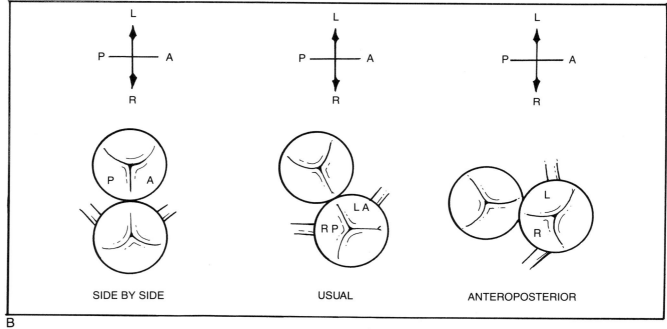

FIGURE 26–1. ☐

The most common types of coronary artery anatomy in transposition of the great arteries. *A* shows a caudal view of the coronary arteries as seen by echocardiographic and angiographic examination (left) and the surgeon's perspective from the right side of the operating table (right). *B,* Origin of coronary arteries depending upon spatial relationship of great arteries. *C,* Most common coronary artery patterns in D-TGA. Insert shows juxtacommissural orifice of left and right coronary arteries. *D,* Single left and right coronary arteries. Insert shows right coronary artery, originating from left coronary artery, coursing between the aorta and pulmonary artery. *E,* Common variations of intramural coronary arteries. A, anterior; L, left; LA, left anterior; LCX, left circumflex coronary artery; P, posterior; R, right; RP, right posterior.

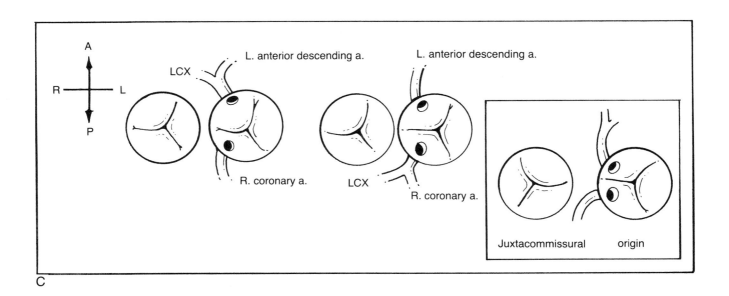

C

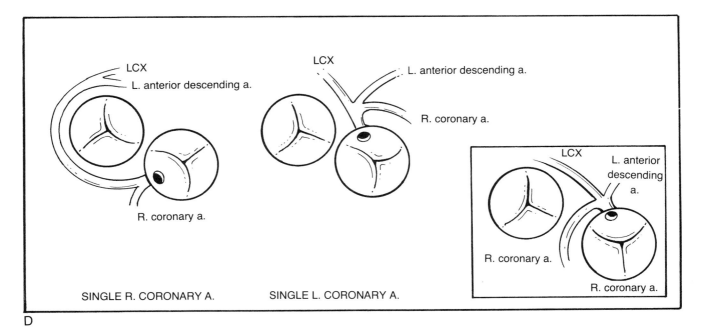

SINGLE R. CORONARY A.   SINGLE L. CORONARY A.

D

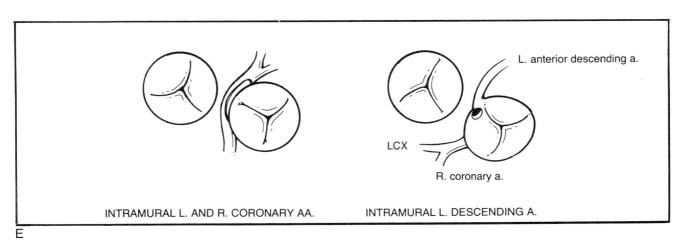

INTRAMURAL L. AND R. CORONARY AA.   INTRAMURAL L. DESCENDING A.

E

FIGURE 26–1. ☐

See legend on opposite page

volume will be transferred into one of the two circuits.

The Fetus With D-Transposition

In the fetus, the only difference from the normal fetal circulation is that in D-TGA the PO_2 is slightly lower than normal in the ascending aorta and slightly higher than normal in the descending thoracic aorta (the reverse of normally related great arteries). Consequently, the heart and the brain receive blood with a somewhat lower PO_2; the effect of this minor difference on these organs is not clear. At the same time, blood coming from the inferior vena cava and the portal vein may have a higher PO_2 than that in the normal fetus. Theoretically, this may maintain a lower than normal pulmonary vascular resistance and, therefore, a somewhat higher pulmonary blood flow in the fetus. The presence of a large VSD could conceivably add blood with a higher PO_2 to the coronary and cerebral circulation, while the presence of an obstruction in the left ventricular outflow tract would channel most of the blood entering the left ventricle through the VSD into the right ventricle. Pulmonary blood flow would be provided mostly by retrograde flow from the aorta through the ductus arteriosus, and the placental and systemic flow would be derived from the right ventricle.

Postnatal Circulation in D-Transposition

D-Transposition With an Intact Ventricular Septum. According to Rudolph,[41] bidirectional shunting through the foramen ovale occurs during variations in atrial pressures, depending on the phases of the cardiac and respiratory cycles. In normally related great arteries, the postnatal right atrial pressure is less than the postnatal left atrial pressure. In patients who have D-TGA with an IVS along with an atrial communication, the right atrium connects with the systemic right ventricle, and during atrial systole, blood shunts from the right atrium to the left atrium through the foramen ovale. During the rapid-filling phase of the atria, the height of the left atrial v wave exceeds that in the right atrium, producing left-to-right atrial shunting. However, unless the atrial communication is large, mixing is inadequate to sustain life; insufficient oxygenation leads to metabolic acidosis and early death. A large atrial communication, either natural or secondary to atrial balloon septotomy or surgical septectomy, usually affords adequate palliation early in life.

D-Transposition With a Ventricular Septal Defect. In the presence of a large VSD, mixing between the pulmonary and systemic circuits is more effective. Occasionally there is only minimal arterial hypoxemia, and the increased pulmonary blood flow can lead to symptoms of severe congestive heart failure. After birth (and the consequent decrease in pulmonary vascular resistance), pulmonary blood flow increases, with a resultant increase in pulmonary venous return and an elevation in left atrial pressure. The increased pulmonary venous return is channeled almost exclusively through the mitral valve into the left ventricle. In the presence of a large septal defect, pressure in the two ventricles remains the same, and because the pulmonary vascular resistance is less than the systemic resistance, during systole systemic venous blood flows by preference into the lower-resistance pulmonary circuit. During ventricular diastole, the increased venous return to the left atrium and ventricle temporarily elevates left ventricular end-diastolic pressure above that in the right ventricle, favoring passage of oxygenated blood to the systemic circuit. Thus, there is a right-to-left shunt at the septal defect during systole, with an equal left-to-right shunt (at the atrial and ventricular level) during diastole.

As mentioned before, a large VSD causes systemic pulmonary artery hypertension, which tends to retard normalization of pulmonary vascular resistance after birth, leading to the development of early pulmonary vascular obstructive disease.

D-Transposition With a Patent Ductus Arteriosus. In D-TGA with an IVS, ductal patency is essential to maintain adequate oxygenation during the first few days of life, or at least until a balloon atrial septostomy is done. After the first few days of life, as pulmonary vascular resistance drops, the flow becomes unidirectional at the ductal level from the aorta to the pulmonary artery. Occasionally, a large patent ductus may cause low cardiac output syndrome and pulmonary edema. In these cases an emergency balloon atrial septostomy should be performed to "decompress" the left atrium and improve mixing; this should be followed by a reparative operation. If the patient is significantly premature, emergency ligation of the ductus may prove the safest course of action, provided there is an adequate atrial septal defect (ASD) or VSD.

D-Transposition With a VSD and Left Ventricular Outflow Tract Obstruction. The hemodynamics and symptomatology of this complex form of D-TGA depend on the size of the VSD and the degree of LVOTO. In patients with severe obstruction, blood within the left ventricle passes preferentially through the septal defect into the right ventricle and hence to the systemic circulation. The critical issue is the degree of obstruction and the adequacy of pulmonary blood flow. While the ductus arteriosus is still patent, the aorta-to–pulmonary artery flow increases as pulmonary vascular resistance falls. As long as pulmonary flow is maintained, sufficient systemic oxygenation is secured, because intracardiac mixing is usually extensive. Once the ductus arteriosus closes, however, systemic hypoxemia and metabolic acidosis may develop rapidly when there is severe LVOTO. Aortopulmonary collaterals may develop, but this compensatory mechanism requires time. The physiology in these patients basically mimics that of tetralogy of Fallot. However, in D-TGA, oxygenated blood tends to recirculate within the pulmonary circuit rather than reaching the arterial system.

Ventricular Muscle Mass

The transition from fetal to neonatal extrauterine circulation in the normal heart results almost immediately in a 25% increase in left ventricular volume load and a 30% decrease in right ventricular volume load. In fact, the postnatal left ventricle growth is presented with a combination of volume overload and a sustained pressure load, which leads to a rapid increase in left ventricular mass. Without these stimuli, there is a much slower increase in right ventricular mass[7] (Fig. 26–2). By 1 month of age, the left ventricle substantially outweighs the right ventricle in normal infants. In D-TGA with an IVS, the postnatal left ventricle ejects blood into the low-resistance pulmonary vasculature and, therefore, does not increase its muscle mass relative to the right (systemic) ventricle (or relative to a normal left ventricle). Consequently, within weeks the left ventricular myocardium loses its capacity to maintain an adequate cardiac output against a systemic afterload. In D-TGA with an IVS, the fall of pulmonary arteriolar resistance postnatally is similar to that observed in the infant with normally related great arteries. Although pulmonary blood flow in patients with D-TGA and an IVS is much greater than the systemic flow, left ventricular muscle growth is retarded because the afterload (pulmonary resistance) is low. Instead, the right ventricle assumes the function, and also the necessary muscle mass, to overcome systemic resistance. These significant differences in left and right ventricular muscle mass progress over time and may assume considerable importance if the left ventricle is suddenly required to perform against systemic resistance, as in the arterial switch operation.

The hemodynamic load to which the ventricle is subjected has a strong influence on its wall stiffness

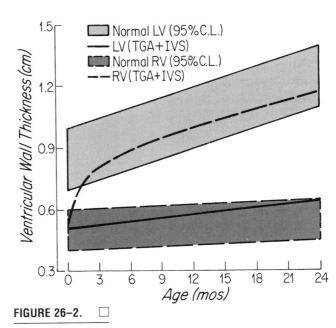

FIGURE 26–2. ☐

In transposition of the great arteries with an intact ventricular septum (TGA-IVS), the left ventricular wall thickness is normal at birth. The rapidly decreasing pulmonary vascular resistance results in a drop of peak left ventricular (LV) pressure and, hence, decreased development of LV muscle mass *(solid line)*. The upper bar shows an increase in LV free-wall thickness in normally related great arteries and a similar increase *(dashed line)* in right ventricular (RV) muscle mass in TGA-IVS. LV muscle mass in TGA-IVS follows the pattern of RV muscle mass in normally related great arteries *(lower bar)*.

and function. Ventricular wall stress is an index of its anatomic and functional responses to any given pressure or volume load. Ventricular wall stress (WS) is directly proportional to intracavitary pressure (P) and diameter (D) and is inversely proportional to wall thickness (WT). Simplistically, WS = P × D/WT. In D-TGA, the left ventricle may work under different hemodynamic conditions, depending on the presence of a patent ductus arteriosus (PDA), a VSD, or LVOTO, and its anatomic and functional features vary accordingly. In D-TGA with an IVS, the left ventricle faces a volume overload and a relatively low afterload. In D-TGA with a VSD or a large PDA, there is both volume and pressure overload in the left ventricle, and in D-TGA with LVOTO and without a VSD, there is predominantly a left ventricular pressure overload. As a general rule, thickness of the left ventricular free wall is dependent on a pressure load to levels of more than 50% of the systemic pressure, but is much less influenced by a pure volume load.[20]

Pulmonary Vascular Obstructive Disease in D-Transposition

Unoperated patients with D-TGA typically develop, early and rapidly, progressive pulmonary vascular obstructive disease. Although the precise etiology of these lesions in D-TGA is not well understood, contributing factors probably include increased pulmonary blood flow, elevated pulmonary artery pressure (both of which together result in increased shear stress), high pulmonary arterial Po_2, systemic hypoxemia and reduced oxygen saturation (with reduced oxygen supply to the pulmonary arterial wall by the bronchial arterial circulation), increased blood viscosity, enlarged aortopulmonary collaterals, and development of microthrombi. Also, pulmonary arterial vasospasm is believed to aggravate endothelial shear stress, thereby favoring the rapid progression of medial and intimal changes.

In a group of infants at Children's Hospital in Boston, who had D-TGA and a VSD, Heath-Edwards grade III lesions were found in approximately 20% of those less than 3 months of age and in almost 80% of those more than 1 year of age. In infants who had D-TGA and an IVS, grade III lesions occurred in less than 1% within the first 3 months of age and in fewer than 20% within the first year of life. Awareness of the accelerated development of pulmonary vascular obstructive disease in patients with D-TGA, even in patients who have D-TGA with an IVS, is particularly important because of the unreliability of calculations for pulmonary blood flow and pulmonary vascular resistance in this disease.

DIAGNOSIS OF D-TRANSPOSITION

Clinically, neonates who have D-TGA and an IVS are usually fairly cyanotic but otherwise well developed. Arterial Po_2 commonly remains between 25 and 40 mm Hg and does not increase substantially with the administration of 100% oxygen. Clinical deterioration usually occurs within the first 24 to 48 hours, presumably as the patent ductus closes. If there is no ASD or only a small atrial communication, progressive acidemia rapidly develops in these neonates if they are untreated. If a large VSD or PDA coexists, the diagnosis of D-TGA may be missed during the first few days or weeks after birth. Because there may be only mild cyanosis, the heart remains small, and murmurs are rarely heard within the first 48 hours after birth. As pulmonary vascular resistance falls, cardiac failure manifests itself, usually within the first 2 to 3 weeks of life. Heart failure is characterized by dyspnea, tachypnea, irritability, diaphoresis, and hepatomegaly. The electrocardiogram reveals right ventricular hypertrophy, and the chest radiograph demonstrates biventricular enlargement and pulmonary overcirculation. Blood gas analysis usually reveals decreas-

ing Po_2 and an increase in Pco_2 with a concomitant fall in pH.

In patients who have D-TGA, VSD, and LVOTO, signs and symptoms are similar to those in patients with tetralogy of Fallot. The neonate is usually mildly cyanotic after birth but remains otherwise asymptomatic until the ductus starts to close. Then cyanosis may increase rapidly, depending on the degree of pulmonary stenosis.

Echocardiography

Because of the rapidly deteriorating clinical course of neonates with D-TGA, particularly those with an IVS, early diagnosis and treatment are extremely important. In most cases, urgent cardiac catheterization with a balloon atrial septostomy (Rashkind procedure) is the initial treatment of choice.[38] In critically ill neonates, the Rashkind procedure can be accomplished at the bedside using two-dimensional echocardiographic guidance. In fact, with improved two-dimensional echocardiography, cardiac catheterization is becoming more and more restricted to neonates with special problems. In the presence of severe hypoxemia and metabolic acidosis, prostaglandin E_1 may be administered to maintain ductal patency and improve oxygenation, although this should not decrease the urgency with which balloon septostomy is performed.

At Children's Hospital in Boston, two-dimensional echocardiography, particularly with pulsed Doppler and color Doppler techniques, has been extremely accurate in defining D-TGA and in outlining the origin and epicardial course of coronary arteries, including the less common variants of coronary artery patterns.[42] In fact, echocardiography has proved more precise in diagnosing intramural coronary arteries than have selective aortic root injections. Of our first 193 patients who underwent an arterial switch operation, the echocardiogram described the coronary anatomy correctly in 190. In the three remaining patients, limited windows (owing to anterior extension of lung tissue) precluded adequate visualization of the coronary arteries. Of the 114 patients with the most common form of coronary artery anatomy, 113 were correctly diagnosed by two-dimensional echocardiography. An unusual coronary artery pattern was detected correctly by two-dimensional echocardiography in 68 of 76 patients with such a pattern. In five of the remaining eight patients, there was a single right coronary artery; in two, both coronary arteries originated from a single sinus; and the eighth patient had an intramural coronary artery with dual left anterior descending coronary arteries. Two-dimensional echocardiography is also effective in identifying and characterizing associated lesions such as LVOTO and abnormalities of the atrioventricular valves.

Currently, in the arterial switch operation for D-TGA, two-dimensional echocardiography offers the additional advantage of providing physiologic data regarding the capacity of the left ventricle to support the systemic circulation, especially in infants who have D-TGA with an IVS and who are beyond the neonatal period. For example, it seems that the left ventricular mass-to-volume ratio will become an important predictor of the postoperative course of infants undergoing the arterial switch operation.

In a more recent review of 260 echocardiograms obtained at Children's Hospital in Boston[53] on neonates with D-TGA, arterial and ventricular alignment and venous and atrial anatomy were diagnosed correctly in all patients. Ninety-two of these patients had one or more VSDs. Only a small, hemodynamically insignificant, 2-mm perimembranous defect was missed in one patient thought to have an aneurysm of the membranous septum. LVOTO was correctly diagnosed in 22 patients. Accessory atrioventricular valve tissue or abnormal attachments into the left ventricular outflow tract were identified in six patients, and a hypertrophied muscle of Moulaert was correctly identified (and subsequently resected at the time of the arterial switch). Anomalies of the aortic arch (e.g., coarctation, hypoplastic aortic arch, and interrupted aortic arch [type A]) were also all correctly diagnosed by two-dimensional echocardiography. Over the years, the accuracy of echocardiography has continued to improve. At present, we believe that echocardiography can provide sufficient detailed anatomic information to make an anatomic repair of D-TGA possible in the great majority of infants without previous cardiac catheterization. Currently, cardiac catheterization is used primarily in patients with D-TGA and an IVS who require surgery after the neonatal period; catheterization is useful to assess the suitability of the left ventricle to support the systemic circulation. The criteria needed for carrying out a preliminary, rapid, two-stage arterial switch operation (i.e., banding of the pulmonary artery plus a systemic-to-pulmonary shunt, followed within 7 to 10 days by debanding, closure of the shunt, and an arterial switch operation) are not yet clearly defined. Factors favoring a two-stage approach include a left ventricle–to–right ventricle ratio < 0.6 or a left ventricle pressure < 50 mm Hg in patients more than 1 month of age.

Helpful, but not yet clearly defined, echocardiographic indices of a left ventricle suitable for an arterial switch operation include ventricular septal position and left ventricular wall thickness, volume, and muscle mass.

SURGICAL HISTORY

Basically there are two options for the repair of D-TGA: redirection of ventricular outflow and redirection of venous inflow. The obvious disadvantage of redirecting venous inflow is that the left ventricle continues as the pulmonary ventricle, while the anatomic right ventricle and tricuspid valve must continue to function as the systemic ventricle and atrioventricular valve.

Preliminary Palliative Operations

Lillehei and Varco[31] first anastomosed the right pulmonary veins to the right atrium and the inferior vena cava to the left atrium. Baffes[4] modified this operation by interposing an aortic homograft between the inferior vena cava and the left atrium. Blalock and Hanlon[9] introduced the ingenious closed atrial septectomy operation, which was subsequently modified by Edwards and associates,[22] who transferred the atrial septum to the left of the right pulmonary veins, thus creating an obligatory pulmonary vein–to–right atrium shunt. An extremely important contribution was balloon atrial septostomy, developed by Rashkind and Miller in 1966.[38]

Reparative Operations

In 1954, Albert[1] described an experimental technique for intra-atrial redirection of all pulmonary and systemic venous return. In the same year, Mustard et al. attempted an arterial switch operation in seven patients, using monkey lungs as oxygenators.[36] This technique included transfer of the left coronary artery only, and none of the patients survived. Before the widespread use of cardiopulmonary bypass, other experimental and clinical attempts at switching the great arteries without coronary transfer also failed. A modification of the Albert procedure was first successfully accomplished clinically in 1959 by Senning.[43] In 1964, Mustard[35] reported his successful modification of the atrial-level repair, using a pericardial baffle to redirect pulmonary venous return toward the tricuspid valve and systemic venous return toward the mitral valve. Anatomic correction—connecting the left ventricle with the aorta and the right ventricle with the pulmonary artery—was first accomplished by Rastelli and coworkers in 1969 in a patient with D-TGA, a VSD, and LVOTO.[39] The first successful intraventricular repair in a patient with D-TGA and a VSD was carried out by McGoon.[34]

Despite the excellent results with the atrial inversion operations (Mustard or Senning), which accomplish physiologic repair, a few investigators continued to explore the possibility of switching the great arteries, together with the coronary arteries. In 1959, Senning[43] described three patients with D-TGA treated by a technique involving en bloc transferral of the pulmonary valve and artery and diversion of the left ventricle to the aorta through a VSD. In 1961, Idriss et al.[24] translocated a segment of the ascending aorta, including both coronary arteries, into the proximal pulmonary artery. However, none of these patients survived. Other experimental techniques were reported by Baffes and coworkers[5] and by Anagnostopoulos.[2]

In 1975, Jatene and associates[26] reported the first successful arterial switch operation in a patient with D-TGA and a large VSD. Many of the technical advances learned from coronary artery bypass surgery in the adult, along with a clear understanding of the need for a left ventricle capable of supporting the systemic circulation, contributed to the success of this first operation. In fact, patients with D-TGA and a VSD (or a large PDA or LVOTO) retain a left ventricular pressure at (or close to) systemic levels after birth; therefore, Jatene initially limited the arterial switch operation to this subset of patients.

Because the early high operative mortality of the arterial switch operation was in part attributed to technical difficulties related to the transfer of the coronary arteries, alternative techniques avoiding mobilization of the coronary arteries were developed. These included (1) baffling of aortic blood to the coronary arteries through a surgically created aortopulmonary window by Aubert et al. in 1978[3]; (2) translocation of the entire aortic root, including the proximal coronary arteries, by Bex and coworkers in 1980[8]; and (3) end-to-side anastomosis of the proximal pulmonary artery to the ascending aorta, with placement of a conduit from the right ventricle to the distal pulmonary artery by Damus,[19] Kaye,[29] and Stansel[44] between 1972 and 1976. However, the arterial switch operation with coronary artery transfer (Jatene) retained its original appeal. In 1981, Lecompte and coworkers[30] added the important technical modification of transferring the distal pulmonary artery anterior to the ascending aorta, thus facilitating direct anastomosis of the neopulmonary artery without the need for a conduit.

Because approximately 75% of the patients with D-TGA have an intact (or virtually intact) ventricular septum, application of the arterial switch principle to this largest subset of patients became of interest to several investigators. To prepare the left ventricle to handle systemic pressure, Yacoub et al.[54] introduced a two-stage approach to D-TGA with an IVS by first banding the pulmonary artery (with or without a systemic pulmonary artery shunt) to stimulate the development of left ventricular muscle mass, followed by an arterial switch procedure many months later. The principle of performing the arterial switch as a primary repair in neonates with D-TGA while the left ventricle is still capable of systemic pressure work was successfully introduced at Children's Hospital in Boston in 1983.[15] In 1988, we also introduced the concept of a rapid, two-stage arterial switch operation for D-TGA with an IVS; this consisted of banding the pulmonary artery and adding a systemic-to–pulmonary artery shunt in preparation for the arterial switch, limiting the interval between the first and second operation to an average of 7 days.[28]

SURGICAL CONSIDERATIONS

Why the Arterial Switch Operation Is Preferred

Primarily, there is increasing concern about late results of the atrial or physiologic type of repair. Although the hospital mortality rate for both the Mustard and the Senning operations is low, the long-term outcome of these procedures is affected by a number of late complications, the most important being a high incidence of atrial dysrhythmias (more than 50% within 10 years) and a less clearly established incidence of late right ventricular (systemic ventricular) dysfunction (approximately 10%). A variety of theoretical considerations support the assumption that the left ventricle is more suitable than the right to serve the systemic circulation. The left ventricle (with its cylindric shape, its concentric contraction pattern, and both the inlet and the outlet orifices situated in close proximity) seems ideally adapted to work as a pressure pump, whereas the right ventricle (with its crescent-shaped cavity, its large internal surface area–to-volume ratio, its bellows-like contraction pattern, and its more separated inlet and outlet segments) seems better suited to serve as a low-pressure-volume pumping chamber. Also, the left ventricle has two coronary arteries (left anterior descending and left circumflex), while the right ventricle has one (right coronary). Developmentally, the stratum compactum of the myocardium is thicker in the left ventricle than in the right, and phylogenetically, the left ventricular sinus is derived from the primitive ventricle at the stage of ventricular looping (the "original pump" of our phylum Chordata), while the conus and much of the right ventricle are derived from the bulbus cordis.[46] Furthermore, the papillary muscles of the right ventricle are small and numerous, originating both from the septum and from the right ventricular free wall (septophylic), in contrast to the two papillary muscles of the left ventricle. This architecture allows the tricuspid valve to be pulled apart as the right ventricle dilates, leading to tricuspid regurgitation. The arterial switch operation recruits the left ventricle as a systemic pump, and because atrial manipulation is essentially limited to closure of an atrial communication, it is also anticipated that after the arterial switch, atrial dysrhythmias should be significantly reduced.

At Children's Hospital in Boston, our policy in cases of D-TGA with an IVS is to perform the arterial switch during the neonatal period when the left ventricle is still "prepared" to support the systemic circulation by the intrauterine physiology. Ideally, the repair should be performed within the first weeks of life. Later, there is increasing likelihood that the left ventricle will be unable to accommodate the increased workload. A number of circumstances can arise that cause postponement of surgery beyond the "safe" period for an arterial switch. For example, a neonate may be seriously ill with necrotizing enterocolitis, renal or hepatic failure, or a hemorrhage in the central nervous system. Also, the neonate may be geographically distant from a center offering the arterial switch operation, or occasionally a patient with D-TGA and a VSD awaiting "elective" repair may experience spontaneous partial closure of the VSD, resulting in a low left ventricular pressure.

Because of these possibilities, we have developed some empiric criteria for predicting postoperative left ventricular performance. Before the age of 2 weeks, every patient with D-TGA and an IVS is repaired, regardless of preoperative left ventricular pressure measurements. As mentioned in Chapter 1, laboratory studies in rats have demonstrated surprisingly rapid induction (within 48 hours) of the genes responsible for the isozyme adaptation of the myocardial myosin, actin, and tropomyosin in response to an acute pressure load.[25] Furthermore, various proto-oncogenes involved in the regulation of cell growth accumulate in rat cardiac cells within 1 hour of an acute pressure load. Stress protein (HSP70) is also seen at high levels within 2 to 3 hours of an acute pressure load. Coincident to these developments has been further refinement of echocardiographic techniques to assess left ventricular mass and volume more accurately. Based on these

criteria, we have successfully performed arterial switch operations 7 to 10 days after preliminary pulmonary artery banding and placement of a modified Blalock-Taussig shunt.[28]

In patients who have D-TGA with a VSD, we also recommend repair shortly after the diagnosis is made. Although the left ventricle remains "prepared" when a large septal defect maintains systemic left ventricular pressure, a delay in surgery may result in pulmonary vascular obstructive disease, failure to thrive, or pulmonary infections, and, in some cases partial closure of the VSD results in an "unprepared" left ventricle. We see no advantage in delaying corrective surgery. Palliative pulmonary artery banding is indicated only in patients with multiple muscular defects, to allow time for growth and spontaneous closure of the less surgically accessible VSDs. Also, transcatheter closure of the muscular VSDs (avoiding a ventriculotomy) can currently be accomplished when infants reach a weight of 5 kg.

Arterial Switch Operation Technique

Cardiopulmonary bypass can be conducted in a number of ways, depending on the surgeon's preference or the time required to accomplish complete repair, particularly in the presence of a VSD or other anomalies such as coarctation of the aorta or a hypoplastic or interrupted aortic arch.[13, 14, 32] In patients with D-TGA and an IVS, we prefer to perform the operation with the patient under either total circulatory arrest or continuous low-flow (50 ml/kg/min) hypothermic perfusion, limiting circulatory arrest time to the few minutes necessary to close the ASD. In the presence of a VSD or other complex associated lesions, we have used two periods of deep hypothermic circulatory arrest, interposing 10 to 15 minutes of hypothermic reperfusion between them, or the arterial switch itself may be performed under continuous low-flow cardiopulmonary bypass, with profound hypothermic circulatory arrest for closure of the VSD and other procedures such as repair of an interrupted aortic arch.

Through a midline sternotomy, a segment of pericardium is first harvested and prepared with 0.6% glutaraldehyde solution. The coronary arteries and great vessels are inspected. The ascending aorta is then cannulated as far distally as possible to allow adequate length for the aortic anastomosis (Fig. 26–3A). A single venous cannula is placed within the right atrium, and cooling to profound hypothermia (18°C rectal temperature) is begun. Before initiating cardiopulmonary bypass, the ductus arteriosus is dissected free, as are the left and right pulmonary

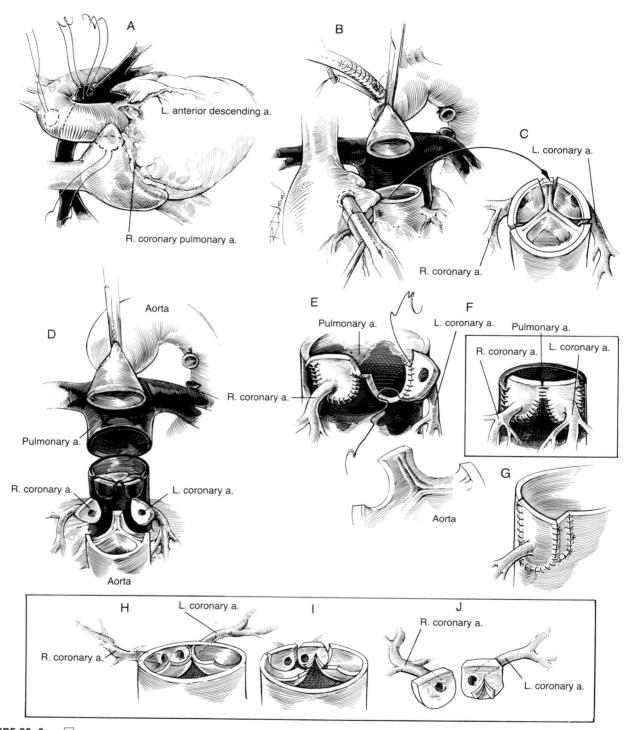

FIGURE 26–3. ☐

A, Cannulation sites for cardiopulmonary bypass. Note the pursestring on the distal ascending aorta and base of the right atrial appendage. The patent ductus arteriosus has been dissected and surrounded by a suture on each end. *B,* Aortic and venous return cannula in place. The aortic crossclamp is placed proximal to the arterial cannula. Transection of the aorta allows inspection of the stoma of the left and right coronary arteries. *C,* Excision of the left and right coronary arteries, including a large flap of aortic wall; the incision is extended well into the base of the sinus of Valsalva. *D,* Equivalent segments of neoaortic wall and proximal pulmonary artery are excised. *E,* The aortocoronary flap is sutured into the proximal neoaorta. *F,* Completed anastomosis of left and right coronary arteries to neoaorta. *G,* Additional pericardial patch augmentation of the coronary aortic anastomosis is sometimes necessary to avoid kinking of (mostly the right) coronary arteries. *H,* In case of juxtacommissural origin of either the left or both coronary arteries from one of the facing sinuses, excision of a segment of the posterior commissure of the native aortic valve (neopulmonary valve) is necessary *(I). J,* Whenever possible, the two coronary ostia are separated for easier implantation.

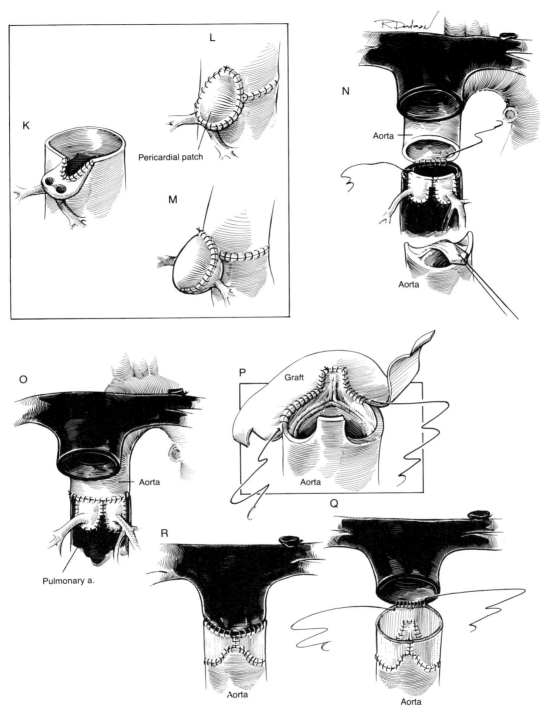

FIGURE 26–3. □

Continued. K, Right and left combined intramural coronary arteries. To avoid torsion and excessive rotation, the aortocoronary flap is left in situ and is sutured along its cephalic border to a counterincision in the anterior wall of the proximal neoaorta. A glutaraldehyde-pretreated pericardial patch is then sutured to the remaining caudal free edge of the aortocoronary flap and the distal ascending aorta (*L* and *M*). *N,* Anastomosis of the proximal neoaorta to the distal aorta. Note the pulmonary artery positioned anteriorly to the ascending aorta (Lecompte maneuver). *O,* Completed anastomosis. *P,* Suture of a pantaloon-shaped pericardial patch into the proximal neopulmonary artery with the purpose of filling the area of explanted coronary arteries and decreasing tension on pulmonary anastomoses. *Q,* Anastomosis of distal pericardial circumference to the distal pulmonary artery. *R,* Completed reconstruction of pulmonary outflow tract.

arteries, including the first pulmonary artery branches in the hilum of each lung. Immediately after beginning cardiopulmonary bypass, the ductus arteriosus is doubly ligated with sutures and divided, and the ascending aorta is dissected free from the main pulmonary artery. At 18°C rectal temperature, the distal ascending aorta is clamped, and cold cardioplegic solution is delivered into the proximal ascending aorta. The aorta is then divided approximately 1 cm distal to the origin of the coronary arteries (Fig. 26–3B). At this point, the ostium, the initial course of the left and right coronary arteries, and the presence of conal branches are identified. If the coronary ostia are distant from the commissures, the left and right coronary ostia (or in the case of a single coronary artery, the corresponding ostium) are excised along with a large segment of surrounding aortic wall, extending the incision well into the base of the sinus of Valsalva (Fig. 26–3C). The proximal coronary arteries are mobilized sufficiently to avoid tension or kinking, while conal branches are very rarely sacrificed.

At this point, the pulmonary artery is divided just proximal to its bifurcation (Fig. 26–3D). The distal pulmonary artery is then brought anterior to the aorta (Lecompte maneuver) and held in position anterior to the ascending aorta by rubber loops or by moving the aortic clamp. An equivalent U-shaped segment of arterial wall is then removed from both the left and right anterior aspects of the native proximal pulmonary artery to prepare the coronary implantation sites. The exact positions of the implantation sites are easily identified by juxtaposing the explanted coronary arteries or by placing marking sutures before cardiopulmonary bypass, when the aortic and pulmonary roots are distended (Fig. 26–3E, F). The coronary ostia are then transferred by sewing the coronary flap to these incisions with a continuous 7-0 monofilament absorbable suture (polydioxanone) or 7-0 nonabsorbable suture material (Prolene). When the circumflex coronary artery arises from the right coronary artery, the site of right coronary implantation must be placed either higher than usual on the proximal neoaorta or, occasionally, above the suture line on the distal ascending aorta to avoid kinking of the circumflex artery. Adequate mobilization of the right coronary artery is frequently necessary to avoid distortion of the circumflex coronary artery. If the two coronary arteries originate from the same sinus, they can often be included in the same aortic flap (provided there is not an intramural course for one of the coronaries). In the presence of an intramural segment, we try to separate the two ostia, if at all possible. If the coronary ostia are located closely adjacent (paracommissural) to the posterior com-

missure, excision of a segment of the posterior commissure of the native aortic valve (neopulmonary valve) is often necessary (Fig. 26–3G–I); the resultant neopulmonary regurgitation is generally mild and well tolerated. Occasionally, with either single (more so with a single right coronary artery) or intramural coronary arteries, to avoid excessive rotation and torsion, the aortocoronary flap is left in situ after excision from the proximal aorta. The cephalic border of the flap is sutured to an appropriate incision made within the anterior wall of the proximal neoaorta (Fig. 26–3J), and a glutaraldehyde-pretreated pericardial patch is sutured to the remaining caudal free edge of the aortocoronary flap and to the opening made within the distal ascending aorta (Fig. 26–3K, L). In other instances, where the aortocoronary segment can be mobilized sufficiently to reach the neoaorta but at a risk of causing a kink, it may also be necessary to interpose a small segment of pericardium into the coronary-neoaortic anastomosis (Fig. 26–3M). Using these various technical modifications, essentially any coronary artery pattern lends itself for the arterial switch operation, excluding perhaps bilateral intramural coronary arteries with a common ostium located deep within one of the facing sinuses. In such rare cases, seen only once in our experience, an Aubert operation may be considered.[3] However, it is not yet clear whether the increased risks that may attend the transfer of some of these rare and complex patterns are warranted in patients with TGA and an IVS.

The distal aorta is anastomosed to the proximal neoaorta with a continuous 6-0 absorbable monofilament suture (polydioxanone) (Fig. 26–3N). Portions of the coronary flaps may be incorporated into this anastomosis anteriorly to compensate for discrepancies in circumference between the ascending aorta and the neoaorta (Fig. 26–3O). At this point, the atrial communication is closed through a right atriotomy. As a rule, this can be accomplished by primary closure after balloon septostomy, as there is usually no tissue deficiency. After closure of the right atriotomy, cardiopulmonary bypass is restarted. The aortic crossclamp can be removed at this point, provided the left side of the heart is fully vented through a stab incision in the ascending aorta. The coronary explantation sites in the neopulmonary artery are then filled, using a single, long, inverted bifurcated patch of 0.6% glutaraldehyde-pretreated, autologous pericardium (Fig. 26–3P). An incision is made into the pericardium to fit into the posterior commissure, and the free pericardial edge is sutured to the area of the aorta (neopulmonary artery) corresponding to the explanted coronary flaps, using a continuous 6-0 Prolene suture. When the anterior remnant of the aortic wall is reached, the pericardium, at this point cylindrically shaped (Fig. 26–3Q), is tailored to bridge the distance between the proximal neopulmonary artery and the distal pulmonary artery without tension. Discrepancies in caliber between the proximal neopulmonary artery and the distal pulmonary artery are also easily reconciled with this pericardial extension (Fig. 26–3R). Alternatively, two separate pericardial patches can be used, one for the site of each coronary donor. The relationship of the great vessels will require certain modifications. With side-by-side great vessels or the more rare posterior aorta, a Lecompte maneuver is not usually performed, and the central stoma in the transverse pulmonary artery is moved to the right pulmonary artery. The proximal neopulmonary artery is then anastomosed to this stoma. In these cases, it is also sometimes technically easier to place the bifurcated pericardial patch as the first maneuver after removing the coronary arteries from the aorta and before coronary reimplantation.

Rewarming, generally initiated when the aortic clamp is released, is continued during bypass until a rectal temperature of 36°C is reached. During weaning from cardiopulmonary bypass, the heart rate, systemic blood pressure, and left atrial pressure are closely monitored. Left atrial, right atrial, and pulmonary artery lines are placed for postoperative measurements, as are atrial and ventricular temporary pacemaker wires. Systemic blood pressure is maintained at about 60 mm Hg; calcium and inotropic agents, usually dopamine, are added if necessary. We have observed that systemic hypertension (systemic blood pressure > 80 mm Hg) may be poorly tolerated by the newly systemic left ventricle, resulting in distention, left atrial hypertension, and mitral regurgitation. Hypertension also promotes bleeding from the extensive suture lines. Abnormalities of cardiac rhythm during rewarming or after bypass, or of myocardial performance after bypass, are strongly suggestive of a coronary perfusion problem. Should this be the case, the cause must be clearly identified at this moment and aggressively corrected.

Postoperative management is similar to that for other neonates undergoing repair of complex cardiac lesions. Neuromuscular blockade, continuous fentanyl sedation, mechanical ventilation, and moderate inotropic support are customarily maintained during the first 12 to 18 hours or until hemodynamic stability is achieved.

D-Transposition With a Ventricular Septal Defect

Techniques for closure of VSDs are discussed in Chapter 11. In the majority of patients with D-TGA,

as in those with normally related great arteries, paramembranous, malalignment, atrioventricular, and midmuscular VSDs are exposed through the right atrium. Some of the paramembranous or malalignment defects can also be closed through the anterior semilunar valve; for some malalignment VSDs coexisting with multiple muscular defects, a combined transatrial and transneoaortic approach may be necessary. In the first 140 patients with D-TGA and a VSD operated on at Children's Hospital in Boston, a right ventriculotomy was used in only four patients, two of whom had infundibular or subarterial VSDs and two of whom had anterior muscular defects. Of the latter two patients, one also had an overriding tricuspid valve, and the other had hypoplasia of both the right ventricle and the tricuspid valve. A right ventricular incision may be necessary in patients with right ventricular infundibular hypoplasia and a VSD (often associated with hypoplasia or interruption of the aortic arch). All large septal defects were closed with a patch. An additional patient required a reduction arterioplasty of a massively dilated main pulmonary artery that had been causing significant compression of the airway. To avoid a left ventriculotomy in patients with apical muscular defects, we currently prefer to close such defects in the catheterization laboratory with a clamshell device,[10] followed within hours by an arterial switch operation and closure of any additional VSDs. Alternatively, a clamshell device can be positioned under direct vision in the operating room. Excellent visualization of the seating of the device is obtained when both great arteries have been divided.

In 27 of 470 patients (5.7%) undergoing this technique at Children's Hospital in Boston, the sternum was not closed primarily; instead, the sternotomy was covered with a Silastic sheet without reapproximation of the bone edges, followed by secondary sternal closure 2 to 26 days (median, 4 days) after surgery. Most of these patients had significant myocardial edema; some of them required intraoperative revision of the coronary anastomosis or closure of a residual VSD and prolonged cardiopulmonary bypass.

Techniques for simultaneous repair of other associated defects (e.g., coarctation, interrupted aortic arch, and hypoplastic aortic arch) in conjunction with the arterial switch operation are discussed in chapters dealing with those lesions. However, it should be noted that in patients with D-TGA and hypoplasia or coarctation of the aortic arch, there is a strong likelihood of subvalvar obstruction of the right ventricular outflow tract (RVOT). This obstruction may not be apparent preoperatively with an open VSD and a PDA when less than full cardiac output is crossing the RVOT, but it may result in right ventricular hypertension and obstruction after repair. Liberal use of a patch on the RVOT is recommended in these cases. In the occasional case in which D-TGA with a VSD is accompanied by extreme diffuse aortic hypoplasia, including the aortic valve, a Damus-Kaye-Stansel approach may be warranted.[29, 44]

Rapid Two-Stage Repair of D-Transposition With an IVS

The First Stage. Through either a right thoracotomy or a midline sternotomy, a 3.5- or 4-mm polytetrafluoroethylene (Gore-Tex) graft is used to connect the right subclavian artery to the right pulmonary artery. Subsequently, and after minimal dissection, a Dacron-reinforced Silastic band is tightened around the main pulmonary artery to achieve a left ventricular pressure that is approximately 75% of systemic pressure. The pericardium is then loosely closed after thoroughly irrigating the pericardial space with heparinized saline to flush out any residual blood or fibrin clots.

The Second Stage. The only modifications required relative to our standard operative approach for the arterial switch are to first divide and oversew the modified Blalock-Taussig shunt and to remove the pulmonary artery band. Because the second stage is carried out an average of 7 days after the first stage, adhesions do not usually present a problem. There was only one patient in whom the origin of the left coronary artery could not be visualized after the banding. Surgery for that patient was deferred for 12 months, at which time there was found to be an intramural and intramyocardial left coronary artery.

In all patients undergoing a rapid two-stage arterial switch operation, the Lecompte maneuver with direct pulmonary artery anastomosis was performed without difficulty.

D-Transposition With a VSD and Obstruction of the Left Ventricular Outflow Tract

The conventional treatment for neonates and infants with D-TGA, a VSD, and hemodynamically significant LVOTO has been an initial Blalock-Taussig shunt. However, we prefer either to attempt direct relief of the obstruction, accompanied by VSD closure and an arterial switch operation, or, in the case of a long-segment hypoplastic LVOTO or valvar pulmonary stenosis, to carry out a Rastelli[39] operation using a cryopreserved valved aortic or pulmonary homograft (particularly in the neonate or young infant in whom the severe cyanosis is due in part to poor mixing, in spite of the possibility of adequate or even overcirculation of the pulmonary vascular bed).

Direct Resection of LVOTO in Addition to an Arterial Switch Operation and Repair of a VSD

The occasional discrete subpulmonary membrane or excrescence of endocardial cushion tissue is easily resected through the posterior (pulmonary) semilunar valve. More common, and surgically more demanding, is LVOTO caused by a posteriorly deviated infundibular septum.

Once the ascending aorta and main pulmonary artery are divided in the course of an arterial switch operation, the obstructing muscle is more safely exposed through the pulmonary semilunar valve. Although exposure of the infundibular septum is often easier through the anterior (aortic) semilunar valve, in patients with D-TGA, incision and excision of the infundibular septum via the aortic valve run the risk of damaging the pulmonary valve, because the pulmonary semilunar valve originates at a lower level than the aortic semilunar valve. Therefore, the transpulmonary approach allows a more aggressive excision of the posteriorly deviated infundibular septum, at the same time leaving sufficient muscle to anchor the ventricular septal patch. It helps to engage the infundibular septum with a skin hook and to deliver it further into the left ventricular outflow tract before excising the muscle mass.

Rastelli Operation for D-Transposition With a VSD and LVOTO

Often, in the case of a long, hypoplastic left ventricular outflow tract, resection is not feasible. In such cases we prefer to carry out a Rastelli operation rather than a palliative shunt operation, regardless of the patient's age. After opening the chest through a midline sternotomy, an appropriate-size valved homograft (aortic or pulmonary) is selected, usually varying in size from 9 mm for a neonate to 14 mm for an older infant. In addition, a patch of pericardium is harvested and pretreated with 0.6% glutaraldehyde for later use to augment the anastomosis from the right ventricle to the homograft. Depending on the age and size of the child, either circulatory arrest or cardiopulmonary bypass with low-flow hypothermic perfusion is used. The main pulmonary artery commonly lies posterior and to the left of the ascending aorta, and its branches are dissected and the ligamentum arteriosum divided. If continuous cardiopulmonary bypass is used, the aorta is crossclamped at 25°C, and cold cardioplegic solution is injected. A vertical right ventriculotomy is then made to expose the aortic valve, the VSD, and the tricuspid valve (Fig. 26–4A, B). Unless the malaligned septal defect is larger than the diameter of the aortic valve, it is enlarged by making two incisions (at 2 o'clock and 4 o'clock) into the antero-superior limb of the septal band (Fig. 26–4C). The intervening muscle is excised (Fig. 26–4D). This maneuver is important to achieve an unobstructed pathway between the left ventricle and the aorta. Interrupted horizontal mattress sutures, reinforced with Teflon pledgets, are placed first along the posteroinferior rim of the defect in a manner similar to the technique used for closure of a malaligned VSD in tetralogy of Fallot (Fig. 26–4E). Additional interrupted stitches are then placed within the remaining circumference of the pathway from the left ventricle to the aortic valve. A baffle is then tailored from a tubular Dacron conduit (retaining approximately 50% of the circumference of the conduit), measuring the distance from the enlarged VSD to the aortic valve rim (Fig. 26–4F). The sutures placed along the anterior border of the VSD and the posteroinferior aspect of the ventricular defect are first threaded through the Dacron baffle and then tied in place (Fig. 26–4G). This partial fixation of the baffle offers the opportunity for adjustments in its length or width. The remainder of the sutures are then passed through the Dacron patch and tied (Fig. 26–4H). The Dacron baffle should contribute approximately 50% to the circumference of the pathway from the left ventricle to the ascending aorta, the remainder being composed of the patient's own tissue. Next, either the aortic or the pulmonary valve homograft is prepared to cover the distance between the distal main and proximal left pulmonary artery and the right ventriculotomy. To avoid extrinsic compression of the homograft, the conduit is aligned along the left heart border; the left mediastinal pleura is opened to gain additional space for the conduit. After doubly ligating the main pulmonary artery proximally (Fig. 26–4I), the distal conduit–to–pulmonary artery anastomosis is fashioned with a 6-0 continuous Prolene suture (Fig. 26–4J). At this point the aortic crossclamp is removed. During rewarming, the anastomosis between the right ventricle and the homograft is begun at the most distal part of the ventriculotomy incision and is extended to include approximately 50% of the circumference of the proximal homograft stoma (Fig. 26–4K). At that point, the glutaraldehyde-preserved pericardial patch is sewn to the remaining part of the right ventriculotomy and to the free edge of the proximal homograft (Fig. 26–4L). This technique eliminates kinking of the anastomosis and ensures unobstructed flow through the homograft. After the air is vented and effective cardiac action has re-

sumed, the infant is weaned from cardiopulmonary bypass. Catheters are routinely placed in the left and right atria and also in the transhomograft pulmonary artery for postoperative monitoring.

Atrial Inversion Operation

Although there are few circumstances in which an arterial switch operation cannot be carried out, there are, as discussed earlier, a few occasions when an arterial switch is not possible and a physiologic repair becomes necessary. Because of a higher incidence, in our experience, of late caval obstructions when the Mustard operation is performed in neonates and young infants, we prefer a modified Senning technique in the very young.

Senning Operation

Deep hypothermic circulatory arrest is used by preference for all neonates and young infants. After a median sternotomy, cardiopulmonary bypass is instituted by cannulating the aorta and placing a single venous cannula through the right atrial appendage. At 18°C rectal temperature, the aorta is crossclamped, cardioplegic solution is infused, and cardiopulmonary bypass is stopped. The right atrial cannula is removed, and the right atrium is opened approximately 5 mm anterior and parallel to the sulcus terminalis; cephalad, the incision is curved slightly anterior toward the atrial appendage (Fig. 26–5A). Through the open right atrium, both the crista terminalis and the eustachian valve are identified, and the atrial incision is extended toward both of these landmarks (Fig. 26–5B). A large atrial communication is made. Most patients already have a large ASD (after a balloon atrial septostomy); therefore, resection of only the limbic portion of the atrial septum is required (Fig. 26–5C).

The roof of the pulmonary-venous pathway is fashioned by suturing a properly tailored Gore-Tex patch, starting above the entrance sites of the left pulmonary veins, then along a line leading to the posterolateral angle of both the superior and inferior venae cavae, and then to the remnant of the atrial septum or the interatrial groove (Fig. 26–5D). The incision into the left atrium is then extended into the right superior pulmonary vein and toward the back wall of the left atrium inferiorly to create as large a pulmonary venous outlet as possible (Fig. 26–5E). The lateral right atrial wall flap is sutured at its superior angle around and over the orifice of the superior vena cava until it reaches the midpoint of the intervalvar septal remnant (Fig. 26–5F). Inferiorly, the roof of the vena caval pathway is

Text continued on page 430

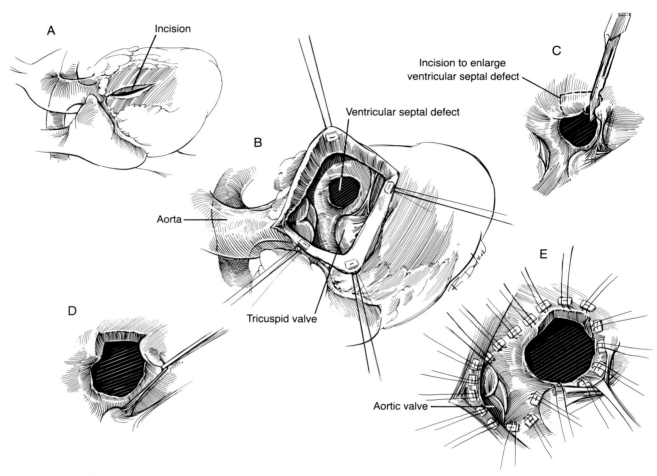

FIGURE 26–4. ☐

Rastelli repair for D-TGA with a ventricular septal defect (VSD) and left ventricular outflow tract obstruction (LVOTO). *A,* On cardiopulmonary bypass, and after crossclamping the ascending aorta, the right ventricle is entered through a vertical incision. *B,* Exposure of ventricular septal defect, tricuspid valve, and aortic valve. *C,* Enlargement of the VSD by incising the anterosuperior limb of the septal band. *D,* Excision of the intervening muscle. *E,* Interrupted horizontal mattress sutures reinforced with Teflon pledgets are placed around the anterosuperior and posteroinferior borders of the VSD and within the remaining circumference of the pathway between the left ventricle and the aorta. A baffle tailored from a tubular Dacron graft *(F)* is sutured first to the anterior and posteroinferior aspects of the pathway to allow adjustments in either length or width of the baffle *(G).* *H,* Baffle in place. *I,* Double ligation of the proximal main pulmonary artery and incision into the main and left pulmonary arteries. *J,* Anastomosis of the distal homograft to the pulmonary incision. *K,* Anastomosis of the proximal homograft to the right ventriculotomy. Only 50% of the circumference of the proximal homograft stoma is sewn directly to the ventriculotomy. *L,* A pericardial hood sewn to the remaining part of the right ventriculotomy and the free edge of the proximal homograft.

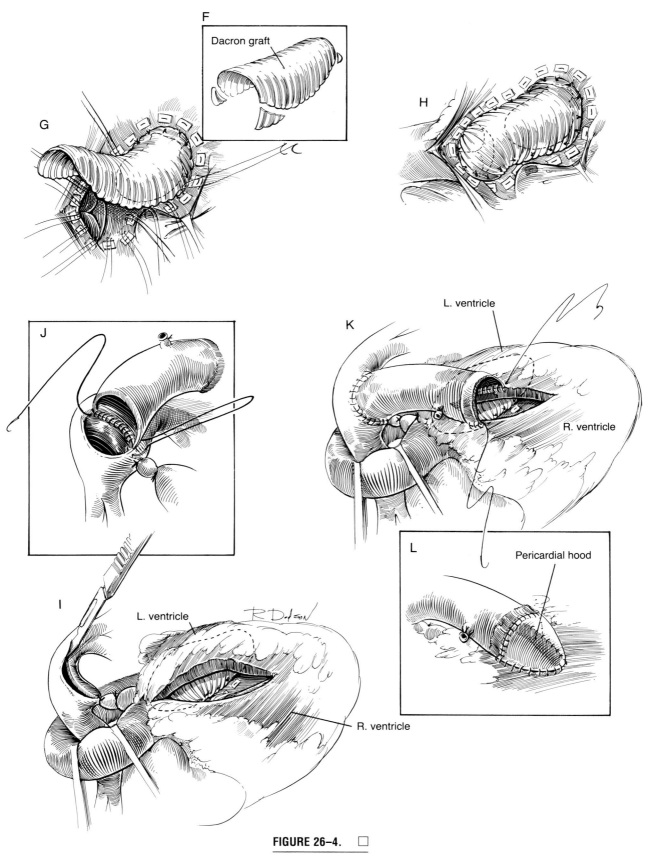

See legend on opposite page

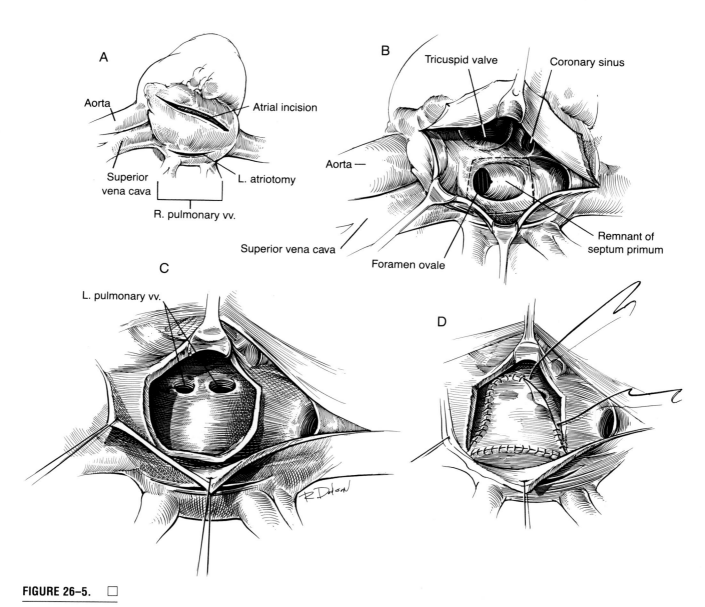

FIGURE 26–5. ☐

Modified Senning operation for D-transposition of the great arteries with an intact ventricular septum. *A*, Right and left atrial incisions. *B*, Inside view of the right atrium. Note the remnant of septum primum after balloon atrial septotomy. *C*, Excised septum primum with exposure of left pulmonary vein entrance site. *D*, Construction of the roof of the pulmonary venous pathway. A Gore-Tex patch is sutured above the entrance site of the left pulmonary veins and along the line leading to the posterolateral angle of both the superior and inferior venae cavae and the remnant of the interatrial groove.

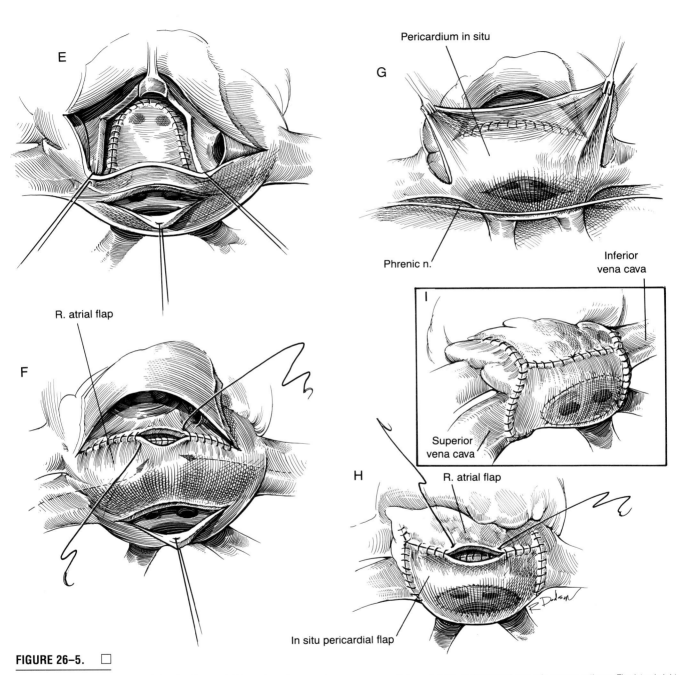

FIGURE 26–5. □

Continued. E, The incision into the left atrium is extended to create as large a pulmonary venous outlet as possible. *F,* Completed systemic venous pathway. The lateral right atrial wall flap is sutured around the superior and inferior venae cavae and along the ligament of Todaro. The coronary sinus is left to drain into the neo–left atrium. *G,* Construction of the pulmonary venous pathway. The pericardial flap in situ is sutured first around the superior and inferior venae cavae and the right atrial wall. Then the free edge of the medial right atrial flap is sutured to the free edge of the pericardium *(H* and *I).*

constructed by continuously suturing the lateral right atrial wall flap to the free edge of the eustachian valve (if present and firm) or, otherwise, around the orifice of the inferior vena cava and then along the tendon of Todaro until meeting the superior suture line. The coronary sinus is left to drain into the neo–left atrium.

Once the caval pathway is completed, the pulmonary venous pathway is constructed. In some patients, it is possible to primarily suture the free edge of the remaining medial right atrial flap around the superior and inferior venae cavae and onto the free edge of the incision in the right pulmonary vein. However, if there is any doubt as to whether the size of the atrial flap will create undue tension or obstruction of either the systemic or pulmonary venous pathway, we prefer to augment the pulmonary venous pathway by interposing a free patch of pericardium or Gore-Tex, or, preferentially, by using pericardium *in situ* (Fig. 26–5G). Using a continuous 5-0 Prolene suture, the pericardium *in situ* is sutured first to the triangle where the pericardial reflection meets the junction between the superior vena cava and the right atrium and also the most cephalad portion of the left atrial incision (Fig. 26–5H). The suture line then attaches the pericardium around the superior vena cava and right atrium, taking shallow bites to avoid damaging the sinoatrial node. Similarly, the pericardium *in situ* is attached along the junction of the inferior vena cava and the right atrium. Finally, the free edge of the medial right atrial flap is sutured to the pericardium, allowing ample space for pulmonary venous blood to pass from the pulmonary veins through the tricuspid valve and into the right ventricle (Fig. 26–5I). It is important also to visualize the right phrenic nerve to avoid injury. For rewarming on cardiopulmonary bypass, the venous cannula is repositioned through the "right" atrial appendage into what has become at this point the functional left atrium. Sufficient venous return indicates unobstructed systemic and pulmonary venous pathways, while an inadequate venous return demands that any possible obstruction within either the systemic or pulmonary venous pathways be identified and repaired at this point.

RESULTS OF THE ARTERIAL SWITCH OPERATION

From January 1983 through December 1992, 500 patients underwent the arterial switch operation at the Children's Hospital in Boston for D-transposition of the great arteries. In 294 patients (58.8%), the ventricular septum was intact; the remaining

206 (41.2%) had VSDs (this included 14 patients with double-outlet right ventricle and subpulmonary VSDs). Of the 294 patients with an intact ventricular septum, 262 (89.6%) had a primary repair, while 30 (9.6%) had a rapid two-stage repair; three patients (1.0%) had had a previous Blalock-Taussig shunt, and two (0.8%) had had a previous coarctation repair. Of the 206 patients with VSDs, 150 (74.5%) underwent a primary arterial switch operation with closure of the VSD; of these 150 patients, three (2.1%) underwent simultaneous repair of an interrupted aortic arch, and 12 (8.5%) underwent coarctation repair. Before the arterial switch operation and closure of the VSD, 11 patients (7.8%) had had coarctation repair, 19 (13.4%) had had coarctation repair and pulmonary artery banding, and another 11 patients (7.8%) had had a pulmonary artery band placed. Another five patients (3.5%) had had early pulmonary artery banding followed by a Blalock-Taussig shunt, and two patients (1.4%) had had a rapid two-stage arterial switch operation. Preoperative findings included a left superior vena cava in seven patients, a straddling mitral valve in three, a straddling tricuspid valve in one, dextrocardia in two, coronary fistula in one, an aberrant right subclavian artery in one, and a double aortic arch in one. There was also necrotizing enterocolitis in four patients and a tracheoesophageal fistula in one.

Hospital and Late Mortality

The overall hospital mortality rate for the arterial switch operation was 5.2% (26/500). In patients considered at higher risk—which includes those with multiple VSDs, coarctation or interruption of the aortic arch, abnormalities of the atrioventricular valves, or unusual coronary artery patterns—the hospital mortality rate was 10.8% (18/166), while in the low-risk group—those with intact ventricular septum, single VSD, normal aortic arch, normal atrioventricular valves, and type 1 or 2 coronary arteries—the hospital mortality rate was 2.4% (8/334). In fact, in the subgroup of patients with D-TGA and IVS or D-TGA and VSD, the hospital mortality rate was reduced to 0.5% among the last 208 consecutive patients operated on between 1989 and 1992 (Table 26–1).

Fifteen of the 26 hospital deaths were due to inadequate coronary blood flow; all 15 patients died either in the operating room or within the first 24 hours after surgery. Usually, coronary-related hospital death is more likely to occur in patients with a single right coronary artery, an intramural left coronary artery, or inverted coronary arteries. Early in our experience the arterial switch operation was

TABLE 26–1. □ HOSPITAL AND LATE MORTALITY AFTER THE ARTERIAL SWITCH OPERATION FOR D-TGA, JANUARY 1983 TO DECEMBER 1992

	NO. OF PATIENTS	HOSPITAL DEATHS (%)	LATE DEATHS (%)	TOTAL (%)
Low risk, 1983–1992	334	8 (2.4)	3 (0.9)	11 (3.2)
1989–1992 subset	208	1 (0.5)	0	1 (0.5)
High risk	166	18 (10.8)	7 (4.2)	25 (15.0)
TOTAL	500	26 (5.2)	10 (2.0)	36 (7.2)

abandoned and a Senning operation done instead in seven of 28 patients (25%) with the above mentioned complex coronary artery abnormalities.[33] However, because these less common coronary artery patterns occur more frequently in patients with an associated VSD and because the long-term results of the atrial inversion operations in patients with D-TGA and VSD have been poor, we have become much more aggressive in our treatment and have found that with more experience in handling the more complex coronary patterns, we have improved our results; the number of aborted arterial switch operations has decreased significantly—two in the last 95 patients with these complex patterns (2.1%). Deaths caused by other associated conditions are outlined in Table 26–2.

In the 475 postoperative survivors, there were 10 late deaths (2.1%) (Table 26–2). Five of these deaths were related to coronary problems, two to pulmonary vascular obstructive disease, one to aspiration, one to a residual VSD and aortic regurgitation, and one to severe aortic regurgitation after balloon valvotomy. The coronary-related late deaths occurred in one patient with a single right coronary artery, in another with a single left coronary artery, and in three patients with inverted coronary arteries. In both single right and inverted coronary arteries, the entire coronary flow to the left ventricle originated from an ostium in the rightward and posterior aspect of the neoaorta and then passed behind the neoaorta to reach the left ventricle. Conceivably, in this position, ventricular distention can either distort the ostium or narrow the artery itself. More extensive mobilization of the proximal portion of the coronary arteries may overcome some of these problems, but residual tension or injury to the wall of the artery during the dissection can also lead to diffuse narrowing of the proximal several millimeters of the coronary artery (a finding in the hearts of two of the three patients with inverted coronary arteries who died from coronary insufficiency within a few months of surgery). Analysis of long-term survival after the arterial switch operation is provided in Figures 26–6 and 26–7.

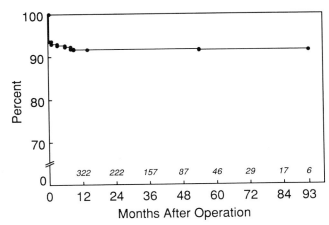

FIGURE 26–6. □

Life table (including hospital death) of all 470 patients receiving an arterial switch operation from 1983 to 1991 at Children's Hospital in Boston. The numbers below the curve represent the number of patients followed beyond that time interval.

Postoperative Hemodynamic Studies

Two hundred and forty-four of the 475 late survivors (51.3%) underwent cardiac catheterization a mean 11.9 ± 6.7 months (range, 2 to 58 months) after the arterial switch operation (Table 26–3).

The most frequent postoperative hemodynamic abnormality identified at cardiac catheterization was supravalvular pulmonary stenosis. In 22 patients the gradient exceeded 40 mm Hg at rest, and the right ventricular pressure was either systemic or suprasystemic and therefore warranted reintervention. Balloon angioplasty was successful in

TABLE 26–2. □ HOSPITAL MORTALITY AFTER THE ARTERIAL SWITCH OPERATION FOR D-TGA (*N* = 500)

CAUSES OF DEATH	INTACT VENTRICULAR SEPTUM	VENTRICULAR SEPTAL DEFECT	TOTAL (%)
Inadequate coronary blood flow	8	7	15 (3.4)
Normal CAs	3	1	
Circumflex from RCA	2	1	
Single RCA	2	2	
Intramural LCA/ADCA	1	2	
Inverted CAs	0	1	
Multiple VSDs	0	2	2 (0.6)
Left-sided obstructive lesions			3 (0.6)
Coarctation	0	2	
Interrupted aortic arch	1	0	
Hemorrhage			3 (0.85)
Mediastinal	1	1	
Pulmonary	1	0	
Left ventricle failure, noncoronary	1	0	2 (0.4)
Straddling atrioventricular valves			2 (0.4)
Mitral		1	
Tricuspid		1	
TOTAL	12	14	26 (5.2)

ADCA, Anterior descending coronary artery; CA, coronary; LCA, left coronary artery; RCA, right coronary artery.

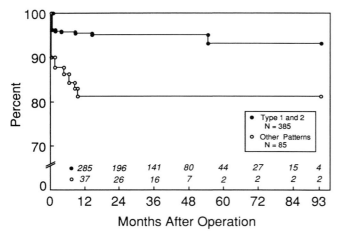

FIGURE 26–7. □

Life table (including hospital death) of all 470 patients receiving an arterial switch operation between 1983 and 1991 at Children's Hospital in Boston. The solid circles represent 385 patients with both the left anterior descending and circumflex coronary arteries originating from the left facing sinus and patients in whom the circumflex coronary artery originates from the right coronary artery (types 1 and 2). The open circles represent 85 patients with all other types of coronary artery patterns. The two rows of numbers below the curves represent the number of patients followed beyond that time interval.

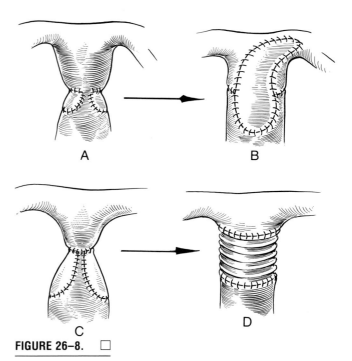

FIGURE 26–8. □

Supravalvar pulmonary stenosis. The upper panel (A, B) shows a patch plasty of a narrowed anastomotic site. In the lower panel (C, D), the narrowed anastomosis is excised, and a conduit is interposed.

seven. In 13 patients a patch plasty was carried out at the anastomotic site, while in the remaining two patients the narrowed anastomosis was excised and a conduit interposed (Fig. 26–8).[15, 16] Three mechanisms for the supravalvular pulmonary stenosis were identified: tension on the anastomosis with anteroposterior flattening of the main pulmonary artery and its branches, circumferential cicatricial narrowing at the suture line, and isolated branch stenosis. Stenosis of the pulmonary artery branches was usually amenable to balloon angioplasty. It should be noted that the incidence of supravalvar pulmonary stenosis has decreased from 16% (seven of the first 42 survivors) to 3.4% (15 of the last 433 survivors). More extensive dissection of the distal pulmonary arteries and more liberal enlargement of the coronary donor sites and anastomotic area with autologous pericardium are mostly responsible for

TABLE 26–3. □ HEMODYNAMIC FINDINGS AFTER CARDIAC CATHETERIZATION (N = 244)

	MEAN (±SD)	RANGE
Peak pressure (mm Hg)		
RV-PA	18 (16)	2–100
LV-Ao	5 (9)	0–50
Mean pressure (mm Hg)		
PA	14 (6)	9–70
RVEDP	5 (2)	1–12
LVEDP	8 (2)	4–18
Cardiac index (L/min/m²)	4.1 (1.1)	2.6–8.0

Ao, Aorta; LV, left ventricle; LVEDP, left ventricular end-diastolic pressure; PA, pulmonary artery; RV, right ventricle; RVEDP, right ventricular end-diastolic pressure.

this improvement. Supravalvar aortic stenosis was not common; only two patients had a transaortic gradient of more than 25 mm Hg, thereby requiring reoperation.

Semilunar Valve Regurgitation. Aortic root angiography revealed trivial aortic regurgitation in 20% of the patients.

Coronary Anastomosis. The proximal coronary arteries were well visualized in all patients at catheterization. Four patients were found to have proximal occlusion of the left coronary artery, but there was visible retrograde perfusion via collaterals from the right coronary system. In two of these four, the right coronary artery gave rise to the circumflex coronary artery, with a separate origin of the left anterior descending coronary from the left facing sinus. All four patients were asymptomatic, with normal electrocardiograms, ventricular end-diastolic pressures, ejection fractions, and cardiac and global indices of ventricular function at echocardiography.

Intracardiac Shunting. Residual shunts greater than 1.5/1.0 were measured at the ventricular level in four patients. Two of these required reoperation for closure of an additional VSD, and two patients had transcatheter closure of residual apical VSDs. One other patient required closure of a residual ASD, and in two others residual ASDs were closed using a transcatheter clamshell device. In all remaining patients the mean pulmonary artery saturation was 75% (range, 61% to 80%), and all had at least 95% saturation in the left ventricle or aorta. Clamshell devices were also placed under direct vision at the time of surgery in three patients with multiple or complex muscular ventricular defects.

Pulmonary Vascular Obstructive Disease. Five patients who had D-TGA with a VSD had persistent pulmonary artery hypertension and progression to pulmonary vascular obstructive disease. Their age at operation ranged from 6 to 28 months (mean, 16 months). Three of these patients had had no previous pulmonary banding to protect the pulmonary arterioles, whereas in the other two, the pulmonary artery bands proved to be ineffective at preoperative cardiac catheterization. In one patient who had D-TGA with an IVS and a large nonrestrictive PDA, pulmonary vascular obstructive disease developed despite an arterial switch operation at 7 weeks of age.

Systemic-to-Pulmonary Collaterals. In 119 patients with suitable postoperative angiographic studies at Children's Hospital in Boston, 55 (46%) had significantly enlarged bronchial collateral vessels. Five of these required coil embolization of the enlarged collateral vessels during postoperative catheterization, because after injection of contrast material in the descending thoracic aorta, there was dense opacification of lung parenchyma and return of contrast to the left atrium.[49] Each of the five had an intact ventricular septum, was seen in early infancy, and had a preoperative balloon atrial septostomy. In four of these five infants, the enlarged bronchial collaterals were not suspected before angiography, although three had continuous murmurs in the infrascapular region. In the majority of patients, flow through these bronchial collaterals is trivial to mild; however, the presence of cardiomegaly, continuous murmurs, prompt visualization of the pulmonary veins and the left atrium after contrast injection into the aorta or left ventricle, elevated left ventricular end-diastolic pressure, and pulmonary artery hypertension may indicate significant flow into the pulmonary vascular bed. In such cases, embolization of these vessels seems indicated. Why these bronchial collaterals persist after repair of transposition of the great arteries, particularly after an arterial switch operation in the neonatal period, remains unexplained.

Echocardiographic Examination. Left ventricular dimensions; wall thickness; wall stress; and indices of afterload, preload, contractility, and early diastolic function, as well as regional wall motion, were determined by echocardiographic methods. Patients evaluated as late as 4 years after repair were found to have normal regional wall motion with no evidence of regional dysfunction as might be seen with regional ischemia. Ventricular size, wall thickness, systolic function, afterload, preload, contractility, and early diastolic function were also normal.[18]

Mild mitral regurgitation was diagnosed in one patient and moderate aortic and pulmonary regurgitation in two. Trivial aortic regurgitation was common, seen in 58.9% of patients.[27]

Arrhythmias and Conduction Disturbances. Sinus rhythm (normal P-wave rate and axis) was present in 98% of patients on their most recent electrocardiograms or Holter records. Electrophysiologic studies on 114 patients revealed normal sinus node recovery times in 96%. The A-H and H-V intervals and atrioventricular node response to rapid atrial pacing were also normal in all patients. Five patients who had D-TGA with a VSD had permanent postoperative complete heart block (2.5%).

RESULTS OF THE RAPID TWO-STAGE ARTERIAL SWITCH OPERATION

Between January 1987 and December 1991, 29 patients underwent a preparatory procedure, including banding of the pulmonary artery and a modified right Blalock-Taussig shunt. A balloon atrial septostomy had been performed during the neonatal period in 28 of the 29. Two had also had blade atrial septostomies. One neonate had had a coarctation repaired when his body weight was 1600 gm. The mean age was 4.9 ± 4.1 months (median, 3.3; range, 0.8 to 18.9). The mean weight was 5.5 ± 1.9 kg (median, 5.0; range, 3.0 to 11.3). At the preparatory procedure a pulmonary artery band was placed in each patient; one also had an atrial septectomy. In 26 patients, a right subclavian pulmonary shunt was placed simultaneously; in two patients, urgent shunting was required 12 to 18 hours after pulmonary artery banding because of severe progressive hypoxemia.

There was one death after the preparatory procedure. This was a child (one of twins), born at term weighing 1600 gm, who had D-TGA, multiple small VSDs, and a severe coarctation. Balloon atrial septostomy and coarctation repair were performed in the neonatal period. In the ensuing 7 months, the weight reached 4.3 kg, but the multiple VSDs had almost completely closed, and left ventricular pressure had decreased to 50% of systemic pressure. Severe stenosis of the left pulmonary veins was also noted at catheterization. After pulmonary artery banding and shunt placement, progressive tachycardia, oliguria, and metabolic acidosis developed over the ensuing 6 hours, associated with an arterial oxygen saturation of 92% to 95%. A sudden episode of bradycardia and hypotension occurred, and the child died despite prolonged resuscitative efforts which included the takedown of both the band and the shunt in the intensive care unit. Autopsy revealed nearly complete occlusion of the left pulmonary veins and no residual coarctation.

One other child required emergency takedown of the pulmonary artery band and the shunt. After the preparatory operation, in the intensive care unit, the oxygen saturation was 93%. Nevertheless, the child became oliguric and acidotic 12 hours after the operation. After a cardiac arrest, followed by successful resuscitation (which included the emergency shunt and band takedown in the intensive care unit), the child recovered. Within days the pulmonary artery band and shunt were replaced. Subsequently the child had a successful arterial switch operation.

Eighteen of 28 patients required inotropic support, mostly dopamine (5 to 10 μg/kg/min); six of the patients needed additional epinephrine. The echocardiographically determined left ventricular ejection fraction before the preparatory procedure averaged 77% ± 11% and decreased to 55% ± 19% on the first postoperative day, while before the arterial switch, left ventricular ejection fraction had again increased to 73% ± 14%. The left ventricular mass index increased from a prepreparatory average of 46 ± 17 gm/m² (range, 24 to 87 gm/m²) to 72 ± 23 gm/m² (range, 36 to 122 gm/m²) before the arterial switch ($P < .001$).

Cardiac catheterization performed at a median of 6 days after pulmonary artery banding and shunting revealed a mean left ventricle–to–right ventricle pressure ratio of 98% ± 19% compared with a value of 48% ± 8% before the pulmonary artery banding.

Two of the 28 patients who received the rapid two-stage arterial switch operation died. In one child, thrombi associated with an indwelling central venous catheter were identified in the inferior vena cava, after the preparatory procedure. At the cardiac catheterization before the arterial switch, this patient had the lowest left ventricular–to–right ventricular pressure ratio of the entire group (54%). Sudden bradycardia associated with an acutely elevated left atrial pressure developed 36 hours after the arterial switch operation and was followed by cardiac arrest. The patient could not be resuscitated. At autopsy the coronary and great vessel anastomoses were widely patent. A large antemortem thrombus, lodged within the ductal diverticulum, extended into the aortic arch and descending thoracic aorta. No other cause of death could be determined. The second child who died after the arterial switch procedure developed severe pneumonia after the preparatory procedure, with profound cyanosis and poorly compliant lungs. He was difficult to ventilate on weaning from cardiopulmonary bypass and also had suprasystemic pulmonary artery pressures and continued hypoxemia. Despite extracorporeal membrane oxygenation instituted 9 hours after surgery, there was progressive clinical deterioration, and the child died.

In all of the other children, the second-stage arterial switch operation was well tolerated. The mean hospital stay after the operation was 12 ± 5 days.

The combination of acute right ventricular volume overload (from the shunt) and acute left ventricular pressure load (from the pulmonary artery band) may result in biventricular dysfunction and low systemic cardiac output after the preparatory operation for D-TGA with low left ventricular pressure. In addition, the patients are still hypoxemic after this procedure. Therefore, as opposed to most other cardiac operations, the patient's postoperative condition is frequently more precarious than the preoperative state. Consequently, an initial low cardiac output should be anticipated, especially when the patient has a relatively high oxygen saturation or metabolic acidosis after the preparatory procedure. Systemic cardiac output must be augmented, and the metabolic acidosis must be treated.[51] It is important to provide adequate ventilation and oxygen carrying capacity to maintain sufficient ventricular filling pressure, and if shunt flow is high, measures must be taken to increase pulmonary vascular resistance. It may be necessary to surgically decrease the size of the shunt if these maneuvers prove inadequate.

Comments

At this time it is still premature to categorically assert that the arterial switch operation is superior to the atrial inversion operation for the treatment of D-TGA with an IVS, as the different lengths of the respective follow-up studies do not yet allow adequate comparison. It appears, however, that in the long run the risk of death is less with the arterial switch operation. The arterial switch procedure presents a single phase of rapidly declining risk, while the atrial inversion repair shows a constant hazard phase that extends indefinitely.[16, 45] This difference becomes even more impressive if the hazard function for death in a protocol of routine early arterial switch operations is compared with that in a protocol of initial balloon atrial septostomy and atrial inversion operations after 2 months of life.

The early and intermediate-term results of the arterial switch procedure have been good. The favorable intermediate echocardiographic and hemodynamic measures of left ventricular function and the electrocardiographic and electrophysiologic data showing a 98% incidence of regular sinus mechanism after the in patients with D-TGA and an IVS are likewise encouraging.[50, 52] At Children's Hospital in Boston, the hospital mortality rate has decreased with increasing experience and is currently less than 1% in patients with low-risk anatomy. Some complex coronary artery patterns, particularly the intramural variant, continue to increase the risk of the operation, but fortunately their overall incidence is relatively low, and the surgical results are improving even in this subset of patients.

The incidence of the most common postoperative complication—namely, supravalvular pulmonary stenosis—has also decreased significantly over time and is currently less than 3%. So far, the late mortality rate is also low (2%) and is mostly a result of unusual coronary artery patterns (which hopefully can be prevented by technical improvements) and to pulmonary hypertension and pulmonary vascular obstructive disease (which also should be preventable by doing the arterial switch in patients with all types of D-TGA—D-TGA with an IVS, D-TGA with a VSD, and D-TGA with an IVS and a PDA—during the neonatal period). Continued close follow-up is imperative for all patients who have had arterial switch operations until truly long-term data are available.

In patients with D-TGA and a VSD, the arterial switch operation has already proved to be significantly better than either of the atrial inversion operations. As mentioned before, we believe that no type of coronary anatomy is an absolute contraindication for the arterial switch procedure in D-TGA with a VSD. Preferably the operation is carried out within the first month of life to avoid the risk of developing early pulmonary vascular obstructive disease and the risk of spontaneous closure of the septal defect, leading to an "unprepared" left ventricle.

Because we believe that the arterial switch operation will continue to yield superior early and long-term results in comparison with the atrial inversion operations, we plan to continue with the rapid two-stage arterial switch operation for those patients beyond the safe period for a primary arterial switch (left ventricle–to–right ventricle pressure < 0.6). We feel committed to substantiating the validity of this treatment strategy and therefore plan to continue to pursue detailed and systematic postoperative studies, including cardiac catheterization, echocardiography, and collection of electrophysiologic data.

For anyone who has witnessed or participated in the earlier struggles to improve the tragic outlook for children born with transposition of the great arteries, the advancements since the 1970s have been spectacular indeed. Who would have predicted two decades ago that children born with D-TGA, with or without a VSD, could be anatomically corrected within the first few days of life at a low risk and with an excellent chance to lead an active life and, hopefully, to have a normal life expectancy?

RESULTS OF SENNING OPERATION

The results of 19 Senning operations at Children's Hospital in Boston in neonates with D-TGA and an IVS were reported in 1984.[21] Ages ranged from 2 to 24 days (mean, 12 days). The hospital mortality rate was 11% (two patients). The two patients who died in the hospital were the first in this series. The causes of early death were overwhelming sepsis (*Pseudomonas* and *Klebsiella*) in one patient and recurrent severe obstruction of the superior vena cava with thrombotic occlusion, despite extensive augmentation of the vessel, in the other. There was one late death that was caused by pulmonary venous obstruction; this was documented by cardiac catheterization and confirmed by postmortem examination.

Postoperative cardiac catheterization in the 16 survivors revealed that pulmonary venous obstruction was present in one patient 6 months after the initial surgery; he underwent a successful reoperation. Dynamic subvalvar pulmonary stenosis occurred in five patients 8 to 20 months after operation. Only one of these had a gradient greater than 45 mm Hg. Two patients had residual shunts at the atrial level; one required closure 1 year after surgery. One patient had mild tricuspid regurgitation, but there was no right ventricular dysfunction in any patient.

Postoperative Electrocardiographic Assessment

All 16 survivors had 24-hour Holter studies, and seven underwent electrophysiologic studies. Fifteen patients had normal sinus rhythm at hospital discharge and at follow-up. One patient was noted to have sinoatrial node dysfunction 28 months after surgery, documented electrophysiologically, with an increased sinus node recovery time (1700 ms) and predominant junctional rhythm on the echocardiogram.

Postoperative Clinical Follow-Up

All 16 patients have continued to do well. Growth and development are normal, and all are active, asymptomatic children. The patient with sinoatrial node dysfunction remains asymptomatic, is not taking any medication, and is without a pacemaker.

Both early and late complications in this group of neonates were related to technical difficulties and therefore should be avoidable. The only case of obstruction of the superior vena cava was severe, and the obstruction recurred despite reoperation; this infant died.

Late pulmonary venous obstruction occurred in two more patients. One of these infants has had successful reoperation followed by an uneventful late postoperative course. The other infant died before any surgical intervention could be attempted.

Comments

One of the advantages of the Senning operation over the Mustard procedure for neonates or infants is that it requires either no prosthetic material or only a very small amount of it, thereby decreasing the risk of late systemic or pulmonary venous pathway obstruction. Augmentation of the atrial septum with a small Gore-Tex patch, almost uniformly necessary in our experience because of septal deficiency caused by atrial balloon septostomy, has not resulted in any early or late complications. The use of pericardium in situ (pedicled) to augment the neo–left atrium also avoids the cicatricial narrowing of that atrium occasionally seen after the use of a free pericardial patch. Despite the relatively good results with elective Senning operations in neonates with D-TGA and an IVS (the last 17 consecutive neonates survived the operation), our experience with Senning operations in neonates after aborting a planned arterial switch operation has been much less satisfactory. The hospital mortality rate in this group was 23% (6/26 patients). Part of the explanation for this increased risk of hospital death was that 18 of the 26 patients (69.2%) had D-TGA with a VSD; 4 of the 6 deaths occurred in patients who had D-TGA with a VSD.

Although the hospital mortality rate for the Senning operation in older infants with D-TGA and a VSD had been reduced to 15% by 1982,[37] the late results continue to be disappointing. Severe late postoperative complications include significant tricuspid valve (systemic atrioventricular valve) regurgitation in approximately 30% of patients and right ventricular (systemic ventricle) failure in approximately 5%. Because of these late sequelae of atrial

switch operations, five patients have required cardiac transplantation, and another five patients have had the atrial inversion operation converted to an arterial switch operation.[17] Therefore, we believe that we must make every possible effort to perform an arterial switch operation in patients with D-TGA and a VSD, regardless of the coronary artery anatomy.

Alternative, less desirable options for children in whom the coronary arteries cannot be transferred include either a Damus-Kaye-Stansel–type repair or an Aubert operation.

RESULTS OF THE RASTELLI OPERATION

From March 1987 through December 1991, 11 infants ranging in age from 2 weeks to 11 months (median age, 4 months) underwent a Rastelli repair. Eight of the infants were male, and three were female. Four of the 11 (36.3%) had had previous modified Blalock-Taussig shunts. All patients, including the three with previous shunts, were operated on because of increasing cyanosis and hypoxemia.

One patient, who was 7 months of age at the time of operation, had a direct anastomosis of the pulmonary artery to the right ventricle. After 32 months, significant obstruction developed at the right ventricle–pulmonary artery anastomosis, which was easily corrected by a Gore-Tex patch augmentation of the area (Table 26–4). Carpentier-Edwards Dacron aortic xenografts containing conduits were used in three patients, and the remaining seven patients received cryopreserved valved aortic homografts ranging in size from 8 to 15 mm. The only patient in this group who has required reoperation had a 9-mm aortic homograft placed at 6

TABLE 26–4. ☐ RASTELLI OPERATION FOR D-TGA WITH A VSD AND LVOTO IN NEONATES AND INFANTS

AGE AT OPERATION	TYPE OF CONDUIT	SIZE OF CONDUIT (mm)	LENGTH OF FOLLOW-UP (mo)	TIME AND TYPE OF REOPERATION
2 wk	Homograft*	12	12	0
1 mo	Xenograft†	12	27	0
3 mo	Homograft	8	33	0
3 mo	Homograft	15	2	0
3 mo	Xenograft	12	19	0
6 mo	Homograft	9	32	19 mo—onlay patch plasty
7 mo	Direct RV-PA graft	—	40	32 mo— anastomotic patch plasty
8 mo	Xenograft	12	19	0
9 mo	Homograft	15	41	0
10 mo	Homograft	16	1	0
11 mo	Homograft	14	24	0

*Cryopreserved valved aortic homograft.
†Carpentier-Edwards Dacron valved xenograft.
PA, Pulmonary artery; RV, right ventricle.

months of age. Within 9 months, an 80–mm Hg right ventricle–to–homograft gradient developed; this was effectively repaired with an onlay Dacron patch 13 months after surgery.

Despite the fact that the VSD was enlarged in seven of the 11 patients (63.6%), none developed permanent complete heart block postoperatively.

The number of patients is not large, and the length of follow-up is not long enough to warrant actuarial analysis of these data. At present, most institutions recommend postponing Rastelli repair of D-TGA with a VSD and LVOTO until the patient is 4 or 5 years old. A modified Blalock-Taussig shunt (Gore-Tex interposition graft) or classic Blalock-Taussig shunt is preferred in neonates, infants, and younger children. Because of the disadvantages of systemic-to–pulmonary artery shunts (e.g., systemic ventricular volume overload and distortion of pulmonary artery branches), we have opted since 1987 to carry out a Rastelli operation instead of an initial shunt operation, regardless of patient age. In our experience the risk of either conduit replacement or patch augmentation of the conduits is extremely low. Because there have been no early or late deaths in this group of neonates and infants, and also because of the low incidence of early reoperations during a follow-up time extending up to 41 months, we intend to continue to evaluate this more aggressive policy of using the Rastelli operation in symptomatic neonates or infants who have D-TGA with a VSD and LVOTO.

Although a Rastelli operation in neonates or infants must be considered a palliative procedure (i.e., conduit replacement will eventually be necessary), this approach leads to an "in-series" circulation with normal oxygen saturation and loading conditions, unlike a palliative shunt, which leads to parallel circulation, persistent cyanosis, right ventricular volume overload, poor mixing, and the risk of pulmonary vascular obstructive disease.

REFERENCES

1. Albert HM. Surgical correction of transposition of the great arteries. Surg Forum 5:74, 1954.
2. Anagnostopoulos CE. A proposed new technique for correction of transposition of the great arteries. Ann Thorac Surg 15:565, 1973.
3. Aubert J, Pannetier A, Couvelly JP, et al. Transposition of the great arteries: New technique for anatomical correction. Br Heart J 40:204, 1978.
4. Baffes TG. A new method for surgical correction of transposition of the aorta and pulmonary artery. Surg Gynecol Obstet 102:227, 1956.
5. Baffes TG, Ketola HK, Tatooles CJ. Transfer of coronary ostia by "triangulation" in transposition of the great vessels and anomalous coronary arteries. Dis Chest 39:648, 1961.
6. Baillie M. The Morbid Anatomy of Some of the More Important Parts of the Human Body. London, Johnson and Nichol, 1797, p 38.
7. Bano-Rodrigo A, Quero-Jimenez M, Moreno-Granado F. Wall thickness of ventricular chambers in transposition of the great arteries: Surgical implications. J Thorac Cardiovasc Surg 79:592, 1980.
8. Bex JP, Lecompte Y, Baillot F, Hazan E. Anatomical correction of transposition of the great arteries. Ann Thorac Surg 29:86, 1980.
9. Blalock A, Hanlon CR. The surgical treatment of complete transposition of the aorta and the pulmonary artery. Surg Gynecol Obstet 90:1, 1950.
10. Bridges ND, Perry S, Keane JF, et al. Preoperative transcatheter closure of congenital muscular ventricular septal defects. N Engl J Med 324:1312, 1991.
11. Castaneda AR. Reoperations after arterial switch operation. In Stark J, Pacifico AD (eds). Reoperations in Cardiac Surgery. London, Springer-Verlag, 1989.
12. Castaneda AR. Management of complications related to surgery for transposition of the great arteries: Arterial switch operation. In Waldhausen JA, Orringer MB (eds). Complications in Cardiothoracic Surgery. St. Louis, Mosby-Year Book, 1991.
13. Castaneda AR, Mayer JE Jr. Neonatal repair of transposition of the great arteries. In Long WA (ed). Fetal & Neonatal Cardiology. Philadelphia, WB Saunders, 1990.
14. Castaneda AR, Mayer JE Jr, Jonas RA, et al. Transposition of the great arteries: The arterial switch operation. Cardiol Clin 7:369, 1989.
15. Castaneda AR, Norwood WI, Lang P, et al. Transposition of the great arteries and intact ventricular septum: Anatomical repair in the neonate. Ann Thorac Surg 38:438, 1984.
16. Castaneda AR, Trusler GA, Paul MH, et al. The early results of treatment of simple transposition in the current era. J Thorac Cardiovasc Surg 95:14, 1988.
17. Chang AC, Wernovsky G, Wessel DL, et al. Late right ventricular failure after Mustard/Senning repair: Surgical management and outcome. Circulation. 86(suppl II):140, 1992.
18. Colan SD, Trowitzsch E, Wernovsky G. Myocardial performance after arterial switch operation for transposition of the great arteries with intact ventricular septum. Circulation 78:132, 1988.
19. Damus PS. Letter to the editor. Ann Thorac Surg 20:724, 1975.
20. Danford DA, Huhta JC, Gutgesell HP. Left ventricular wall stress and thickness in complete transposition of the great arteries. J Thorac Cardiovasc Surg 89:610, 1985.
21. DeLeon VH, Hougen TJ, Norwood WI, et al. Results of the Senning operation for transposition of the great arteries with intact ventricular septum in neonates. Circulation 70(suppl I):21, 1984.
22. Edwards WS, Bargeron LM, Lyons C. Reposition of right pulmonary vein in transposition of the great vessels. JAMA 188:522, 1964.
23. Gittenberger-DeGroot AC, Sauer U, Oppenheimer-Dekker A, et al. Coronary arterial anatomy in transposition of the great arteries: A morphologic study. Pediatr Cardiol 4(suppl I):15, 1983.
24. Idriss FS, Goldstein IR, Grana L, et al. A new technique for complete correction of transposition of the great vessels. Circulation 24:5, 1961.
25. Izumo S, Nadal-Ginard B, Mahdavi V. Protooncogene induction and reprogramming of cardiac gene expression produced by pressure overload. Proc Natl Acad Sci 85:339, 1988.
26. Jatene AD, Fontes VF, Paulista PP, et al. Successful anatomic correction of transposition of the great vessels: A preliminary report. Arq Bras Cardiol 28:461, 1975.
27. Jenkins KJ, Hanley FL, Colan SD, et al. Function of the anatomic pulmonary valve in the systemic circulation. Circulation 84(5):173, 1991.
28. Jonas RA, Giglia TM, Sanders S, et al. Rapid, two-stage arterial switch for transposition of the great arteries and intact ventricular septum beyond the neonatal period. Circulation 80(suppl I):203, 1989.
29. Kaye MP. Anatomic correction of transposition of the great arteries. Mayo Clin Proc 50:638, 1975.

30. Lecompte Y, Zannini L, Hazan E, et al. Anatomic correction of transposition of the great arteries. A new technique without use of prosthetic conduit. J Thorac Cardiovasc Surg 82:629, 1981.

31. Lillehei CW, Varco RL. Certain physiology, pathologic and surgical features of complete transposition of the great vessels. Surgery 34:376, 1953.

32. Mayer JE, Jonas RA, Castaneda AR. Arterial switch operation for transposition of the great arteries with intact ventricular septum. J Cardiovasc Surg 1:97, 1986.

33. Mayer JE, Sanders SP, Jonas RA, et al. Coronary artery pattern and outcome of arterial switch operation for transposition of the great arteries. Circulation 82(suppl IV):139, 1990.

34. McGoon DC. Intraventricular repair of transposition of the great arteries. J Thorac Cardiovasc Surg 64:430, 1972.

35. Mustard WT. Successful two-stage correction of transposition of the great vessels. Surgery 55:469, 1964.

36. Mustard WT, Chute AL, Keith JD, et al. A surgical approach to transposition of the great vessels with extracorporeal circuit. Surgery 36:39, 1954.

37. Penkoske PA, Westerman GR, Marx GR, et al. Transposition of the great arteries and ventricular septal defect: Results with the Senning operation and closure of the ventricular septal defect in infants. Ann Thorac Surg 36:281, 1983.

38. Rashkind WJ, Miller WW. Creation of an atrial septal defect without thoracotomy: A palliative approach to complete transposition of the great arteries. JAMA 196:991, 1966.

39. Rastelli GC, Wallace RB, Ongley PA. Complete repair of transposition of the great arteries with pulmonary stenosis: A review and report of a case corrected by using a new surgical technique. Circulation 39:83, 1969.

40. Rosenthal A, Fyler DC. The effect of red cell volume reduction on pulmonary blood flow in polycythemia of cyanotic congenital heart disease. Am J Cardiol 33:410, 1974.

41. Rudolph AB. Congenital Diseases of the Heart. St. Louis, Year Book Medical, 1974.

42. Sanders SP, Mayer JE Jr, Wernovsky G, et al. The role of two-dimensional and Doppler echocardiography in the preoperative evaluation of D-transposition of the great arteries. Cardiovasc Imag 1:71, 1989.

43. Senning A. Surgical correction of transposition of the great vessels. Surgery 45:966, 1959.

44. Stansel HC Jr. A new operation for D-loop transposition of the great vessels. Ann Thorac Surg 19:565, 1975.

45. Trusler GA, Castaneda AR, Blackstone EH, et al. Current results of management in transposition of the great arteries, with special emphasis on patients with associated ventricular septal defect. J Am Coll Cardiol 10:1061, 1988.

46. Van Praagh R, Jung WK. The arterial switch operation in transposition of the great arteries: Anatomic indications and contraindications. Thorac Cardiovasc Surg 39:138, 1991.

47. Van Praagh R, Van Praagh S. Isolated ventricular inversion: A consideration of the morphogenesis, definition and diagnosis of nontransposed and transposed great arteries. Am J Cardiol 17:395, 1966.

48. Van Praagh R, Van Praagh S, Vlad P, et al. Anatomic types of congenital dextrocardia: Diagnostic and embryologic implications. Am J Cardiol 13:510, 1964.

49. Wernovsky G, Bridges ND, Mandell VS, et al. Persistent bronchial collaterals following early repair of transposition of the great arteries. J Am Coll Cardiol 21:465, 1993.

50. Wernovsky G, DiDonato RM, Lang P, et al. Early results of the arterial switch operation in 195 consecutive patients. In Parenzan L, Anderson RH (eds). Perspectives in Pediatric Cardiology. Vol 2. Mount Kisco, NY, Futura, 1989, pp 20–24.

51. Wernovsky G, Giglia TM, Jonas RA, et al. Course in the intensive care unit after "preparatory" pulmonary artery banding and aortopulmonary shunt placement for transposition of the great arteries with low left ventricular pressure. Circulation 86(suppl II):133, 1992.

52. Wernovsky G, Hougen TJ, Walsh EP, et al. Midterm results after the arterial switch operation for transposition of the great arteries with intact ventricular septum: Clinical, hemodynamic, echocardiographic and electrophysiologic data. Circulation 77:1333, 1988.

53. Wernovsky G, Jonas RA, Colan SD, et al. Results of the arterial switch operation in patients with transposition of the great arteries and abnormalities of the mitral valve or left ventricular outflow tract. J Am Coll Cardiol 16:1446, 1990.

54. Yacoub MH, Radley-Smith R, MacLaurin R. Two-stage operation for anatomical correction of transposition of the great arteries with intact interventricular septum. Lancet 1:1275, 1977.

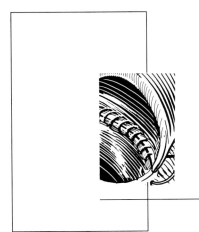

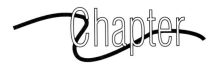

27

Chapter

Corrected Transposition of the Great Arteries

In 1875, von Rokitansky[9] first noted that transposed arteries could be "corrected by the position of the ventricular septum." Corrected transposition of the great arteries (C-TGA) has since been the most commonly used term to describe this condition in which there are both atrioventricular and ventriculoarterial discordant connections. Although C-TGA may rarely exist without other intracardiac malformations, there is a high incidence of associated intracardiac anomalies such as single ventricle, ventricular septal defect, obstruction of the pulmonary outflow tract, and anatomic regurgitation of the tricuspid valve. In addition, these patients are prone to the development of rhythm disturbances, including first-, second-, and third-degree heart block. The largest subgroup of C-TGA patients have single-ventricle anatomy (see Chapter 15). This chapter will focus on C-TGA exclusive of single-ventricle anatomy.

ANATOMY

C-TGA most often occurs with situs solitus of the atria and abdominal viscera with {S,L,L} segmental anatomy, but it also can occur in situs inversus with {I,D,D} segmental anatomy.[5] In situs solitus C-TGA, the right atrium connects through a morphologic mitral valve with a rightward and anteriorly positioned morphologic left ventricle. This finely trabeculated ventricle connects with an outflow tract and

then with a somewhat posteriorly positioned pulmonary artery. The left atrium connects through the tricuspid valve with a coarsely trabeculated right ventricle. The right ventricular outflow tract is located anteriorly and leads to a leftward-positioned aortic valve and ascending aorta (Fig. 27–1A). The outflow tracts in C-TGA are parallel, and the ventricular septum is oriented anteroposteriorly.

In C-TGA the coronary arteries are inverted; that is, the right-sided coronary artery gives rise to the anterior descending coronary artery and also to the circumflex coronary artery, which travels in the atrioventricular groove behind the right-sided mitral valve. The pattern of the left-sided coronary artery resembles that of the usual right coronary artery. The origin and distribution of this coronary artery are quite constant in this malformation.

Although ventricular septal defects can occur within all segments of the ventricular septum, they are most often conoventricular, located within the membranous portion of the septum, and commonly extend either anteriorly or inferiorly toward the atrioventricular canal. A ventricular septal defect is the most frequent associated anomaly, occurring in approximately 75% of hearts with C-TGA.

Hemodynamically significant obstruction of the pulmonary outflow tract is present in about 40% of patients with C-TGA, particularly when there is an associated ventricular septal defect. The obstruction is mostly subpulmonary and may consist of a fibro-

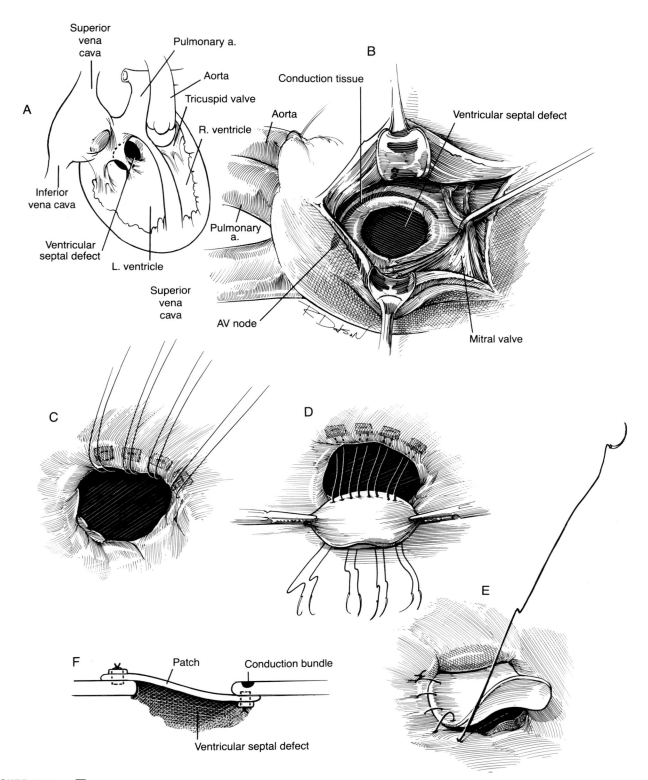

FIGURE 27–1. ☐

Congenitally corrected transposition {SLL} and ventricular septal defect. *A,* Schema of anatomic relationship in {S, L, L}. *B,* Transatrial exposure of ventricular septal defect (VSD). Note the anterior location of the AV node between the right AV valve and stoma of right atrial appendage. The conduction bundle travels near the anterior wall of the left ventricular outflow tract, just beneath the right-sided ventricular surface anterosuperiorly, the pulmonary valve, and the annulus and continues descending along the left side of the ventricular septum. Often the bundle lies subendocardially and can be seen. *C,* To avoid damage to the conduction tissue, interrupted horizontal mattress sutures reinforced with Teflon pledgets are guided through the defect and anchored approximately 4 mm from the edge of the VSD within the left-sided ventricular surface, particularly along the anterior and inferior rim of the defect. *D,* These interrupted sutures are passed through a Dacron patch. *E,* The remainder of the patch is sewn to the rim of the VSD with a continuous suture. *F,* Schematic representation of anchoring of the patch within the right ventricular surface anteriorly and on the left ventricular surface posteriorly.

muscular ridge, excrescences of endocardial cushion tissue, or, more commonly, a long, narrow, fibromuscular tunnel. Isolated pulmonary valvar stenosis is rare.

Malformations of the anatomic tricuspid valve (functional left-sided or systemic atrioventricular valve) are also common accompaniments of C-TGA. The valvular lesion frequently resembles an Ebstein deformity with short, thick chordae anchoring the septal and posterior leaflets of the tricuspid valve to the posterior ventricular wall. However, unlike in true Ebstein's anomaly, atrialization of part of the anatomic right ventricle and stenosis of the tricuspid valve are not common.

Atrioventricular Node and Conduction Bundle

In {S,L,L} C-TGA, the functional atrioventricular node arises anteriorly and superiorly and is usually lodged between the annulus of the mitral valve and the ostium of the right atrial appendage. After penetrating the fibrous triangle that produces mitral pulmonary fibrous continuity, the elongated, nonbranching portion of the atrioventricular bundle traverses the anterior wall of the anatomic left ventricular outflow tract just over the pulmonary valve annulus. It then continues subendocardially to descend within the left side of the ventricular septum, where it trifurcates into the left, anterior, posterior, and right bundle branches. When there is a membranous ventricular septal defect, the proximal conduction system is in close proximity to its anterosuperior and anteroinferior borders, unlike the usual relationship in {S,D,S} hearts, in which the proximal conduction system travels along the posteroinferior margin of the septal defect. Often there is a posterior atrioventricular node in its usual position within the triangle of Koch, but it is usually disconnected from the remainder of the conduction tissue. However, in {I,D,D} C-TGA hearts, the atrioventricular bundle arises from the posterior atrioventricular node to follow a conventional path along the posteroinferior margin of the ventricular septal defect if one is present. The conduction system in C-TGA is more tenuous than that of normal hearts. Fibrosis of the junction between the atrioventricular node and the atrioventricular bundle has been related to the high incidence of spontaneously occurring complete heart block in patients with this anomaly.

SURGICAL HISTORY

After von Rokitansky's first report in 1875[9] and Monckeberg's description in 1913[8] of the anteriorly positioned atrioventricular node, the next most surgically relevant report on C-TGA came in 1957 when Anderson and colleagues[1] described the clinical, radiologic, electrocardiographic, and cardiac catheterization features of this syndrome and reviewed their surgical experience with 10 patients with C-TGA and suggested, among other things, closure of the ventricular septal defect through the right atrium and mitral valve. deLeval et al.[7] added an important technical innovation designed to avoid damaging the conduction tissue during closure of the ventricular septal defect. Although isolated reports of the differences in the conduction system in patients with {S,L,L} C-TGA had been published before, much is owed to Lev and Anderson and their colleagues, who substantiated and carefully documented the position of the anteriorly located atrioventricular node and the anterosuperior trajectory of the conduction bundle.[2, 3, 6] Later, Dick and associates,[4] through intraoperative mapping, further outlined the anatomy of the conduction system in cases of {I,D,D} C-TGA.

CLINICAL FEATURES AND DIAGNOSIS

Unlike the conventional isolated ventricular septal defect, C-TGA with a ventricular septal defect only rarely causes symptoms during the first year of life. The reason for this difference is not entirely clear; one explanation is that these patients have additional mild functional or organic subpulmonary stenosis. In our experience with C-TGA since the early 1980s at Children's Hospital in Boston, it has been equally unusual to find a neonate or infant with C-TGA and subpulmonary stenosis sufficiently severe to warrant operation. It is much more common for symptoms of congestive heart failure, pulmonary stenosis, or incompetence of the left-sided atrioventricular valve to become manifest after the first few years of life. Often the diagnosis of C-TGA is first suggested by a chest radiograph that reveals the typically leftward-positioned ascending aorta.

Echocardiography

In general, the diagnosis of C-TGA can be made with echocardiography. Subxiphoid and long-axis views with Doppler color flow mapping add importantly to qualitative and quantitative analysis of atrioventricular valve function and aid in locating and quantitating left ventricular outflow gradients, as well as in anatomically defining ventricular septal defects and measuring pulmonary flow velocities. Cardiac catheterization is indicated only if the degree of pulmonary hypertension or pulmonary vascular resistance is in question or if visualization of possible distortions of peripheral pulmonary arteries secondary to previous shunt operations is desired.

SURGICAL CONSIDERATIONS

As mentioned previously, repair of lesions associated with C-TGA (i.e., closure of a ventricular septal defect, bypass of significant subpulmonary stenosis, or repair or replacement of an insufficient tricuspid valve) is rare in infancy. Since the early 1980s, only one neonate and one infant with C-TGA, a ventricular septal defect, and subpulmonary stenosis and one other infant with C-TGA and an isolated ventricular septal defect have been referred to Children's Hospital in Boston for repair. Whether this truly represents the limited need for reparative surgery in this age group or instead reflects long-held concerns about a high incidence of permanent complete heart block and its sequelae after reparative surgery is not clear at this time.

Closure of Ventricular Septal Defects in C-TGA {S,L,L}

Ventricular septal defects associated with C-TGA offer a special problem. Although conal septal defects, atrioventricular canal defects, or muscular defects (single or multiple) may coexist with {S,L,L} C-TGA, by far the most common ventricular septal defect in this condition is the malalignment type of conoventricular defect in which the pulmonary valve overrides the septum, arising partially over the anatomic right ventricle. If viewed through the right-sided ventricle (anatomic left ventricle), the conoventricular septal defect tends to extend posterior to the septal leaflet of the mitral valve. It is limited anteriorly and inferiorly by the infundibular and muscular interventricular septum and superiorly by the pulmonary valve annulus. Commonly, the posteroinferior edge is contiguous with the mitral valve annulus, forming part of the pulmonary, mitral, and tricuspid fibrous continuity. When viewed through the left-sided ventricle (anatomic right ventricle), the conoventricular septal defect is rimmed characteristically by the superior and inferior limbs of the septal band and the conal septum above. However, from a surgical point of view, the important differences between L-loop and D-loop transposition are the origin of the atrioventricular node and the course pursued by the atrioventricular bundle and its branches. As mentioned previously,

the atrioventricular bundle arises from the anteriorly positioned atrioventricular node and travels along the right-sided anatomic left ventricular surface, anterosuperiorly over the pulmonary valve annulus and the left-sided ventricular septum. The ventricular septal defect can best be approached either through the aortic valve (which permits placement of sutures into the anatomic "right" ventricular surface, thereby avoiding the conduction bundle) or through the right atrium and right-sided atrioventricular valve. Figure 27–1B depicts transatrial closure of the ventricular septal defect as recommended by deLeval and associates.[7] After the septal leaflet of the mitral valve is retracted, the conoventricular septal defect can be easily identified. To avoid damage to the conduction bundles, interrupted horizontal mattress sutures, reinforced with Teflon pledgets, are guided through the septal defect and anchored approximately 4 mm from the edge of the defect within the left-sided anatomic right ventricular surface, particularly along its superior and anterior rim (Fig. 27–1C, D). The remainder of the patch is sutured to the right-sided surface of the ventricular septal defect (Fig. 27–1E, F).

When the aortic annulus is sufficiently large to allow exposure of the ventricular septal defect—as is common when it is associated with pulmonary stenosis or pulmonary atresia—we prefer to close conoventricular defects in L-loop hearts through the aorta, placing all sutures directly on the left side of the infundibular and ventricular septum and surrounding the ventricular septal defect, away from the right-sided conduction tissue.

Use of Valved Extracardiac Conduits in {S,L,L} C-TGA With Subpulmonary Stenosis

When subpulmonary stenosis exists as an isolated lesion, or if it coexists with a ventricular septal defect, a valved extracardiac conduit is usually necessary to effectively eliminate the subpulmonary obstruction unless there is a resectable obstructing excrescence of endocardial cushion tissue. Otherwise, attempts at direct relief of subpulmonary stenosis by obstructing muscle are contraindicated because of (1) the risk of causing permanent heart block and (2) inadequate relief of the obstruction. The use of allograft conduits has been described in Chapter 6. The only special feature related to the use of an allograft in C-TGA is that when the left ventriculotomy is made, injury to the papillary muscles must be avoided. We prefer to explore the left ventricular free wall digitally through the mitral valve. This maneuver allows direct location of the papillary muscles and selection of a safe area for the ventriculotomy. Also, to avoid compression of the conduit by the sternum, the right pleura should be opened to permit the conduit to curve toward the right, away from the undersurface of the sternum.

Rhythm Disturbances in C-TGA

Perhaps the most common clinical features that may demand attention in patients with C-TGA during the neonatal period or infancy are disturbances of rhythm. First-, second- or third-degree heart block is common. If permanent, complete, third-degree heart block is present, whether spontaneous or iatrogenic, permanent pacing is indicated. Complete atrioventricular block has occurred during cardiac catheterization or after placement of a Blalock-Taussig shunt, which suggests that intraoperative or postoperative complete atrioventricular block can result from a mechanism unrelated to closure of the ventricular septal defect itself. For these patients, we prefer a DDD-mode atrioventricular sequential pacemaker that can sense both atrial and ventricular depolarization and also initiate or inhibit a pacing impulse. This pacemaker mode tends to improve both cardiac output and left atrioventricular valve function. There is a suggestion that complete atrioventricular block may accentuate tricuspid valve regurgitation in patients who have {S,L,L} TGA with an Ebstein-like deformity of the left atrioventricular valve. Because complete atrioventricular block results in a fixed heart rate, cardiac output varies mostly as a result of changes in stroke volume. Conceivably, increased left ventricular volume caused by a slow, fixed heart rate may render the marginally compensated, abnormal atrioventricular valve incompetent.

RESULTS OF REPARATIVE OPERATIONS FOR C-TGA IN NEONATES AND INFANTS

Since the early 1980s, only three patients (one neonate and two infants) have undergone repair of C-TGA at Children's Hospital in Boston. The first patient was a 3-day old neonate with severe hypoxemia who underwent successful transaortic closure of a ventricular septal defect and interposition of a nonvalved 6-mm Gore-Tex conduit. At 13 months of age, this child required patch augmentation of the previous conduit and distal anastomosis. The second patient was 1 year old and had a ventricular septal defect with significant obstruction of the left ventricular outflow tract. This patient, who also underwent transaortic closure of the ventricular

septal defect and interposition of a 14-mm valved aortic allograft, remained in regular sinus rhythm and was alive and well 3 years after the operation. The third patient, who was 5 months old, had C-TGA with a large conoventricular ventricular septal defect. Cardiac catheterization revealed systemic pressures in the pulmonary artery and a QP/QS ratio of greater than 3:1. The conoventricular septal defect was closed through the right atrium and mitral valve. The patient remained in regular sinus rhythm and continued to do well 6 years after the operation.

SUMMARY

C-TGA is a complex malformation. Surgical indications are related to associated lesions such as ventricular septal defect, subpulmonary stenosis, left atrioventricular valve regurgitation, and permanent third-degree atrioventricular block. Repair of the associated intracardiac lesions during the neonatal period or infancy has been undertaken only rarely in the past. However, a clearer understanding of the atrioventricular conduction system has led us to be more aggressive and to recommend primary repair of C-TGA with a ventricular septal defect and subpulmonary stenosis during infancy. So far, our limited experience with only three infants who had this constellation of defects has been encouraging. Neonates or young infants with significant tricuspid (left atrioventricular valve) regurgitation, severe subpulmonary stenosis, or hypoplasia of the systemic right ventricle and an unrestrictive ventricular septal defect require either a cardiac transplant or a Norwood operation, as is used for the hypoplastic left heart syndrome. In older infants and children, a primary or staged Fontan approach may be preferable.

REFERENCES

1. Anderson RC, Lillehei CW, Lester RG. Corrected transposition of the great vessels of the heart. Pediatrics 20:626, 1957.
2. Anderson RH, Arnold R, Wilkinson JL. The conduction tissue in congenitally corrected transposition. Lancet 1:1286, 1973.
3. Anderson RH, Becker AE, Arnold R, et al. The conducting tissues in congenitally corrected transposition. Circulation 50:911, 1974.
4. Dick M, Van Praagh R, Rudd M, et al. Electrophysiological delineation of the specialized atrioventricular conduction system in two patients with corrected transposition of the great arteries with situs inversus {I,D,D}. Circulation 55:896, 1977.
5. DiDonato RM, Wernovsky G, Jonas RA, et al. Corrected transposition in situs inversus: Biventricular repair of associated cardiac anomalies. Circulation 84(suppl III):193, 1991.
6. Lev M, Fielding RT, Zaeske D. Mixed levocardia with ventricular inversion (corrected transposition) with complete A-V block. Am J Cardiol 12:875, 1963.

7. de Leval MR, Bastos P, Stark J, et al. Surgical technique to reduce the risks of heart block following closure of ventricular septal defects in atrioventricular discordance. J Thorac Cardiovasc Surg 78:515, 1979.

8. Monckeberg JG. Zur Entwicklungsgeschichte des Atrioventrikularsystems. Verh Dtsch Pathol 16:228, 1913.

9. von Rokitansky CF. Die Defekte der Scheidewande des Herzens. Vienna, Wilhelm Braumuller, 1875.

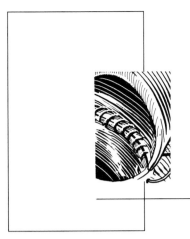

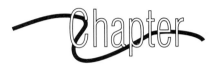

28

Chapter

Double-Outlet Right Ventricle

Whereas the majority of congenital heart anomalies consist of a wide quantitative spectrum of severity (e.g., the hypoplastic left heart syndrome ranges from critical neonatal aortic valve stenosis to aortic atresia with mitral atresia), double-outlet right ventricle (DORV) spans a wide qualitative spectrum of pathophysiology from tetralogy of Fallot to transposition of the great arteries. Surgical management is completely different at the two ends of the spectrum, because physiologically and anatomically, the tetralogy and transposition ends of the DORV spectrum *are* completely different. However, the nomenclature currently used to classify DORV fails to easily distinguish the two surgically relevant ends of the spectrum.

There are some types of DORV in which both ventricles are adequate to allow biventricular repair, but DORV may also be associated with severe underdevelopment of the left ventricle. In these circumstances, a single ventricle/Fontan pathway must be pursued. This is a particularly common cardiac anomaly in patients with heterotaxia and asplenia who have a common atrioventricular valve and transposed great arteries. DORV is also seen in conjunction with mitral atresia; in this setting the great vessels are usually normally related. Single-ventricle forms of DORV are discussed in detail in Chapter 15.

PATHOLOGIC ANATOMY

Defined simply, DORV is an anomaly in which both great vessels arise from the right ventricle. However, to some extent this is also true of tetralogy of Fallot, as, by definition, the tetralogy includes override of at least some of the aorta over the right ventricle. Thus, how can tetralogy of Fallot and DORV be differentiated? Once again, a simple definition would be that in DORV, at least 50% of the aortic annulus overlies the right ventricle. For the surgeon this is probably as practically relevant as any definition, although in view of the curved nature of the ventricular septum and the presence of the subaortic ventricular septal defect that accompanies DORV at the tetralogy end of the spectrum, whether the aortic override is 40% or 60% may not be entirely clear. Pathologists have argued that the distinction between tetralogy of Fallot and DORV can be made by the presence of aortic-to-mitral fibrous continuity in tetralogy of Fallot and its absence (and, therefore, the presence of a subaortic conus) at the tetralogy end of the DORV spectrum. This is not something a surgeon can determine with the usual surgical exposure for DORV. Furthermore, in view of the variable length of the subaortic fibrosa, even in a normal heart, definition of the fibrous continuity by two-dimensional echocardiogra-

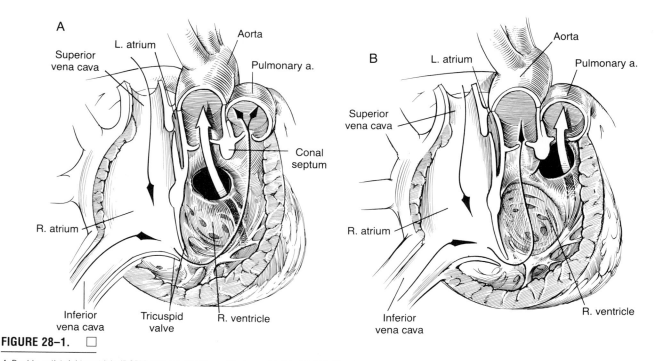

FIGURE 28-1. ☐

A, Double-outlet right ventricle (DORV) with a subaortic ventricular septal defect (VSD). Flow from the left ventricle preferentially enters the aorta. This is similar to what occurs in tetralogy of Fallot. *B,* DORV with a subpulmonary VSD. Left ventricular blood preferentially enters the pulmonary artery, resulting in physiology similar to that seen in transposition of the great arteries.

phy or angiography is only slightly more precise than assessment of the percentage of override by the surgeon. In any event, the definition is of little relevance to the surgical procedure, which is essentially the same for both tetralogy of Fallot and the tetralogy form of DORV, regardless of the terminology used. Nevertheless, the definition is relevant when the results of surgery for DORV are analyzed.

At the transposition end of the DORV spectrum, the aorta completely arises from the right ventricle, and the same problem regarding definition must be contemplated for the degree of override of the pulmonary artery over the left ventricle. If more than 50% of the pulmonary artery arises from the left ventricle, then by the "50% rule," this is transposition and not DORV. Alternatively, fibrous continuity between the pulmonary valve and the mitral valve can also serve to distinguish transposition from DORV.

Classification of DORV by Anatomy of the Ventricular Septal Defect

DORV is virtually always associated with a ventricular septal defect. The classic pathologic classification of DORV centers on the location of the ventricular septal defect relative to the great vessels.[10] Although this is of some relevance to the surgeon, it

does not focus on the critical anatomic features that determine the type of surgical procedure to select. Lev et al.[10] classified the ventricular septal defects associated with DORV as subaortic, subpulmonary, doubly committed, or noncommitted (Fig. 28–1). The anatomy and physiology of the DORV patient with a subaortic ventricular septal defect are likely to be similar to those of the patient with tetralogy of Fallot, who is also likely to have a *subaortic* ventricular septal defect (i.e., the ventricular septal defect is positioned immediately below the aortic valve). At the tetralogy end of the DORV spectrum, there is no subaortic conus, so the superior margin of the ventricular septal defect is the aortic annulus itself (Fig. 28–2). Moving through the spectrum of DORV toward transposition, there is progressive development of the subaortic conus so that the aortic valve moves cephalad, away from the ventricular septal defect, and the pulmonary valve becomes more intimately associated with the ventricular septal defect. Therefore, at the transposition end of the spectrum, the ventricular septal defect is usually *subpulmonary*. Although this definition was originally designed as an anatomic definition, it probably more accurately serves as a physiologic definition in that left ventricular blood is directed to the aorta after passing through a subaortic ventricular septal defect (i.e., pulmonary artery saturation will be lower than aortic saturation), while left ventricular

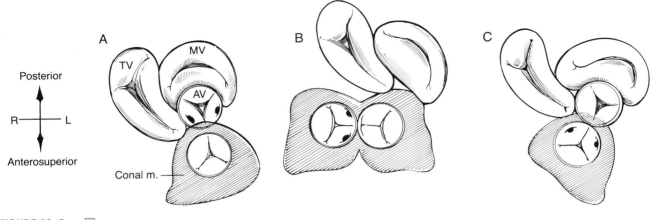

FIGURE 28–2. ☐

The spectrum of conus development between the tetralogy and transposition ends of the DORV spectrum. *A,* In tetralogy of Fallot, there is a subpulmonary conus with fibrous continuity between the aortic and mitral valve. *B,* In the middle of the DORV spectrum, there are both subpulmonary and subaortic coni. *C,* At the transposition end of the DORV spectrum, there is a subaortic conus with fibrous continuity between the pulmonary and mitral valves. In all diagrams, the aortic valve is indicated by the coronary ostia, the tricuspid valve by three leaflets, and the mitral leaflets by two leaflets; hatching indicates conal myocardium. AV, Aortic valve; MV, mitral valve; TV, tricuspid valve.

blood is directed to the pulmonary artery by a sub-pulmonary ventricular septal defect (i.e., pulmonary artery saturation will be higher than aortic saturation, as in transposition).

At the midpoint of the spectrum, a ventricular septal defect may appear to be equally committed to both the aorta and the pulmonary artery; this can be termed a *doubly committed* ventricular septal defect. As already stated, this does not help the surgeon determine the type of repair. Although this term implies that the surgeon might reasonably choose to use either a tetralogy or transposition type of repair, it is highly unlikely that the two forms of repair would be equally satisfactory.

Any ventricular septal defect that is not situated either within the conal septum (subpulmonary) or at the junction of the conal and muscular interventricular septa (conoventricular or subaortic) is likely to be so remote from the aorta that it will be difficult, if not impossible, to direct left ventricular blood to the aorta. Lev et al. termed such ventricular septal defects *noncommitted.* They frequently occur in the inlet septum (atrioventricular canal type); therefore, the surgeon must deal not only with the distance separating the aorta from the ventricular septal defect, but also with the problem of negotiating a left ventricular baffle pathway around multiple tricuspid valve chordae. Midmuscular and apical muscular ventricular septal defects are also included in the category of noncommitted defects.

Anatomic Determinants of Method of Repair

Despite the definition problems encountered at both ends of the DORV spectrum, the transition from DORV to transposition, like the transition from tetralogy to DORV, does not interfere with the choice of surgical technique of repair. However, within the DORV spectrum, there are points of transition in surgical technique. As stated previously, the type of ventricular septal defect does not help the surgeon select the optimal method of repair. The judgment as to which type of repair is best in a specific anatomic situation constitutes the fundamental complexity of the surgical management of DORV.

Separation of Pulmonary and Tricuspid Valves (Fig. 28–3). As one progresses from tetralogy into DORV, the repair is identical, whether 49% or 51% of the aorta overlies the right ventricle. The repair is *intraventricular* (i.e., entirely within the right ventricle); a baffle is constructed that creates a pathway from the left ventricle to the aorta, and the right ventricular outflow tract passes around the left ventricular baffle, but within the right ventricle.[13] Farther into the spectrum, the aorta lies ever farther from the left ventricle as it moves cephalad, carried by the subaortic conus. This alone does not exclude an intraventricular repair, although a longer tunnel baffle must be constructed, but there is an associated anatomic shift that eventually precludes an intraventricular repair. As the aortic valve moves superiorly from the tricuspid valve, the pulmonary valve moves ever closer to the tricuspid valve. Because both the tricuspid and pulmonary valves must, by definition, be within the right ventricle if there is to be an intraventricular repair, and because the baffle pathway from the left ventricle to the aorta must pass *between* the tricuspid and pulmonary valves, there is a point of transition where

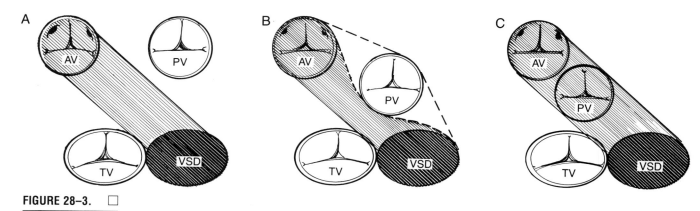

FIGURE 28–3. ☐

Separation between the tricuspid and pulmonary valves is critical in determining anatomic suitability for an intraventricular baffle repair. *A,* There is adequate separation of the pulmonary and tricuspid valves so that the pathway from the VSD to the aorta is unobstructed. *B,* The separation of the tricuspid and pulmonary valve is less than the diameter of the aortic annulus. An intraventricular repair is highly likely to result in subaortic stenosis either immediately or postoperatively. *C,* When the pulmonary valve is very close to the tricuspid valve, a Rastelli repair must be performed. The pulmonary valve lies within the baffle pathway, necessitating division and oversewing of the main pulmonary artery. AV, Aortic valve; PV, pulmonary valve; TV, tricuspid valve; VSD, ventricular septal defect.

the tricuspid-to-pulmonary distance is significantly less than the diameter of the aortic annulus. Beyond this point, more than 50% of the pathway from the left ventricle to the aorta is made up of the baffle, and although a satisfactory initial result can be achieved, there is a risk that the growth potential with such a repair will be insufficient. Late subaortic tunnel stenosis of the baffle is a difficult problem that should be strenuously avoided.

Prominence of the Conal Septum. The length of the conal septum is largely determined by the degree of development of the subaortic conus, although it is also influenced by the development of the subpulmonary conus. If the ventricular septal defect is more leftward and anterior (i.e., more a subpulmonary than a subaortic ventricular septal defect), it will be necessary for the baffle pathway to follow a longer course around the inferior margin of the conal septum to reach the aortic annulus. A prominent conal septum, per se, does not exclude a tunnel repair, because it may be resected (Fig. 28–4) as long as there are not important chordal attachments of the mitral valve (tricuspid chordae may be detached and reattached). However, a long conal septum may be associated with a shorter distance between the tricuspid and pulmonary valves, and this may exclude intraventricular repair. A long conal septum—and, therefore, a long subaortic conus—may be associated with subaortic stenosis, which in turn is often associated with hypoplasia of the aortic arch and coarctation.[18]

Presence of Subpulmonary Stenosis. At the tetralogy end of the DORV spectrum, there is commonly some degree of subpulmonary stenosis. Intraventricular repair must include relief of this stenosis, usually by division of hypertrophied extensions of the septal and parietal bands, as well as by place-

ment of an infundibular outflow patch and, if necessary for pulmonary annular hypoplasia, a transannular patch. As one progresses toward the middle of the spectrum, there is less likely to be severe subpulmonary stenosis, although the left ventricular baffle pathway will protrude to some extent into the right ventricular outflow tract, necessitating at least an infundibular outflow patch in the right ventricle to prevent iatrogenic obstruction of the right ventricle outflow tract.

When an intraventricular repair is no longer possible because of the proximity of the pulmonary valve to the tricuspid valve, and when there is important hypoplasia of the pulmonary annulus, a repair similar to the Rastelli repair for transposition (see Chapter 26) must be undertaken. The baffle pathway passes around the pulmonary annulus, which is incorporated within the left ventricular pathway. The main pulmonary artery must be divided, and a conduit is placed from the right ventricle to the distal divided main pulmonary artery.

If there is no important subpulmonary or pulmonary annular hypoplasia and the distance between the pulmonary and tricuspid valves excludes an intraventricular repair, an arterial switch procedure should be performed, regardless of the relationship of the great vessels to one another (i.e., whether side by side or more anteroposterior) and regardless of coronary artery anatomy.

Coronary Artery Anatomy. There is an important difference between the coronary artery anatomy of tetralogy and that of transposition. In transposition, the left main coronary artery and the left anterior descending coronary artery usually pass anterior to the pulmonary root. Conversely, in tetralogy, the left anterior descending coronary usually passes posterior to the pulmonary artery. The

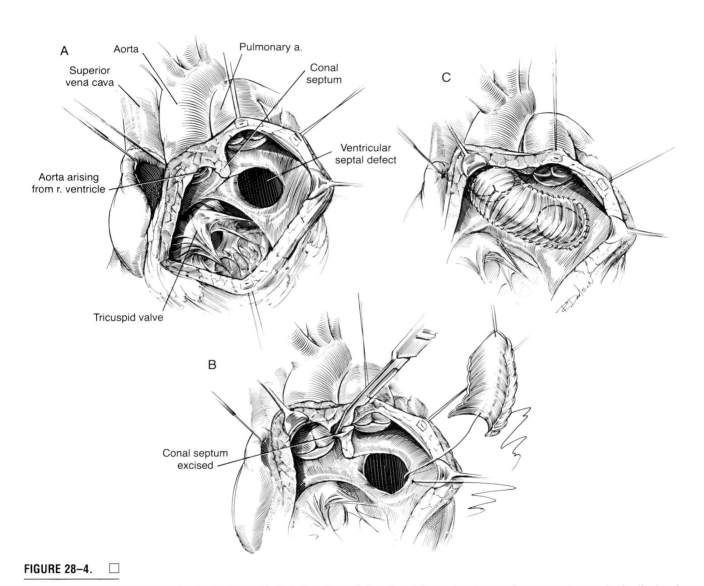

FIGURE 28–4. □

A, A prominent conal septum may project into the intraventricular baffle pathway. *B,* Resection of the conal septum may be necessary to prevent subaortic stenosis. *C,* Completion of intraventricular repair with a baffle.

presence of a left anterior descending coronary anterior to the pulmonary outflow will generally exclude an intraventricular repair without a conduit, and in any event, it is likely to signify that the defect is closer to the transposition end of the spectrum and that either an arterial switch (if there is no subpulmonary or pulmonary annular hypoplasia) or a Rastelli procedure should be selected.

The Taussig-Bing Anomaly

The term *Taussig-Bing* DORV is applied in at least two different ways and therefore may be confusing. When applied in a physiologic sense, it is a broad term that covers any form of DORV that is physiologically similar to transposition (i.e., the saturation is higher in the pulmonary artery than in the aorta because of a preferential flow pattern from the left ventricle to the pulmonary artery). If used in an anatomic sense, the term *Taussig-Bing* is restricted by most authors to a more limited entity that is similar to that originally described by Taussig and Bing in 1949.[19] Van Praagh summarized the anatomic definition in 1968.[20] Subaortic and subpulmonary coni separate both the aortic and the pulmonary valves from the atrioventricular valves. The semilunar valves lie side by side and are at the same height. There is a large subpulmonary ventricular septal defect above the septal band and the muscular ventricular septum. The ventricular septal defect, although subpulmonary, is not confluent with the pulmonary valve, the defect being somewhat separated from the valve by the subpulmonary conal free wall. There is a "true" DORV, in that the aorta arises entirely above the right ventricle, while the pulmonary valve overrides the ventricular septum but does not override the left ventricular cavity.

PATHOPHYSIOLOGY

At the tetralogy end of the DORV spectrum, patient physiology is similar to that in tetralogy. If there is only a mild degree of obstruction in the right ventricular outflow tract, there may be a left-to-right shunt, as in "pink tetralogy." If there is severe, fixed pulmonary stenosis, there will be a consistent right-to-left shunt, and the child may be severely cyanosed. Infundibular stenosis raises the possibility of intermittent, severe obstruction of the right ventricular outflow tract, causing spells similar to those seen with tetralogy.

Of course, at the transposition end of the DORV spectrum, patient physiology resembles that in transposition (i.e., there are two parallel circula-

tions, and the systemic saturation is determined by the degree of mixing between these circulations). Because there is almost always a nonrestrictive ventricular septal defect, the systemic arterial oxygen saturation is usually not a problem unless there is associated pulmonary stenosis. The presence of subaortic stenosis or coarctation will exacerbate the elevated pulmonary blood flow.

Just as for transposition with a nonrestrictive ventricular septal defect, there is a significant risk at the transposition end of the DORV spectrum of accelerated development of pulmonary vascular disease during the first year of life. At the tetralogy end of the spectrum, the degree of subpulmonary stenosis will determine the risk of pulmonary vascular disease, which will clearly be low if the degree of obstruction is severe.

PREOPERATIVE EVALUATION

The type of symptoms and the age at which they appear are largely determined by the degree of pulmonary stenosis. In most cases it will be evident that the child has a congenital heart anomaly during the neonatal period. Echocardiography can almost always provide adequate diagnostic information in the neonate and young infant.[17] Only in the older infant or young child may catheterization be necessary to exclude the presence of pulmonary vascular disease. At the transposition end of the spectrum, it may be useful to undertake a balloon atrial septostomy preoperatively to improve mixing and, therefore, the oxygen saturation and stability of the child. Also, intraoperative management of the child with transposition physiology is made easier if a preoperative balloon septostomy has been performed, as described in Chapter 7. The atrial septal defect allows decompression of the left side of the heart by placement of a single venous cannula in the right atrium; this provides a surgical field free from left heart return if the procedure is performed with continuous, low-flow hypothermic bypass.

Preoperative studies should accurately determine the surgically relevant features that have already been described. At the tetralogy end of the spectrum, the separation of the pulmonary valve from the tricuspid valve must be measured relative to the diameter of the aortic annulus. The location of the ventricular septal defect, including the degree of development of the conal septum, should be determined. Chordal attachments to the conal septum should be visualized, and the degree of subpulmonary and pulmonary stenosis should be assessed. A judgment should be made as to whether the subpulmonary stenosis might be dynamic rather than fixed. Coronary anatomy should be defined (by echocardiography), and the relative sizes of the great vessels and their relationship (whether side by side or anteroposterior) should be determined. The aortic arch should be inspected for the presence of hypoplasia or coarctation. Of course, preoperative studies should also exclude associated anomalies such as multiple ventricular septal defects and atrioventricular valve anomalies.

MEDICAL MANAGEMENT

If pulmonary stenosis is minimal so that pulmonary blood flow is increased, it may be useful to begin giving the child decongestive medication and digoxin. However, there seems little point in aggressively pursuing medical therapy when surgical repair can be effectively undertaken early in infancy (see "Indications for Surgery").

SURGICAL MANAGEMENT

History

Repair of a DORV with a subaortic ventricular septal defect (tetralogy type) was first described by Kirklin and associates in 1957[8] and shortly thereafter by Barratt-Boyes and coworkers.[1] For some time the transposition end of the DORV spectrum was confused with transposition; therefore, it is difficult to determine when the first repairs of this anomaly were undertaken. Early reports include those by Kirklin, Kawashima, and Patrick and their associates.[5, 7, 14] More recent contributors to the understanding of the surgical management of DORV are Pacifico and Sakata and their colleagues.[13, 16]

Indications for Surgery

Because DORV does not resolve spontaneously, the diagnosis is sufficient indication for surgery. The usual arguments regarding the timing of surgery can be applied and have been described in detail in Chapters 13 and 26. Currently we prefer to undertake repair during the neonatal period, regardless of the specific form of DORV. This also applies in situations where a conduit will be necessary—as, for example, when there is pulmonary annular hypoplasia and an intraventricular repair is not feasible. A systemic-to-pulmonary shunt is a reasonable alternative, although it does not reduce the total number of operations that will be necessary, and it does impose a period of abnormal physiology that

has been demonstrated, in some circumstances, to prejudice the quality of the final outcome.[2]

Technical Considerations

Intraventricular Repair of Tetralogy-to–Mid-Spectrum DORV. The general setup and approach to this form of DORV are the same as those used for tetralogy of Fallot. After a median sternotomy, a patch of anterior pericardium is harvested and treated with 0.6% glutaraldehyde solution for 20 to 30 minutes. Either circulatory arrest or continuous bypass may be selected, although for more complex intraventricular baffles, it is generally wise to use continuous bypass to avoid an excessively long period of circulatory arrest. After application of the aortic crossclamp and administration of cardioplegic solution, an infundibular incision is made. As in tetralogy, great care is taken to preserve as many coronary arteries as possible. Often, there is a long conal coronary artery that may reach well toward the apex of the heart. With a carefully planned incision, this may be preserved.

The relationship of the aortic annulus to the ventricular septal defect is carefully defined, and the length of the conal septum is assessed with respect to both the aortic and pulmonary valves. The presence of tricuspid chordal attachments to the conal septum is noted. The anatomy of the subpulmonary stenosis is also defined. Usually, excision of the conal septum helps to relieve the subpulmonary stenosis to some degree. If there are chordal attachments, these may be reattached to the patch on the ventricular septal defect at a later time. Close to the tetralogy end of the spectrum, simple division of the septal and parietal extensions of the conal septum will relieve subpulmonary stenosis when performed with subsequent placement of an infundibular outflow patch. Until reaching the mid-point of the DORV spectrum, there should be a sufficient distance separating the pulmonary and tricuspid valves to allow a tunnel repair to be constructed.

Sutures are placed around the circumference of the baffle pathway using the standard pledgetted, horizontal mattress technique that we generally prefer in neonates and infants. In older children the circumference of the baffle is so great that it is generally impractical to use all interrupted sutures, and a continuous suture technique is necessary. In infants the friability of the muscle may result in an unacceptable incidence of residual ventricular septal defect if a continuous suture technique is used, and in any event, the circumference is very much shorter than in the older child.

Although a flat patch of knitted Dacron velour is

used when the ventricular septal defect is closely related to the aortic annulus, consideration should be give to the use of a synthetic tube graft rather than a flat patch on the part of the circumference where the patch becomes more of a tunnel (Fig. 28–5). Particular care must be taken at the mid-point of the baffle tunnel to ensure that a "waist" is not created where the pulmonary valve begins to approach the tricuspid valve. Care must also be taken at the site of excision of the conal septum, where lack of the endocardium may increase the risk that sutures will tear out of the raw muscle surface.

As is the case with closure of the anterior, malalignment ventricular septal defect of tetralogy, great care should be taken with the placement of sutures as one passes around the aortic annulus. Muscle trabeculations often extend up to the annulus, creating "ridges and valleys." Failure to place sutures virtually in the annulus (taking great care not to injure the leaflets) may result in a residual ventricular septal defect through the "valleys."

Relief of subpulmonary stenosis is largely achieved by division of the septal and parietal extensions of the conal septum with or without excision of the conal septum itself. The ventricular incision should virtually never be closed by direct suture, as such closure will necessarily consume some of the circumference of the right ventricular outflow tract. A patch of pericardium is used to close the incision, employing a continuous Prolene suture. If the pulmonary annulus is too small, it may be necessary to place a transannular patch. The decision process used for DORV is the same as that used for tetralogy (see Chapter 13).

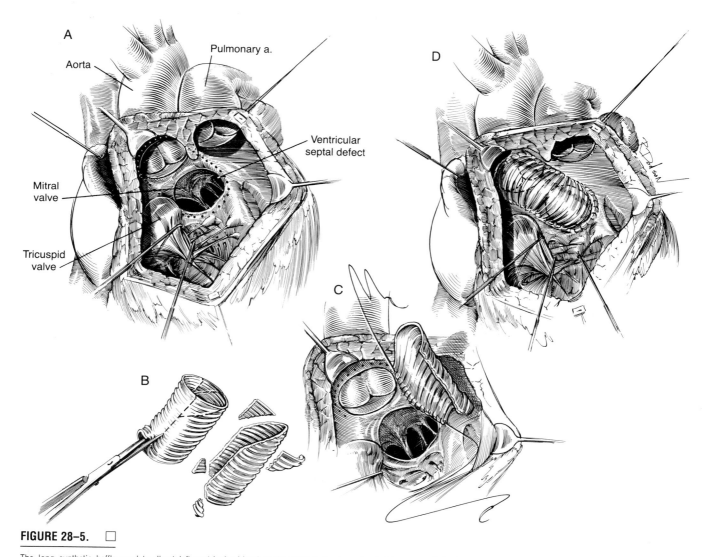

FIGURE 28–5. □

The long synthetic baffle used to direct left ventricular blood to the aorta is best constructed from a partial tube graft. *A,* The suture line is indicated by a dotted line. *B,* Tailoring of the baffle from a tube graft. *C,* A continuous suture technique may be necessary for a very long baffle. *D,* Completion of intraventricular baffle repair of tetralogy type DORV.

The Rastelli Repair and Réparation à l'Étage Ventriculaire

Subpulmonary Stenosis and Inadequate Pulmonary-to–Tricuspid Valve Separation.

When the pulmonary valve is so close to the tricuspid valve that there is a significant risk that either early or late subaortic stenosis may be created within a tunnel repair, it is necessary to place the baffle over both the pulmonary and aortic valves, as described by Rastelli[15] for transposition with a ventricular septal defect and pulmonary stenosis (Fig. 28–6). The main pulmonary artery should be divided (not ligated) and may be connected to the right ventricle using either a pulmonary or aortic allograft conduit (Rastelli repair).

An alternative to the use of an allograft or synthetic conduit for the Rastelli type of repair is wide mobilization of the pulmonary arteries, as for the arterial switch repair, followed by direct suture of the main pulmonary artery to the right ventriculotomy. This technique was first described by the French group from Hôpital Laénnec, Paris,[3] and has been termed *Réparation à l'étage ventriculaire* (REV). Anteriorly the repair is completed by placement of a generous patch of pericardium (Fig. 28–

7). To achieve the Lecompte maneuver as part of the REV repair, it is necessary to divide the ascending aorta. The aorta is reconstituted by direct anastomosis with continuous polydioxanone sutures. When the great arteries are related directly anterior and posterior, it is useful to bring both pulmonary artery branches anterior to the aorta, as described by Lecompte et al.[9] If this is not done, either the right or the left pulmonary artery must traverse an excessively long course around the aorta, depending on whether the main pulmonary artery is brought around the left side or the right side of the aorta once the aorta has been moved posteriorly. The advantage of the Lecompte maneuver—less distance that the pulmonary artery branch must reach—is considerable for anteroposterior great arteries, being at least

$$\pi/2 \times \text{aortic diameter.}$$

When the great vessels take up a more side-by-side relationship (as one moves from the transposition end of the DORV spectrum toward the tetralogy end), the advantage of the Lecompte maneuver decreases, but it is probably still useful until the aorta

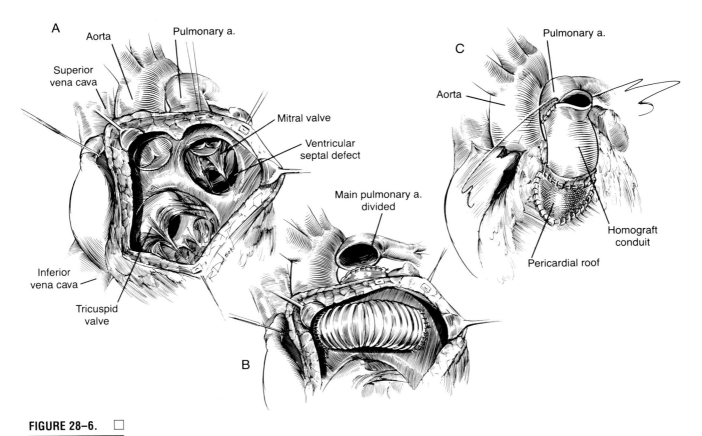

FIGURE 28–6. □

A, Taussig-Bing type of DORV with subpulmonary stenosis necessitating repair by the Rastelli technique. *B,* Main pulmonary artery is divided and oversewn proximally. The pulmonary valve lies within the baffle pathway. *C,* Completion of the Rastelli repair with a right ventricle–to–pulmonary artery allograft conduit.

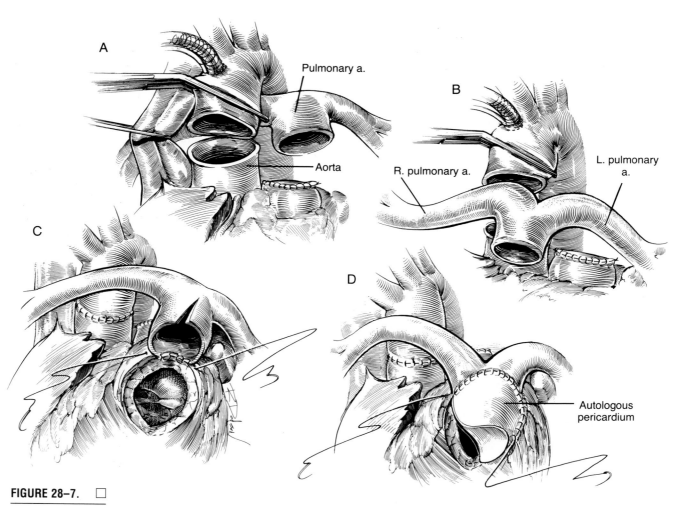

FIGURE 28–7. ☐

The REV procedure. *A*, Division of the ascending aorta and main pulmonary artery and overscoring of the proximal pulmonary artery. *B*, Anterior translocation of the distal pulmonary arteries. *C*, Direct suture of the mobilized distal main pulmonary artery to a right ventricular infundibular incision. *D*, Completion of the anastomosis of the pulmonary artery to the right ventricle with a generous roof of autologous pericardium.

lies in a plane posterior to the main pulmonary artery. It is not possible to establish a rule as to when to apply the Lecompte maneuver, because not only are the pulmonary arteries being translocated in an anteroposterior direction, but there is also translocation in a superoinferior plane onto the anterior right ventricular free wall. The amount of superoin

%exferior movement necessary will be determined by the development of the right ventricular infundibulum, as well as the distribution of the coronary arteries, which will determine the location of the right ventriculotomy. In addition, careful consideration must be given to the relationship of the anterior coronary artery (usually the right coronary artery as it arises from the aorta) to the main pulmonary artery. Because the pulmonary artery will be under some degree of tension, it must not lie directly on the coronary artery, as this may cause unacceptable compression. In a report of 40 cases of REV by Vouhe et al.,[21] the mortality rate was 12.5%, highlighting the additional risks that may be inherent in this procedure.

Coronary Artery Anterior to the Infundibulum. If the anterior descending coronary artery passes across the infundibulum at its narrowest point, this may also present a contraindication to the standard intraventricular repair without a conduit. The right ventricular incision must be placed lower in the right ventricular free wall. Continuity between the right ventricle and the pulmonary arteries is generally established by the placement of a conduit—preferably an aortic allograft, as a pulmonary allograft is unlikely to be sufficiently long. The REV procedure usually is not feasible in this setting because of the long distance separating the ventriculotomy from the pulmonary arteries. In addition, the severe tension that would result from the distance required for translocation might cause serious compression of the anteriorly placed coronary.

Aortic Translocation (Nikaidoh Procedure). An operation that we have had no experience with but that has been described in the setting of DORV or transposition with pulmonary stenosis, including pulmonary annular hypoplasia, is aortic translocation with reconstruction of the right ventricular outflow tract.[12] The aortic root, including the aortic valve, is excised from the right ventricular outflow tract in a manner analogous to that applied for the pulmonary autograft operation. In addition, it is necessary to mobilize the coronary arteries, as is done for an arterial switch procedure. The pulmonary root is divided at the level of the pulmonary valve, which is excised. The conal septum is excised, thereby removing the superior margin of the ventricular septal defect. The aortic root is translocated posteriorly so that it lies primarily over the left ven-

tricle. The ventricular septal defect is closed with a patch, which is anchored to the aortic root at its superior margin. The pulmonary artery is connected to the right ventriculotomy with an anterior patch of pericardium. No large series using this procedure have been reported, so its practicability remains to be determined. Nevertheless, with increasing experience with the arterial switch and the pulmonary autograft aortic root operations, the necessary steps will be familiar to surgeons who contemplate using this innovative procedure.

Arterial Switch and Atrial Inversion Procedures. In view of the almost constant association of DORV with a ventricular septal defect, as well as the known poor results of atrial inversion procedures such as the Senning and Mustard operations when combined with ventricular septal defect closure (see Chapter 26), it is highly unlikely that circumstances could arise in which an atrial inversion procedure would be indicated for the management of DORV. In contrast to the poor results achieved with atrial inversion procedures, excellent results have been achieved with the arterial switch procedure for DORV, although many institutions experienced a learning curve in translating this procedure to the specific anatomic requirements of DORV.[11]

An arterial switch procedure is indicated at the transposition end of the DORV spectrum when there is little or no pulmonary or subpulmonary stenosis. It may be possible to resect muscular or fibrous tissue from the subpulmonary region as long as there are no important chordal or direct attachments of the mitral valve to the narrow area, thereby allowing an arterial switch even when moderate subpulmonary stenosis is present. Similarly, a bicuspid pulmonary valve should not be considered an absolute contraindication to an arterial switch, particularly if the alternative procedures carry significant short-term or long-term risks, such as a high early and late mortality risk for the atrial inversion or the lesser quality of life dictated by the use of a conduit.[22]

The general principles of the arterial switch operation for DORV are identical to those employed in the operation for transposition. The procedure is generally performed using low-flow hypothermic bypass for the extracardiac portion of the procedure while the intracardiac steps (i.e., closure of the atrial and ventricular septal defects) are conveniently performed during a period of circulatory arrest, which can be kept to less than 45 minutes. Division of the great arteries is followed by inspection of the pulmonary valve and left ventricular outflow tract to ensure that there is no important outflow tract obstruction that might increase the risks from an arterial switch. Coronary mobilization and transfer are performed, followed by the aortic anastomosis. It is preferable not to undertake closure of the intracardiac communications before these steps are taken, as they will allow venting of left heart return to the single right atrial cannula. The single cannula is preferred to two caval cannulae for the same reason, as well as for the improved exposure provided by one cannula as compared with two.

The ventricular septal defect may be approached through the anterior semilunar valve, through the right atrium, or through a right ventriculotomy, as determined by the specific anatomic situation. Often there is some element of subaortic narrowing, so a right ventricular infundibular incision serves a dual purpose: access for closure of the ventricular septal defect and access for placement of an infundibular outflow patch to relieve outflow tract obstruction. Approach through the semilunar valve or ventriculotomy often allows continuation of bypass throughout closure of the ventricular septal defect. The atrial septal defect is closed through a short, low, right atriotomy, with the left heart filled with saline to exclude air before tying the suture.

With bypass re-established, the aortic crossclamp is released. Perfusion of all areas of the myocardium is checked. A single large pericardial patch is used to reconstruct the coronary donor areas, although to obtain optimal exposure, this step may be performed before the intracardiac steps. It is important that the pericardial patch actually supplement the neopulmonary artery (i.e., the patch needs to be quite a bit larger than the excised coronary buttons, because the aorta is frequently somewhat smaller than the pulmonary artery, particularly if there is a long and somewhat narrow subaortic conus). The pulmonary anastomosis is fashioned, and the patient is weaned from bypass.

Variations of the Arterial Switch Operation for DORV

Coronary Patterns. Unusual coronary patterns are much more common with side-by-side great arteries than in standard transposition with anteroposterior great arteries. A common pattern is an anterior origin of the right and left anterior descending coronary arteries from a single ostium, with the circumflex originating from a posterior facing sinus. Extensive mobilization of the right coronary is necessary to prevent tethering of the anterior coronary, which must be transferred directly away from the line of the right coronary. Conal and right ventricular free wall branches of the right and anterior descending coronaries should be extensively mobilized from their epicardial beds to prevent tension on the arteries and on the anastomosis. On occasion, we have used an autologous pericardial tube extension of the coronary artery to avoid excessive tension. Excessive tension will be manifested by persistent bleeding from the coronary anastomosis and early or late coronary insufficiency. Another common coronary pattern with side-by-side great arteries is origin of the right and circumflex coronaries from the posterior sinus, with the left anterior descending artery originating from the anterior-facing sinus. As will be discussed later (see "Pulmonary Artery Anastomosis"), it is important to guard against compression of the anteriorly transferred coronary by the posterior wall of the main pulmonary artery.

Closure of the Ventricular Septal Defect. Exposure of the ventricular septal defect associated with DORV may present special difficulties. The defect may be quite leftward and anterior in what almost appears, from the surgeon's perspective, to be a separate, leftward, blind-ending infundibular recess. Exposure through the anterior semilunar valve and right atrium is particularly difficult, and even through a right ventriculotomy it may not be easy. Although exposure may be achieved through the original pulmonary valve, this is usually not recommended because of the risk of damage to the conduction system and the neoaortic valve. An additional complication to ventricular septal defect closure in this setting is the tendency for the very leftward ventricular septal defect to extend into the anterior trabeculated septum—that is, there appears to be no clear leftward and anterior margin to the defect. By taking large bites with pledgetted sutures, the size of any residual ventricular septal defect can be minimized. Catheter-delivered devices have been useful for ultimate closure of residual ventricular septal defects in this area.[4]

Multiple Ventricular Septal Defects. Surgical closure of multiple muscular ventricular septal defects as well as of the large subpulmonary ventricular septal defect may be difficult and may consume an excessive amount of circulatory arrest time. One approach to this problem is intraoperative delivery of a double-clamshell device.[6] After division of the two great vessels, an excellent view is obtained of both sides of the ventricular septum. The sheath loaded with the device is introduced through the right atrium and tricuspid valve into the right ventricle. A right-angled instrument is passed through the original pulmonary valve into the left ventricle, through the ventricular septal defect, and into the right ventricle, where it grasps the delivery pod. The pod is drawn into the left ventricle, and the left ventricular arms are released under direct vision. The pod is then carefully pulled back into the right ventricle, and, viewing through the original aortic valve into the right ventricle, the right ventricular arms are released. If necessary, multiple devices

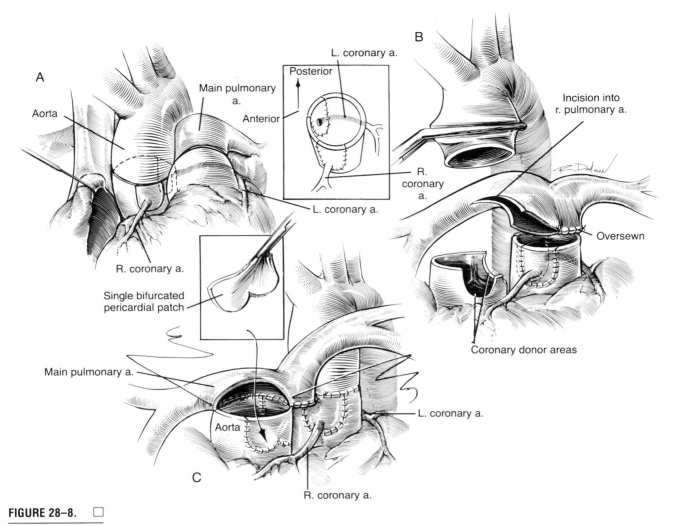

FIGURE 28–8. □

When the great vessels are side by side, it may be necessary to move the pulmonary artery anastomosis rightward as indicated, to avoid compression of the more anterior coronary artery. *A,* Mobilization of the coronary arteries. In this case, the right coronary artery arises from the anterior facing sinus *(insert)* and the left coronary artery arises posteriorly. *B,* The left end of the divided distal main pulmonary artery is closed by direct suture (or with a pericardial patch) and the right end is extended into the right pulmonary artery. A Lecompte maneuver is performed, bringing the pulmonary artery anterior to the aorta. *C,* The coronary donor areas are closed with a patch of autologous pericardium, and the pulmonary anastomosis is completed. The transferred right coronary artery is clear of the main pulmonary artery.

may be placed. Although this system has worked well for children weighing more than 4 to 5 kg, the delivery pod requires further modification for neonates and infants weighing less than 4 kg.

Pulmonary Artery Anastomosis. Although the Lecompte maneuver is uniformly useful for patients with standard transposition in which the great arteries are positioned anteroposteriorly (or relatively close to this), for side-by-side great arteries judgment is required in deciding whether translocation of the right pulmonary artery anterior to the aorta will be useful in decreasing tension on the right pulmonary artery. In general, if the aorta is the slightest bit anterior to the pulmonary artery, a Lecompte maneuver should be performed. Another consideration in this decision, other than just the

tension on the right pulmonary artery, is the relationship of the transferred coronary arteries to the pulmonary artery. Care must be taken to ensure that there is no compression of the coronary arteries.

A useful maneuver to minimize the risk of coronary compression, as well as to decrease the tension on the pulmonary artery anastomosis, is to shift the anastomosis somewhat from the original distal divided main pulmonary artery into the right pulmonary artery. The leftward end of the main pulmonary artery is closed (usually by direct suture, although the pericardial patch used to fill the coronary donor areas may be extended here), and the orifice is extended into the right pulmonary artery (Fig. 28–8). In other respects the anastomosis is

TABLE 28–1. □ RESULTS OF BIVENTRICULAR REPAIR FOR DOUBLE-OUTLET RIGHT VENTRICLE DURING THE FIRST MONTH OF LIFE

LOCATION OF VSD	n	ASSOCIATED LESIONS			TYPE OF REPAIR				
		SAS	SPS	AAO	IVR	ASO	Rastelli	DKS	Sen/Mus
Subaortic	0 (0)	—	—	—	—	—	—	—	—
Subpulmonary	4 (1)	—	—	4 (1)	—	3 (1)	—	1 (0)	—
Doubly committed	0 (0)	—	—	—	—	—	—	—	—
Noncommitted	2 (1)	2 (1)	—	2 (1)	1 (1)	—	—	1 (0)	—
Total	6 (2)	2 (1)	0 (0)	6 (2)	1 (1)	3 (1)	0 (0)	2 (0)	0 (0)

VSD, ventricular septal defect; SAS, subaortic stenosis; SPS, subpulmonary stenosis; AAO, aortic arch obstruction; IVR, intraventricular rerouting; ASO, arterial switch operation; DKS, Damus-Kay-Stansel type procedure; Sen/Mus, Senning or Mustard operation.
Numbers in ( ) refer to hospital deaths.

performed in the usual fashion. This maneuver has the effect of shifting the main pulmonary artery rightward so that it will not lie anterior to the aorta, where it would likely cause compression of the anteriorly transferred coronary artery.

Repair With Noncommitted Ventricular Septal Defect. The most common form of noncommitted ventricular septal defect is the atrioventricular canal type, which extends under the septal leaflet of the tricuspid valve. Several authors[8a] have suggested that when this defect occurs with pulmonary stenosis (which precludes an arterial switch), the procedure of choice is patch closure of the ventricular septal defect with creation of a generous anterior and superior extension. The ventricular septal defect extension is then baffled to the aorta as for the standard intraventricular repair described previously. In view of the known tendency for surgically created ventricular septal defects to close spontaneously, as well as the inherent risk of creating subaortic stenosis with the tunnel repair, we have generally avoided this approach. If the child's hemodynamics are ideal for a Fontan procedure—as they usually are, because of the presence of natural pulmonary stenosis—we often choose that approach rather than atrial-level repairs or other complex biventricular repairs employing conduits.

Repair of Associated Subaortic Stenosis and Arch Anomalies. The long subaortic conus associated with DORV toward the transposition end of the spectrum may cause some degree of subaortic stenosis. Not surprisingly, aortic arch hypoplasia and coarctation often accompany such subaortic stenosis. There is likely to be considerable disparity between the diameters of the great vessels. During the preliminary phase of the arterial switch procedure, tourniquets should be loosely applied around the head vessels. The coronary transfer should be undertaken in the usual fashion, using low-flow bypass. The circulation is then arrested, the tourniquets are tightened, and the aortic crossclamp is removed. An incision is made along the lesser curve of the ascending aorta and arch, extending across the coarctation. A long patch of pericardium is sutured into this aortotomy, which serves to minimize the disparity between the proximal neoaorta and the distal ascending aorta. The aortic crossclamp is reapplied, and bypass may be recommended. The remainder of the procedure is undertaken as described previously. We do not favor coarctation repair and pulmonary artery banding as preliminary maneuvers.

RESULTS

Between 1981 and 1991 at Children's Hospital, Boston, six patients underwent biventricular repair of DORV (defined by the 50% rule) with atrioventricular concordance during the first month of life.

TABLE 28–2. □ RESULTS OF BIVENTRICULAR REPAIR FOR DOUBLE-OUTLET RIGHT VENTRICLE DURING THE FIRST YEAR OF LIFE

LOCATION OF VSD	n	ASSOCIATED LESIONS			TYPE OF REPAIR				
		SAS	SPS	AAO	IVR	ASO	Rastelli	DKS	Sen/Mus
Subaortic	20 (3)	3 (0)	7 (0)	1 (0)	20 (3)	—	—	—	—
Subpulmonary	13 (2)	4 (1)	2 (0)	6 (0)	3 (0)	3 (0)	2 (1)	2 (1)	3 (0)
Doubly committed	4 (0)	2 (0)	1 (0)	1 (0)	4 (0)	—	—	—	—
Noncommitted	2 (0)	1 (0)	—	1 (0)	—	1 (0)	—	—	1 (0)
Total	39 (5)	10 (1)	10 (0)	9 (0)	27 (3)	4 (0)	2 (1)	2 (1)	4 (0)

VSD, ventricular septal defect; SAS, subaortic stenosis; SPS, subpulmonary stenosis; AAO, aortic arch obstruction; IVR, intraventricular rerouting; ASO, arterial switch operation; DKS, Damus-Kay-Stansel type procedure; Sen/Mus, Senning or Mustard operation.
Numbers in ( ) refer to hospital deaths.

Bilateral conus was documented in three patients. There were two hospital deaths (33%) and no late deaths, and one patient required reoperation during 15 patient-years of follow-up in four survivors. The anatomic findings and methods of repair are shown in Table 28–1.

During the same period 39 patients 1 month to 1 year of age underwent biventricular repair of DORV. Bilateral conus was documented in 27 patients. There were five hospital deaths (13%) and late deaths, and seven patients required reoperation over 135 patient-years of follow-up obtained from 30 of 34 survivors. The anatomic findings and method of repair are shown in Table 28–2.

REFERENCES

1. Barratt-Boyes BG, Lowe JB, Watt WJ, et al. Initial experiences with extracorporeal circulation in intracardiac surgery. Br Med J 2:1826, 1960.
2. Borow KM, Green LH, Castaneda AR, et al. Left ventricular function after repair of tetralogy of Fallot and its relationship to age at surgery. Circulation 61:1150, 1980.
3. Borromee L, Lecompte Y, Batisse A, et al. Anatomic repair of anomalies of ventriculoarterial connection associated with ventricular septal defect. J Thorac Cardiovasc Surg 95:96, 1988.
4. Bridges ND, Perry SB, Keane JF, et al. Preoperative transcatheter closure of congenital muscular ventricular septal defects. N Engl J Med 324:1312, 1991.
5. Daicoff GR, Kirklin JW. Surgical correction of Taussig-Bing malformation. Report of three cases. Am J Cardiol 19:125, 1967.
6. Fishberger SB, Bridges ND, Hanley FL, et al. Intraoperative device closure of ventricular septal defects. Circulation 86(suppl I):181, 1992.
7. Kawashima Y, Fujita T, Miyamoto T, et al. Intraventricular rerouting of blood for the correction of Taussig-Bing malformation. J Thorac Cardiovasc Surg 62:825, 1971.
8. Kirklin JW, Harp RA, McGoon DC. Surgical treatment of origin of both vessels from right ventricle, including cases of pulmonary stenosis. J Thorac Cardiovasc Surg 48:1026, 1964.
8a. Kirklin JW, Barratt-Boyes BA. Cardiac Surgery. 2nd ed. New York, Churchill Livingstone, 1993.
9. Lecompte Y, Neveux JY, Leca F, et al. Reconstruction of the pulmonary outflow tract without prosthetic conduit. J Thorac Cardiovasc Surg 84:727, 1982.
10. Lev M, Bharati S, Meng CCL, et al. A concept of double outlet right ventricle. J Thorac Cardiovasc Surg 64:271, 1972.
11. Musumeci F, Shumway S, Lincoln C, et al. Surgical treatment for double outlet right ventricle at the Brompton Hospital, 1973 to 1986. J Thorac Cardiovasc Surg 96:278, 1988.
12. Nikaidoh H. Aortic translocation and biventricular outflow tract reconstruction. J Thorac Cardiovasc Surg 88:365, 1984.
13. Pacifico AD, Kirklin JK, Colvin EV, et al. Intraventricular tunnel repair for Taussig-Bing heart and related cardiac anomalies. Circulation 74(suppl I):153, 1986.
14. Patrick DL, McGoon DC. Operation for double outlet right ventricle with transposition of the great arteries. J Cardiovasc Surg 9:537, 1968.
15. Rastelli GC. A new approach to "anatomic" repair of transposition of the great arteries. Mayo Clin Proc 44:1, 1969.
16. Sakata R, Lecompte Y, Batisse A, et al. Anatomic repair of anomalies of ventriculoarterial connection associated with ventricular septal defect. J Thorac Cardiovasc Surg 95:90, 1988.
17. Sanders SP, Bierman FZ, Williams RG. Conotruncal malformations: Diagnosis in infancy using subxiphoid two-dimensional echocardiography. Am J Cardiol 50:1361, 1982.
18. Sondheimer HM, Freedom RM, Olley PM. Double outlet right ventricle: Clinical spectrum and prognosis. Am J Cardiol 39:709, 1977.
19. Taussig HB, Bing RJ. Complete transposition of the aorta and a levoposition of the pulmonary artery. Am Heart J 37:551, 1949.
20. Van Praagh R. What is the Taussig-Bing malformation? Circulation 38:445, 1968.
21. Vouhe P, Tamisier D, Leca F, et al. Transposition of the great arteries, ventricular septal defect, and pulmonary outflow obstruction. J Thorac Cardiovasc Surg 103:428, 1992.
22. Wernovsky G, Jonas RA, Colan SD, et al. Results of the arterial switch operation in patients with abnormalities of the mitral valve or left ventricular outflow tract. J Am Coll Cardiol 16:1446, 1990.

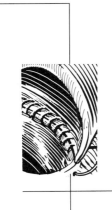

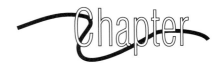

29

Cardiac Masses

Space-occupying lesions within or adjacent to the heart include neoplasms and thrombus. These lesions, although rare, are occasionally encountered in infants. Surgical removal is often, but not exclusively, an important aspect of management, and the opinion of the pediatric cardiac surgeon is of critical importance in formulating the overall management of these frequently complex conditions.

TUMORS

Cardiac tumors are rare in infancy, with an incidence of less than three per 10,000 according to the autopsy series reported by Nadas and Ellison.[28] A wide variety of histopathologic features has been found in primary cardiac tumors, and the relative frequency of each type is highly dependent on patient age. In infancy, the most common tumors are rhabdomyomas and fibromas,[3] although myxomas,[29] teratomas,[32] and various forms of sarcoma[22] and angioma[5, 10] have also been reported.

Rhabdomyomas

Morphology. Rhabdomyomas are discrete, nodular, gray masses that usually occur in the ventricular myocardium but may be found in the atria as well.[4, 21] These lesions are benign; however, there is no true tumor capsule. They may be isolated, al-

though they are multiple in about 90% of cases.[14] The tumor cells have been described histologically as "spider cells"[25] and consist of glycogen-filled protoplasm with filament-like strands extending radially to the periphery of the cell. These lesions are thought to be hamartomas.

Pathophysiology and Natural History. The pathophysiology of rhabdomyoma is that of a space-occupying lesion; therefore, the total mass of tumor as well as its location determine its exact nature. There may be discrete inflow or outflow obstruction of either ventricle or, in cases of multiple tumors, more general interference with ventricular function. Rhythm disturbances may occur and can be related to primary involvement of conduction tissue or secondary to obstructive phenomena.[14]

The natural history of these tumors is variable. The traditional thinking has been that the majority of neonates and infants who have rhabdomyomas will die either from congestive heart failure or sudden death.[1, 7, 28] The true natural history, however, is somewhat questionable, as many asymptomatic tumors may go undetected early in life. A number of cases of spontaneous tumor regression have been described.[31, 36, 38] The use of noninvasive techniques such as echocardiography and magnetic resonance imaging has provided a new perspective on the natural history of these lesions. One study suggests that the true natural history is favorable, with spontaneous resolution occurring in approximately 85% of cases.[35]

Rhabdomyomas account for about 60% of cardiac tumors found in neonates and infants[25] and have been diagnosed in utero,[20] but they account for a much smaller percentage of cardiac tumors in older children. They are associated with the multiple, noncardiac hamartomatous lesions of tuberous sclerosis in 50% to 86% of cases.[18]

Diagnosis and Indications for Surgery. The diagnosis is usually made in the infant or neonate with symptoms of cardiac obstruction, congestive heart failure, or rhythm disturbance, although other types of symptoms are becoming more frequent. Fetal diagnosis is not uncommon when hydrops or a rhythm disturbance is present. The diagnosis can also be made in patients with noncardiac symptoms (typically neurologic) related to tuberous sclerosis. The primary modalities for diagnosis are the noninvasive imaging techniques, including echocardiography, magnetic resonance imaging, and computed tomography.[33, 40] Cardiac catheterization may be important to obtain hemodynamic and electrophysiologic data in patients with obstructions or rhythm disturbances.

Indications for surgery are the presence of significant symptoms in combination with a resectable mass. The more recent information regarding favorable natural history suggests that asymptomatic, and even mildly symptomatic, infants should not undergo surgery. Because these tumors are not particularly mobile or friable, sudden obstruction or embolization is unlikely in the asymptomatic patient.

Surgical Management

Historical Perspective. Understandably, the earliest surgical approaches to intracardiac tumors involved resection of atrial myxomas in older patients. In 1952, Bahnson and Newman excised an atrial myxoma using normothermic caval inflow occlusion, without success.[2] In 1954, Crafoord successfully removed a myxoma using continuous cardiopulmonary bypass.[12] Both Foster et al.[15] and Corono et al.[11] reported successful removal of rhabdomyomas in neonates in 1984.

Surgical Technique. Although not encapsulated, rhabdomyomas are well circumscribed, and therefore, they lend themselves to surgical resection. Technical difficulties arise when the tumor distorts or impinges on a vital structure such as a major coronary artery branch, a valve annulus, or the conduction system.

The surgical approach uses cardiopulmonary bypass. For right ventricular, free-wall lesions a single venous cannula is sufficient, often with only moderate hypothermia (28°C) and without crossclamping the aorta. For ventricular septal or left ventricular lesions, bicaval venous cannulation is often helpful, with colder core temperatures (25°C), aortic crossclamping, and myocardial protection with cardioplegic solution.

The cardiac incision is dictated by the position of the tumor. Complete removal of the tumor is attempted; however, for large tumors impinging on other vital cardiac structures or for multiple tumors, this is often not advisable, and removal limited to the obstructing portion of the lesion may represent the best treatment. This is especially true in light of the knowledge that these lesions may regress spontaneously. The defect that results may require a patch for reconstruction.

Fibromas

Morphology. Fibromas are solitary benign neoplasms that are almost always limited in location to the left, right, or septal ventricular myocardium. On gross examination they are white, nodular lesions that appear to have a border distinct from the surrounding myocardium. Their size and position may distort surrounding structures such as major coronary artery branches. Histologically they are made up of fibroblasts, collagen, smooth muscle, and endothelial-lined spaces.[19] There is no true tumor capsule.

Pathophysiology and Natural History. The pathophysiology is similar to that of rhabdomyomas—i.e., essentially that of a benign, space-occupying lesion. The rarity of fibromas limits the reliability of attempts to characterize their natural history; however, they are thought to be slow-growing neoplasms. Fibromas account for about 15% to 20% of neoplasms in infants (representing the second most common neoplasm in this age group).[39] Most are seen during infancy or the first few years of life.

Diagnosis and Indications for Surgery. The diagnosis is made by imaging studies, usually in a patient with symptoms of obstruction[16] or rhythm disturbance.[13]

The major indication for excision is the presence of symptoms. An asymptomatic fibroma may be considered for excision if it is large and in a position that allows safe removal, as the natural history of this lesion is uncertain.

Surgical Management. The surgical approach to fibromas is similar to that for other benign, well-circumscribed masses in the heart, as outlined earlier for rhabdomyomas. For lesions that are adjacent to critical cardiac structures, partial excision has produced good long-term results.[9]

Other Neoplasms

Primary sarcoma of the heart is predominantly a disease of older individuals, although rare cases have been reported as early as the first year of life.[6] Primary pericardial sarcoma has been reported in the neonate, and combined surgical and chemotherapeutic management has been successful.[22] Intrapericardial teratoma can occur in the fetus and neonate and typically causes pericardial effusion and compression.[8, 32] Early diagnosis (prenatal) and neonatal resection can result in successful outcome. Atrial myxoma, the most common cardiac neoplasm, is rare in infants.[17, 29] Successful surgical management is possible. Various forms of angiomas have been reported with successful surgical and nonsurgical management.[5, 10]

Various cardiac tumors have been associated with structural heart lesions, and although these are poorly understood, it has been suggested that in certain cases the tumor may be responsible for the structural congenital heart lesion.[34, 37]

Results of Surgical Management of Cardiac Tumors in Infants

Between January 1983 and January 1992, six neonates and infants underwent surgical resection of cardiac tumors at Children's Hospital in Boston. Three patients had multiple rhabdomyomas; two of these had tuberous sclerosis. One was diagnosed by intrauterine echocardiography, and the other two had murmurs and heart failure at birth. All three underwent partial surgical resection in the neonatal period. One of these patients had subvalvar obstruction of the left ventricular outflow tract, one had the equivalent of mitral stenosis from a tumor originating at the mitral annulus, and one had the equivalent of tricuspid stenosis from a tumor originating in the right side of the inlet ventricular septum. The patient with the mitral stenosis equivalent had biventricular failure from multiple tumors and died on the first postoperative day from low cardiac output. The other two patients were doing well 1 year later, with no further obstructive problems. At that time echocardiography showed no progression of the remaining tumors.

Another patient had a solitary rhabdomyoma of the right side of the ventricular septum causing obstruction of the right ventricular outflow tract. This tumor was successfully "enucleated" through an incision in the right ventricular outflow tract, with no evidence of recurrence at 1 year of follow-up.

Another patient had a solitary fibroma in the free wall of the right ventricular outflow tract that was causing obstruction. This was excised at 6 months of age, and the defect was reconstructed with a pericardial patch. At follow-up 1 year later, there was no evidence of obstruction or tumor recurrence.

The final patient had congestive heart failure and pericardial effusion at 11 days of life. A mediastinal tumor was diagnosed by echocardiography and computed tomography. At exploration, an intrapericardial tumor arising from the external surface of the right atrial appendage was found. This was completely excised, with the right atrial closure accomplished using a pericardial patch. The pathologic diagnosis was low-grade spindle cell sarcoma. At 1 year of follow-up there was no evidence of recurrence.

Conclusions

Primary tumors of the heart are rare in the neonate and infant. Rhabdomyomas, considering their tendency to regress, should be treated expectantly unless significant symptomatology is present. Fibromas and other lesions should be considered for resection when diagnosed, especially if symptoms are present. Complete resection is desirable; however, partial excision of both obstructive rhabdomyomas and fibromas can provide long-term survival without recurrence of symptoms.

INTRACARDIAC THROMBUS

Intracardiac thrombus formation is primarily an iatrogenic problem. This lesion has become more frequent with the increased use of indwelling cardiac catheters. Recognition has also probably increased with the development and use of diagnostic echocardiography. Although patients with intracardiac thrombi may have associated heart disease, they frequently are neonates and infants with structurally normal hearts who are chronically ill and require long-standing central venous catheters for intravenous nutrition or prolonged intravenous antibiotics.[27]

Neonatal aortic thrombosis has also been described.[26] This rare condition may be idiopathic or related to diseases such as perinatal sepsis or maternal diabetes.

Morphology

Thrombus formation is typically stimulated by an indwelling right atrial catheter. The thrombus becomes organized and adheres to the endothelium of the right atrium or to the cavoatrial junction. Even after removal of the responsible catheter, the nidus for thrombus will remain. Often a cast of the catheter is all that is present. This lesion may continue to organize, remodel, and become an insignificant lesion, or it may stimulate further thrombus formation, which may result in a clinically significant lesion. The factors that determine the development of a significant thrombus in this setting are not well documented; however, hypercoagulability, stasis, inflammation, infection, and continued presence of a foreign body are likely to be important. The thrombus may eventually enlarge to fill the right atrial cavity, attached only by a relatively tenuous mural connection.

Neonatal aortic thrombus is defined as occlusive fresh thrombus in the ascending aorta, transverse arch, or ductal remnant.

Pathophysiology and Natural History

Many small and moderate-size thrombi are of no clinical consequence. When pathophysiology is present, it is related to one of three possible mechanisms: obstruction, embolism, or refractory infection. As an atrial thrombus enlarges, it usually grows in the direction of flow (i.e., toward the tricuspid valve orifice). Obstruction of tricuspid valve inflow or caval inflow may occur. Mobile lesions may actually move back and forth across the tricuspid valve with cardiac activity. This mobility and friability, especially of actively forming lesions, may result in an embolus. These emboli can range from small fragments to the entire thrombus. Infection of a thrombus constitutes endocarditis. Prolonged antibiotic therapy is indicated but may not be effective because of the size of the infected mass.

The natural history of asymptomatic but significant thrombi is not well characterized, although spontaneous resolution by reorganization and remodeling is likely to occur in many cases. One screening study showed that the incidence of thrombus formation was 1.8% in 56 neonates followed for an average of 30 ($\pm$ 24 SD) days with indwelling central venous catheters.[24]

A neonatal aortic thrombus may cause an acute left ventricular afterload resulting in severe left ventricular dysfunction. Signs and symptoms may be similar to those in neonatal coarctation. The natural history is obscure.

Diagnosis and Indications for Surgery

Diagnosis of an intra-atrial thrombus is made by echocardiography, usually in a chronically ill neonate or infant with a long-standing central venous catheter.[23] The echocardiographic study may be precipitated by ongoing sepsis, hemodynamic compromise, or evidence of venous obstruction, or it may be performed simply as a screening procedure in a high-risk setting.[24]

The indications for surgery are refractory sepsis, embolism, and hemodynamically significant obstruction. Large thrombi, especially if they appear mobile on the echocardiogram, should probably be removed, even if the patient is asymptomatic.

Diagnosis of a neonatal aortic thrombus may be difficult. Echocardiography and cardiac catheterization may suggest coarctation or interrupted aortic arch.

Surgical Management

Historical Perspective. Surgical management of catheter-related atrial thrombi in infants is a relatively recent phenomenon. In 1979, Pliam et al. reported the surgical removal of a "ball valve" right atrial thrombus in an infant receiving long-term central venous alimentation.[30]

Surgical Technique. Venous cannulation for an intra-atrial thrombus must be carefully planned and executed because of the possibility of disruption of the thrombus. After opening the pericardium, the right atrial appendage and free wall are carefully inspected. Induration can often be discerned in the area of attachment of the thrombus, and this information, in combination with a careful review of the preoperative echocardiogram, is useful in formulating the cannulation technique. If the infant weighs less than 3 to 4 kg and the right atrial appendage is free of thrombus, single venous cannulation through the right atrial appendage, along with routine aortic cannulation, is the preferred approach. Deep hypothermic circulatory arrest is then used to expose the lesion. In larger infants or in those in whom the right atrial appendage is involved with the thrombus, bicaval cannulation with moderate hypothermia (28°C) and continuous cardiopulmonary bypass is preferred. In either case, after the target core temperature has been achieved, the aorta is crossclamped, and cardioplegic solution is administered.

The right atrial appendage is opened in an area not involved with the thrombus. Typically, the mass is relatively well organized and, therefore, densely adherent to the right atrial wall. If the point of attachment is on the free wall, it may be best to simply excise that segment of right atrial wall that contains the base of the thrombus. More often the mass is attached in a relatively complex manner (e.g., either to the cavoatrial junction or to the tricuspid valve leaflets). The thrombus must then be carefully removed from the endothelial surface without resecting cardiac tissue. This usually leaves a somewhat disrupted endothelial surface, and care must be taken to remove all remaining strands of thrombus. The right atrium and right ventricle are then carefully inspected for the presence of any remaining thrombus, either adherent or free standing. The right atriotomy is then closed, and the remainder of the cardiopulmonary bypass is managed routinely.

For neonatal aortic thrombosis, the surgical approach varies with the site of obstruction. If the ascending aorta or proximal arch is involved, a median sternotomy along with cardiopulmonary bypass and deep hypothermic circulatory arrest will be required for exploration of the aorta and removal of the thrombus. If the distal arch or isthmus is the site of thrombosis, exposure by a left thoractomy, as for coarctation, is optimal.

Results

Between January 1983 and January 1992, 121 patients had echocardiographic diagnoses of intracardiac thrombi at Children's Hospital in Boston. In 98 of these patients (81%), the thrombus was an incidental finding, usually in a patient undergoing echocardiography after surgical repair of congenital heart disease. In 23 patients (19%), because of symptoms of obstruction or refractory infection, or because of thrombus size, surgical resection was a consideration.

Surgical resection was actually performed in eight of these 23 patients (35%). Ages ranged from 2 to 9 months. The heart was structurally normal in six of these eight, and the thrombus was related to chronic, indwelling central venous catheters. Excision was successful in all of these patients. In one of the two remaining patients, thrombus developed after repair of a complex congenital heart lesion. This patient underwent successful excision but died 1 month later from multisystem failure. The other patient was referred to Children's Hospital in Boston at 6 weeks of age with unrepaired hypoplastic left heart syndrome (aortic and mitral atresia), a restrictive patent foramen ovale, and a massively dilated left atrial chamber that was essentially filled with thrombus. This patient had been placed on a waiting list for cardiac transplant at birth at another institution and was urgently transferred to us after he became progressively cyanotic over a 48-hour period. He underwent successful removal of the thrombus at the time of stage 1 palliation for hypoplastic left heart syndrome.

No episodes of perioperative embolism or recurrent thrombus formation were evident on postoperative echocardiographic examination in any of the eight patients. Long-term follow-up in six of the seven survivors (mean, 45 months) revealed no evidence of recurrent infection or thrombus.

In the 15 patients in whom surgical resection was not undertaken (65%), there was one notable event related to the thrombus. This was in a critically ill neonate with a structurally normal heart who had undergone repair of a congenital diaphragmatic hernia and required 10 days of extracorporeal membrane oxygenation (ECMO) after surgery. Approximately 2 weeks after removal from ECMO, the patient became hemodynamically unstable. An echocardiogram revealed a mobile thrombus, 1 cm × 1 cm, in the right atrium, attached just below the superior cavoatrial junction. The patient was treated with intravenous streptokinase and, 24 hours later, became acutely hypoxic and died. Postmortem examination revealed that the thrombus had embolized to the pulmonary artery supplying the right lung.

At Children's Hospital in Boston, we have had experience with two cases of spontaneous aortic thrombus. In one, the ascending aorta was occluded by a clot. This patient underwent a thrombectomy using cardiopulmonary bypass and deep hypothermic circulatory arrest. After a successful procedure, the thrombosis of the aorta redeveloped, and the patient died on the second postoperative day. The second patient had a thrombus within an aneurysm of the ductus diverticulum; the clot extended to occlude the aortic isthmus. This patient underwent exploration of the upper descending aorta via a left thoracotomy, thrombectomy, and ligation of the ductus. After a successful procedure with hemodynamic documentation of relief of this obstruction, this patient died suddenly on the first postoperative day. Diffuse microemboli and infection of the adrenal glands were noted at postmortem examination.

Conclusions

The number of neonates and infants with significant intracardiac thrombi who are seen by the pediatric cardiac surgeon is likely to increase in coming years as neonatal and pediatric specialists continue to rely on indwelling central venous catheters as part of their management of complex lesions and as diagnostic imaging is used more frequently in screening these patients. Surgical judgment may be difficult in these complex and chronically ill patients; however, our relatively small experience suggests that surgical excision of the thrombus is beneficial.

REFERENCES

1. Arciniegas E, Hakimi M, Farooki ZO, et al. Primary cardiac tumors in children. J Thorac Cardiovasc Surg 79:582, 1980.
2. Bahnson HT, Newman EV. Diagnosis and surgical removal of intracavitary myxoma of the right atrium. Bull Johns Hopkins Hosp 93:150, 1953.
3. Bertolini P, Meisner H, Paek SU, et al. Special considerations on primary cardiac tumors in infancy and childhood. Thorac Cardiovasc Surg 38:164, 1990.
4. Bogren HG, DeMaria AN, Maston DT. Imaging procedures in the detection of cardiac tumors with emphasis on echocardiography. A review. Cardiovasc Intervent Radiol 3:107, 1980.
5. Burke A, Johns JP, Virmani R. Hemangiomas of the heart. A clinicopathologic study of ten cases. Am J Cardiovasc Pathol 3:283, 1990.
6. Burke AP, Cowan D, Virmani R. Primary sarcomas of the heart. Cancer 15:387, 1992.
7. Burke AP, Virmani R. Cardiac rhabdomyoma: A clinicopathologic study. Mod Pathol 4:70, 1991.
8. Castanon M, Mayol J, Mulet Melia J, et al. Neonatal intrapericardial teratoma. Circ Pediatr 2:38, 1989.
9. Ceithaml EL, Midgley FM, Perry LW, et al. Intramural ventricular fibroma in infancy: Survival after partial excision in 2 patients. Ann Thorac Surg 50:471, 1990.
10. Chang JS, Young ML, Chuu WM, et al. Infantile cardiac hemangioendothelioma. Pediatr Cardiol 13:52, 1992.
11. Corono A, Catena G, Marcelletti C. Cardiac rhabdomyoma: Surgical treatment in the neonate. J Thorac Cardiovasc Surg 87:725, 1984.
12. Crafoord C. Discussion on mitral stenosis and mitral insufficiency. In Lam CR (ed). Proceedings of the International Symposium on Cardiovascular Surgery. Philadelphia, WB Saunders, 1955, p 202.
13. Filiatrault M, Beland MJ, Neilson KA, et al. Cardiac fibroma presenting with clinically significant arrhythmias in infancy. Pediatr Cardiol 12:118, 1991.
14. Fine G. Neoplasms of the pericardium and heart. In Gould SE (ed). Pathology of the Heart and Blood Vessels. Springfield IL, Charles C Thomas, 1968, p 851.
15. Foster ED, Spooner EW, Farina MA, et al. Cardiac rhabdomyomas in the neonate: Surgical management. Ann Thorac Surg 37:249, 1984.
16. Groppo AA, dos Santos GG, Beyruti R, et al. Surgical treatment of right ventricular fibroma in infants. Report of 2 cases. Arq Bras Cardiol 54:137, 1990.
17. Hals J, Ek J, Sandnes K. Cardiac myxoma as the cause of death in an infant. Acta Paediatr Scand 79:999, 1990.
18. Harding CO, Pagan RA. Incidence of tuberous sclerosis in patients with cardiac rhabdomyoma. Am J Med Genet 37:443, 1990.
19. Heath D. Pathology of cardiac tumors. Am J Cardiol 21:315, 1968.
20. Kidder LA. Congenital glycogenic tumors of the heart. Arch Pathol 49:55, 1950.
21. Kilman JW, Craenen J, Hosier DM. Replacement of entire right atrial wall in an infant with cardiac rhabdomyoma. J Pediatr Surg 8:317, 1973.
22. Lazarus KH, D'Orsogna DE, Bloom KR, et al. Primary pericardial sarcoma in a neonate. Am J Pediatr Hematol Oncol 11:343, 1989.
23. Mahoney L, Snider AR, Silverman NH. Echocardiographic diagnosis of intracardiac thrombi complicating total parenteral nutrition. J Pediatr 98:469, 1981.
24. Marsh D, Wilkerson SA, Cook LN, et al. Right atrial thrombus formation screening using two-dimensional echocardiograms in neonates with central venous catheters. Pediatrics 81:284, 1988.
25. McAllister HA Jr. Primary tumors and cysts of the heart and pericardium. Curr Prob Cardiol 4:8, 1979.
26. McFaul RC, Keane JF, Nowicki ER, et al. Aortic thrombosis in the neonate. J Thorac Cardiovasc Surg 81:334, 1981.
27. Mendoza JB, Soto A, Brown EG, et al. Intracardiac thrombi complicating central total parenteral nutrition: Resolution without surgery or thrombolysis. J Pediatr 108:613, 1986.
28. Nadas AD, Ellison RC. Cardiac tumors in infancy. Am J Cardiol 21:363, 1968.
29. Pasaoglu I, Demircin M, Ozkutlu S, et al. Right atrial myxoma in an infant. Jpn Heart J 32:263, 1991.
30. Pliam MB, McGough EC, Nixon GW, et al. Right atrial ball-valve thrombus: A complication of central venous alimentation in an infant: Diagnosis and successful surgical management of a case. J Thorac Cardiovasc Surg 78:579, 1979.
31. Prichard RW. Tumors of the heart: Review of the subject and report of 150 cases. Arch Pathol 51:98, 1951.
32. Rheuban KS, McDaniel NL, Feldman PS, et al. Intrapericardial teratoma causing nonimmune hydrops fetalis and pericardial tamponade: A case report. Pediatr Cardiol 12:54, 1991.
33. Rienmuller R, Tiling R. MR and CT for detection of cardiac tumors. Thorac Cardiovasc Surg 28:168, 1990.
34. Russell GA, Dhasama JP, Berry PJ, et al. Coexistent cardiac tumours and malformations of the heart. Int J Cardiol 22:89, 1989.
35. Smythe JF, Dyck JD, Smallhorn JF, et al. Natural history of cardiac rhabdomyoma in infancy and childhood. Am J Cardiol 15:1247, 1990.
36. Soria F, Valdes M, Garcia A, et al. The spontaneous regression of a rhabdomyoma of the right ventricle. Rev Esp Cardiol 44:203, 1991.
37. Watanabe T, Hojo Y, Kozaki T, et al. Hypoplastic left heart syndrome with rhabdomyoma of the left ventricle. Pediatr Cardiol 12:121, 1991.
38. Watson GH. Cardiac rhabdomyomas in tuberous sclerosis. Ann NY Acad Sci 615:50, 1991.
39. Williams WG, Trusler GA, Fowler GS, et al. Left ventricular myocardial fibroma: A case report and review of cardiac tumors in children. J Pediatr Surg 7:324, 1972.
40. Yamashita K, Togashi K, Minami S, et al. Primary intracardiac tumors in magnetic resonance imaging. Radiat Med 9:127, 1991.

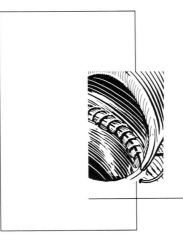

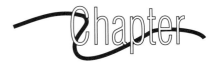

30

Chapter

Cardiac Transplantation

Cardiac transplantation is a tantalizing therapeutic option for patients with either severely myopathic ventricles or severe structural congenital defects that preclude restoration of normal cardiovascular physiology by conventional techniques. The prospect of implanting a structurally normal heart that could function in a nearly normal fashion for a lifetime is extraordinarily attractive, but clearly there are a multitude of problems that remain to be solved before this ideal can become a consistent reality. The most important of these problems is the lack of any donor-specific immunosuppressive techniques to prevent rejection of the transplanted heart. As a result, the risks of generalized immunosuppression, including rejection of the transplanted organ, infection, and neoplasia, are always present. Because of these immunologic limitations, cardiac transplantation has continued to be an expensive, labor-intensive undertaking that requires a lifetime of medication and surveillance for rejection and for the complications of immunosuppression. A second, and equally important, problem is the chronic shortage of allograft donor organs, which affects transplantation of all organs. For transplantation to become widely available to children with all forms of incurable heart disease, these problems must be addressed. In the interim, decisions to embark on transplantation must be made by weighing the not-inconsiderable risks of the post-transplant management of immunosuppression versus the risks of either continued medical therapy or conventional surgical approaches. As knowledge and experience with both transplant and nontransplant approaches continue to progress, the relative risks and benefits of these treatments will be unlikely to remain static, and continuing reassessment will be necessary.

HISTORY

The first human-to-human cardiac transplant operation was carried out in 1967 by Barnard,[7] but it is not widely appreciated that the second human transplant was carried out a few days later, when the heart of an anencephalic child was unsuccessfully transplanted into a 17-day-old infant with Ebstein's malformation by Kantrowitz.[17] These clinical efforts followed the extensive experimental work of Lower and colleagues.[23, 24] Despite initial world-wide enthusiasm for heart transplantation, the problems of rejection and infection soon reduced active cardiac transplantation to a few specialized centers. Until 1981, few, if any, transplants were undertaken in pediatric patients. However, with the introduction of cyclosporine in that year, the number of heart transplants rapidly increased, and within a few years, the number of pediatric patients undergoing cardiac transplantation began to increase as well. This expansion into the pediatric population continued into the neonatal age group with the pioneering efforts of Bailey in the mid-1980s.[4] However, the total experience, even in the centers that have been the most aggressive in offering transplantation, remains relatively small when compared with that in older children and adults.

PATHOPHYSIOLOGY

The majority of patients who are candidates for cardiac transplantation have acute or chronic congestive heart failure. The exceptions are patients who are offered transplantation in the newborn period because of the type and severity of structural heart disease or because of medically uncontrollable arrhythmias that are not amenable to treatment with the automatic implantable cardioverter defibrillator (AICD). Current technology makes the AICD impractical for neonates or small infants because of the size of the generator.

The clinical manifestations of heart failure vary somewhat by the age of the patient, but they are generally due to depressed function of one or both of the ventricles. (Congestive heart failure caused primarily by left-to-right shunts should rarely be an issue for the transplant patient, as these shunts should be amenable to surgical or catheterization laboratory interventions.) The heart is generally enlarged, and wall thickness is increased, although the hypertrophy is frequently inadequate to normalize the wall stress on the ventricle.[12] The ejection velocity and peak acceleration of flow from the left ventricle are subnormal. Normal levels of cardiac output may be preserved in the early stages of congestive heart failure, although this maintenance of systemic output may occur at the expense of elevated ventricular filling pressures, with congestion and interstitial edema in the pulmonary or systemic venous beds.[15] There may be reduced reserve to increase cardiac output when demands are increased. Therefore, common early symptoms in infants include feeding difficulties, with tachypnea and inability to take in normal amounts of nutrition.[15] Excessive perspiration during feeding is likely due to catecholamine release, which in turn is due to an inadequate cardiac output response to the increased demands imposed by feeding. In the later stages of heart failure, even resting cardiac output falls below normal. Tachypnea is frequently present, particularly during feeding or other stress, and is presumed to result from increased pulmonary interstitial fluid, which increases the stiffness of the lungs.[15] Frequent pulmonary infections may also result from chronic interstitial pulmonary edema. Because feeding is a major cardiovascular stress for the neonate or infant, it is not surprising that failure to gain weight at a normal rate (i.e., failure to thrive) is frequently seen in infants with heart failure.[15]

In patients with hypertrophic cardiomyopathy, the primary defect is one of diastolic dysfunction.[12] Several mechanisms may be involved in this phenomenon, including asynchronous ventricular activation and deactivation, abnormalities in cellular calcium homeostasis, and ischemia.[12] The hypertrophy itself leads to decreased ventricular compliance, and frequently there is also an element of fibrosis, which can increase chamber stiffness. The resultant elevation of ventricular filling pressures leads to clinical manifestations of heart failure similar to those seen in patients with other forms of myopathy, except that normal levels of cardiac output are usually present until the end stages of this disorder.[12]

DIAGNOSIS

Anatomic Diagnosis

The single most important piece of diagnostic information that must be obtained when evaluating the patient for cardiac transplantation is the exclusion of a surgically or medically remediable cause for the congestive heart failure. In the neonatal and infant age group, in particular, anomalous origin of the left coronary artery from the pulmonary artery must be excluded (see Chapter 19), along with inherited, treatable metabolic defects and nutritional or endocrine abnormalities.[12] Rhythm disorders with chronic tachycardia must also be excluded as a cause of depressed ventricular function. In patients who have had previous palliative or reparative cardiovascular surgical procedures, the evaluation should exclude residual anatomic problems that are amenable to reintervention (e.g., a residual left-to-right shunt or an obstruction to ventricular emptying). Evaluation by echocardiography and catheterization are mandatory in these patients to exclude surgically remediable problems. Biopsy when ventricular dysfunction and congestive heart failure have occurred relatively acutely, and biopsy of the ventricular myocardium should be carried out at the time of catheterization to determine whether active myocarditis is present.[12] Anecdotal reports suggest that immunosuppressive therapy may sometimes be helpful in patients with certain forms of myocarditis. Acute and convalescent viral titers, particularly for coxsackievirus type B, may also be helpful in establishing the etiology of a new onset of cardiomyopathy.[12] Echocardiography may also reveal endocardial fibroelastosis in the newborn if the endocardial surfaces are more echogenic than normal. Echocardiography will also reveal the presence of hypertrophic cardiomyopathy (also known as asymmetric septal hypertrophy or idiopathic hypertrophic subaortic stenosis) or structural forms of congenital heart disease that are not amenable to reparative surgery (e.g., a left ventricular diverticulum). Echocardiography clearly delineates the anatomy of most forms of structural heart disease, allowing the selection of transplantation as the best therapeutic option in certain circumstances (e.g., the hypoplastic left heart syndrome with diminutive ascending aorta; see Chapter 23).

The most significant anatomic information for a potential transplant operation concerns the locations of the great arteries, the anatomy of the central and peripheral pulmonary arteries, and the points of connection of the systemic and pulmonary veins. The combination of echocardiography and angiography should be able to provide this information. Techniques for dealing with almost all known variations in these anatomic structures at the time of transplantation have been described,[1, 13, 26] but information about the recipient's anatomy must be known before transplantation so that appropriate donor tissue, particularly extra lengths of the great arteries and systemic veins, can be harvested with the donor heart.

PHYSIOLOGIC DIAGNOSIS

Congestive heart failure caused by primary disease of the cardiac muscle (i.e., cardiomyopathy) produces no characteristic hemodynamic findings at catheterization other than elevated ventricular filling pressures and depressed cardiac output, as noted previously.[12] Calculated wall stress is almost always elevated in patients with dilated cardiomyopathy. Patients with primarily restrictive myopathies may have well-preserved systolic function but abnormal diastolic function, which results in elevated filling pressures.[12] Those with hypertrophic myopathy frequently have normal cardiac output, but the arterial waveform may show a characteristic "spike-and-dome" appearance that reflects the midsystolic obstruction to left ventricular emptying.[12] Arterial pressure will generally fall during the beat after an extrasystole. Mean atrial and atrial a wave pressures are elevated because of the diastolic dysfunction associated with hypertrophic myopathy. In cases of hypertrophic myopathy, angiography shows systolic cavity obliteration. Right ventricular outflow obstruction may also occur because of septal hypertrophy resulting in a pressure gradient between the right ventricle and the pulmonary artery.[12]

The single most important physiologic measurement in the evaluation of the patient for cardiac transplantation is the calculation of pulmonary vascular resistance (PVR). This measurement is important, because the donor heart is likely to be accustomed to a low PVR and will potentially fail if implanted into a patient with a significant fixed elevation in PVR.[20] There are numerous potential pitfalls in the calculation of PVR, as outlined in Chapter 15. Briefly, these pitfalls include problems with measurement of oxygen consumption (from which pulmonary blood flow is calculated) and pulmonary venous oxygen content (which may vary between individual pulmonary veins if there is pulmonary parenchymal disease). It is also important to ensure that transient factors that may elevate PVR, such as hypercarbia or acidosis, are not present. Acute trials with pharmacologic agents that may affect PVR should be carried out during the catheterization to determine whether PVR is fixed or is amenable to pharmacologic manipulation. Inotropic agents (e.g., dobutamine) or vasodilators (e.g., nitroprusside, amrinone, and inhaled oxygen) should be used. Because of the extremely short half-life of inhaled nitric oxide, which acts as a selective pulmonary vasodilator when administered via the airway, we at Children's Hospital in Boston have begun to acquire some experience with it. (See Chapter 5.)

MANAGEMENT

Medical Management

The most important aspects in the medical management of the patient with cardiomyopathy and congestive heart failure are: (1) to be certain that conventional forms of medical and surgical therapy are not likely to be useful and (2) to maximize the chances for patient survival until a donor heart becomes available. The importance of excluding surgically or medically treatable forms of heart disease has been noted earlier, but it is also important to be aware of the natural history of different forms of cardiomyopathy in neonates and infants.

The clinical course in obstructive cardiomyopathy is highly age dependent and appears to carry a much worse prognosis for infants than for older patients. In one series, 10 of 20 infants with obstructive cardiomyopathy died during a mean follow-up of 5.5 years.[25] Symptomatic infants who have congestive heart failure and cyanosis have a particularly poor prognosis, with nine of 11 patients in Maron et al.'s series dying before 5 years of age.[25] In contrast, patients seen at our institution at less than 2 years of age with congestive cardiomyopathy not caused by metabolic defects or toxic drugs (e.g., doxorubicin) had a much better prognosis, with 70% surviving and 60% recovering normal ventricular function.[12] The mechanisms responsible for the improvement (which clearly can occur) are unknown, but anecdotally, we have seen similar improvements in ventricular function in children in the first year of life who have undergone palliative operations for various forms of single ventricle (including the hypoplastic left heart syndrome) and who have had sufficiently severe ventricular dysfunction to be considered for transplantation (see indications below). Therefore, a period of medical therapy seems justified for infants with some forms of congestive cardiomyopathy but not for infants with hypertrophic cardiomyopathy.

Medical therapy for congestive cardiomyopathy generally consists of digoxin, diuretics, and, most importantly, afterload reduction.[15] There is evidence of increased levels of renin and angiotensin in these patients with congestive heart failure,[14] and therefore, therapy with angiotensin-converting enzyme inhibitors (i.e., captopril or enalapril) has seemed logical and has in fact proved to be of significant benefit in our experience.[12, 15] In contrast, medical therapy for hypertrophic myopathy is directed toward maintaining normal levels of preload and afterload while reducing ventricular contractility, generally with calcium channel antagonists such as verapamil.[12] Arrhythmias are a significant risk to patients with dilated or hypertrophic myopathy; approximately half of the deaths in series of adults with congestive heart failure are sudden and probably related to ventricular arrhythmias.[27] However, most antiarrhythmic medical therapy has failed to show any improvement in survival, and some medications, such as quinidine and procainamide, may actually have some proarrhythmic effects.[30]

Indications for Transplant

In simplest terms, the indication for cardiac transplantation is cardiac disease that has a poor patient prognosis for short-term survival (<1 year) and that is not treatable by "conventional" therapy. Clearly, the difficulties lie in accurately defining the 1-year prognosis for a given patient and in deciding what the prognosis will be with conventional therapy, particularly when transplantation is being considered for patients with complex forms of single ventricle, including the hypoplastic left heart syndrome. These decisions may vary among institutions, depending on previous experience with both conventional surgical therapy and transplantation for patients in whom structural heart disease, not myopathy, is the indication for transplantation. As noted earlier, the prognosis for patients with individual forms of cardiomyopathy is variable and may

depend on the age of the patient and the etiology of the myopathy.

There are a number of contraindications to transplantation for neonates and infants. First, severe and life-limiting coexisting medical problems, such as uncontrolled malignancy or significant renal or hepatic dysfunction unrelated to the heart failure, make transplantation unlikely to be successful. The renal and hepatic toxicity of cyclosporine makes the use of this agent hazardous in those with pre-existing renal and hepatic disease, and active immunosuppression is likely to make it impossible to control a malignancy. Second, any active bacterial or viral infection will be exacerbated by immunosuppression and should be viewed as a contraindication to transplantation. Third, a psychosocial family situation that is incompatible with care for the child after transplantation contraindicates this form of therapy, although the precise criteria for determining which families will be able to care for a child with a transplant are not completely defined. In retrospect, perhaps the most useful criterion in our program's experience has been the reliability with which parents have kept clinic appointments, administered medication, and been in attendance when the child was hospitalized. Parental socioeconomic or marital status has not been related to parents' success as caregivers. Fourth, the presence of severely elevated PVR (>8 Wood units) is a contraindication to transplantation for the reasons outlined previously. In marginal cases, it is important to attempt pharmacologic manipulation of PVR during the pretransplant evaluation to determine whether PVR is labile. As outlined earlier, trials of inotropic agents or vasodilators should be considered during the initial catheterization before excluding a particular patient from consideration. Repeating right heart catheterization after chronic therapy (particularly with oxygen administered at home) may demonstrate that some patients can meet the PVR criterion for transplantation. Finally, there is some evidence from a review of predominantly adult cardiac transplant experience that the immunologic status of the recipient will have an impact on the short- and long-term outcome after transplantation and therefore should be considered in the transplant evaluation.[22] Patients with elevated panel-reactive antibodies (PRA) (i.e., preformed antibodies that react with lymphocytes from a random "panel" from the general population) have a reduced 5-year actuarial survival probability that correlated in a linear fashion with the level of PRA. Thus, patients with a PRA >25% had a rate of freedom from death caused by all forms of rejection of only 57%, while those with a PRA from 0% to 10% had a rate of 5-year freedom from death owing to rejection of 85%. Interestingly, there was no correlation between survival and the outcome of lymphocyte crossmatching between the specific donor and recipient.[22] Most centers have required ABO compatibility between donor and recipient, and there have been anecdotal reports of severe hyperacute rejection when ABO barriers have been crossed.

If these indications and contraindications are followed, patients can be accurately selected for transplantation. However, families and patients must be prepared for a potentially long wait for a suitable donor.

Donor Selection

Under current U.S. law, patients must meet criteria for irreversible brain death to be considered suitable for organ donation (except for living organ donation [e.g., kidneys]). The definition of brain death is relatively well established and includes the following clinical findings in the absence of sedative medication or hypothermia: lack of response to painful or other stimuli, lack of brain stem reflexes, and lack of spontaneous respiratory effort for at least 3 minutes while off the ventilator. There are some differences among the three most commonly used definitions of brain death concerning the use of electroencephalographic and cerebral blood flow criteria and the duration over which the observations must be made (12 vs. 24 hours). The situation with the neonatal and infant donor is somewhat more controversial because of the difficulties in arriving at an accurate neurologic prognosis in this age group.[2] In fact, a multidisciplinary task force specifically declined to define criteria for brain death for neonates less than 7 days old. In infants up to 2 months of age, two clinical examinations and electroencephalograms (EEGs) 48 hours apart are recommended before declaration of brain death.[2] After the age of 1 year, two clinical examinations showing apnea, coma, and absence of brain stem function are thought to be necessary. In a retrospective review of 18 neonates <30 days old, Ashwal and Schneider found that electrocerebral silence (flat EEG) over 24 hours confirmed brain death if clinical criteria were met, as did absence of cerebral blood flow by radionuclide scan. However, term infants who met clinical criteria for brain death over 48 hours also did not survive, regardless of electroencephalographic or cerebral blood flow status.[2] Therefore, the electroencephalographic and cerebral blood flow examinations were thought to be of value only because they could shorten the period of observation necessary to make the diagnosis of brain death.[2] The question of the anencephalic donor remains problematic, because many of these children initially have some brain stem function that prevents them from meeting brain death criteria.

From a cardiac standpoint, the infant or neonatal donor should have a normal blood pressure with relatively low-dose inotropic support (e.g., dopamine at 10 μg/kg/min), should not have had a prolonged cardiac arrest or intracardiac injections, and should have a normal electrocardiogram except for ST and T wave changes, which may occur with cerebral injury. However, often these criteria are not fulfilled, but the heart may still be acceptable for donation. An echocardiogram is not mandatory, but it can help in marginal situations by providing additional data about global and regional ventricular function, atrioventricular and semilunar valve function, and the presence of major structural abnormalities in the heart. The presence of a minor defect (e.g., a small atrial septal defect) should not signify that the heart cannot be used. The use of invasive monitoring lines to monitor central venous pressure and right atrial or pulmonary artery saturation allows the maximization of filling pressures and provides an index of cardiac output. If the cardiac output is high (as reflected by an elevated mixed venous saturation), hypotension may simply reflect an abnormally low systemic vascular resistance rather than inadequate ventricular function and may be treated with alpha-adrenergic agents. Also, in some cases, ventricular function may improve as the interval from the initial insult increases. At Children's Hospital in Boston, we have observed remarkable improvements in ventricular function in neonates over several days after an episode of asphyxia resulted in severe permanent damage to the central nervous system. More commonly, however, there is deterioration of cardiac function when brain death occurs, particularly when brain herniation occurs. Furthermore, frequently there is pressure from the donor family to bring matters to a conclusion, and the time necessary for recovery of a myocardium "stunned" by an ischemic insult is not known.

Other aspects of donor evaluation include exclusion of active bacteremia and screening for viral disease such as the human immunodeficiency virus and hepatitis B and C. The donor blood type must be determined, and a search should be made for evidence of previous cytomegalovirus and toxoplasmosis infections. The height and weight of the donor should be determined; donors ranging from 50% below to 150% above the height and weight of the recipient may be suitable for a given recipient. If pulmonary hypertension exists in the recipient, the standard wisdom has been to attempt to use donors who are larger than the recipient to avoid right heart failure in the early post-transplant phase.

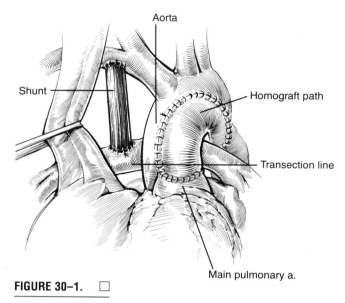

FIGURE 30–1.   □

The appearance of the heart after a stage 1 palliative operation for hypoplastic left heart syndrome with the pulmonary artery–to-aorta anastomosis and arch augmentation and right-sided modified Blalock-Taussig shunt.

Surgical Management of the Recipient

In the patient without significant anatomic abnormalities of systemic or pulmonary venous return or of the great arteries, the technique for transplantation of the heart is not significantly different from that described by Lower and Shumway.[24] Despite the need for vascular anastomoses to grow, at Children's Hospital in Boston we have used fine monofilament nonabsorbable suture for these anastomoses and have not observed anastomotic stenoses with growth. We have also paid particular attention to avoiding high aortic root pressures during the initial 5 to 10 minutes after removal of the aortic cross-clamp, based on observations of a deleterious effect of elevated reperfusion pressures made in the experimental laboratory.[16, 29]

In patients with certain types of congenital heart disease, these techniques must be altered. In the neonatal patient with the hypoplastic left heart syndrome, the transplant operation must also include reconstruction of the hypoplastic aortic arch; this is best accomplished by harvesting the entire aortic arch of the donor and using this donor tissue to substitute for the arch of the recipient. Thus, the descending aorta of the donor is anastomosed to the descending aorta of the recipient below the ductus arteriosus, and the brachiocephalic vessels of the recipient are anastomosed as a single Carrel patch to the aortic arch of the donor aorta. The remainder of the transplant operation can be carried out using the usual techniques for the atrial and pulmonary

artery anastomoses. Bypass can be established with a single right atrial venous cannula or with two small venous cannulas, as described by Allard and Backer and colleagues.[1, 3] Deep hypothermia and circulatory arrest are necessary to allow the arch reconstruction, but after completion of the left and right atrial anastomoses, bypass can be resumed and rewarming started during the pulmonary artery anastomosis. The technique of bicaval cannulation allows resumption of bypass after the aortic arch and left atrial anastomoses are completed. The technique for transplantation after stage 1 palliation for hypoplastic left heart syndrome is shown in Figures 30–1 through 30–4.

In patients with either D- or L-transposition of the great arteries, no special modifications of the transplant operation are necessary, although it is useful to have extra length in both donor and recipient pulmonary arteries and aortas. It has been necessary to move the pulmonary artery anastomotic site leftward of the natural main pulmonary artery orifice, particularly with an L-transposed aorta. However, in the patient with a previous atrial-level repair of D-transposition, some technical modifications of the transplant operation are necessary. Cannulation for bypass is done with a single arterial and two venous cannulas, which are inserted into

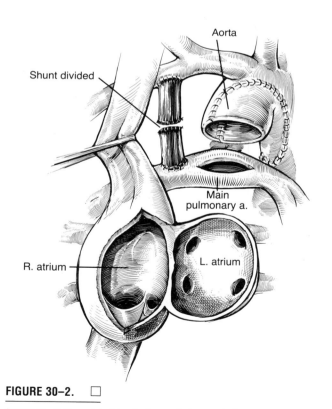

FIGURE 30–2.   □

Appearance of the recipient heart after cardiectomy and division of the Blalock-Taussig shunt. The left atrium may be significantly smaller than the right atrium.

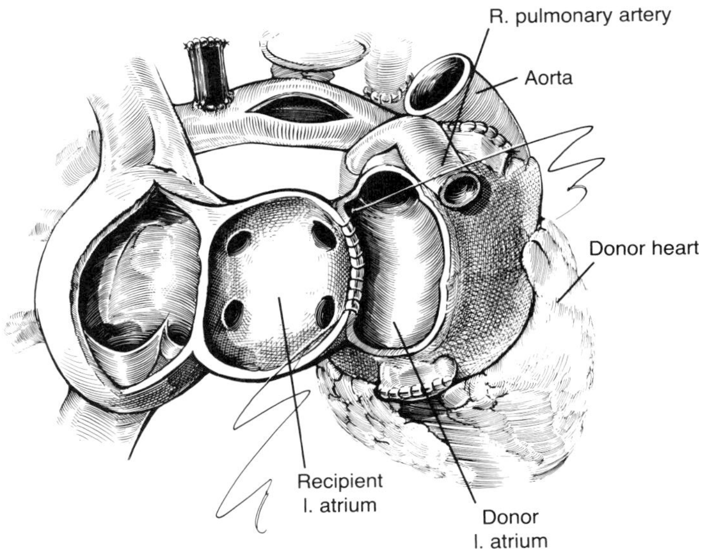

FIGURE 30-3. □

The donor left atrium is being sewn to the recipient left atrium. Note the incision in the recipient main pulmonary artery, which will be the point for anastomosis of the donor pulmonary artery. The donor branch pulmonary arteries have been left intact so that they may be used in the repair of residual stenoses in the recipient pulmonary arteries.

the superior vena cava and the junction of the inferior vena cava and right atrium (Fig. 30–5). After bypass is established, the ventricles are removed at the level of the atrioventricular groove, and the great arteries are transected just above the semilunar valves. This resection leaves the pathways from the venae cavae to the left atrium and from the pulmonary vein to the right atrium intact, and these must be converted to normal systemic and pulmonary venous connections. The roof of the systemic venous pathway (right atrial flap in a Senning repair) is detached from its connection to the atrial septum and excised (Fig. 30–5), and the floor of the systemic venous pathway is excised. The superior and inferior venae cavae are detached from their connections to the atrial mass. Thus, all that remains attached to the atrium are the pulmonary veins, and the entire remaining rim of atrium (including the pericardial augmentation of the pulmonary venous atrium in the modification of the Senning operation used at Children's Hospital in Boston[28]) can then be sewn to the donor left atrium (Fig. 30–6). The donor venae cavae are then directly anastomosed to the recipient venae cavae, and the arterial connections are made in end-to-end fashion (Fig. 30–7). This technique avoids the problem of the leftward displacement of the vena caval orifices that results from atrial-level repairs (Fig. 30–5) and that can complicate the atrial connections in a standard transplant operation.[9]

In patients with anomalies of systemic or pulmonary venous return, most problems can be solved by harvesting extra lengths of donor superior vena cava and innominate vein and making direct cavocaval anastomoses or by using techniques, such as those described by Allard and coworkers,[1] in which

intra-atrial baffling of anomalous systemic venous return or actual translocation of the systemic venous return was carried out.

Surgical Management of the Donor

In general, the donor operation in infants and neonates is similar to that described in texts on cardiac surgery and transplantation. It is worthy of emphasis that ventricular distention must be

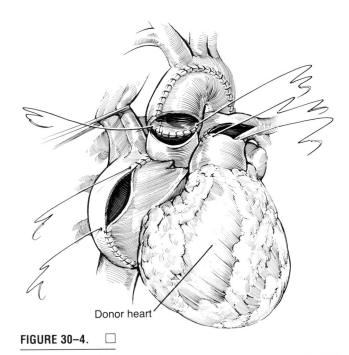

FIGURE 30-4. □

The transplant operation is completed with aortic, pulmonary artery, and right atrial anastomoses.

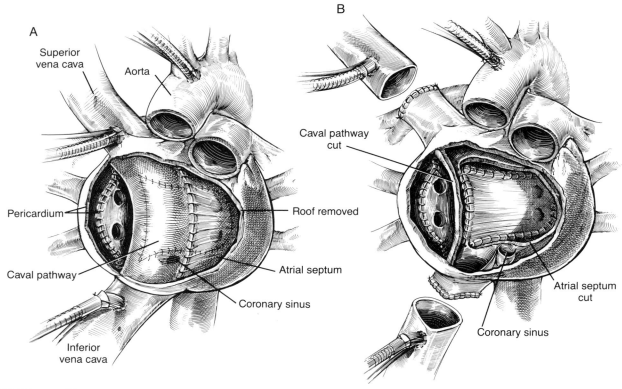

FIGURE 30–5. ☐

The appearance of the recipient heart (post atrial repair of D-TGA) after resection of the recipient's ventricles just above the atrioventricular valves and after division of the great arteries. The systemic venous pathway to the mitral valve is still intact. The leftward displacement of the superior and inferior venae cavae, shown in the figure, has been consistently present in patients after atrial level repairs. Direct cannulation of the superior and inferior venae cavae allow direct cavocaval anastomoses.

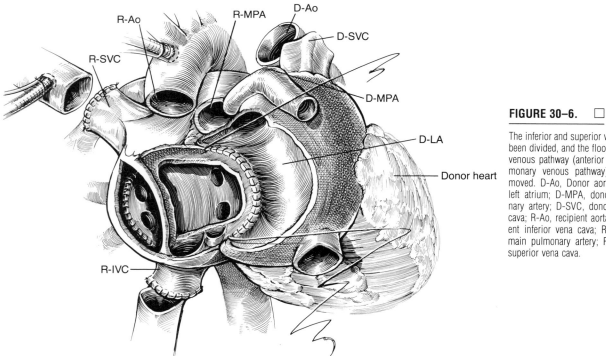

FIGURE 30–6. ☐

The inferior and superior venae cavae have been divided, and the floor of the systemic venous pathway (anterior wall of the pulmonary venous pathway) has been removed. D-Ao, Donor aorta; D-LA, donor left atrium; D-MPA, donor main pulmonary artery; D-SVC, donor superior vena cava; R-Ao, recipient aorta; R-IVC, recipient inferior vena cava; R-MPA, recipient main pulmonary artery; R-SVC, recipient superior vena cava.

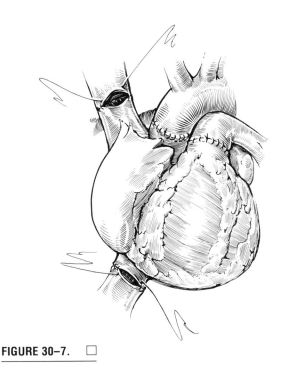

FIGURE 30–7. ☐

Completion of the transplant operation with anastomoses of the donor superior and inferior venae cavae to the recipient venae cavae.

avoided, and therefore the donor inferior vena cava and left atrium must be widely incised immediately after placement of the clamps on the aorta and superior and inferior venae cavae. Myocardial preservation has consisted of oxygenated cardioplegia St. Thomas solution or glucose-potassium cardioplegia (see Chapter 3) combined with transportation in a cooler filled with ice. As noted in the previous sections, additional lengths of donor veins and aorta should be harvested to accommodate the anatomic variations in the recipient. In situations where additional lengths of the right/left pulmonary artery branches are necessary to accommodate pulmonary artery stenoses in the recipient, the donor may not be able to be used as a lung donor. These considerations must be delineated when the recipient is enrolled with the local organ procurement organization.

Postoperative Management

The postoperative hemodynamic management of the recipient is relatively similar to that used for a typical nontransplant patient after an open cardiac procedure. However, the patients generally have required some chronotropic support in the form of atrial pacing or low-dose isoproterenol (0.02 to 0.05 µg/kg/min). Additional inotropic support with dopamine is also frequently necessary. Attempts are

made to wean the infant from ventilatory support within the first 24 hours, if the hemodynamic status is satisfactory, to minimize the risk of pulmonary infection and allow oral administration of medication for immunosuppression. In patients with known preoperative pulmonary hypertension, monitoring of pulmonary artery and right atrial pressures is essential. If there is evidence of severe right ventricular failure, consideration should be given to the use of an assist device for the right ventricle. At Children's Hospital in Boston, we have had only one case (an older patient) in which a right ventricular assist device was needed, but the placement of right atrial and pulmonary arterial cannulas with connections to a centrifugal pump allowed complete or partial support for the right ventricle. Alternatively, venoarterial bypass (extracorporeal membrane oxygenation) [ECMO] can be used, but this technique requires greater levels of anticoagulation with an associated increased risk of bleeding. Mechanical assistance for the left ventricle should rarely be necessary if donor selection and management are appropriate.

Management of Immunosuppression

Triple-drug immunotherapy (azathioprine, cyclosporine, and prednisone) has generally been employed in our patients. Administration of cyclosporine is started preoperatively, and a dose of 6 to 8 mg/kg is given orally as soon as the recipient reaches the hospital after a suitable donor has been identified. Intraoperatively, methylprednisolone (30 mg/kg) is given at the start of bypass and azathioprine (2 mg/kg) is given intravenously at the conclusion of bypass. Postoperatively, prednisone (1 mg/kg/day) is started on the day of surgery. Cyclosporine is given initially in two daily doses of 1 mg/kg intravenously over 8 hours, and the dosage is adjusted to provide whole blood "trough" levels (just before the next dose) of approximately 200 ng/ml. Dosage is also adjusted for renal function as assessed by urine output and serum levels of urea nitrogen and creatinine. As soon as gastrointestinal function returns, cyclosporine is administered orally. It has been our experience that infants require a more frequent cyclosporine dosing regimen than older patients; frequently a schedule of three times per day is used. In addition, higher total daily doses are also often necessary. Azathioprine is continued at 2 mg/kg/day, either intravenously or orally, adjusted to maintain the leukocyte count at >4000. Immunosuppression with either rabbit antithymocyte globulin (ATG) or the T cell–specific murine antibody OKT3 has been reserved for those patients with significant pre-existing renal dysfunction or for those who develop renal insufficiency postoperatively. Studies have shown that OKT3 may have no significant advantage over other forms of antilymphocyte antibody therapy (e.g., ATG or antilymphoblast globulin [ALG]), and patients can become immunized against OKT3, rendering future therapy with this agent ineffective.[5] Therefore, we have not used OKT3 as part of the routine rejection prophylaxis after transplantation and have reserved its use for steroid-refractory rejection. At Loma Linda University, where the largest neonatal cardiac transplant experience has been acquired, corticosteroid therapy is not routinely used except in the treatment of rejection,[5] and cyclosporine and azathioprine are given as antirejection therapy.

Monitoring for Rejection. We have relied primarily on endomyocardial biopsy for the definitive diagnosis of rejection. Other noninvasive indicators of rejection, such as the electrocardiogram or echocardiogram, have lacked both sensitivity and specificity for the diagnosis of rejection, although other centers have used these techniques with some success.[11] However, when there is a significant change in either the myocardial wall thickness or the echocardiographic indices of left ventricular function,[18] biopsy is generally undertaken. In our catheterization laboratory, biopsy in children as young as 3 months has been performed via the femoral or subclavian veins, with a low risk of complication; two patients who initially weighed less than 6 kg at the time of transplantation each had more than 15 biopsies in the first 2 years after transplant without significant problems. Similar results have been reported by Kawauchi and coworkers from Loma Linda University using two-dimensional echocardiography to guide the biopsy.[18]

Management of Rejection. Pulse administration of either oral prednisone (1 mg/kg/day for 3 days) or intravenous methylprednisolone (30 mg/kg/day) has been the first-line treatment of rejection, but in refractory patients, either OKT3 or rabbit ATG has been used with success. One older patient who had recurrent rejection despite OKT3, rabbit ATG, and total lymphoid irradiation was treated with a relatively new agent, FK 506, which stabilized her rejection for 1 year.

RESULTS

Between January 1986 and July 1991, a total of 38 neonates and infants under the age of 2 years were evaluated for cardiac transplantation at Children's Hospital in Boston. Of the entire group of 38 patients, 17 are alive, and 21 have died. Twenty

patients were listed for transplantation, but only five have received hearts, including one who underwent transplant at another institution after the family relocated. There was one early post-transplant death from respiratory syncytial virus, and there have been two late deaths, each more than 2 years after transplant. One of the late deaths was due to chronic rejection, and the second was sudden (at home) and occurred during a presumed viral illness. Two patients are alive with transplanted hearts.

The outcome of the remaining patients who were listed for transplantation is shown in Figure 30–8. Nine patients died while awaiting a donor heart, and two others died during transplant evaluation before enlisting with the organ procurement organization. Interestingly, six patients were initially listed for transplantation but had notable improvement in ventricular function with the passage of time and went on to conventional forms of surgical or medical therapy. Four had hypoplastic left heart syndrome or single-ventricle physiology with aortic arch obstruction, one had myocarditis, and one had coronary artery disease secondary to Kawasaki's disease. Two of these six were patients with complex single ventricle who had had successful Fontan operations. Six families declined transplantation, and all five infants with structural variants of the hypoplastic left heart syndrome died. One patient with cardiomyopathy has survived. Ten other patients were evaluated but not listed for transplantation; two of these were believed to have medical contraindications to transplantation, and both have died. However, the other eight patients were judged to be manageable by conventional means, and all are still alive.

These small numbers of infants transplanted at our institution make it difficult to reach any conclusions regarding transplantation in neonates and infants, other than noting the major difficulties in obtaining donor hearts for this age group. The combined experience of all institutions reporting to the registry maintained by the International Society for Heart Transplantation through 1990 was reported by Kriett and Kaye.[21] From 1980 through 1990, the operative mortality rate for patients undergoing transplantation within the first year of life has been higher than for patients undergoing transplantation after the first year of life;[19] as late as 1989, this rate remained higher than 20%.[19] Once the initial operative mortality risk was accounted for, the subsequent survival curves were comparable to those for adult recipients.[19] In 1989, 39% of the transplants reported in children were performed in patients less than 1 year of age, and most of these were in patients less than 2 months old.[1] At Loma

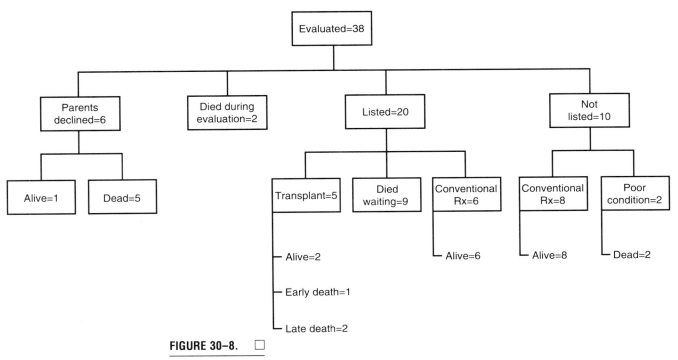

FIGURE 30–8. ☐

Results of cardiac transplantation at Children's Hospital, Boston, between 1986 and 1991.

Linda University, 34 of 40 newborns survived transplantation between 1985 and 1990.[6] Despite the theoretical possibility that, from an immunologic standpoint,[10] the neonate may be more likely to accept a transplant, rejection has not been eliminated as a threat to the neonatal transplant recipient in the Loma Linda experience,[8] and approximately 50% of children undergoing transplantation at less than 6 months of age developed serious infections in the postoperative period.[8] Although only two of these infections proved to be fatal, the overall survival rate in 63 infants less than 6 months old was 78%. These figures for the incidence of rejection seem to be lower than those for older patients, although routine surveillance endomyocardial biopsies were not carried out. More recently, the experience at Loma Linda has been expanded to include 111 patients with the hypoplastic left heart syndrome who were listed for cardiac transplantation (L. Bailey, personal communication, September 1992). Eighty-four actually underwent transplantation, with 11 early deaths (13.1%) and four late deaths (4.8%). Of the 111 patients listed for transplantation, 27 died while waiting for a donor heart (24.3%).

SUMMARY

Transplantation has clearly become a viable option for neonates and infants with cardiomyopathy or with some forms of congenital heart disease that are not amenable to conventional medical or surgical therapy. The most obvious limitations to the application of this form of "replacement" therapy have been the shortage of donor hearts and the uncertainties about the long-term effects of chronic immunosuppression. Therefore, it has been difficult for us at Children's Hospital in Boston to consider transplantation for most forms of complex congenital heart disease when more conventional palliative options exist, even if those options (such as stage 1 palliation for the hypoplastic left heart syndrome) carry a significant mortality risk. As noted earlier, continued review of the experience with these palliative options may help to identify those patients who are at prohibitive risk with conventional palliation, and transplantation can then be offered to this more select group of neonates and infants. Transplantation can still be offered under less urgent circumstances to those patients who are failing after initial palliation in the short to intermediate term, although as noted previously, some patients experience remarkable improvement in the function of their single ventricles with medical management and the passage of time. Only additional experience with both transplantation and conventional therapy will resolve the issue of which approach, or combination of approaches, will result in the greatest patient survival and the best quality of life.

REFERENCES

1. Allard M, Assaad A, Bailey LL, et al. Surgical techniques in pediatric heart transplantation. J Heart Lung Transplant 10:808, 1991.
2. Ashwal S, Schneider S. Brain death in the newborn. Pediatrics 84:429, 1989.
3. Backer CL, Zales VR, Idriss FS, et al. Heart transplantation in neonates and in children. J Heart Lung Transplant 11:311, 1992.
4. Bailey LL, Assaad AN, Trimm RF, et al. Orthotopic transplantation during early infancy as therapy for incurable congenital heart disease. Ann Surg 208:279, 1988.
5. Bailey LL, Gundry SR. Hypoplastic left heart syndrome. Pediatr Clin North Am 37:137, 1990.
6. Bailey LL, Kahan BD, Nehlsen-Cannarella SL, et al. The neonatal immune system: Window of opportunity? J Heart Lung Transplant 10:828, 1991.
7. Barnard CM. A human cardiac transplant: An interim report of a successful operation performed at Groote Schuur Hospital, Capetown. S Afr Med J 41:1271, 1967.
8. Behrendt DM, Billingham ME, Boucek MM, et al. Rejection/infection: The limits of heart transplantation success. J Heart Lung Transplant 10:841, 1991.
9. Chang AC, Wernovsky G, Wessel DL, et al. Surgical management of late right ventricular failure after Mustard or Senning repair. Circulation 86(suppl II):II-1, 1992.
10. Chiavarelli M, Boucek MM, Nehlsen-Cannarella SL, et al. Neonatal cardiac transplantation. Arch Surg 127:1072, 1992.
11. Colan SD. Assessment of ventricular and myocardial performance. In Fyler DC (ed). Nadas' Pediatric Cardiology. 21st ed. Philadelphia, Hanley & Belfus, 1992, pp 225–248.
12. Colan SD, Spevak PJ, Parness IA, et al. Cardiomyopathies. In Fyler DC (ed). Nadas' Pediatric Cardiology. Philadelphia, Hanley & Belfus, 1992, pp 329–361.
13. Doty DB, Renlund DG, Caputo GR, et al. Cardiac transplantation in situs inversus. J Thorac Cardiovasc Surg 99:493, 1990.
14. Francis FS, Pierpont GL. Pathophysiology of congestive heart failure secondary to congestive and ischemic cardiomyopathy. In Shaver JA (ed). Cardiomyopathies: Clinical Presentation, Differential Diagnosis, and Management. Philadelphia, FA Davis, 1988, pp 57–74.
15. Freed MD. Congestive heart failure. In Fyler DC (ed). Nadas' Pediatric Cardiology. Philadelphia, Hanley & Belfus, 1992, pp 63–72.
16. Fujiwara T, Kurtts T, Silvera M, et al. Physical and pharmacological manipulation of reperfusion conditions in neonatal myocardial preservation. Circulation 78(suppl II):II-444, 1988.
17. Kantrowitz A, Haller JD, Joos H, et al. Transplantation of the heart in an infant and an adult. Am J Cardiol 22:782, 1968.
18. Kawauchi M, Gundry SR, Boucek MM, et al. Real-time monitoring of the endomyocardial biopsy site with pediatric transesophageal echocardiography. J Heart Lung Transplant 11:306, 1992.
19. Kaye MP, Kriett JM. Pediatric heart transplantations: The world experience. J Heart Lung Transplant 10:856, 1991.
20. Kirklin JK, Naftel DC, McGiffin DC, et al. Analysis of morbid events and risk factors for death after cardiac transplantation. J Am Coll Cardiol 11:917, 1988.
21. Kriett JM, Kaye MP. The registry of the International Society for Heart and Lung Transplantation: Eighth official report—1991. J Heart Lung Transplant 10:491, 1991.
22. Lavee J, Kormos RL, Duquesnoy RJ, et al. Influence of panel-reactive antibody and lymphocytotoxic crossmatch on survival after heart transplantation. J Heart Lung Transplant 10:921, 1991.
23. Lower RR, Dong E, Shumway NE. Long-term survival of cardiac homografts. Surgery 58:110, 1965.
24. Lower RR, Shumway NE. Studies on the orthotopic homotransplantation of the canine heart. Surg Forum 11:18, 1960.
25. Maron BJ, Tajik AJ, Ruttenberg HD, et al. Hypertrophic cardiomyopathy in infants: Clinical features and natural history. Circulation 65:7, 1982.
26. Mayer JE Jr, Perry S, O'Brien P, et al. Orthotopic heart transplantation for complex congenital heart disease. J Thorac Cardiovasc Surg 99:484, 1990.
27. Nestico PF, Morganroth J. Congestive heart failure and ventricular arrhythmias. In Shaver JA (ed). Cardiomyopathies: Clinical Presentation, Differential Diagnosis, and Management. Philadelphia, FA Davis, 1988, pp 253–262.
28. Otero-Coto E, Norwood WI, Lang P, et al. Modified Senning operation for treatment of transposition of the great arteries. J Thorac Cardiovasc Surg 78:721, 1979.
29. Sawatari K, Kadoba K, Bergner KA, et al. Influence of reperfusion pressure after hypothermic cardioplegia on endothelial modulation of coronary tone in neonatal lambs: Impaired coronary vasodilator response to acetycholine. J Thorac Cardiovasc Surg 101:777, 1991.
30. Walsh EP, Saul JP. Cardiac arrhythmias. In Fyler DC (ed). Nadas' Pediatric Cardiology. 2nd ed. Philadelphia, Hanley & Belfus, 1992, pp 377–433.

3

Part

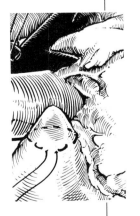

Future Developments

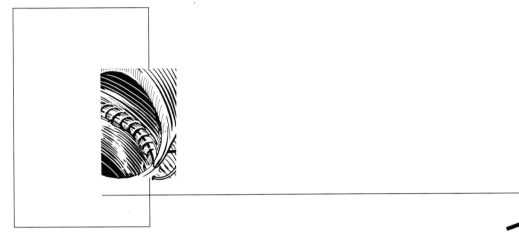

31

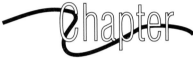

Myocardial Preservation

Until the early 1990s, investigations into myocardial preservation focused on the protection of the *myocyte* during both ischemia and reperfusion. However, there has been increasing interest in the effects of ischemia and reperfusion on the coronary vascular bed. It is intuitively obvious that recovery of the heart after a period of ischemia requires that blood flow be re-established at both the macro- and microvascular levels, and there is growing evidence that interventions that have their primary effects in the vascular bed play an important role in determining the recovery of the entire organ after a period of ischemia and reperfusion. This discussion will focus on relatively recent investigations in our laboratory at Children's Hospital in Boston and in other laboratories that have begun to consider the effects of ischemia and reperfusion on the coronary vasculature in general, and on the endothelium and endothelial-neutrophil interactions in particular.

Although blood flow must be restored after ischemia for organ function to recover, additional reperfusion injury can occur in conjunction with this restoration of blood flow.[6] There is increasing evidence that the damage that results from ischemia or reperfusion involves not only injury to the parenchymal cells in the previously ischemic tissue, but also injury to the vasculature, particularly at the microcirculatory level.[3] The term *no-reflow phenomenon* has been used to describe the inability of the vascular bed to carry blood flow to the parenchymal cells after a period of ischemia or reperfusion.[19] The en-

dothelium, in particular, seems to be the target of this ischemia-reperfusion injury, and studies in isolated organs[4, 34] and isolated blood vessels[40, 41] have demonstrated endothelial dysfunction after ischemia. These functional changes include reduction or loss of endothelial-mediated vasodilatation[4, 34, 40] and increases in capillary permeability.[27] Abnormalities in endothelial function have been shown to occur as early as 2.5 minutes after starting reperfusion. The endothelial abnormalities seem to precede parenchymal cell injury,[40] implying that the events affecting the vascular bed have an important impact on the recovery of the parenchymal cells. Morphologic changes in endothelial cells after ischemia or reperfusion have been noted by some investigators,[3, 20] but others[40] have not found ultrastructural changes, despite alterations in endothelial function. At Children's Hospital in Boston, we have demonstrated a correlation between endothelial dysfunction and the extent of mechanical dysfunction after hypothermic ischemia in the isolated, blood-perfused, neonatal lamb heart,[14, 34] and we,[15, 34] as well as others,[17, 31, 35] have found that postischemic interventions that primarily affect the vasculature favorably influence the effects of ischemia on the function of both the vasculature and the organ as a whole.

The mechanisms of this endothelial injury resulting from ischemia or reperfusion are incompletely defined, but they almost certainly involve neutrophils.[10, 12, 13, 26, 27, 29, 31, 45, 46] Neutrophil adherence to the capillary and venular endothelium, with capillary "plugging," has been well described after ischemia followed by reperfusion,[1, 3] and several experiments have shown that either neutrophil depletion or administration of agents that inhibit neutrophil function will ameliorate this damage to the vascular bed, as well as improve the recovery of whole organ function after ischemia.[7, 11, 18, 21, 45] The mechanisms by which the neutrophils can induce endothelial damage remain under investigation but likely involve the generation of highly reactive oxygen free radicals as well as the proteolytic enzymes myeloperoxidase and elastase.[12, 23, 25, 26, 44]

For neutrophils to interact with and damage the endothelium, they must first adhere to the endothelial cells.[15, 44] Leukocyte adherence to the endothelium has been shown to be an integral part of a number of inflammatory processes, and this adherence depends on specialized adhesion molecules on the surfaces of the leukocyte and the endothelial cells.[37] There is good reason to believe that ischemia followed by reperfusion is an "inflammatory" process, based on the demonstration of an activated complement in tissues reperfused after ischemia[9] and on the demonstration of a protein in cardiac lymph after ischemia and reperfusion, which activates that complement.[33] Platelet-activating factor (PAF), another acute-phase reactant, has also been shown to be released from the heart during reperfusion after ischemia.[30] Many mediators of inflammation, including activated complement C5a, PAF, tumor necrosis factor (TNF), interleukin-1 (IL-1), and leukotriene B$_4$, have been shown to induce the expression of specific adhesion molecules on either endothelial cells[32, 38] or leukocytes,[37, 39] and these adhesion molecules are an integral part of the interaction between leukocytes and endothelial cells.[22, 37] The current understanding of specific binding interactions between the various endothelial and leukocyte adhesion molecules has been reviewed by Springer.[37] Of the currently known endothelial-leukocyte adhesion molecule interactions, the most important seem to involve the integrin family of molecules on the neutrophil (CD11a-CD18, CD11b-CD18, and CD11c-CD18), which interact with ICAM-1 (intercellular adhesion molecule-1) and ICAM-2 on the endothelial cells. These three integrin molecules share the same beta subunit (CD18) with different alpha subunits (CD11a or LFA-1, CD11b or Mac-1, and CD11c or p15095). A second interaction is that between CD62 P-selectin PADGEM (platelet activation–dependent granule external membrane), which is expressed on the surfaces of endothelial cells, and · an incompletely defined leukocyte molecule known as sialyl X. Other endothelial adhesion molecules have been described, including ELAM-1 (endothelial leukocyte adhesion molecule-1) and VCAM-1 (vascular cell adhesion molecule), which may also be involved with the adhesion of leukocytes to endothelium. It seems highly likely that additional molecules will be discovered that influence the interactions between neutrophils and the endothelium, and the precise roles of any or all of these adhesion molecules in the response to ischemia and reperfusion are currently being explored.

Several experiments have suggested that blockade of certain leukocyte adhesion molecules before or during ischemia is associated with improved vascular function and improved whole organ function after normothermic ischemia and reperfusion. Vedder and coworkers showed that in a hemorrhagic shock model, administration of a monoclonal antibody, MAb 60.3, which blocks CD18, leads to reduced mortality and organ injury in both rabbits[43] and rhesus monkeys[2]; in a second model of tourniquet ischemia, they showed that survival of the tissue subjected to ischemia and reperfusion was markedly improved by treatment with this same antibody before reperfusion.[42] In a model of central nervous system ischemia, Clark and associates showed that administration of an anti-CD18 monoclonal antibody (3.3) produced a significant reduction in neurologic deficits after spinal cord ischemia induced by temporary occlusion of the thoracic aorta.[8] In a model of skeletal muscle ischemia, Carden and coworkers showed that administration of the anti-CD18 monoclonal antibody IB4 eliminated the increases in permeability induced by ischemia or reperfusion.[7] In cardiac *normothermic* ischemia models, Dreyer and colleagues demonstrated that neutrophil accumulation in regions exposed to 1 hour of ischemia and then reperfused was reduced by administration of the R15.7 monoclonal antibody to CD18[10]; Lefer and Litt and associates, using the same antibody, found that it prevented postischemic endothelial dysfunction in isolated feline coronary artery segments and also reduced neutrophil accumulation and the extent of myocardial injury after 90 minutes of normothermic ischemia.[23, 24] Simpson and coworkers found similar reductions in neutrophil accumulation and in the extent of infarction using an anti-CD11b/CD18 antibody after 90 minutes of *normothermic* ischemia in the dog.[36] Kubes and colleagues[21] also showed that the monoclonal antibody IB4 prevented the vascular permeability changes induced by infusions of PAF, a chemoattractant known to be released during ischemia and reperfusion. Experiments in our laboratory at Children's Hospital in Boston with a blood-perfused neonatal lamb heart and a monoclonal antibody to the leukocyte adhesion molecule CD18 (R15.7) showed that the inhibition of leukocyte adhesion with this monoclonal antibody results in signifi-

cantly improved recovery of both vascular and myocardial contractile function after 2 hours of hypothermic ischemia. In these experiments, the anti-
CD18 monoclonal antibody R15.7 was added to the
perfusate for nine experimental hearts just before
the start of postischemic reperfusion to yield an antibody concentration of 20 μg/ml of circulating blood
volume. After 30 minutes of rewarming and reperfusion, the monoclonal antibody–treated hearts
showed remarkably improved recovery of mechanical function and of myocardial blood flow and oxygen consumption when compared with a control
group undergoing otherwise identical hypothermic
ischemia and reperfusion (Table 31–1).

These various experiments demonstrate that leukocyte-endothelial interactions play a significant
role in the vascular dysfunction induced by both
normothermic and hypothermic ischemia and reperfusion, and that adhesion molecules on the surfaces
of leukocytes are involved in these deleterious interactions. These vascular events, in turn, also correlate well with the overall functional recovery of both
isolated organs and whole organisms subjected to
ischemic insults followed by reperfusion.

Although various "inflammatory" stimuli—including IL-1, TNF, PAF, leukotriene B$_4$, and C5a—
have been shown to induce the expression of endothelial cell adhesion molecules that serve as ligands
for leukocyte adhesion molecules, the question of
whether ischemia followed by reperfusion has any
effect on the expression of *endothelial* adhesion molecules has not been addressed. The observation that
endothelial dysfunction can be demonstrated as
soon as 2.5 minutes after the start of reperfusion[23,40]
suggests that new protein synthesis is not involved,
but it is also known that at least two endothelial
adhesion molecules (ICAM-1 and ICAM-2) are con-
stitutively expressed on the endothelial cell and
that a second adhesion molecule (PADGEM, CD62)
is stored in granules within the endothelial cell and
can be rapidly expressed[5] in response to complement,[16] histamine,[28] and thrombin.[5] However, the
role of these endothelial cell adhesion molecules, or
of other molecules such as ELAM-1 or VCAM-1, in
the response to ischemia and reperfusion remains
unclear.

Increased knowledge of the molecular processes
by which neutrophils and endothelial cells interact
and the ability to produce monoclonal antibodies
that can block these interactions offer the potential
to use monoclonal antibody therapy to ameliorate
the effects of ischemia and reperfusion in the clinical setting. Experimental evidence suggests that
therapies directed at neutrophil adhesion molecules
are likely to be effective, but these effects are likely
to be generalized and may have deleterious effects
(e.g., increasing the risk of infection) in the setting
of surgically induced ischemia. In contrast, therapies directed at endothelial cells have the potential
advantage that they are directed only at the injured
or activated cells that are expressing the adhesion
molecules. Alternatively, short-acting or rapidly reversible therapies that affect neutrophils or endothelial cells could have similar beneficial effects on
the vasculature while minimizing potential systemic side effects.

Overall, it appears that these new directions in
myocardial preservation, focusing on the coronary
vasculature and on the interactions between the endothelium and the circulating leukocytes, will produce new therapies that will improve the heart's
tolerance of ischemia and reperfusion and therefore
make reparative cardiac operations safer for patients. It is clear that the tools of molecular biology
will play a major role in these advances and that
ongoing close interactions between molecular biolo-
gists and those interested in myocardial preservation will be important.

REFERENCES

1. Ambrosio G, Weisman HF, Mannisi JA, et al. Progressive impairment of regional myocardial perfusion after initial restoration of postischemic blood flow. Circulation 80:1846, 1989.
2. Arfors KE, Lundberg C, Lindbom L, et al. A monoclonal antibody to the membrane glycoprotein complex CD18 inhibits polymorphonuclear leukocyte accumulation and plasma leakage in vivo. Blood 69:338, 1987.
3. Armiger LC, Gavin JB. Changes in the microvasculature of ischemic and infarcted myocardium. Lab Invest 33:51, 1975.
4. Babbitt DG, Virmani R, Forman MB. Intracoronary adenosine administered after reperfusion limits vascular injury after prolonged ischemia in the canine model. Circulation 80:1388, 1989.
5. Bonfanti R, Furie BC, Wagner DD. PADGEM (GMP140) is a component of Weibel-Palade bodies of human endothelial cells. Blood 73:1109, 1989.
6. Braunwald E, Kloner RA. Myocardial reperfusion: A double edged sword? J Clin Invest 76:1713, 1985.
7. Carden DL, Smith JK, Korthuis RJ. Neutrophil-mediated microvascular dysfunction in post-ischemic canine skeletal muscle. Role of granulocyte adherence. Circ Res 66:1436, 1990.
8. Clark WM, Madden KP, Rothlein R, et al. Reduction of central nervous system ischemic injury in rabbits using leukocyte adhesion antibody treatment in rabbits. Stroke 22:877, 1991.

TABLE 31–1. □ EFFECTS OF ANTIBODY TO LEUKOCYTE
ADHESION MOLECULE CD18 ON RECOVERY
AFTER HYPOTHERMIC ISCHEMIA

GROUP	NO.	Max devP	MAX dP/dt	CBF	MVO$_2$
Anti-CD18	9	83.9%	78.4%	159.5%	129.8%
Control	9	73.6%	67.4%	84.4%	71.2%

*All expressed as % of baseline. All differences between the groups were significant
($P < .05$).

9. Crawford MH, Grover FL, Kolb WP, et al. Complement and neutrophil activation in the pathogenesis of ischemic myocardial injury. Circulation 78:1449, 1988.
10. Dreyer WJ, Michael LH, West MS, et al. Neutrophil accumulation in ischemic canine myocardium. Insights into time course, distribution, and mechanism of localization during early reperfusion. Circulation 84:400, 1991.
11. Engler R, Covell JW. Granulocytes cause reperfusion ventricular dysfunction after 15-minute ischemia in the dog. Circ Res 61:20, 1987.
12. Forman MB, Puett DW, Virmani R. Endothelial and myocardial injury during ischemia and reperfusion: Pathogenesis and therapeutic implications. J Am Coll Cardiol 13:450, 1989.
13. Forman MB, Virmani R, Puett DW. Mechanisms and therapy of myocardial reperfusion injury. Circulation 81(suppl IV):IV-69, 1990.
14. Fujiwara T, Kurtts T, Silvera M, et al. Physical and pharmacological manipulation of reperfusion conditions in neonatal myocardial preservation. Circulation 78(suppl II):II-444, 1988.
15. Harlan JM. Leukocyte-endothelial interactions. Blood 65:513, 1985.
16. Hattori R, Hamilton KK, McEver RP, et al. Complement proteins C5b-9 induce secretion of high molecular weight multimers of endothelial von Willebrand factor and translocation of granule membrane protein GMP-140 to the cell surface. J Biol Chem 264:9053, 1989.
17. Johnson G III, Furlan LE, Aoki N, et al. Endothelium and myocardial protecting actions of Taprostene, a stable prostacyclin analogue, after acute myocardial ischemia and reperfusion in cats. Circ Res 66:1363, 1990.
18. Kawata H, Sawatari K, Mayer JE. Evidence for the role of neutrophils in reperfusion injury after cold cardioplegic ischemia in neonatal lambs. J Thorac Cardiovasc Surg 103:908, 1992.
19. Kloner R, Ganote CE, Jennings RB. The "no-reflow" phenomenon after temporary coronary occlusion in the dog. J Clin Invest 54:1496, 1974.
20. Kloner RA, Rude RE, Carlson N, et al. Ultrastructural evidence of microvascular damage and myocardial cell injury after coronary artery occlusion: Which comes first? Circulation 62:945, 1980.
21. Kubes P, Ibbotson G, Russell J, et al. Role of platelet-activating factor in ischemia/reperfusion-induced leukocyte adherence. Am J Physiol 259:G300, 1990.
22. Lawrence MB, Springer TA. Leukocytes roll on a selectin at physiologic flow rates: Distinction from and prerequisite for adhesion through integrins. Cell 65:859, 1991.
23. Lefer AM, Tsao PS, Lefer DJ, et al. Role of endothelial dysfunction in the pathogenesis of reperfusion injury after myocardial ischemia. FASEB J 5:2029, 1991.
24. Litt MR, Jeremy RW, Weisman HF, et al. Neutrophil depletion limited to reperfusion reduces myocardial infarct size after 90 minutes of ischemia. Circulation 80:1816, 1989.
25. Lucchesi BR. Role of neutrophils in ischemic heart disease: Pathophysiologic role in myocardial ischemia and coronary artery reperfusion. In Mehta JL, Conti CR, Brest AN (eds). Thrombosis and Platelets in Myocardial Ischemia. Philadelphia, FA Davis, 1987, pp 35–48.
26. Lucchesi BR. Modulation of leukocyte-mediated myocardial reperfusion injury. Annu Rev Physiol 52:561, 1990.
27. McDonagh PF, Laks H. Use of cold blood cardioplegia to protect against coronary microcirculatory injury due to ischemia and reperfusion. J Thorac Cardiovasc Surg 84:609, 1982.
28. McEver RP, Beckstead JH, Moore KL, et al. GMP-140, a platelet alpha granule membrane protein, is also synthesized by vascular endothelial cells and is localized in Weibel-Palade bodies. J Clin Invest 84:92, 1989.
29. Mehta JL, Dinerman J, Mehta P, et al. Neutrophil function in ischemic heart disease. Circulation 79:549, 1989.
30. Montrucchio G, Alloatti G, Tetta C, et al. Release of platelet-activating factor from ischemic-reperfused rabbit heart. Am J Physiol 256:H1236, 1989.
31. Olafsson B, Forman MB, Puett DW, et al. Reduction of reperfusion injury in the canine preparation by intracoronary adenosine: Importance of the endothelium and the no-reflow phenomenon. Circulation 76:1135, 1987.
32. Pober JS, Cotran RS. The role of endothelial cells in inflammation. Transplantation 50:537, 1990.
33. Rossen RD, Michael LH, Kagiyama A, et al. Mechanism of complement activation after coronary artery occlusion: Evidence that myocardial ischemia in dogs causes release of constituents of myocardial subcellular origin that complex with human C1q in vivo. Circ Res 62:572, 1988.
34. Sawatari K, Kadoba K, Bergner KA, et al. Influence of reperfusion pressure after hypothermic cardioplegia on endothelial modulation of coronary tone in neonatal lambs: Impaired coronary vasodilator response to acetylcholine. J Thorac Cardiovasc Surg 101:777, 1991.
35. Simpson PJ, Mickelson J, Fantone JC, et al. Iloprost inhibits neutrophil function in vitro and in vivo and limits experimental infarct size in canine heart. Circ Res 60:666, 1987.
36. Simpson PJ, Todd RF, Fantone JC, et al. Reduction of experimental canine myocardial reperfusion injury by a monoclonal antibody (Anti-Mo1, Anti-CD11b) that inhibits leukocyte adhesion. J Clin Invest 81:624, 1988.
37. Springer TA. Adhesion receptors of the immune system. Nature 346:425, 1990.
38. Tonnesen MG, Anderson DC, Springer TA, et al. Adherence of neutrophils to cultured human microvascular endothelial cells. J Clin Invest 83:637, 1989.
39. Tonnesen MG, Smedly LA, Henson PM. Neutrophil-endothelial cell interactions. Modulation of neutrophil adhesiveness induced by complement fragments C5a and C5a des arg and Formyl-Methionyl-Leucyl-Phenylalanine in vitro. J Clin Invest 74:1581, 1984.
40. Tsao PS, Aoki N, Lefer DJ, et al. Time course of endothelial dysfunction and myocardial injury during myocardial ischemia and reperfusion in the cat. Circulation 82:1402, 1990.
41. VanBenthuysen KM, McMurtry IF, Horwitz LD. Reperfusion after acute coronary occlusion in dogs impairs endothelium-dependent relaxation to acetylcholine and augments contractile reactivity in vitro. J Clin Invest 79:265, 1987.
42. Vedder NB, Fouty BW, Winn RK, et al. Role of neutrophils in generalized reperfusion injury associated with resuscitation from shock. Surgery 106:509, 1989.
43. Vedder NB, Winn RK, Rice CL, et al. A monoclonal antibody to the adherence-promoting leukocyte glycoprotein, CD18, reduces organ injury and improves survival from hemorrhagic shock and resuscitation in rabbits. J Clin Invest 81:939, 1988.
44. Weiss SJ. Tissue destruction by neutrophils. N Engl J Med 320:365, 1989.
45. Westlin W, Mullane KM. Alleviation of myocardial stunning by leukocyte and platelet depletion. Circulation 80:1828, 1989.
46. Zimmerman BJ, Granger DN. Reperfusion-induced leukocyte infiltration: role of elastase. Am J Physiol 259:H390, 1990.

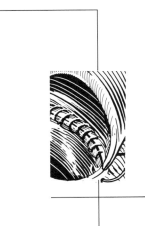

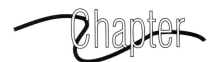

32

Cerebral Protection

Some aspects of the neurologic morbidity associated with repair of congenital heart defects were dealt with in Chapter 2. In this chapter, however, specific mechanisms of neurologic morbidity will be examined in greater detail. Relatively recent insights in this area have suggested lines of research that hold the promise of improving the quality of life for survivors of cardiac surgery during infancy.

INCIDENCE OF NEUROLOGIC MORBIDITY AFTER PEDIATRIC CARDIAC SURGERY

The incidence of neurologic sequelae of pediatric open heart surgery has been delineated in a study commissioned by the National Institutes of Health.[6] The neurologic morbidity rate in that review ranged from 1% to 25%. Protean neurologic sequelae included seizures, mental retardation, cerebral palsy, and lifelong language and learning disorders.

MECHANISMS OF NEUROLOGIC MORBIDITY

General Deleterious Effects of Cardiopulmonary Bypass

As explained in Chapter 2, there are multiple potential mechanisms of organ injury associated with the use of cardiopulmonary bypass. These mechanisms include particulate and gaseous microemboli,

activation of humoral cascades and cellular components of the blood and endothelial cells, and stimulation of a profound catecholamine response. Total systemic perfusion may be reduced for varying periods of time, either deliberately or secondary to anatomic factors related to specific congenital heart anomalies.

Excitotoxicity and Selective Neuronal Vulnerability

A global ischemic insult to the brain does not result in uniform distribution of cellular necrosis.[18, 20] Although some of the heterogeneity of distribution is related to the anatomy of the vascular tree, causing less perfusion in "watershed" areas, the other important cause of selective neuronal vulnerability relates to greater substrate demand by particular cells. Amino acids such as glutamate and aspartate are excitatory neurotransmitters in several pathways of the mammalian brain. They act on at least three different receptors, including N-methyl-D-aspartate (NMDA), kainate (KA), and quisqualate (QA). High concentrations of excitatory amino acids, which have been shown to result from an ischemic insult, result in neuronal cell death, presumably by increasing cellular metabolic demands in excess of substrate supply.[15] This mechanism of neuronal cell injury has been labeled *excitotoxicity*. The CA1 area of the hippocampus in adults, where cells have a

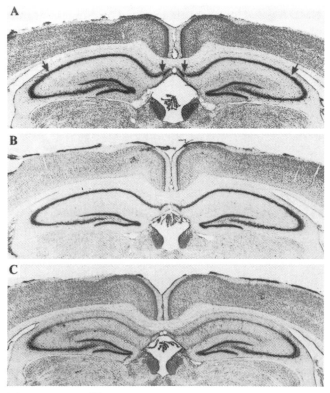

FIGURE 32–1. ☐

A, The CA1 area of the hippocampus (between the two left and right arrows) is selectively vulnerable to cerebral hypoxic/ischemic injury. This area has a high concentration of *N*-methyl-D-aspartate (NMDA) receptors and is therefore susceptible to elevated levels of neurotransmitters such as glutamate that occur after ischemia. *B,* Hypothermia to 33°C protects the CA1 area against 5 minutes of ischemia. *C,* At normothermia, there is selective loss of CA1 neurons after 5 minutes of ischemia (40 μm cresyl violet–stained sections of gerbil brain). (From Corbet D, Evans S, Thomas C, et al. MK-801 reduces cerebral ischemic injury by inducing hypothermia. Brain Res 514:300–304, 1990.)

dense concentration of NMDA receptors, is an area known to be particularly vulnerable to ischemic injury (Fig. 32–1). The hippocampus is involved with short-term memory function. Sensitive neuropsychometric tests of short-term memory have demonstrated deficits after cardiac surgery in adults.[21]

Excitotoxicity and Delayed Neuronal Death

The phenomenon of initial recovery from a cerebral insult followed by subsequent deterioration has been recognized in clinical practice for many years. It has also been clear from many laboratory studies that histologic assessment of neurologic injury will underestimate the extent of injury if it is undertaken less than 1 week from the time of the insult. It is quite probable that at least part of the explanation for this phenomenon may be vascular related, perhaps a result of the no-reflow effect.[1] Ische-

mic injury to endothelial cells may result in inappropriate vasoconstriction as well as leukocyte adhesion to activated intracellular adhesion molecules (ICAMs).[8] However, it is also probable that excitotoxicity plays a role in delayed neuronal cell death. Cells in which metabolic processes continue after the insult, but with borderline reserve, are excessively stressed by the metabolic demands secondary to the elevated levels of excitatory neurotransmitters.[16] Injection of KA, an amino acid neurotransmitter, directly into the brain of experimental animals results in localized cell death. This is also associated with electrical seizure activity. Although the importance of postoperative seizures after hypothermic circulatory arrest has been minimized in the past, it is possible that such seizures represent the phenomenon of excitotoxicity in action. As noted in Chapter 2, electroencephalographic (EEG) monitoring during the Boston Circulatory Arrest Study revealed a 26% incidence of seizures during the first 48 hours after circulatory arrest (mean duration, 55 minutes) and a 13% incidence of seizures after low-flow (50 ml/kg/min) hypothermic bypass. Preliminary analysis suggests a correlation between seizures and impaired psychomotor development.

Excitotoxicity in Neonates and Infants

As described in Chapter 1, much of the human brain's normal development occurs after birth. This development includes formation of synaptic communications between neurons (Fig. 32–2). It has been suggested that expression of NMDA and KA

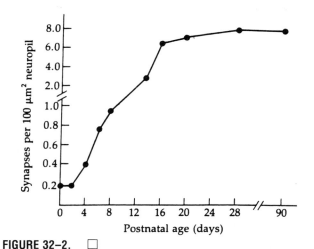

FIGURE 32–2. ☐

There is a rapid increase in the number of synapses in the human brain in the first month of life. This is associated with a parallel increase in the concentration of NMDA receptors. (From Purves D, Lichtman JW. Principles of Neural Development. Sunderland, MA, Sinauer Associates, 1985, p 209.)

receptor sites facilitates synaptogenesis.[22] This might explain the dramatic increase in the concentration of NMDA receptors observed in the first week of life, followed by a decrease over the next 3 weeks to the adult level.[9] Thus, unlike in the adult, where the CA1 area is exquisitely sensitive to hypoxic or ischemic injury, the immature animal is more likely to suffer injury in the CA3 area of the hippocampus, as well as in the dentate gyrus and globus pallidus.[10] The globus pallidus forms part of the basal ganglia, which, when injured, can cause choreoathetoid movements. Choreoathetoid cerebral palsy with preservation of intellectual function is a common result of perinatal hypoxic ischemic insult.

In addition to the changes in receptor density that may influence susceptibility to hypoxic or ischemic injury to the central nervous system, there are also important changes in high-energy phosphate metabolism in the first weeks of life. Respiration of rat cerebral cortical slices stimulated by potassium and dinitrophenol (DNp) increases abruptly during a brief time window between 10 and 15 days after birth.[12] At the same time there is a four-fold increase in the activity of creatine kinase.[11] The latter facilitates much more rapid availability of adenosine triphosphate (ATP) from phosphocreatine, thus "coupling" energy supply more directly with demand. In view of the neonate's known greater resistance to ischemic brain injury when compared with the adult, it is possible that the lower concentration of receptors, the fewer number of synapses, and the less efficient coupling of energy supply and demand are in some way protective.

POTENTIAL NEUROPROTECTIVE STRATEGIES DURING PEDIATRIC CARDIAC SURGERY

As described in Chapter 2, there are many aspects of current techniques of neurologic protection during cardiac surgery that are poorly understood. Currently, researchers at Children's Hospital in Boston and elsewhere are examining issues such as optimal pH strategy during hypothermic bypass, optimal cooling strategy, and safe duration of circulatory arrest. However, in addition to refining current techniques, there are a number of novel approaches to neurologic protection during cardiac surgery in the young that are worthy of attention.

Neurotransmitter Antagonists

Perhaps the most exciting area of contemporary neuroscientific research into pharmacologic methods to decrease cerebral ischemic injury is the po-

tential application of receptor antagonists. By decreasing neuronal metabolic activity, particularly in response to the elevated levels of neurotransmitters seen after ischemia, there is a real possibility that the extent of neuronal injury will be decreased. The noncompetitive NMDA antagonist MK-801[7, 14] has shown promise in a number of rodent models of cerebral ischemia and is currently being studied in other models. In the laboratories at Children's Hospital in Boston, a piglet model of hypothermic circulatory arrest and low-flow bypass[13] has been used to explore pharmacologic methods of brain protection (i.e., neurotransmitter antagonists). In 10 4-week-old piglets treated with MK-801, recovery of cerebral phosphocreatine, ATP, and intracellular pH, as determined by magnetic resonance spectroscopy, was significantly accelerated during reperfusion after 1 hour of circulatory arrest at 15°C when compared with 14 control animals.[4] The cerebral metabolic rate, determined by oxygen extraction recovered to $105\% \pm 30\%$ of baseline in the MK-801 group compared with $94\% \pm 32\%$ in the control animals.

More recently the agent NBQX, which blocks both KA and QA receptors, has shown promise in rodent models in reducing ischemic injury.[19] However, in our piglet model, pretreatment with NBQX was associated with both delayed recovery and diminished final recovery of cerebral phosphocreatine, ATP, and intracellular pH (Fig. 32–3). The cerebral metabolic rate, determined by oxygen consumption, recovered to only $61\% \pm 22\%$ of baseline after 3 hours and 45 minutes of reperfusion compared with $94\% \pm 32\%$ in control animals.[4]

Other Pharmacologic Agents

Apart from specific receptor antagonists, many other agents are being studied for their effects on neurons and on other postischemic tissues. Adenosine is known to inhibit the release of excitatory neurotransmitters. Free radical scavengers, calcium antagonists, and antagonists of the ligands of activated white cells (anti-CD18) and activated endothelial cells (anti-ICAM-1) are all receiving attention at present.

In our piglet model of circulatory arrest, it was found that pretreatment with the monoclonal antibody to the leukocyte adhesion molecule CD18 resulted in a significant improvement in cerebral vascular endothelial function assessed by response to an endothelium-dependent vasodilator (acetylcholine). In addition, the total gain in body weight from fluid accumulation owing to extravascular fluid leak

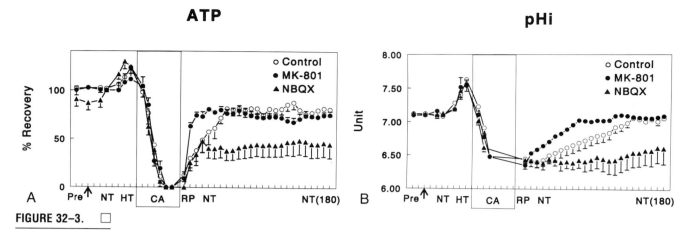

FIGURE 32–3. ☐

Recovery of cerebral adenosine triphosphate (ATP) (*A*) as determined by magnetic resonance spectroscopy is accelerated by pretreatment with the NMDA antagonist dizocilpine maleate (MK-801) after 1 hour of deep hypothermic circulatory arrest at 15°C nasopharyngeal temperature. In contrast, pretreatment with an alternative receptor antagonist, NBQX, is associated with diminished recovery of ATP. Similar findings are seen with recovery of intracellular pH (pHi). *B*, After 1 hour of hypothermic circulatory arrest. CA, Circulatory arrest; HT, after 30 minutes of core cooling to nasopharyngeal temperature of 15°C; NT, baseline measurement after 20 minutes of normothermic cardiopulmonary bypass; NT (180), after 3 hours of reperfusion at normothermia; pre, before cardiopulmonary bypass; RP, commencement of reperfusion/rewarming.

was significantly lower, as was the postoperative water content of the heart and lungs.[3]

One other agent that has been studied in our piglet model, and that shows promise in improving cerebral protection during hypothermic bypass and circulatory arrest, is the protease inhibitor aprotinin.[2] Cerebral ischemia resulting from bilateral carotid artery occlusion in the rat results in increased cerebral water content. This is paralleled by an increase in cerebral tissue bradykinin. Pretreatment of rats with aprotinin, which blocks the kallikrein/bradykinin cascade, resulted in lower levels of cerebral water, bradykinin, and lactate, as well as improved preservation of cerebral ATP. In our piglet model, the cerebral water content was also decreased by pretreatment with aprotinin ($P = .055$). In addition, recovery of cerebral ATP and intracellular pH, as determined by magnetic resonance spectroscopy, was accelerated by aprotinin in the initial 30 minutes of reperfusion. Interestingly, the animals treated with aprotinin also showed improved preservation of endothelial function after reperfusion when compared with control animals, suggesting that vascular protection may play a role in the multiple actions of aprotinin.

Cerebroplegia

It is possible that, analogous to cardioplegia, a single infusion (or perhaps multiple intermittent infusions) of a "cerebroplegic" solution may provide improved cerebral protection when compared with continuous perfusion with cold, dilute blood (low-flow bypass) or complete cessation of circulation (hypothermic circulatory arrest) (see Fig. 32–3).[17] This would be useful not only for the cardiac surgeon undertaking complex reconstructive procedures of the aortic arch (e.g., correction of hypoplastic left heart syndrome or interrupted aortic arch) or dealing with acquired disease (e.g., aortic arch aneurysms), but also for the vascular surgeon (i.e., in carotid artery procedures) and the neurosurgeon. No doubt a similar technique could be extrapolated to spinal cord protection for procedures involving the descending aorta (e.g., correction of coarctation or descending aortic aneurysms). Robbins and associates[17] infused a cardioplegic solution at 4°C into the carotid arteries of juvenile sheep undergoing 2 hours of circulatory arrest. Using magnetic resonance spectroscopy, they found improved preservation of cerebral high-energy phosphates and pH with a more rapid return of the EEG signal. In a more recent study by the same group,[5] five of seven sheep that received a simple crystalloid cerebroplegic solution, administered antegrade, were free of neurologic deficit after 6 hours of recovery. Interestingly, animals in which the cerebroplegic solution was administered retrogradely did poorly as did control animals. However, animals that had their heads packed in ice during the arrest period performed as well as the animals receiving antegrade cerebroplegia.

In our laboratories at Children's Hospital in Boston, in conjunction with the Magnetic Resonance Spectroscopy Laboratory at Massachusetts Institute of Technology, cerebroplegic solutions that incorporate neurotransmitter antagonists such as MK-801 are being examined along with complex buffering solutions incorporating adenosine (e.g., the University of Wisconsin solution). Preliminary results suggest a much greater recovery of cerebral high-energy phosphates and intracellular pH when using such solutions during a 2-hour period of circulatory arrest than when using simple crystalloid cerebroplegia.

CONCLUSION

The 1990s have been designated the "Decade of the Brain," so there is hope that funding for neuroscientific research will expand accordingly. Until fundamental understanding of neurologic processes and neurologic development progresses, neurologic injury, both severe and subtle, is likely to continue to be an unfortunate consequence of cardiac surgery in the young.

REFERENCES

1. Ames A, Wright RL, Kowada M, et al. Cerebral ischemia. II. The no-reflow phenomenon. Am J Pathol 52:437, 1968.
2. Aoki M, Jonas RA, Nomura F, et al. Aprotinin enhances acute recovery of cerebral metabolism after circulatory arrest. Circulation 86(suppl I):I-182, 1992.
3. Aoki M, Jonas RA, Nomura F, et al. Impact of monoclonal antibody to leukocyte adhesion molecule CD18 on deleterious effects of cardiopulmonary bypass and hypothermic circulatory arrest in piglets. Submitted for publication to Anesthesiology.
4. Aoki M, Nomura F, Stromski ME, et al. Impact of MK-801 and NBQX on acute recovery of piglet cerebral metabolism after hypothermic circulatory arrest. J Cereb Blood Flow Metab. In press.
5. Crittenden MD, Roberts CS, Rosa L, et al. Brain protection during circulatory arrest. Ann Thorac Surg 51:942, 1991.
6. Ferry PC. Neurologic sequelae of open heart surgery in children. Am J Dis Child 144:369, 1990.
7. Gill R, Foster AC, Woodruff GN. Systemic administration of MK-801 protects against ischemia-induced hippocampal neurodegeneration in the gerbil. J Neurosci 7:3343, 1987.
8. Gimbrone MA, Buchanan MR. Interactions of platelets and leukocytes with vascular endothelium; in vitro studies. Ann NY Acad Sci 401:171, 1982.
9. Greenamyre JT, Penney JB, Young AB, et al. Evidence for transient perinatal glutamatergic innervation of globus pallidus. J Neurosci 7:1022, 1987.
10. Hagberg H, Andine P, Lehmann A. Excitatory amino acids and hypoxic-ischemic damage in the immature brain. In Schurr A, Rigor BM (eds). Cerebral Ischemia and Resuscitation. Boca Raton, FL, CRC Press, 1990, p 166.
11. Holtzman D, McFarland EW, Jacobs D, et al. Maturational increase in mouse brain creatine kinase reaction rates shown by phosphorous resonance. Dev Brain Res 58:181, 1991.
12. Holtzman D, Olson J, Zamvil S, et al. Maturation of potassium stimulated respiration in rat cerebral cortex slices. J Neurochem 39:274, 1982.
13. Kawata H, Fackler JC, Aoki M, et al. Recovery of cerebral blood flow and energy state after hypothermic circulatory arrest versus low flow bypass in piglets. J Thorac Cardiovasc Surg. In press.
14. Meldrum B. Protection against ischemic neuronal damage by drugs acting on excitatory neurotransmission. Cerebrovasc Brain Metab Rev 2:27, 1990.
15. Olney JW, Ho OL, Rhee V. Cytotoxic effects of acidic and sulphur-containing amino acids on the infant mouse central nervous system. Exp Brain Res 14:61, 1971.
16. Petito CK, Feldmann E, Pulsinelli WA, et al. Delayed hippocampal damage in humans following cardiorespiratory arrest. Neurology 37:1281, 1987.
17. Robbins RC, Balaban RS, Swain JA. Intermittent hypothermic asanguineous cerebral perfusion (cerebroplegia) protects the brain during prolonged circulatory arrest. J Thorac Cardiovasc Surg 99:878, 1990.
18. Rothman SM, Olney JW. Glutamate and the pathophysiology of hypoxic-ischemic brain damage. Ann Neurol 19:105, 1986.
19. Sheardown MJ, Nielson EO, Hansen AJ, et al. 2,3-Dihydroxy-6-nitro-7-sulfamoyl-benzo(F)quinoxaline: A neuroprotectant for cerebral ischemia. Science 247:571, 1990.
20. Simon RP, Swan JH, Griffiths T, et al. Blockade of N-methyl-D-aspartate receptors may protect against ischemic damage in the brain. Science 226:850, 1984.
21. Smith PLC, Newman SP, Ell PJ, et al. Cerebral consequences of cardiopulmonary bypass. Lancet 1:823, 1986.
22. Tremblay E, Roisin MP, Represa A, et al. Transient increased density of NMDA binding sites in the developing brain hippocampus. Brain Res 461:393, 1988.

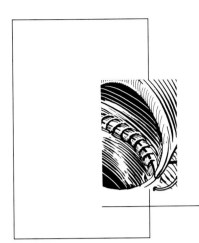

33

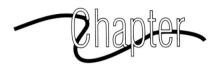
Chapter

Fetal Intervention for Congenital Heart Disease

In principle, it is difficult to find fault with the philosophy that total correction of clinically important structural heart lesions should be performed as early in life as possible. The example that comes most readily to mind in support of this philosophy is the neonatal arterial switch operation for transposition of the great arteries with an intact ventricular septum. The operation provides anatomic and physiologic correction of a lethal condition within days of the onset of morbidity (i.e., birth).

Unfortunately, congenital heart disease is more varied and complex than this example, and under certain conditions neonatal repair may not be ideal. For instance, a truly total correction may not always be performed (e.g., in tetralogy of Fallot requiring a transannular patch). In this case, total correction would involve placement of a nonviable, nongrowing valved conduit; otherwise, pulmonary regurgitation must be accepted in the presence of somewhat elevated pulmonary vascular resistance. With other lesions, the onset of morbidity may not be at the time of birth, as it is in transposition, but at the time of primary morphogenesis (i.e., about the eighth week of gestation). For example, in critical aortic stenosis, not only is it unlikely that total correction will be achieved when the intervention is undertaken in the first days of life, but as many as 7 months of ongoing morbidity will have already occurred (from completion of primary morphogenesis to birth). The prolonged exposure to this morbidity may cause irreversible pathologic cardiac abnormalities.

Given our present understanding of biology, it remains a somewhat remote possibility that therapy involving genetic or other manipulation of hypoplastic or abnormal tissues will allow generation of a normal structure (e.g., creation of a normal right ventricular outflow tract in tetralogy of Fallot). In contrast, the possibility of minimizing the extent of morbidity of certain lesions that cause ongoing pathophysiology throughout fetal development, by intervening before birth, is not so remote. Relatively simple and standardized cardiac surgical and cardiovascular interventional techniques can be applied to various lesions in the fetus, just as they can be applied to the neonate. However, the fetus is a physiologic entity about which we know relatively little when compared with the neonate.

BACKGROUND

Health care of the human fetus has long been recognized as an important concept. However, in more recent years this concept has matured from simple optimization of maternal health to active diagnosis and treatment of fetal diseases, sometimes involving invasive fetal procedures.[9, 16–18] Open fetal surgical correction of lesions such as diaphragmatic hernia and obstructive hydronephrosis have been performed in humans.[13–15] The appropriate use of these therapeutic interventions depends on three critical factors: the ability to diagnose specific lesions in utero, a clear advantage to correcting the lesion before birth, and the technical skills and physiologic knowledge to be able to accomplish the corrections safely. The principles of these three factors can be applied to fetal heart abnormalities as well.

With regard to diagnosis, clinical advances in echocardiography have made it possible to accurately diagnose specific congenital heart defects in utero as early as the tenth or eleventh week of gestation in humans.[10, 22] Advances in imaging have progressed rapidly, and further progress is a certainty. These advances offer the opportunity to identify fetuses with congenital heart diseases that are not amenable to surgical correction after birth.

There are a number of congenital heart defects for which prenatal corrective or palliative surgical procedures offer significant advantages over current postnatal surgical approaches. The reason for this advantage is that many complex congenital heart defects are not fully expressed during primary cardiac morphogenesis but develop gradually throughout fetal development. A primary flow-altering lesion such as a valvar stenosis may occur during primary morphogenesis. This lesion will then cause secondary abnormal patterns of intracardiac blood flow in the developing heart. These flow patterns eventually result in severe secondary lesions such as severe hypoplasia of a heart chamber or great vessel. It is the resulting hypoplastic or dysfunctional heart segment, not the primary lesion, that is largely responsible for the mortality in the postnatal period. In such cases, fetal intervention offers several advantages:

1. Correction of the primary lesion can be performed earlier. This restores normal cardiac flow patterns, which result in less secondary maldevelopment.
2. A period of time after the intervention (i.e., the remainder of gestation) is provided during which the fetal heart can recover and prepare for the change to postnatal circulation. This period provides a critical advantage, as the complex cardiac lesions under discussion are well tolerated within the hemodynamic milieu of the fetal circulation. In essence, the remainder of gestation can be viewed as a period of "natural extracorporeal membrane oxygenation" (ECMO), during which the heart can recover without stress to the overall fetus caused by a struggling heart.

Examples of the type of lesion that might be approached in this way include critical aortic stenosis with a dysfunctional left ventricle, pulmonary atresia with an intact ventricular septum, and some forms of the hypoplastic left heart syndrome. Taken together, these lesions make up an important portion of congenital heart defects.

These concepts can be more clearly delineated by examining pulmonary atresia with an intact ventricular septum in more detail. In this lesion, the obstructed pulmonary valve during early or mid-gestation alters right ventricular pressure and flow patterns, resulting in severely abnormal development of the right ventricle. Intrauterine relief of the obstruction would lead to less right ventricular damage and allow for a period during which the right ventricle could recover from the dysfunction incurred. This would result in better right ventricular development and function at birth.

A historical perspective of the changes in the management philosophy of this lesion provides evidence that supports the validity of this approach. The postnatal approach to this lesion has evolved toward earlier relief of pulmonary atresia. Neonatal systemic-to-pulmonary artery shunting without relief of the right ventricular outflow obstruction results in poor right ventricular salvage, even if a right ventricular outflow patch is performed later in life. This observation has encouraged the practice of neonatal patching of the right ventricular outflow tract, which has correlated with improved right ventricular growth and function. Earlier relief of obstruction can be extrapolated to fetal life, with the promise of further improvement in right ventricular development. Relatively recent fetal echocardiographic documentation of the intrauterine "natural history" of pulmonary atresia indicates that this lesion first develops relatively late in gestation (i.e., in the second and third trimester of pregnancy)[1, 2, 23] and can cause another secondary change: pulmonary parenchymal hypoplasia. These observations add strength to the argument that fetal correction would be beneficial. Intervention can be performed relatively close to the time of initial insult, and pulmonary as well as cardiac benefits might be achieved.

A parallel argument can be made for critical aortic stenosis in which severe left ventricular dysfunction and secondary endocardial fibroelastosis are seen after birth. The high mortality rate associated with this lesion after birth is related more to the left ventricular dysfunction than to the relatively simple surgical or interventional procedure of relieving the aortic valve stenosis. Avoidance or minimization of the severe left ventricular dysfunction by fetal intervention could potentially reduce the mortality rate of this lesion, which is currently approximately 50%.

These arguments indicate that two of the three necessary factors for recommending fetal cardiac intervention already exist: the ability to diagnose in utero, and the advantage over postnatal intervention. The final factor is the ability to perform the corrective procedure in utero. This ability requires not only the development of technical approaches to the fetus but also, more importantly, an understanding of the pathophysiology of the responses of the fetus to surgical stress and to extracorporeal circulatory support.

EXPERIMENTAL STUDIES

Fetal cardiac surgery and its sequelae have not been widely investigated. The earliest work in this area was performed at the University of California at San Francisco between 1982 and 1984.[24] These investigations consisted largely of technical feasibility studies. Beginning in 1988, more rigorous physiologic studies investigating the pathophysiologic sequelae accompanying fetal surgical intervention and fetal cardiopulmonary bypass were initiated.[5–8] These studies indicated that, late in gestation, fetal lambs weighing as little as 1 to 1.5 kg could be placed on and removed from cardiopulmonary bypass quite reliably. However, these studies also showed that the fetuses did not physiologically tolerate cardiopulmonary bypass. After removal of the fetus from cardiopulmonary bypass, severe fetal respiratory acidosis ensued. Additional studies, using techniques to measure regional blood flow, showed that elevated placental vascular resistance during and after cardiopulmonary bypass reduced placental blood flow and accounted for the poor fetal gas exchange (Fig. 33–1). This was shown to be a vasoactive phenomenon in the placenta by the demonstration that intravenous sodium nitroprusside markedly improved fetal gas exchange by reducing placental vascular resistance and increasing placental blood flow. These studies were the first to suggest that the major limitation to successful clinical application of fetal intervention for cardiovascular problems would not be related to technique but instead would be related to the pathophysiologic responses of the fetus to various forms of intervention.

Experimental Work

In the fetal surgical laboratory at Children's Hospital in Boston, we have continued to investigate the pathophysiologic responses of the fetus to surgical intervention and to extracorporeal circulation.*

Placental Response to Fetal Cardiopulmonary Bypass. The most immediate cause of fetal demise after fetal cardiopulmonary bypass is placental dysfunction characterized by the elevation of fetal P_{CO_2}, respiratory acidosis, and terminal ventricular fibrillation. We have further investigated the mechanism of placental dysfunction using a fetal lamb bypass model.

The use of indomethacin to block the arachidonic acid cascade at the cyclo-oxygenase step causes a marked reduction in the unwanted placental response to fetal bypass, implicating eicosanoid products as mediators of placental vasoconstriction in this model (Fig. 33–2).[20] In other work, the use of corticosteroids to block the arachadonic acid cascade at the phospholipase step more specifically implicated either thromboxane or prostaglandin E_2 (PGE_2) as the important mediator.[21] Both of these are known potent placental vasoconstrictors and are locally produced in placental tissue. Studies using a thromboxane synthetase blocker and also a thromboxane competitive inhibitor failed to achieve inhibition of placental vasoconstriction as seen with indomethacin or corticosteroids, suggesting that, in fact, PGE_2 may be the most important mediator of

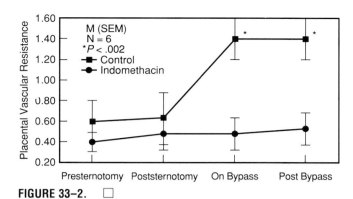

FIGURE 33–2. ☐

Effect of indomethacin on the placental vascular response to fetal cardiac bypass. M (SEM) is defined in Fig. 33–1. Asterisk compares control and indomethacin values at similar time points.

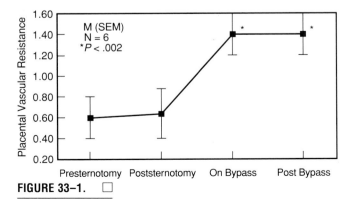

FIGURE 33–1. ☐

Change in placental vascular resistance after fetal cardiac bypass. M (SEM) refers to mean ± standard error of the mean and asterisk compares value to presternotomy value.

---

*This work was supported in part by grant HL-43357-01 from the National Institutes of Health.

this response (unpublished data from Sabik JS and Hanley FL).

Studies specifically manipulating PGE_2 production and action are currently being designed to test this hypothesis. From a clinical perspective, a highly selective inhibition of the mediator is desirable, because a less specific inhibitor, such as indomethacin, may have other unwanted effects (e.g., constriction of the ductus arteriosus).

Without blockage of the placental response to fetal bypass, fetal demise generally occurs within 30 to 60 minutes after separation from bypass, as the blood pH in the fetus approaches 7.0. With administration of indomethacin, placental blood flow is maintained, and fetal gas exchange normalizes, allowing fetal survival for much longer periods. This prolonged survival, however, has uncovered a more subacute problem: progressive fetal metabolic acidosis. A slowly progressive base deficit develops from the time of separation from bypass, eventually causing hemodynamic instability (usually within 6 to 8 hours after bypass) as the increasing base deficit reduces the fetal blood pH to 7.0.

Fetal Stress Response. A number of observations have suggested that the progressive metabolic acidosis might be due to depressed fetal cardiac output. Fetuses of mid and late gestational age can mount a massive stress response, as measured by the elevation of various stress hormones, including endogenous catecholamines. Our studies indicate as much as a tenfold elevation in circulating catecholamines during fetal surgical exposure and during fetal bypass. These levels of catecholamines significantly elevate the total vascular resistance in the fetus.

It is also known that the contractile apparatus of the fetal myocardium is quite immature, and as a result the fetal heart does not tolerate increased hemodynamic afterload.

Experimental surgical studies in the fetal lamb model typically have been performed using halothane anesthesia. Halothane is the anesthetic of choice in both experimental and human fetal interventions, because it crosses the placenta after maternal administration, obviating the need for a direct fetal anesthetic, and because it is a potent uterine muscle relaxant, allowing improved fetal exposure. However, halothane is known to be both a myocardial depressant and a poor blocker of the stress response elicited by pain and surgery.

Based on all of these observations, the hypothesis was formulated that the progressive metabolic acidosis seen after fetal intervention is caused by an unchecked fetal stress response, causing increased afterload in combination with some degree of direct myocardial depression. Figure 33–3 shows the det-

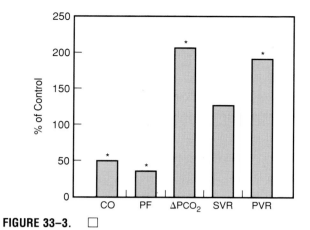

FIGURE 33–3. ☐

Effects of halothane anesthesia during fetal surgery. CO, Cardiac output; controls, control values in chronic resting fetal preparations; PF, placental flow; pCO_2, difference between maternal and fetal CO_2; PVR, placental vascular resistance; SVR, systemic vascular resistance.

rimental effects of halothane anesthesia in the fetus during surgical intervention. Halothane allows a massive stress response, which increases afterload and also causes some degree of direct myocardial depression; these effects markedly reduce fetal cardiac output. In addition, placental vascular resistance is maintained at relatively high levels, while systemic vascular resistance is lowered such that placental blood flow is not only reduced because of the lowered cardiac output, but also is further reduced by the relative changes in placental and systemic vascular resistance as the available cardiac output is shunted away from the placenta.[19] These data suggest that halothane is a poor anesthetic choice for fetal surgery.

The ideal fetal anesthetic should be easy to administer, totally block the stress response, not cause fetal myocardial depression, and not disrupt the balance of resistances in various peripheral beds. The importance of the delicate balance of resistances in various peripheral vascular beds in the fetus is similar to that in a neonate with a single ventricle and shunt-dependent pulmonary blood flow.

Studies have been performed using total spinal anesthesia in the fetus by applying tetracaine to the spinal fluid via the cisterna magna to block all afferent neural signals to the brain. This is a reliable method of blocking the stress response to painful stimuli. These studies demonstrated markedly increased fetal cardiac output and placental blood flow when compared with other anesthetic techniques.[12]

More recently, experiments using a combination of indomethacin to block the specific placental response to bypass and total spinal anesthesia to block the stress response and preserve fetal myocardial function in the standardized fetal lamb bypass model have shown that placental and myocardial function are maintained with excellent gas exchange and cardiac output. A number of fetal lamb bypass models have become chronic survivors, with delivery of normal lambs at full-term gestation.

Experimental Studies Examining Isolation of the Placenta During Bypass. Although the technical aspects of fetal intervention and bypass have not been critical factors in achieving survival in experimental models, technical issues will undoubtedly be of great importance. The unique aspects of the fetal circulation are reviewed in Chapter 1, and the differences in fetal and neonatal circulation will undoubtedly have important implications for bypass circuitry. The high resistance and low flow in the fetal lungs allow continued lung perfusion during bypass without detrimental effects. However, the placenta is the organ of gas exchange, and its function must be preserved after bypass. The ideal manner in which to handle the placenta during bypass remains undetermined. Allowing the placenta to remain in the bypass circuit has the advantage of eliminating an extracorporeal oxygenator from the bypass circuit, as the placenta will act as the gas exchange unit. However, there are two potential disadvantages to this type of circuitry. First, ongoing perfusion of the placenta may cause continuous stimulation of the production of vasoactive substances, which will tend to cause placental vasoconstriction. Second, because the placenta normally requires a very large flow rate (about 40% to 45% of the total cardiac output), perfusion rates using bypass with the placenta in the circuit will be approximately 400 ml/kg/min. These high flow rates can be difficult to achieve in small fetuses because of limitations in the cannula size.

Removal of the placenta from the bypass circuit would potentially decrease stimulation of vasoactive substances and reduce the required flow rates by about 50%. However, an extracorporeal oxygenator would be necessary, and the effects of arresting placental flow for a substantial time during the period of bypass at normothermic temperatures are not known.

These issues have been addressed in a series of experiments using an isolated placental model in which the umbilical arteries and vein were cannulated directly and attached to an extracorporeal circuit, with the fetus itself being completely eliminated (Fig. 33–4). A gas exchanger was placed in the extracorporeal circuit such that CO_2 was added and oxygen extracted, simulating the metabolism of the removed fetus. This isolated placental model allowed precise measurement of umbilical and placental hemodynamic characteristics and placental gas exchange under various conditions. Experiments

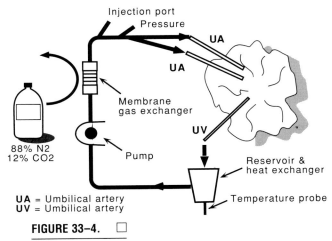

UA = Umbilical artery
UV = Umbilical artery

FIGURE 33–4. ☐

Schematic representation of isolated placental experimental preparation.

using this preparation showed that the placenta will tolerate a 30-minute period of normothermic umbilical and placental circulatory arrest, with resumption of normal gas exchange after reperfusion.[3, 4] Similar experiments in the standardized fetal lamb bypass model, performed by clamping the umbilical vessels during the 30-minute period of bypass and using flow rates up to 200 ml/kg/min and normothermia, verified the findings obtained in the isolated placental model. Normal resumption of placental gas exchange was achieved after umbilical and placental arrest. These experiments on intact animal models also suggested a beneficial effect of arrested placental flow on postbypass placental vasoconstriction,[11] indicating that a major stimulus for placental vasoconstriction is continuous placental perfusion during extracorporeal circulation.

Additional work is necessary in this area. At the present time the ideal circuitry for fetal bypass has not been determined with certainty.

SUMMARY

Any form of fetal intervention for cardiovascular disease requires extensive understanding of the fetal pathophysiologic responses to intervention, whether the intervention involves "closed" interventional techniques or "open" techniques using extracorporeal circulation (Fig. 33–5). Arguments based on the concepts of preventing secondary cardiovascular morbidity and minimizing the length of time that the organism is exposed to a morbid cardiovascular state suggest that fetal therapeutic intervention will be beneficial in selected instances of congenital heart disease.

Continuation of studies addressing the issues presented in this discussion, exploration of pathophys-

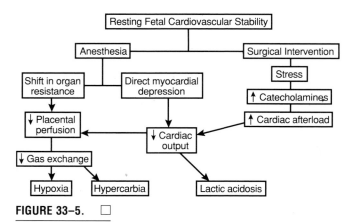

FIGURE 33–5. ☐

Current understanding of the cardiovascular effects of fetal surgical intervention. This diagram does not include the specific effect of fetal bypass on placental vascular resistance.

iologic responses in fetuses at earlier gestational ages, and confirmatory studies in primate models will be necessary before clinical trials are initiated. It is anticipated that these trials may be possible within several years. The many ethical and socioeconomic issues raised by the possibility of clinical application of this line of research, although not discussed here, must also be recognized.

REFERENCES

1. Allan LD, Crawford DC, Tynan MJ. Pulmonary atresia in prenatal life. J Am Coll Cardiol 8:1131, 1986.
2. Allan LD. Development of congenital lesions in mid or late gestation. Int J Cardiol 19:361, 1988.
3. Assad RS, Lee FY, Hanley FL. Extracorporeal circulation in the isolated in situ lamb placenta: Hemodynamic considerations. J Appl Physiol 72:2176–2180, 1992.
4. Assad RS, Lee FY, Sabik J, Hanley FL. Tolerance of the placenta to normothermic umbilical circulatory arrest. J Maternal-Fetal Invest 2:145–150, 1992.
5. Bradley SM, Hanley FL, Duncan BW, et al. Fetal cardiac bypass alters regional blood flows, arterial blood gases and hemodynamics in sheep. Am J Physiol 263(3 Pt. 2):919–928, 1992.
6. Bradley SM, Hanley FL, Duncan BW, et al. Regional myocardial blood flow during cardipulmonary bypass in the fetal lamb. Surg Forum 71:203, 1990.
7. Bradley SM, Hanley FL, Jennings RW, et al. Regional blood flows during cardiopulmonary bypass in fetal lambs: The effect of nitroprusside. Circulation 82(suppl III):413, 1990.
8. Bradley SM, Hanley FL, Jennings RW, et al. The site of increased placental vascular resistance caused by fetal cardiopulmonary bypass in sheep. Surg Forum 72:196, 1991.
9. DeCrespigny L, Robinson HP, Quinn M, et al. Ultrasound guided fetal blood transfusion for severe Rhesus isoimmunication. Obstet Gynecol 66:529, 1985.
10. Dolkart LA, Reimers FT. Transvaginal fetal echocardiography in early pregnancy: Normative data. Am J Obstet Gynecol 165:688, 1991.
11. Fenton KM, Heinemann MK, Hanley FL. Exclusion of the placenta during fetal cardiac bypass allows improved systemic perfusion and provides important information about the mechanism of placental injury. J Thorac Cardiovasc Surg 105:502–512, 1993.
12. Fenton KM, Heinemann MK, Hickey PR, Hanley FL. The stress response during fetal surgery is blocked by total spinal anesthesia. Surg Forum 43:631–634, 1992.
13. Golbus MS, Harrison MR, Filly RA, et al. In utero treatment of urinary tract obstruction. Am J Obstet Gynecol 142:383, 1982.
14. Harrison MR, Filly RA, Golbus MS, et al. Fetal treatment. N Engl J Med 307:1651, 1982.
15. Harrison MR, Golbus MS, Filly RA. Management of the fetus with a correctable congenital defect. JAMA 246:774, 1981.
16. Hobbins JC, Grannum PA, Romero R, et al. Percutaneous umbilical blood sampling. Am J Obstet Gynecol 152:1, 1985.
17. Lynch DC, Rodeck CH, Nicolaides K, et al. Attempted bone marrow transplantation in a 17 week fetus. Lancet 2:1453, 1986.
18. Rodeck CH, Nicolaides KH, Warsof SL, et al. The management of severe Rhesus isoimmunization by fetoscopic intravascular transfusions. Am J Obstet Gynecol 150:769, 1984.
19. Sabik JF, Assad RS, Hanley FL. Halothane as an anesthetic for fetal surgery. J Pediatr Surg 28:542–547, 1993.
20. Sabik JF, Assad RS, Hanley FL. Prostaglandin synthesis inhibition prevents placental dysfunction after fetal cardiac bypass. J Thorac Cardiovasc Surg 103:733, 1992.
21. Sabik JF, Heinemann MK, Assad RS, Hanley FL. High dose steroids prevent placental dysfunction after fetal cardiac bypass. J Thorac Cardiovasc Surg. In press.
22. Silverman NH, Golbus MS. Echocardiographic techniques for assessing normal and abnormal fetal cardiac anatomy. J Am Coll Cardiol 5:20S, 1985.
23. Todros T, Presbitero P, Gaglioti P, et al. Pulmonary stenosis with intact ventricular septum: Documentation of development of the lesion echocardiographically during fetal life. Int J Cardiol 19:355, 1988.
24. Turley K, Vlahakes GJ, Harrison MR, et al. Intrauterine cardiothoracic surgery: The fetal lamb model. Ann Thorac Surg 34:422, 1982.

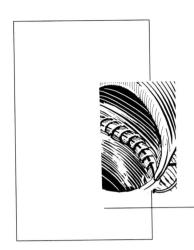

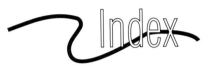

Note: Page numbers in *italics* indicate figures; those followed by t indicate tables.

ISBN 0-7216-4301-9

90038